# CORNEAL Topography

SECOND EDITION

A Guide for Clinical Application in the Wavefront Era

# CORNEAL Topography

SECOND EDITION

## A Guide for Clinical Application in the Wavefront Era

Editor:
Ming Wang, MD, PhD
Director, Wang Vision Cataract and LASIK Center
Clinical Associate Professor of Ophthalmology, University of Tennessee
International President, Shanghai Aier Eye Hospital

Co-Editor:
Tracy Schroeder Swartz, OD, MS, FAAO
Center Director, VisionAmerica
Huntsville, Alabama

SLACK
INCORPORATED

www.slackbooks.com

**ISBN: 978-1-55642-970-5**



Cover images compliments of Ryan Vida, OD, Wang Vision Cataract and LASIK Center, Nashville, TN.



Published by: SLACK Incorporated
6900 Grove Road
Thorofare, NJ 08086 USA
Telephone: 856-848-1000
Fax: 856-853-5991
www.slackbooks.com

Contact SLACK Incorporated for more information about other books in this field or about the availability of our books from distributors outside the United States.

Library of Congress Cataloging-in-Publication Data

Corneal topography : a guide for clinical application in the wavefront era / edited by Ming Wang ; co-editor Tracy S. Swartz. -- 2nd ed.

p. ; cm.

Rev. ed. of: Corneal topography in the wavefront era / edited by Ming Wang ; coordinated by Tracy Swartz. c2006.

Includes bibliographical references and index.

ISBN 978-1-55642-970-5 (alk. paper)

1. Corneal topography. 2. Cornea--Pathophysiology. 3. Cornea--Surgery. I. Wang, Ming X., 1960- II. Swartz, Tracy Schroeder. III. Wang, Ming X., 1960- Corneal topography in the wavefront era.

[DNLM: 1. Corneal Topography--instrumentation. 2. Cornea--anatomy & histology. 3. Cornea--physiology. 4. Corneal Diseases. WW 220]

RE336.C685 2012

617.7'1907545--dc23

2011028147



Printed in the United States of America

Last digit is print number: 10 9 8 7 6 5 4 3 2 1

# Dedication

To: Professor Zhen-Ping Zhang

Professor Zhang, my dear friend and colleague, your untimely departure has left a void in the hearts of all of us who care for you. We miss you, Lao Zhang.

# Contents

# Acknowledgments

I would like to express my sincere appreciation and gratitude toward the co-editor and project manager of this book, Dr. Tracy S. Swartz, for her hard work and dedication. Without Tracy, this book would not have been possible.

I would like to also thank all the staff members of Wang Vision Cataract & LASIK Center: Dr. Helen Boerman, Dora Sztipanovits, Dr. Kevin Jackson, Dr. Ryan Vida, Leona Walthorn, JJ Wang, Suzanne Gentry, Ashley Marlow, Terry Hagans, and the entire team.

I have had the good fortune to have the chance to learn from some great teachers over my professional career, including my PhD thesis advisor, Professor John Weiner; my MD (magna cum laude) thesis advisor and *Nature* paper co-author Professor George Church at Harvard Medical School and Massachusetts Institute of Technology; my ophthalmology residency advisors Professors Larry Donoso and William Tasman at Wills Eye Hospital; my cornea and refractive surgery fellowship mentors Professors Richard Forster, Scheffer Tseng, Eduardo Alfonso, Carol Karp, William Culbertson, and Lori Ventura at Bascom Palmer Eye Institute; my Vanderbilt University colleagues, Professors Dennis O'Day, James Elliott, and Donald Gass; and my colleagues at the University of Tennessee, Professors Barrett Haik, Natalie Kerr, and James Fleming.

I would like thank my national and international colleagues as well, including Professors Arun Gulani, Ilan Cohen, David Chang, Ron Krueger, Aleksandar Stojanovic, Guiseppe D'Ippolito, Francis Muier, Steve Klyce, Marguerite McDonald, Dan Durrie, Steve Slade, George Waring, Terry Kim, Karl Stonecipher, Brian Boxer-Wachler, Terrence O'Brien, Jay Pepose, Guy Guzarin, Noel Alpins, Tong Sun, Min-jun Zhang, Yong Tan, Li Li, Bang Chen, Bao-sung Liu, Michael Zhou, Xiao-bing Wang, Ke-ming Yu, Zhi-yu Du, Qin-mei Wang, David Liu, Arthur Tan, Jin-feng Chai, Hui-yin Liu, Ai-min Li, Ed Peterson, and Henry Zhou.

Often one learns as much from fellows that he trains, and I have been fortunate to have a great group of doctors who have been my fellows over the years: Drs. Shin Kang, Ilan Cohen, Uyen Tran, Walid Haddad, Mouhab Aljaheh, Ke-ming Yu, Yang-zi Jiang, Ray-Ann Lin, Lav Panchal, Lisa Marten, and Lance Kugler. I have learnt a great deal also from our optometry residents over the years, Drs. Helen Boerman, David Coward, Shawna Hill, Tracy Winton, Dora Sztipanovits, Kevin Jackson, Ryan Vida, Mark Raymond, and Michael George.

Finally, I want to thank my family for their unfailing support and love: my wife, Ye-jia "JJ" Wang; my father, Dr. Zhen-sheng Wang; my mother, Dr. A-lian Xu; my brother, Dr. Ming-yu Wang; my godmother, June Rudolph; and my godfather, Misha Bartnovsky.

# About the Editors

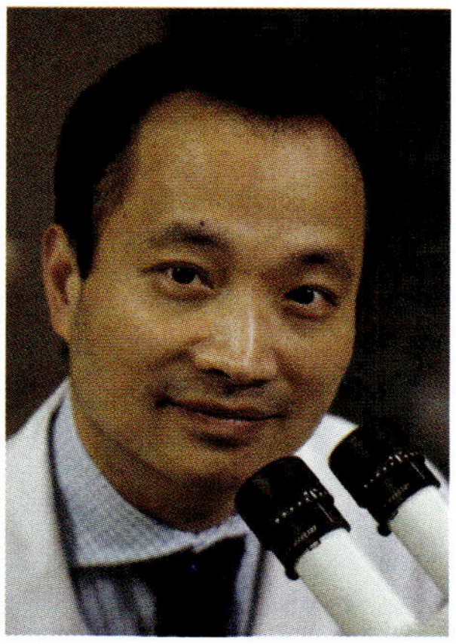

*Ming Wang, MD, PhD* is the Director of Wang Vision Cataract and LASIK Center in Nashville, TN, Clinical Associate Professor of the University of Tennessee, Nashville, TN, and International president of Shanghai Aier Eye Hospital, Shanghai, China.

Dr. Wang graduated from Harvard Medical School and Massachusetts Institute of Technology (MD, magna cum laude) in Boston, MA, holds a doctorate degree in laser spectroscopy, and completed his residency at Wills Eye Hospital in Philadelphia, PA and his corneal and refractive surgery fellowship at Bascom Palmer Eye Institute, Miami, FL. He is an editorial board member of *Cataract and Refractive Surgery Today* and *Refractive EyeCare*.

A former panel consultant to the United States FDA Ophthalmic Device Panel and a founding director of Vanderbilt Laser Sight Center, Nashville, TN, Dr. Wang published a paper in the world-renowned journal *Nature*. This was followed by his editing 4 ophthalmic textbooks: *Corneal Topography in the Wavefront Era: A Guide for Clinical Application* (SLACK Incorporated: Thorofare, NJ; 2006), *Irregular Astigmatism: Diagnosis and Treatment* (SLACK Incorporated: Thorofare, NJ; 2008), *Corneal Dystrophies and Degenerations: A Molecular Genetics Approach* (Oxford University Press: New York, NY; 2003), and *Keratoconus and Keratoectasia: Prevention, Diagnosis and Treatment* (SLACK Incorporated: Thorofare, NJ; 2010). Additionally, he has published over 120 papers and book chapters.

Dr. Wang has several US patents for his inventions of new biotechnologies to restore sight, including an amniotic membrane contact lens, an adaptive infrared retinoscopic device for detecting ocular aberrations, and a digital eye bank for virtual clinical trials. He is currently one of three investigators in the United States conducting an FDA-regulated clinical trial to treat age-related loss of near vision (presbyopia). He introduced the femtosecond laser to China, and performed China's first LASIK procedure using this laser in 2005. He also performed the world's first femtosecond laser-assisted artificial cornea implantation (Alphacor), and the first Intacs procedure in the United States using a new version of Intacs for keratoconus.

Dr. Wang was a recipient of the Academy of Ophthalmology Honor Award, as well as the Lifetime Achievement Award of Association of Chinese American Physicians.

As the founding president of the Tennessee Chinese Chamber of Commerce, and co-owner and international president of Shanghai Aier Eye Hospitals in Shanghai, China, which is the largest private eye hospital group in China today with 28 locations, Dr. Wang founded a 501c(3) nonprofit organization called the Wang Foundation for Christian Outreach to China.

Dr. Wang specializes in refractive cataract surgery; keratorefractive surgery; corneal and external diseases, including keratoconus; and anterior segment reconstructive surgeries with the amniotic membrane, stem cell, and keratoprosthesis. He runs a busy international referral clinic for post-LASIK and postcataract surgery complications. He founded another 501c(3) nonprofit charity, the Wang Foundation for Sight Restoration, which has also helped patients from over 40 states in the United States and 55 countries worldwide with all sight restoration surgeries performed free of charge.

Dr. Wang is a champion amateur ballroom dancer and a former finalist in the world ballroom dance championships in the open pro-am international 10 dance. He plays the Chinese violin (er-hu) and accompanied country music legend Dolly Parton on her CD *Those Were the Days*. Dr. Wang organized an annual classical ballroom dance sight charity event, the EyeBall, which is now in its 6th year, and has drawn attendees from all over the United States and around the world.

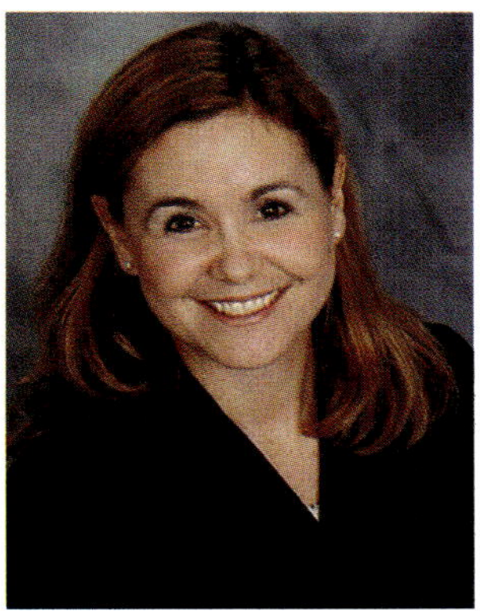

*Tracy Schroeder Swartz, OD, MS, FAAO* currently serves as Center Director of VisionAmerica in Hunstville, AL where she practices consultative optometry, specializing in ocular surface disease and dry eye. Originally from Wisconsin, Dr. Swartz attended Indiana University in Bloomington for her undergraduate education. During optometry school, she served as an assistant instructor for the Biology department and became interested in pediatrics and strabismus.

After completing her doctorate, she pursued a master's degree in Physiological Optics, specializing in pediatrics. She served as faculty at the IU School of Optometry for 4 years, and earned the Indiana Chapter of the American Academy of Optometry Gordon Heath Fellowship in 1996.

After completing her master's, she relocated to Metro DC, where she specialized in refractive and corneal surgery, and earned her Fellowship in the American Academy of Optometry.

She later joined Wang Vision Cataract and LASIK Center in Nashville, TN. Here she served as Director of Clinical Operations, Residency Director for the Optometric Residency Program, and adjunct faculty to Indiana University School of Optometry. While there, she edited 2 textbooks with Ming Wang, MD, PhD: *Corneal Topography in the Wavefront Era: A Guide for Clinical Application* (SLACK Incorporated: Thorofare, NJ; 2006) and *Irregular Astigmatism: Diagnosis and Treatment* (SLACK Incorporated: Thorofare, NJ; 2008), as well as authored numerous book chapters on refractive surgery, topography, aberrometry, and anterior segment disease. She served as Co-Editor for the literature review column for *Cataract and Refractive Surgery Today* from 2003 to 2008, and now serves on the editorial board for *Optometry Times.*

She left Nashville for Huntsville, AL where she became the Center Director for VisionAmerica. She edited 2 textbooks, *Keratoconus and Keratoectasia: Prevention, Diagnosis and Treatment* (SLACK Incorporated: Thorofare, NJ; 2010) followed by *Cornea Handbook* (SLACK Incorporated: Thorofare, NJ; 2010). She is a board member of the Optometric Council for Refractive Technology, is a diplomat of the American Board of Optometery, serves as Adjunct Faculty for the University of Waterloo School of Optometry in Waterloo, Ontario, Canada, and tries to be the best soccer mom she can.

# Contributing Authors

*Ashkan M. Abbey, MD (Chapter 2)*
Miami, Florida

*Amar Agarwal, MS, FRCS, FRCOphth (Chapter 8)*
Chennai, India

*Noel Alpins, FRANZCO, FRCOphth, FACS (Chapter 12)*
Cheltenham, Victoria, Australia

*Renato Ambrósio Jr, MD, PhD (Chapters 5, 6, 11)*
Tijuca, Rio de Janeiro

*Dianne Anderson, OD, FAAO (Chapter 5)*
Naperville, Illinois

*Timothy J. Archer, MA(Oxon), DipCompSci(Cantab) (Chapters 6, 11)*
London, United Kingdom

*Amin Ashrafzadeh, MD (Chapter 6)*
Modesto, California

*Harkaran S. Bains, BSc (Chapter 7)*
Fremont, California

*Michael W. Belin, MD, FACS (Chapter 6)*
Nashville, Tennessee

*Megan Buliano, OD (Chapter 3)*
Media, Pennsylvania

*Phillip M. Buscemi, OD (Chapter 7)*
Greensboro, North Carolina

*Diogo L. Caldas, MD (Chapters 5, 6)*
Tijuca, Rio de Janeiro

*Massimo Camellin, MD (Chapter 7)*
Rovigo, Italy

*Ana Laura C. Canedo, MD (Chapters 5, 6)*
Tijuca, Rio de Janeiro

*Shihao Chen, MD, OD (Chapter 5)*
Wenzhou, Zhejiang, China

*Xiangjun Chen, MD, MS (Chapters 6, 11)*
Oslo, Norway

*Y. Ralph Chu, MD (Chapter 3)*
Bloomington, Minnesota

*Ilan Cohen, MD (Chapter 3)*
New York, New York

*Sonya M. Dakin, COT (Chapter 5)*
Houston, Texas

*Michael J. Endl, MD (Chapter 5)*
Buffalo, New York
Amherst, New York

*Zhengjun Fan, MD (Chapter 11)*
Beijing, China

*Claus M. Fichte, MD (Chapter 5)*
Amherst, New York

*Marine Gobbe, MST(Optom), PhD (Chapters 6, 11)*
London, United Kingdom

*Frederico P. Guerra, MD (Chapter 11)*
Rio de Janeiro, Brazil

*Doug Horner, OD, PhD (Chapter 1)*
Bloomington, Indiana

*Mirko R. Jankov II, MD, PhD (Chapters 5, 6)*
Belgrade, Serbia

*Jason Jedlicka, OD, FAAO (Chapter 9)*
Mankato, Minnesota

*Paul M. Karpecki, OD, FAAO (Chapter 6)*
Lexington, Kentucky

*Stephen S. Khachikian, MD (Chapter 6)*
Rapid City, South Dakota

*Stephen D. Klyce, PhD (Chapter 5)*
Port Washington, New York

*Randy Kojima, OD, FAAO, FOAA (Chapter 9)*
Vancouver, British Columbia, Canada

*Lance J. Kugler, MD (Chapter 13)*
Omaha, Nebraska

*Matthew Lampa, OD, FAAO (Chapter 9)*
Silverton, Oregon

*Sissimos Lemonis (Chapter 5)*
Nürnberg Area, Germany

*Ray-Ann Lin, MD (Chapter 3)*
Taipei, Taiwan, ROC

*Bing Liu, MD (Chapter 11)*
Beijing, China

*David D. Liu, PhD (Chapters 5, 11)*
Winter Park, Florida

*Zuguo Liu, MD, PhD (Chapter 4)*
Xiamen, China

*Naoyuki Maeda, MD (Chapter 7)*
Yamadaoka, Suita, Japan

*Renzo Mattioli, PhD (Chapters 1, 5, 7)*
Roma, Italy

*Murray McFadden, MD, FRCSC, DABO (Chapter 7)*
Langley, British Columbia, Canada

*Cristiana de Moraes Ramalho, MD (Chapter 11)*
Juiz de Fora, Minas Gerais, Brazil

*Katherine E. Paton, MD, FRCSC, DABO (Chapter 7)*
Vancouver, British Columbia, Canada

*Leonardo N. Pimentel, MD (Chapters 5, 6)*
Tijuca, Rio de Janeiro

*Gaurav Prakash, MD (Chapter 8)*
Chennai, India

*Jia Qu, MD (Chapter 5)*
Chashan Gaojiao Campus, Wenzhou, China

*J. Bradley Randleman, MD (Chapters 6, 10)*
Atlanta, Georgia

*Dan Z. Reinstein, MD, MA(Cantab), FRCSC, FRCOphth (Chapters 6, 11)*
New York, New York
Paris, France

*Karolinne Maia Rocha, MD, PhD (Chapter 6)*
Cleveland, Ohio

*George Stamatelatos, BScOptom (Chapter 12)*
Cheltenham, Victoria, Australia

*Aleksandar Stojanovic, MD (Chapters 6, 11)*
Tromsoe, Norway

*Bradford L. Tannen, MD (Chapter 5)*
New York, New York

*Nancy K. Tripoli, MA (Chapters 1, 5, 7)*
Durham, North Carolina

*Bruno F. Valbon, MD (Chapters 5, 6)*
Tijuca, Rio de Janeiro

*Shawna Hill Vanderhoof, OD, FAAO (Chapter 9)*
Denver, Colorado

*Joe S. Wakil, MD (Chapters 5, 7)*
Houston, Texas

*Junhua Xiao, MD (Chapter 11)*
Nanchang, China

*Xiao Yang, MD (Chapter 4)*
Guangzhou, China

*Sonia H. Yoo, MD (Chapter 2)*
Miami, Florida

*Mei Zhang, MD (Chapter 4)*
Guangzhou, China

# Preface

The first edition of the popular textbook, *Corneal Topography in the Wavefront Era*, became SLACK Incorporated's best seller at the American Society of Cataract and Refractive Surgery's annual meeting in 2006 and has since become one of their best-selling ophthalmic books. Since the publication of the first edition, a tremendous amount of advancement has taken place in the field of corneal topography. Hence, we feel that a second edition of this textbook should be published at this time in order to help our readers remain updated about the exciting developments in this field.

In 2011, there has been a resurgence of worldwide interest in the study of corneal topography for the following reasons:

- There has been a growing awareness that in order to improve visual quality of a primary keratorefractive treatment, one does need to be concerned with how much we have altered the cornea.
- It is clear now that the best treatment strategy for a postkeratorefractive complex eye is a corneal topography-driven treatment.
- The rising popularity of cataract surgery with the premium intraocular lens (IOL)—a new field in ophthalmology called *refractive cataract surgery*—brings with it the need for a better understanding of the role played by the cornea in an eye implanted with a presbyopic IOL.
- There has been an emergence of a myriad of new technologies to treat various ocular conditions and, therefore, it is important to attain knowledge about the imaging of the cornea, Intacs and ultraviolet light cross-linking treatments for keratoconus, and corneal intrastromal femtosecond laser technologies.
- New anterior imaging devices have been developed at an increasingly rapid pace, including new corneal tomographers such as Pentacam, optical coherent tomography, ultrasonic biomicroscopy, ocular response analyzer, infrared devices, and ultrasonic devices.

The second edition of this corneal topography textbook has been produced with the goal of helping our colleagues to become current in their knowledge of the tremendous advances in the corneal topography field and should serve as an indispensable reference for all ophthalmologists and optometrists.

Below is my updated Form Fruste Keratoconus (FFKC) Criteria 2011:

2 D rule:

- >2 D difference in superior and inferior K readings outside the central 3 mm
- >2 D difference in the corresponding inferior corneal locations between 2 eyes
- Absolute value of K very high (over 50 D) in one eye

3-point touch:

- Coincidence of location of pathology of anterior and posterior elevation, pachymetry, and anterior curvature
- Displaced apex in all maps

Anterior & posterior elevation:

- Orbscan (best-fit sphere [BFS]):
  - ¤ "Ominous purple" in the posterior surface
  - ¤ Anterior greater than 15 to 20 μm
  - ¤ Posterior greater than 20 to 25 μm (post-LASIK: 40 to 50 μm)
- Pentacam (relative to BFS in an 8-mm zone):
  - ¤ Anterior elevation differences greater than +8 μm
  - ¤ Posterior elevation differences greater than +16 μm
- Holladay Report (Pentacam, toric ellipsoid):
  - ¤ Anterior or posterior elevation greater than 10 μm

Pachymetry:

- Bed 250 to 300 μm
- Normal: 535 μm, SD = 35 μm. No LASIK below 1 D (500 μm), no PRK below 2 D (465 μm)
- Keratoconus (KC): 430 μm, SD = 70 μm
- Thinnest area is more than 15 μm thinner than center
- The difference between thinnest areas between 2 eyes is greater than 15 to 20 μm
- Abrupt and more rapid "out-of-zone" pachymetry increase from thinnest point radially out
- Holladay Report (Pentacam): relative pachymetry that exceeds -5% (with respect to normal)

Irregular astigmatism orientation, amount, pattern:

- >3 D or more dioptic curvature change, in central 3-mm circle
- Asymmetric bowtie, bent or "squeezed," bitemporal outward "hugging"
- Change of astigmatism orientation and amount

- Against-the-rule astigmatism, plus inferior steepening, the “C” pattern, suggesting peripheral marginal degeneration

Topography-based FFKC detectors:

- Tomey: positive KC score with either the KC index or KC suspicion index
- EyeSys: I-S > 1.3
- Pentacam: red indicators
- Humphrey Atlas Pathfinder: red zone

*Ming Wang, MD, PhD*
Wang Vision Cataract & LASIK Center
Nashville, Tennessee

# Foreword

It is with great honor that I have been given the privilege of writing the foreword for the *Second Edition* of *Corneal Topography: A Guide for Clinical Application in the Wavefront Era* edited by Ming Wang, MD, PhD and Tracy Schroeder Swartz, OD, MS, FAAO.

The introduction of wavefront aberrometry by the end of the last century determined a new era for refractive surgery. An upheaval in understanding of optical quality beyond classic sphere and cylinder, and the advent of customized ablations have made the popularity of wavefront sensing to rise significantly over the last decade. However, it is of critical importance to understand the latest developments of corneal topography and its continuous role for corneal, refractive, and anterior segment surgery.

Placido's disc-based corneal topography was introduced in the mid 1980s and represented a true revolution for the diagnosis and management of corneal disease, with critical applications for refractive surgery. In fact, the role of corneal topography for screening, planning, and evaluating the results of refractive procedures was determinant for the acceptance, efficacy, and safety of keratorefractive procedures. Interestingly, refractive surgery also determined the absolute need to evolve the scientific knowledge on other areas related to corneal biology, such as biomechanics and wound healing. In addition, it is important to differentiate topography (from Greek words "to place" [topo] and "to write" [graphein] and tomography (from the Greek words "to cut or section" [tomos] and "to write" [graphein]). Tomography enables the reconstruction of the corneal architecture 3-dimensionaly, providing anterior and posterior elevation maps along with thickness maps. Topography enables the characterization of the front corneal surface curvature. Corneal tomography has been accepted to enhance the sensitivity and specificity for screening refractive candidates, as well as to provide objective parameters to choose and plan the refractive procedure (increasing efficacy and safety) and to evaluate clinical results.

*Corneal Topography: A Guide for Clinical Application in the Wavefront Era, Second Edition* is a book that provides clinicians with a current understanding of state-of-the-art corneal topographic instruments, including 3-dimensional tomographic systems and combined topographers with whole eye aberrometers. The applications for planning topography-guided custom ablations are also covered and illustrated. A last chapter on the future developments of corneal topography is included, which also discusses corneal biomechanics importance and the integration of systems for calculating intraocular lenses.

The editors are to be commended for the efforts to lead and edit the *Second Edition* of such an important book for ophthalmology.

*Renato Ambrósio Jr, MD, PhD*
Instituto de Olhos Renato Ambrósio
Tijuca, Rio de Janeiro

# SECTION I

# BASIC TOPOGRAPHIC PRINCIPLES

Chapter 1

# History

Tracy Schroeder Swartz, OD, MS, FAAO; Renzo Mattioli, PhD; Nancy K. Tripoli, MA; Doug Horner, OD, PhD; and Ming Wang, MD, PhD

The interface of air with the tear layer on the human cornea accounts for approximately two-thirds of the eye's refractive power. The typical cornea is responsible for 43 D of the 60 D of the refractive power of the eye. The average radius of curvature, 7.8 mm, generates the majority of the refractive power of the cornea (about +48.00 D). The posterior surface, with its concave shape and stromal index similar to that of the aqueous, contributes about -5.00 D. In addition, the majority of astigmatism originates from the corneal shape. It is not surprising that great effort has been put forth to measure this surface of the eye.

A normal cornea is not spherical but rather *asphero-torical*, vaguely like a bell with flat sides that have been slightly "squeezed" vertically. "With the rule" (wherein the vertical axis is steeper and horizontal axis flatter) corneal astigmatism from around 0.50 to 1.00 D is usually compensated by the natural tilt of the crystalline lens. The central 6- to 7-mm "apical cap" is ellipsoidal, with nearly constant curvature only at its apex. The surrounding periphery is considerably flatter. Finally, in some corneas, a small steep junction to the limbus (like the bell's edge) can be found.

Corneal curvature measurement has been the subject of study since Father Christoph Scheiner's works on the human eye (1619).[1] Ophthalmologists have tried to measure corneal topographic characteristics for more than 150 years, when A. Placido designed the keratoscopy target still in use today.

Two techniques, *keratometry* and *keratoscopy*, were used during the past century before merging into the present-day computer-assisted video keratography or, as it is commonly called, *corneal topography* (CT). A comprehensive review can help us to understand the real meaning of keratometric readings and topographic color maps.

## History of Keratometry

In 1796, Ramsden created a telescope to magnify images reflected off the cornea to measure corneal curvature. Magnification of the reflected images also magnifies the normal instability of eye movements that becomes a serious issue in making accurate measurements. Ramsden is credited with developing a doubling device that eliminates the problems arising from normal instability of eye movements.

Not until 1839 was another such instrument used, when Kohlrausch used a telescope with adjustable mires. In 1881, Javal and Schiotz improved the instrument by using mires that were adjustable in size, and this model is still used clinically as the Haag-Streit ophthalmometer (Haag-Streit USA, Mason, OH). The modern configuration is shown in Figure 1-1. Since this and similar instruments measure the curvature and astigmatism of the cornea, they were renamed "keratometers." Bausch & Lomb (Rochester, NY) improved on the keratometer in 1932 by adding a Scheiner's disk



Wang M. *Corneal Topography: A Guide for Clinical Application in the Wavefront Era, Second Edition (pp. 3-10)*

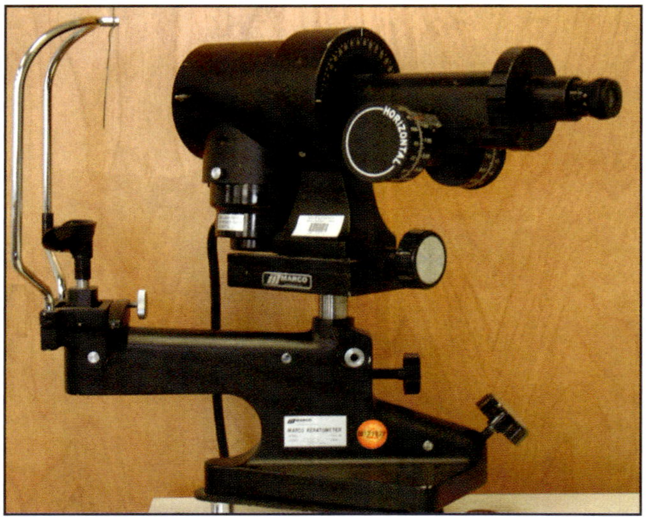

**Figure 1-1.** A modern keratometer.

to improve focusing mechanisms, circular mires, and the ability to measure 2 meridians simultaneously, and this model has essentially remained unchanged since that time in the form of the Bausch & Lomb and Reichert (Depew, NY) models. Such instruments are designed to measure the size of an image reflected off a convex surface using illuminated mires, a magnifying telescope, and a doubling prism.

Keratometry measurements are typically written in diopters (D). However, keratometers do not actually measure refractive power. They measure radius of curvature of the central 3 mm of the cornea. The formula for calculating the corneal radius treats the cornea as a spherical reflecting surface:

$$\frac{h'}{h} = \frac{-f}{x}$$

where $h'$ is the linear image size, $h$ is the linear object size, $f$ is the focal length, and $x$ is the distance from mires to convex mirror focal plane. Note that the focal length, $f$, of a spherical refracting surface is $r/2$, and the equation then becomes:

$$\frac{h'}{h} = \frac{-r}{2x}$$

where $r$ is the mirror radius of curvature. The distance from the mires to the image approximates the distance from the mires to the focal plane of the spherical convex mirror ($x$), resulting in the following formula:

$$\frac{h'}{h} = \frac{-r}{-2d}$$

The distance, $d$, is fixed in most instruments. For example, it is 75 mm for the Reichert keratometer. In Reichert and similar keratometers, the mire separation ($h$) is constant, and the size of the image ($h'$) is measured. Microscopic eye movements make this measurement problematic, so a doubling system is employed. A moveable prism is used to form a doubled image of the mires such that one image is displaced from the other and then manually aligned. The distance required to align the images is equal to the size of one image ($h'$), allowing calculation of $r$. Eye movements are minimized because they affect both mires equally.

The radius-to-diopter conversion requires the following equation:

$$F = \frac{(n' - n)}{r}$$

where $F$ is the corneal surface power in D; $n'$ is the corneal index of refraction; $n$ is the refractive index surrounding medium (for air, n = 1.0); and $r$ is the corneal radius of curvature in meters.

Javal's index of 1.3375 has become the standard corneal refractive index used. Note that the anterior tear film surface index is closer to 1.376. Because the Javal ophthalmometer as well as Bausch & Lomb's keratometer were designed to measure the total corneal power, this reduced index accounts for the negative power contribution of the posterior corneal surface.

Keratometers acquire data from a central annular zone of the cornea, which may vary in size depending on the curvature and instrument. In the Reichert keratometer, the annulus is approximately 0.1-mm wide, and the diameter varies from 2.8 mm (in a 48.0-D cornea) to 3.5 mm (in a 37.0-D cornea). It is important to remember the following assumptions related to keratometry[2]:

- The formula used is based on spherical geometry. The cornea, however, is not spherical but is a prolate (flattened) ellipsoid. Thus, the central radius is slightly steeper than actually measured.
- Keratometry is based on 4 data points within the central 3 mm of the cornea. It provides no insight into the area inside or outside of the 3-mm ring.
- Keratometry theory assumes paraxial optics. While the approximation may be clinically acceptable for fitting contacts or estimating corneal astigmatism, it may not be when measuring peripheral curvature.
- Keratometers assume alignment of the corneal apex, line of sight, and instrument axis. However, this rarely occurs during actual measurement.
- The formula used to calculate the radius (r) approximates the distance to the convex focal point, which, in the case of the Reichert keratometer, may introduce up to 0.12 D of error. This error may increase if the instrument is not correctly focused or the operator accommodates during measurement.
- Because the indices may differ between manufacturers, one must be careful when comparing the readings in D between different instruments.
- Reichert and similar keratometers are "one position" instruments, able to measure 2 meridians 90 degrees apart without moving the instrument position. While this allows for quick measurement, it decreases the clinician's ability to measure irregular astigmatism. The Haag-Streit ophthalmometer must be rotated to measure each meridian, allowing the clinician to better detect irregular astigmatism at the price of efficiency.

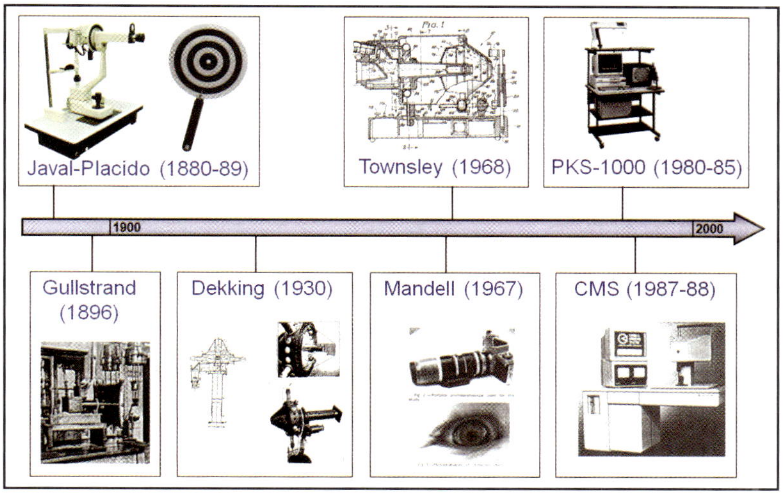


**Figure 1-2.** Topography timeline.

Modern corneal topographers calculate a simulated keratometry reading that incorporates the same paraxial assumptions of traditional keratometry. These "simulated K" readings have been enriched by reporting curvature along "semi-meridians" of the steepest and flattest meridians at different zones (usually 3, 5, and 7 mm) to evaluate irregular astigmatism in the peripheral cornea.

## Keratoscopy, Corneal Topography, and Its Color Maps

In 1880, A. Placido devised his keratoscopy target, a flat disk with alternating black and white rings. Soon after in 1889, Javal attempted to give a quantitative measure of the corneal shape by placing Placido disks into his ophthalmometer, behind the arc that carried the ophthalmometric mires.[3] Although the actual inventor of the first photokeratoscope is still a matter of discussion,[4] it was Allvar Gullstrand who developed the algorithms for the first description of CT based on quantitative measurements. In a paper published in 1896, part of the work that earned him a Nobel prize in 1911, Gullstrand[5] illustrated how, following Javal's suggestion, he developed a method of using a measuring microscope described as a "dividing engine" to determine the distance between 2 points on a keratoscopic photograph. Instantaneous radius of curvature was deduced from Gullstrand's measurement through an arc-step algorithm, and the corneal meridian profiles that he was able to plot are surprisingly similar to those from modern computerized CT.

It took about 90 years for photokeratoscopy to enter the computer age. A timeline is shown in Figure 1-2. During those 90 years, several people contributed to the development of modern CT. These include Dekking,[6] who in 1930 devised the first "cone," and Bonnet,[7] who in 1964 edited a book on CT, reporting elevation maps obtained by stereo-photographic measurement of eyes sprayed with talcum, a technique more recently replaced by fluorescein.[8] Mandel published several works on corneal shape models and contact lens fitting in the 1960s.[9-11] In 1979, Kuyama[12] made 3-dimensional isometric computerized maps, which were subsequently adopted by Sun/Nidek PKS-1000 (Fremont, CA).

A major step in the clinical utility of CT was the introduction of color-coded power maps. Several early maps are shown in Figure 1-3. The first 2-dimensional, color-coded map was published by Maguire and colleagues,[13] and this is shown in Figure 1-3A. Following the introduction of Maguire's map, fully integrated commercial computer-assisted videokeratoscopes such as the Corneal and Topographic Modeling Systems (CMS and TMS-1, respectively; Computed Anatomy, New York, NY; Figure 1-3B), the CT System (CTS; EyeSys Vision, Inc, Houston, TX; Figure 1-3C), and the VISIO (Visioptic, Inc, Houston, TX; Figure 1-3D) introduced maps in which each point in the cornea was assigned a color according to its power (Figure 1-4).

As CT moved from a scientific curiosity to a clinical tool, disputes arose over what quantities were scientifically logical, most valuable for applications, most easily understood by clinicians, and ultimately most useful. A parallel set of disputes concerned the terminology for types of instruments, measurements, maps, and algorithms. It is not surprising that eye professionals confused types of maps with the algorithms that created them. False theoretical limits on some methodologies were assumed because of the limited computing power of earlier PCs. Much of the confusion could have been avoided by an earlier understanding of the relationship between measuring corneal shape and measuring corneal optics and by recognizing the clinical potential of keratoscopy.

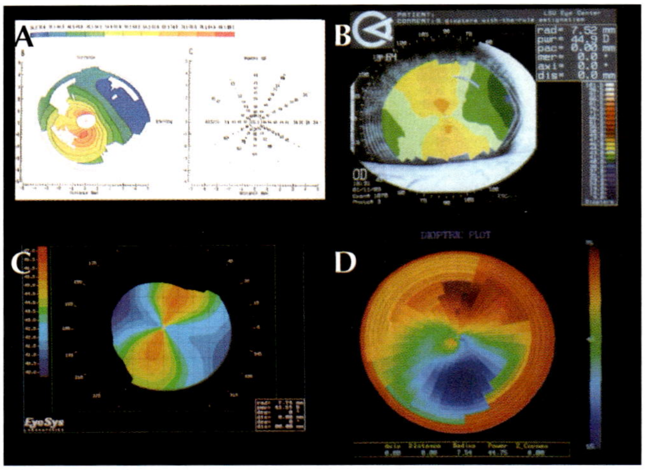


Figure 1-3. Early topographic maps.

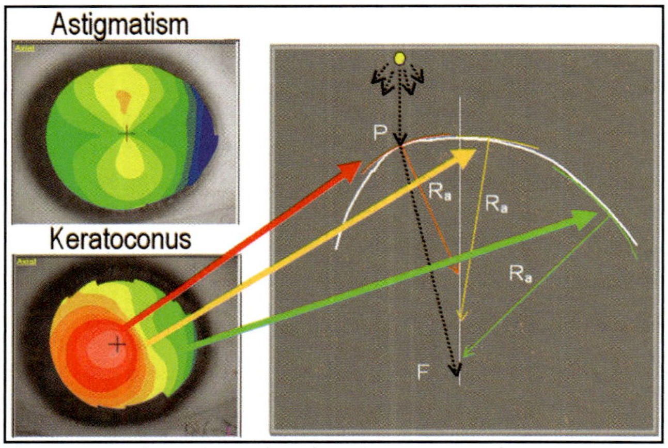


Figure 1-4. The colors of each point in an axial map represent the power associated with a sphere centered on the VK axis.

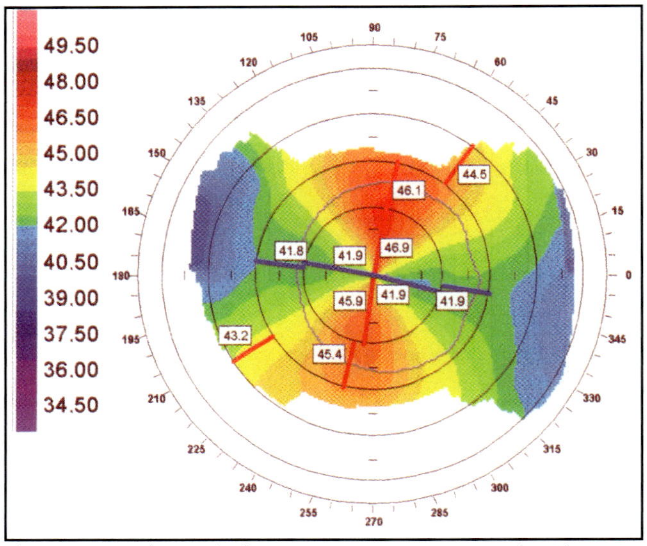


Figure 1-5. Classical "bow-tie" image associated with astigmatism.

## The Axial Map

For many keratoscopes designed in the mid-1980s, axial power was the primary quantity extracted from the raw data. As seen in Figure 1-4, the values and colors of each point, P, in an axial map represent the power associated to a sphere, Ra, having the same slant as the cornea and, therefore, refracting a ray of light in the same way at each point, P. The assumption regarding the index used (1.3375) is similar to that of keratometry. The axial map is more a descriptor of corneal optics than shape.

The axial map is a traditional but poor descriptor of corneal refraction because it does not take into account spherical aberration,[14,15] nor is the axial map a descriptor of shape. At each point, P, in Figure 1-4, the curvature and height of the centered sphere are not the same as the curvature and height of the cornea, and the discrepancy increases toward the periphery. Therefore, the axial map distorts shape. For example, in the map at the bottom-left, the wide red area indicates a keratoconic cone. However, the size of the cone is exaggerated, and increasing the resolution of the depiction would not increase the map detail.

The axial map has some utility as a simple descriptor of corneal astigmatism, including cylinder, axis, and irregularity. The example at the top-left in Figure 1-4 and in Figure 1-5 shows the classical "bow-tie" or "hourglass." The vertical "yellow-orange" axis of symmetry of the hourglass is the steeper meridian.

Despite its limitations, the axial map became known as "the CT map" because of 2 factors. First, keratoscopes were thought of as merely Javal ophthalmometers or keratometers newly capable of measuring a larger corneal area with greater precision. In other words, they were used to assess the need for simple optical correction of optics. They were not intended to measure more sophisticated optical aberrations, much less the physical shape of the cornea. Second, the calculation of axial power from reflective data required only simple algorithms.[16-18]

## The "Revolution" Around Years 1993–1996: New Algorithms and Maps

The calculus required for data analysis was the limiting factor for several years following the introduction of computer-assisted CT. Because axial power was computed by algorithms[16,18] that did not reconstruct the physical surface of the cornea, it was thought impossible to extract accurate corneal height and instantaneous curvature from Placido disk images.[19] There were authors who proposed alternative algorithms. El Hage used a differential equation whose coefficients were fitted by polynomials.[20] Doss and colleagues proposed an algorithm that attempted to overcome some of the spherical bias.[21] Wang and colleagues proposed the first arc-step method,[22] van Saarloos and Constable proposed an alternative arc-step,[23] and Klein's more sophisticated algorithm[14] used parabolas instead of arcs. The 3 arc-step algorithms demonstrated that long-forgotten Gullstrand methods could not only approximate axial power, but also measure corneal shape. Unfortunately, these approaches could not be practically implemented without further technical developments. The major challenge to implementing an arc-step algorithm was to calculate "local" quantities with high resolution while controlling the "noise" that made maps inaccurate and nonreproducible and confining the calculus complexity to stay within the limits of available computer power.[22]

In the early to the mid-1990s, the explosion of excimer laser refractive surgery necessitated more accurate instruments and more detailed representation of the corneal surface. The previous evaluation of keratoscopes on spheres[18,24-26] did not reflect their suitability for use in surgical design. The first evaluations made on aspheric test surfaces by Roberts,[27] Cohen, Tripoli, and colleagues,[28-31] and Carones and colleagues[32] in 1993 through 1995 revealed the inadequacy of spherically biased methods for measuring height and curvature, especially in the periphery. It also became evident that the use of an appropriate arc-step algorithm on Placido disk images, rather than being impossible, was quite accurate (less than or around 1 μm) for measuring corneal height and curvature.

Once released from the over-simplicity of axial power, instrument makers quickly developed new, useful quantities. An instantaneous curvature map, calculated by an arc-step algorithm, was introduced[33-35] by the Keratron (Optikon 2000, Rome, Italy). An example is shown in Figure 1-6. Curvature maps were soon adopted by most keratoscopes under different names (eg, instantaneous, true, instantaneous radius of curvature, local, tangential, or meridional).*

After the curvature map was introduced in keratoscopes, it quickly revealed its role as an accurate descriptor of corneal shape.[33] Along a meridional section of the cornea (Figure 1-7), as shown on the right, each zone has a center of curvature that is not on the corneal axis, except at the vertex. Without axial constraints, the curvature map can track and display all transitions between flat and steep zones and can reveal any local distortions, from the center to the extreme periphery.**

The maps in Figure 1-7 illustrate the clinical value of the curvature map's depiction of detail. In both maps, the

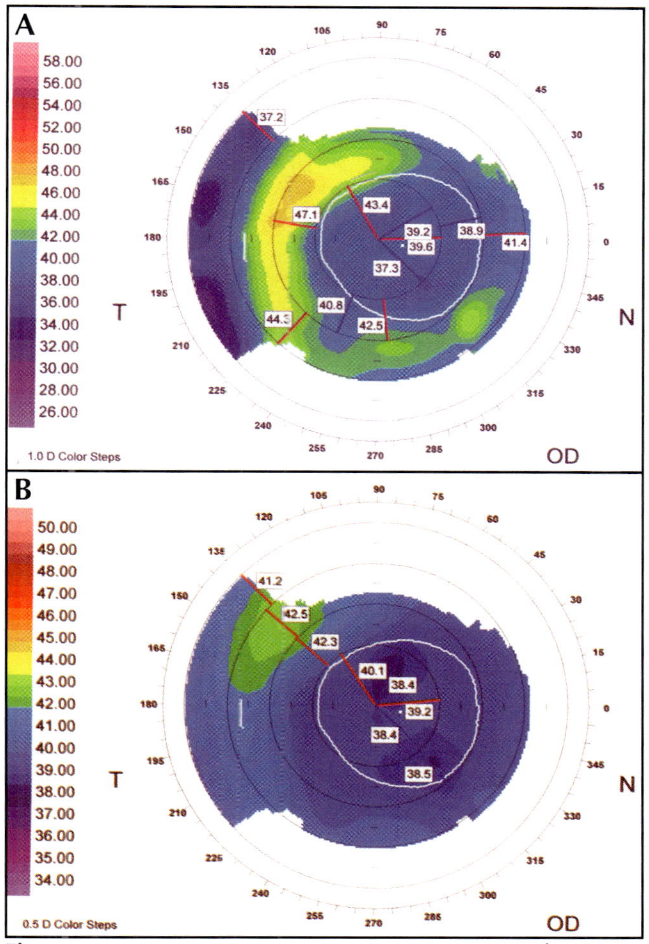


**Figure 1-6.** (A) An instantaneous curvature map showing a patient S/P myopic LASIK. (B) An axial map showing the same in Figure 1-6A.

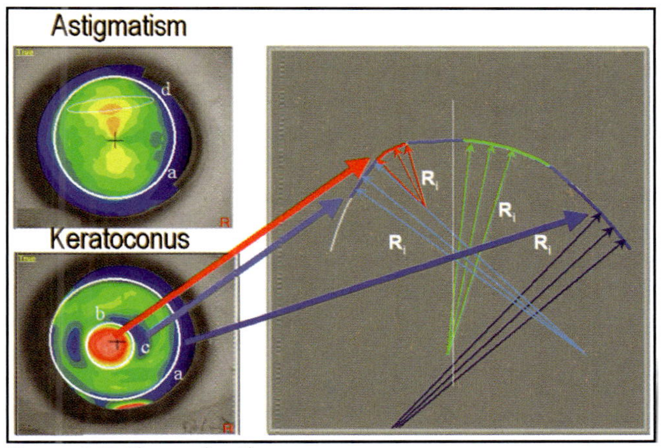


**Figure 1-7.** Shape detail.

*In their proposed standards, the ANSI committee has recently qualified the curvature map as "meridional curvature" to distinguish it from Gaussian and other nondirectional measures. Unfortunately "meridional," besides being an uncommon term, neglects a more important distinction between curvature and axial power, both of which are measured along meridians. Therefore, while waiting for an eventual acceptance by CT manufacturers and by ISO, we will refer only to "curvature" in this text.

**Although the precise boundaries and terminology of the "zones" are controversial among authors in the clinical literature, they are usually referred to as a change in the corneal curvature.

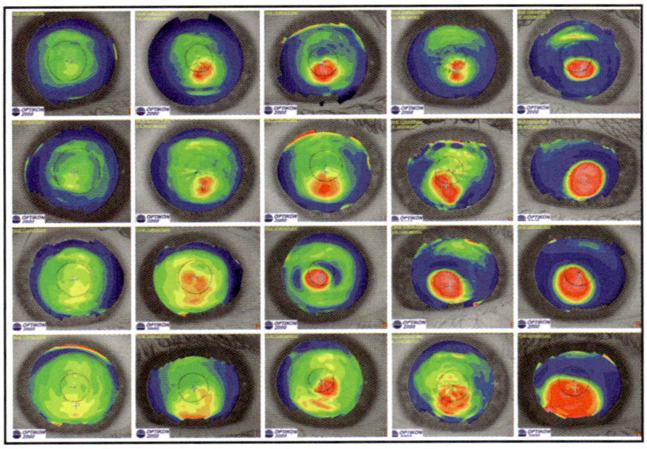

**Figure 1-8.** Progression of keratoconus shape in a number of different patients.

green-blue transition (circle a, about 7 to 8 mm in size) reveals an abrupt change of curvature delimiting the "apical zone"[36] or "optical cap." Bier's primitive cornea model described this zone in 1955[37] and defined the periphery around it as "negative zone" in curvature. Actually, this annular region may be very flat, but never goes to concavity. Information about corneal shape that cannot be seen in the axial map is revealed: (a) indicates the size of "corneal cap," (b) the size of keratoconus apex, (c) the surrounding flat zone, and (d) a mild warpage induced by normal lid pressure.

Curvature maps in Figure 1-8 show the degeneration of the cap with increasing keratoconus.

A power or refractive map, where power is calculated according to ray tracing (Figure 1-9), was proposed at the same time by Roberts and was first introduced by EyeSys in the Holladay diagnostic summary.[38] In 1996, Barsky and others proposed a Gaussian curvature map[39,40] similar to that shown in Figure 1-10. Its purpose was to overcome a limit of both axial and instantaneous curvature maps. Because axial and instantaneous maps were based on a center, they did not retain the same appearance on eccentric corneas if the patient changed fixation. Unfortunately, the Gaussian map hides astigmatism, a clinically important feature. For this reason, Barsky proposed overlaid arrows to represent the amount and direction of astigmatism at each point (as seen in the bottom left map in Figure 1-9). Though the Gaussian map is not common on commercial keratoscopes, it might yet find a useful application, for example, in intraoperative situations when the patient cannot fixate.

Corneal surface reconstruction algorithms also made accurate measurement of corneal height feasible. Because a representation of absolute height from a plane would have little meaning, the quantity is generally shown in "spherical offset" maps. Construction is illustrated in Figure 1-11. The colors represent the height of the cornea with respect to a reference sphere, measured in a direction parallel to the axis. The points that are above the sphere appear in

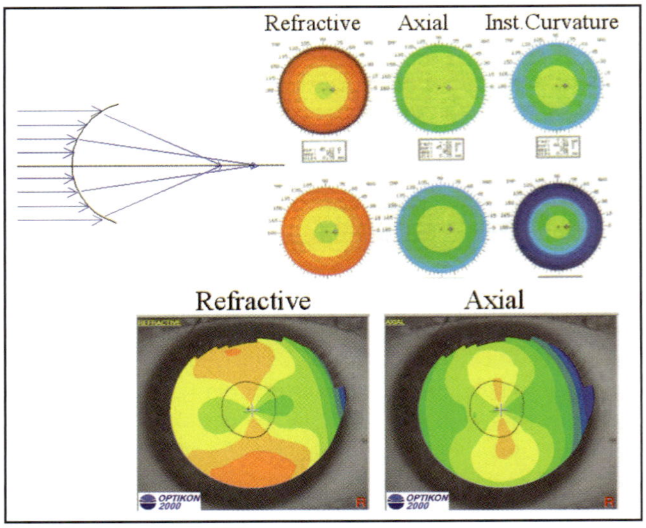


**Figure 1-9.** The refractive map. Power is calculated according to ray tracing.

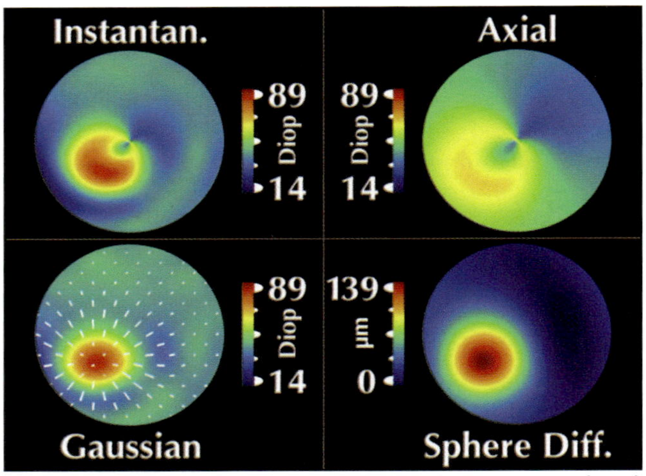


**Figure 1-10.** Gaussian map. (Reprinted with permission of Prof. B. Barsky.[39,40])

orange-red, and those below the sphere are green-blue. This universally accepted color convention in CT was inspired by geographic topography, in which warm colors represent hills and mountains and blue shades are sea depth.

## Corneal Tomography

True elevation-based systems were developed to directly measure the shape of the cornea, and allowed evaluation of the posterior surface for the first time. The first system, the Orbscan (Bausch & Lomb), used slit-scanning technology. This was followed by the use of Scheimpflug imaging (Figure 1-12), and anterior segment ocular coherence tomography (AS-OCT; Figure 1-13) Elevation-based

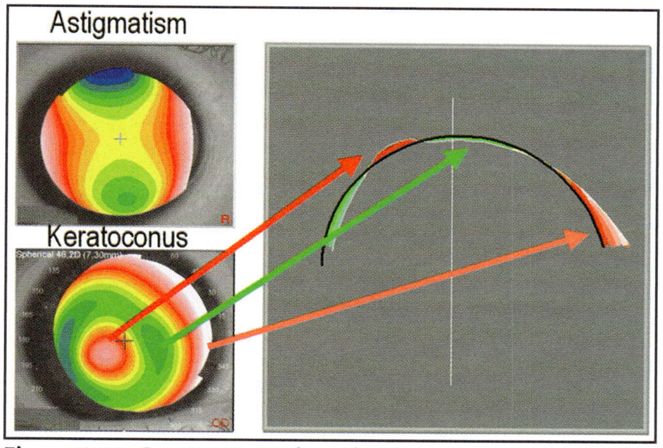


**Figure 1-11.** Construction of an elevation map.

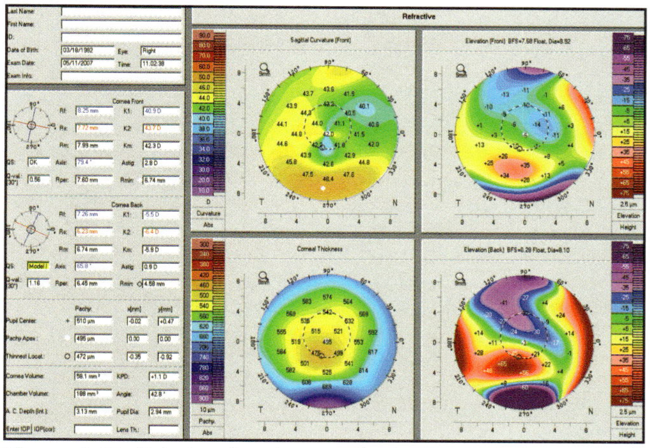

**Figure 1-12.** Scheimpflug image of a keratoconic cornea with scarring.

systems capture 2-dimensional images, and create a 3-dimensional model; hence, the term *tomographer* rather than *topography* is used to describe these systems. Some systems incorporate a Placido disc for curvature measurement, allowing direct measurement of both curvature and elevation. Pachymetry quickly became associated with topography due to the capability of these systems to create maps of the corneal thickness.

# CONCLUSION

CT has become an invaluable tool in ophthalmology, due to advancements in technology and its application to refractive surgery. Newest advances include indices for diagnosis of corneal diseases such as keratoconus, evaluation of posterior cornea and other anterior segment structures, pachymetry measurement, and calculations for intraocular lens (IOL) measurements. Interpretation of maps such as those reviewed briefly in this chapter is a learned skill, and

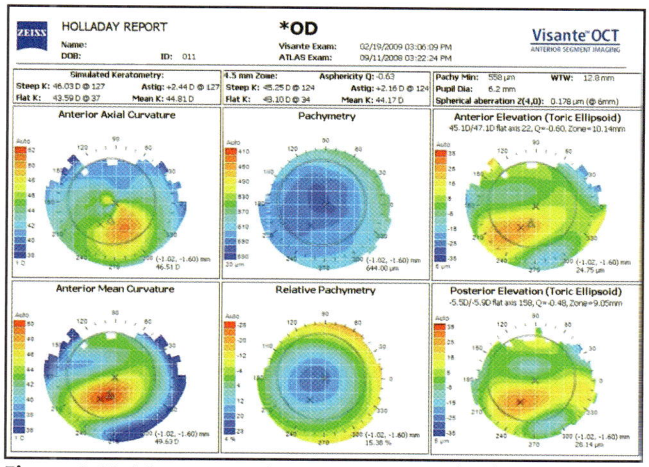


**Figure 1-13.** Visante anterior segment optical coherence tomographer combined with the Atlas topographer enables measurement of curvature, elevation, and pachymetry. (Reprinted with permission of Carl Zeiss Meditec, Jena, Germany.)

it is the goal of this book to educate the reader to better understand topography and its value in clinical decision making. What follows is a review of corneal anatomy and optical properties, a technical review of the technology, map presentation and scaling, and in-depth information on system-specific parameters, including using topography in refractive surgery.

# REFERENCES


1. Scheiner C. *Oculus, Hoc Est. Fundamentum Opticum.* Innsbruck, Austria: Danielem Agricola (Oeniponti); 1619:12-17. http://gallica2.bnf.fr/ark:/12148/bpt6k95041m.modeAffichageimage.langEN.f251.vignettesnaviguer. Accessed July 11, 2011.
2. Horner DG, Salmon TO, Soni PS. Corneal topography. In: Benjamin WJ, Borish, IM, eds. *Borish's Clinical Refraction.* 2nd ed. St. Louis, MO: Butterworth Heinemann Elsevier; 2010:645-681.
3. Reynolds A. Introduction: history of corneal measurement. In: Schanzlin D, Robin J, eds. *Corneal Topography Measuring and Modifying the Cornea.* New York, NY: Springer-Verlag; 1991:vii-x.
4. Levene JR. The true inventors of the keratoscope and photo-keratoscope. *The British Journal for the History of Science, Vol. 2.* 1965;8:324-342.
5. Gullstrand A. Photographic-ophthalmometric and clinical investigations of corneal refraction. *Am J Optom Arch Am Acad Optom.* 1966;43:143-214.
6. Dekking HM. Zur photographie der hornhautoberfläche. *Albert Von Graefe Archiv für Ophtalmologie.* 1930;124(4):708-730.
7. Bonnet R, Le Grand Y, Rapilly C. *La Topographie Corneenne*, Paris, France: N. Desroches; 1964.
8. Warnicki JW, Rehkopf PG, Arrfa RC, Stuart JC. Corneal topography using a projected grid. In: Schanzlin D, Robin J, eds. *Corneal Topography Measuring and Modifying the Cornea.* New York, NY: Springer-Verlag; 1991:25-32.
9. Mandell RB. Keratometry and contact lens practice. *The Optometric Weekly.* 1965;May 6:69-75.
10. Mandell RB. Corneal contour of the human infant. *Arch Ophthalmol.* 1967;77:345-348.

11. Mandell RB. Mathematical model of the corneal contour. *Brit J Physiol Opt.* 1971;26(3):183-197.
12. Kuyama H, Sasamoto K, Maruyama S, Itoi M. A new photokeratometer for contact lens in clinic. *J Jpn C L Soc.* 1979;21(3):80-84.
13. Maguire LJ, Singer DE, Klyce SD. Graphic presentation of computer-analyzed keratoscope photographs. *Arch Ophthalmol.* 1987;105:223-230.
14. Klein SA. A corneal topography algorithm that produces continuous curvature. *Optom Vis Sci.* 1992;69:829-834.
15. Roberts C. The accuracy of "power" maps to display curvature data in corneal topography systems. *Invest Ophthalmol Vis Sci.* 1994;35:3524-3532.
16. Gersten M, Mammone RJ, Brunswick NJ, Larchmont NY. System for topographical modeling of anatomical surfaces. US patent 4,863,260. September 5, 1989.
17. Olsen T. On the calculation of power from curvature of the cornea. *Br J Ophthalmol.* 1986;70:152-154.
18. Koch DD, Foulks GN, Moran CT, Wakil JS. The corneal EyeSys system: accuracy analysis and reproducibility of first-generation prototype. *J Refract Corneal Surg.* 1989;6:423-429.
19. Wilson SE, Wang JY, Klyce SD. Quantification and mathematical analysis of photokeratoscopic images. In: Shanzlin DJ, Robin JB, eds. *Corneal Topography: Measuring and Modifying the Cornea.* New York, NY: Springer-Verlag; 1991:1-9.
20. El Hage SG. The computerized corneal topographer EH-270. In: Shanzlin DJ, Robin JB, eds. *Corneal Topography: Measuring and Modifying the Cornea.* New York, NY: Springer-Verlag; 1991:11-24.
21. Doss JD, Hutson RL, Rowsey JJ, Brown R. Method for calculation of corneal profile and power distribution. *Arch Ophthalmol.* 1981;99:1261-1265.
22. Wang J, Rice DA, Klyce SD. A new reconstruction algorithm for improvement of corneal topographical analysis. *J Corneal Refract Surg.* 1989;5:379-387.
23. van Saarloos PP, Constable IJ. Improved method for calculation of corneal topography for any photokeratoscopic geometry. *Optom Vis Sci.* 1991;68:957-965.
24. Hannush SB, Crawford SL, Waring GO III, Gemmill MC, Lynn MJ, Nizam A. Accuracy and precision of keratometry, photokeratoscopy and corneal modeling on calibrated steel balls. *Arch Ophthalmol.* 1989;107:1235-1239.
25. Maguire LJ, Wilson SE, Camp JJ, Verity SM. Evaluating the reproducibility of topography systems on spherical surfaces. *Arch Ophthalmol.* 1993;111:259-262.
26. Wilson SE, Verity SM, Conger DL. Accuracy and precision of the corneal analysis system and the topographic modeling system. *Cornea.* 1992;11:28-35.
27. Roberts C. Characterization of the inherent error in a spherically-biased corneal topography system in mapping a radially aspheric surface. *J Refract Corneal Surg.* 1994;10:103-116.
28. Cohen KL, Tripoli NK, Holmgren DE, Coggins JM. Assessment of the height of radial aspheres reported by a computer-assisted keratoscope. *Invest Ophthalmol Vis Sci* (suppl). 1993;34:1217.
29. Cohen KL, Tripoli NK, Holmgren DE, Coggins JM. Assessment of the power and height of radial aspheres reported by a computer-assisted keratoscope. *Am J Ophthalmol.* 1995;119:723-732.
30. Tripoli NK, Cohen KL, Holmgren DE, Coggins JM. Assessment of radial aspheres by the Keratron keratoscope using an arc-step algorithm. *Am J Ophthalmol.* 1995;120:658-664.
31. Tripoli NK, Cohen KL, Obla P, Coggins JM, Holmgren DE. Height measurement of astigmatic test surfaces by a keratoscope that uses plane geometry reconstruction. *Am J Ophthalmol.* 1996;121;668-676.
32. Carones F, Gobbi PG, Brancato R, Venturi E. Comparison between two computer-assisted keratoscopes in measuring aspheric surfaces. *Invest Ophtalmol Vis Sci* (suppl). 1994:3748.
33. Brancato R, Carones F. *Topografia corneale computerizzata.* Milan, Italy: Fogliazza; 1994.
34. Mattioli R, Carones F, Cantera E. New algorithms to improve the reconstruction of corneal geometry on the Keratron videokeratographer. *Invest Ophthalmol Vis Sci* (suppl). 1995;36:1400.
35. Mattioli R, Tripoli N. Corneal geometry reconstruction with the Keratron Videokeratographer. *Optom Vis Sci.* 1997;74:881-894.
36. Kraff CR, Robin JB. Normal corneal topography. In: Shanzlin DJ, Robin JB, eds. *Corneal Topography: Measuring and Modifying the Cornea.* New York, NY: Springer-Verlag; 1991:33-38.
37. Bier N. A study of the cornea in relation to contact lens practice. *Am J Optom.* 1956;33(6):291-304.
38. Holladay JT. Corneal topography using the Holladay diagnostic summary. *J Cataract Refract Surg.* 1997;23:209-221.
39. Barsky BA, Klein SA, Garcia DD. Gaussian power, mean sphere, and cylinder representations for corneal maps with applications to the diagnosis of keratoconus. *Invest Ophthalmol Vis Sci.* 1996;37(suppl):558.
40. Barsky B, Klein S, Garcia D. Gaussian power with cylinder vector field topography maps. *Optom Vis Sci.* 1997;74:917-925.

Chapter 2

# Corneal Anatomy and Optics

Ashkan M. Abbey, MD and Sonia H. Yoo, MD

The cornea is the transparent, avascular anterior portion of the eye that covers the iris, pupil, and anterior chamber. It comprises the external layer of the eye along with the sclera, with which it is continuous. The transition area between the cornea and sclera is the limbus, a highly vascularized area of pluripotent stem cells. Fluid covers both its anterior (tear film) and posterior (aqueous) surfaces. The average horizontal diameter of the oval-shaped cornea is 11.7 mm, while the vertical diameter is 10.6 mm, providing an overall area equivalent to one-sixth of the circumference of the eyeball.[1] The cornea is thinnest at its center and undergoes progressive thickening toward the periphery. On average, corneal thickness ranges from 0.5 mm centrally to 1 mm peripherally.[2] The overall corneal thickness tends to increase with age.

With respect to shape, the cornea is aspheric. The central one-third (optic zone) of the cornea is almost spherical, and asymmetric flattening occurs with extension to the periphery. The nasal superior portion of the cornea displays more extensive flattening than the temporal inferior portion.

The cornea serves 2 primary functions in the eye: vision and protection. With respect to vision, the cornea acts as a transparent tissue to allow light to be transmitted to the lens and the retina. Its transparency is dependent on several factors, including regularity and smoothness of the epithelium, its avascularity, and the size and arrangement of extracellular and cellular components in the stroma, which are dependent on the state of hydration, metabolism, and nutrition of the stromal elements.[3] Furthermore, the cornea provides significant refractive power so that light may be appropriately focused upon the retina. In fact, the anterior surface of the cornea and its associated tear film account for 44 D of the total 64 D of refractive power in the eye.[4] With respect to protection, the cornea provides both a barrier to fluid loss through tight junctions in apical epithelial cells and a barrier to pathogens through membrane-spanning mucins at the apical surface. The cornea's rigidity and ability to quickly regenerate from mitotically active basal epithelial cells make it well-suited to act as a natural physical shield against ocular trauma.

## *Anatomy and Physiology*

The normal cornea consists of 5 layers, listed from anterior to posterior: the epithelium, Bowman's layer, stroma, Descemet's membrane, and endothelium (Figure 2-1).

### Epithelium

The corneal epithelium is composed of 5 to 7 layers of stratified, squamous epithelial cells and has an overall thickness of 50 to 52 µm.[5,6] It is a smooth, regular surface to which the tear film adheres, and it plays an integral role as a barrier to pathogens and fluid and solute loss.



Wang M. *Corneal Topography: A Guide for Clinical Application in the Wavefront Era, Second Edition* (pp. 11-20)

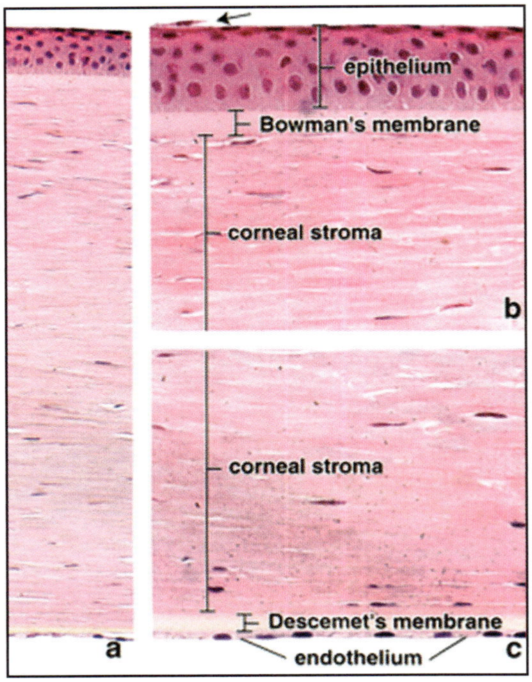


**Figure 2-1.** Normal histology of the cornea: epithelium, Bowman's layer, stroma, Descemet's membrane, and endothelium. (Reprinted with permission from Wang M, ed. *Keratoconus and Keratoectasia: Prevention, Diagnosis, and Treatment.* Thorofare, NJ: SLACK Incorporated; 2010.)

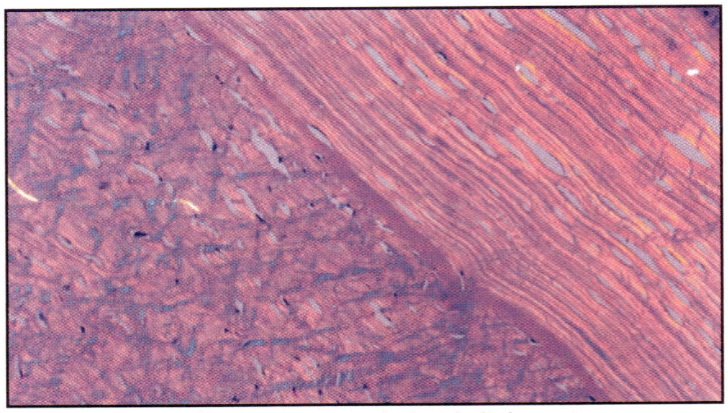

**Figure 2-2.** Color-contrast polarized light microscopy at the boundary of a keratoconus epikeratoplasty. The normal (donor) human cornea is seen at the top, demonstrating the lamellar structure. The keratoconic host cornea is at the bottom (magnification 100×). Notice the disorganization of the keratoconic lamellae.

The corneal epithelium can be divided into 3 distinct sections based on cell type. Flattened superficial epithelial cells ("squames") compose the outer 3 to 4 layers of the epithelium. Below the superficial epithelial cells are 1 to 3 layers of wing cells, aptly named for their thin wing-like extensions that project laterally from the cell body. The final layer is composed of basal cells, which are the mitotically active cells of the epithelium. These cells replicate and differentiate to form all layers of the corneal epithelium. The basal cell layer is anchored to the basement membrane and stroma through an anchoring complex. In this complex, a hemidesmosome located on the cytoplasmic side of the basal cell membrane adheres to the basement membrane and is attached to the stroma through anchoring fibrils composed of Type VII collagen.

The corneal basement membrane is an extracellular matrix that lies beneath the basal cell layer. Basal cells are responsible for secreting its components, which include Type IV collagen, laminin, and other glycoproteins. The basement membrane separates the epithelium from the stroma and provides a scaffold for the organization of the epithelium.[7]

## Bowman's Layer

Bowman's layer is an acellular condensation of randomly oriented collagen fibrils and proteoglycans that does not regenerate after injury. It is attached anteriorly to the basement membrane and blends into the more organized anterior stroma. Its function remains unclear, but many have hypothesized that it plays a role in the maintenance of epithelial uniformity and structure and thereby helps to uphold the refractive power of the cornea.

## Stroma

The corneal stroma lies between the Bowman's layer and Descemet's membrane and composes approximately 90% of the corneal thickness. It is primarily composed of flattened bundles of Type I collagen fibrils arranged in parallel, known as lamellae. These collagen fibrils are embedded within a matrix of glycoproteins and proteoglycans that maintain adhesion between cells of the stroma and allow for transport of nutrients and oxygen. Keratoconus produces compaction and a loss of the typical arrangement of collagen fibrils in the anterior stroma (Figure 2-2). Proteoglycans also play a significant role in the regulation of spacing between collagen fibrils.

The diameter of each collagen fibril ranges from 27 to 35 nm, and the distance between each fibril is between 41.4 and 60 nm.[8,9] The diameter of the collagen fibril is considered too small to result in significant scattering of light.[10] It has been proposed that stromal transparency will be maintained if the following 2 conditions are met: 1) collagen fibrils maintain a fairly uniform small size and 2) collagen fibrils are not spaced apart greater than approximately $\lambda/2n$, in which $\lambda$ is the wavelength and n is the refractive index of the medium. Unlike the orientation of collagen fibrils in other parts of the body, both the diameter of and the distance between each collagen fibril in the corneal lamellae are highly uniform. This regular arrangement is thought to play a significant role in the establishment of the shape, strength, and transparency of the cornea.

The primary cell type found within the corneal stroma is the keratocyte, which is a type of fibroblast or specialized cell of connective tissue. The keratocyte is a flattened cell that is interposed between lamellae, and its elongated processes often attach through gap junctions to those of other keratocytes. Keratocytes secrete and maintain the collagen and proteoglycans that form the majority of the corneal stroma. They also produce enzymes that are able to degrade older collagen fibrils in need of replacement. Furthermore, keratocytes migrate to areas of stromal injury in order to assist with scar formation and collagen repair.[11]

In normal corneal stroma, collagen fibrils are arranged along the vertical and horizontal meridians, orthogonal to one another.[12-15] Furthermore, stromal collagen mass progressively increases from the center of the cornea to the periphery. Both of these characteristics of the corneal stroma are integral to the maintenance of appropriate corneal shape.

### Descemet's Membrane

Descemet's membrane is the basement membrane of the corneal endothelium. It is synthesized by endothelial cells and is assembled at the basal surface of the cell layer. This membrane is primarily composed of Type IV and VIII collagen, and it does not regenerate after injury. Its primary functions include filtering of solutes passing to and from epithelial cell layers and serving as a substrate for the induction of polarity and differentiation of the overlying epithelium.

### Endothelium

The corneal endothelium is a single layer of hexagonal cells adherent to the posterior aspect of Descemet's membrane. Their abundant organelles demonstrate the high level of metabolic and synthesizing activity of these cells. Endothelial cells in an adult are arrested in the G1 phase of the mitotic cell cycle, meaning that they do not replicate despite their capacity to do so.[16] A major function of the endothelium is the maintenance of corneal transparency through the regulation of stromal hydration. The endothelial cells provide a "leaky barrier" to aqueous humor and contain numerous specialized ion transport systems to transfer excess water out of the cornea. These 2 functions of the endothelium facilitate its regulation of the amount of water within the corneal stroma.

### Tear Film

The tear film of the eye covers the anterior surface of the cornea. It is composed of 3 separate layers: an anterior lipid layer, a middle aqueous layer, and a posterior mucin layer. The average thickness of the tear film is approximately 7 μm, the majority of which is the aqueous layer.[17] The tear film serves the following functions: lubricates the anterior surface of the eye; acts as a smooth, transparent refractive surface for the transmission of light; transfers nutrients and oxygen to the corneal epithelium; protects against infection; and removes desquamated epithelial cells from the surface of the eye.[18] The lipid layer is produced by meibomian glands as a means by which to increase surface tension and therefore prevent evaporation of the aqueous layer. The aqueous layer is secreted by the main lacrimal glands and the accessory lacrimal glands of Wolfring and Krause and primarily serves to lubricate the corneal epithelium. The mucin layer is manufactured by the goblet cells of the conjunctiva and serves to reduce the surface tension of the aqueous tear layer so that it may adsorb to the epithelium and remain intact between blinks.

### Corneal Innervation

The cornea has an extensive supply of sensory nerve fibers, making it one of the most highly innervated tissues in the body. Corneal sensory nerves are derived from the ophthalmic division of the trigeminal nerve (cranial nerve V). Nerve branches enter the anterior corneal stroma from an annular nerve plexus near the limbus. At this entry point, myelination of the nerve axons is lost, which is essential for the maintenance of corneal transparency.[19] The nerve fibers then proceed to run parallel to the epithelium, forming a sub-basal nerve plexus. From this plexus, axons without Schwann cells penetrate Bowman's layer and extend into the epithelium. The corneal nerves serve 2 main functions. First, they provide protection by serving as the afferent portion of an aversion reflex in response to any contact with the corneal surface. Second, corneal nerves secrete trophic factors for the preservation of corneal health. If corneal nerves are damaged either by disease or trauma, the lack of adequate production of trophic factors could lead to neurotrophic keratitis, which is characterized by epithelial sloughing and impaired healing.

## Corneal Optics

The cornea is the first structure that interacts with light as it is being transferred into the eye and contributes the greatest amount of refractive power. The cornea can be treated like an ophthalmic lens created from 3 different interfaces: tears, corneal tissue, and the aqueous humor. To calculate the power of the cornea, a thin lens formula can be used 3 times, one for each interface. The thin lens formula is as follows:

$$F = \frac{(n-n^1)}{r}$$

where F is the total refractive power at the surface of the cornea; n is the refractive index of the air; and $n^1$ is the refractive index of the tear film. r is the radius of curvature of the cornea in meters. For the average human cornea, the central anterior corneal radius of curvature is 7.8 mm, and the posterior corneal radius of curvature is 6.5 mm. The indices of refraction are as follows: air, 1.00; tears, 1.336; cornea, 1.376; aqueous humor, 1.336.

When using the above thin lens equation, the tear-air interface power is 43.00. This first interface accounts for the majority of corneal power because the change in density from air to tears has the greatest differential. Using the thin lens equation for the tear-cornea interface and the cornea-aqueous humor interface, the resulting refractive powers are +5.1 D and -6.2 D, respectively. The total cornea power, calculated by combining these dioptric powers, is approximately +42.00 D for the average human cornea.[20]

## Physical Considerations That Reduce Visual Aberrations

The majority of a patient's visual complaints arise from lower-order aberrations, commonly known as refractive errors. Defocus is considered absent when the punctum remotum of the eye is at infinity in a situation where the eye is not accommodating and a congruent image is perfectly focused on the retina.[21] A hyperopic patient can use accommodation to focus the image on the retina, while a myopic patient has to move the object closer than infinity to focus the image.

Even when lower-order refractive errors are corrected with spectacles or contact lenses, uncorrected higher-order aberrations may decrease visual quality.[22] Aberrations relevant to the cornea are spherical aberration, coma, and oblique astigmatism.

Spherical aberration is an expression of the difference in refracting power for peripheral rays relative to central rays. This occurs when a point source of light is refracted by a large-aperture optical system. Different zones of the aperture have different focal lengths and, therefore, do not focus the point source of light to the same location. Normally, spherical aberration is not important in the human eye because the pupil is sufficiently small. Figure 2-3 shows the effect of spherical aberration on the Snellen E.

Coma occurs when an object is located off axis or if the apex of the cornea is not properly aligned with the other optical elements of the eye. Similar to spherical aberration, it has little effect due to the pupil being relatively small. Coma can be thought of as a type of off-axis spherical aberration. It creates a series of images superimposed on each other with the brightest image being the smallest one. Figure 2-4 shows the effect of coma on the Snellen E.

Oblique astigmatism is independent of pupil size and cornea. It is induced when rays pass through the cornea, obliquely inducing astigmatism. This phenomenon explains how a spherical cornea may register astigmatism when measured obliquely.

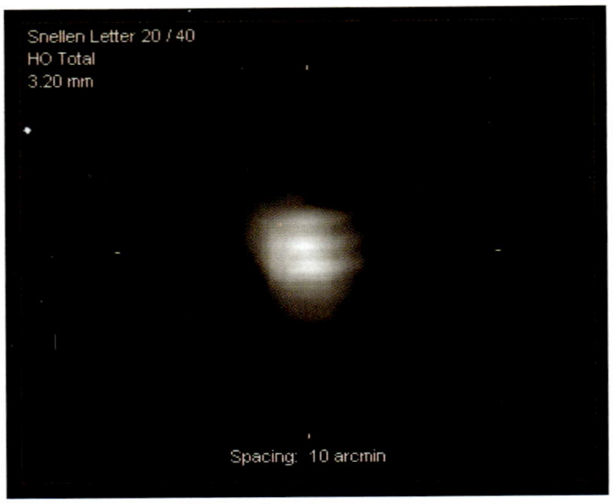


**Figure 2-3.** Effect of spherical aberration on a Snellen E.

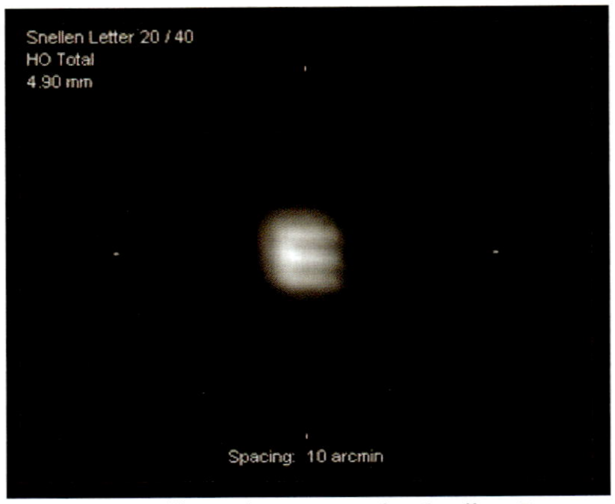


**Figure 2-4.** Effect of coma on the Snellen E.

Corneal structure is such that aberrations are minimized. This is accomplished by the prolate shape and small angle Kappa. The cornea is not spherical, but rather aspheric. The curve flattens toward the periphery as you move away from the center, and the shape is described as prolate. Natural asphericity decreases the power of the peripheral parts of the cornea, resulting in decreased spherical aberration and coma.[23] The asphericity of the human cornea is described by factor Q, which represents the difference in curvature from the center to the periphery of the cornea. The average value for a human's cornea is -0.26. A perfect value for Q would be -0.50, but the junction of the cornea and sclera at the limbus prohibits this in nature.

Aberrations are further minimized by the location of the corneal apex. If the apex of the cornea aligns with the pupil center, it would naturally intercept the visual axis. When this does not occur, light rays get redirected and meet with the retina at oblique angles. These redirected rays result in a lessened retinal response, producing what is known as the "Stiles-Crawford Effect." The pupil normally reduces

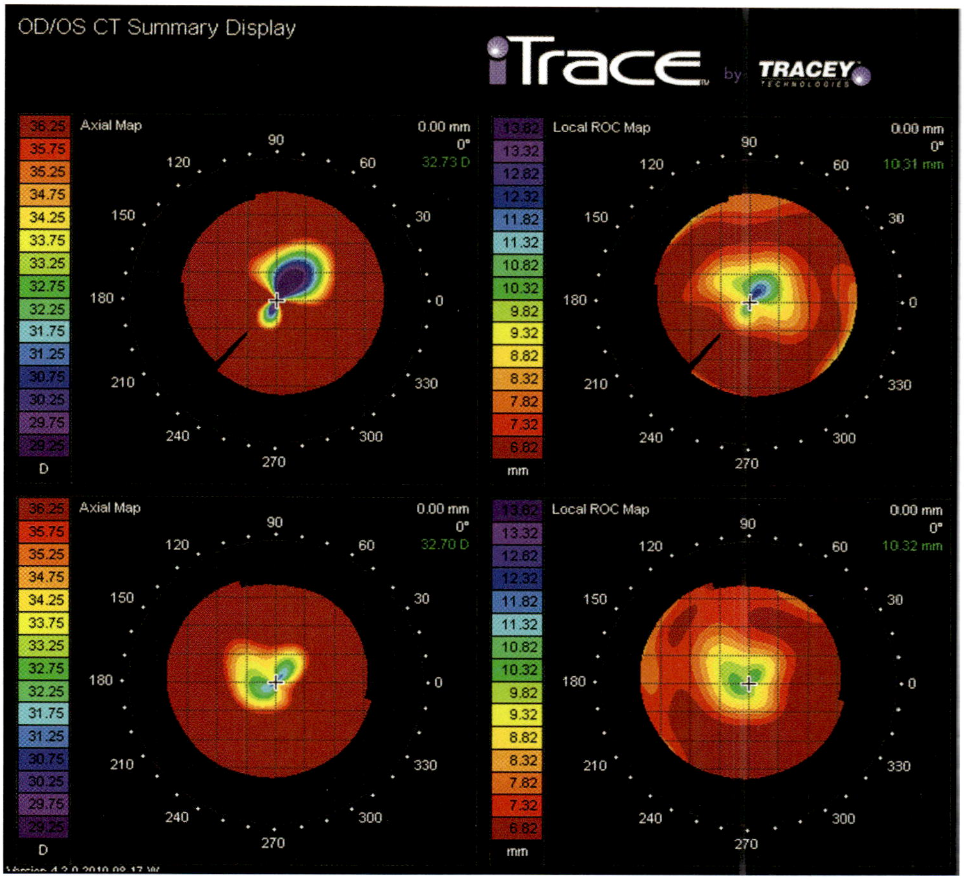


**Figure 2-5.** Radial keratotomy creates a central flattening, and optic zones are often smaller than the pupil size, resulting in halos and night vision problems.

aberrant rays, which decreases the effect of oblique rays. Essentially, the same problem occurs if the pupil is not centered.[20]

Pupil size is uniquely suited to limited aberrations, such as spherical aberration and diffraction. The pupil size that is best for limiting higher-order aberrations and minimizing diffraction is 2.5 mm. The average pupil size is 5 mm, with younger patients naturally having larger pupils.[24]

## Corneal Optics After Keratorefractive Surgery

Keratorefractive surgery changes the natural shape of the cornea, typically decreasing the natural safeguards against aberrations. Keratorefractive surgeries are successful because the optical properties of the eye can be manipulated by changing the shape of the cornea. With radial keratotomy, the central cornea is flattened due to relaxing incisions (Figure 2-5). When using excimer procedures, the prolate structure of the cornea is changed by the removal of a convex positive meniscus for myopic ablations (Figure 2-6), a concave positive meniscus for hyperopic corrections (Figure 2-7), and a toric positive meniscus in astigmatic corrections.

The size of angle Kappa in reference to the ablation zone becomes important when this angle is large (Figure 2-8). If the visual axis is far from the geometric center of the cornea, the ablation will be effectively decentered. This is most often problematic with a hyperopic treatment where the central cornea is steeped around the visual axis.[25] With a refractive surgery, pupil size related to the treatment zone remains important. Patients with pupil sizes greater than 8 mm should be identified and appropriately educated about visual side effects before undergoing keratorefractive surgical correction.

Physiologically, the response of the cornea is complex following ablative procedures. The amount of tissue removed can be predicted by Munnerlyn's formula:

$$T = \frac{S^2D}{3}$$

where S is the diameter of the treatment optical zone, D is the refractive correction, and T is the maximum amount of corneal tissue removed in microns. Clinically, for every diopter of correction, approximately 12 µm of tissue are removed when using a 6-mm ablation.

Ablative, incisional, and INTACS all change keratometric readings. A 0.8-D change in K is associated with a 1-D change in refraction.[23] This is important for surgical planning because creating a cornea that is too flat (less than 35 D) or too steep (more than 52 D) can result in a disabling loss of visual quality.[22]

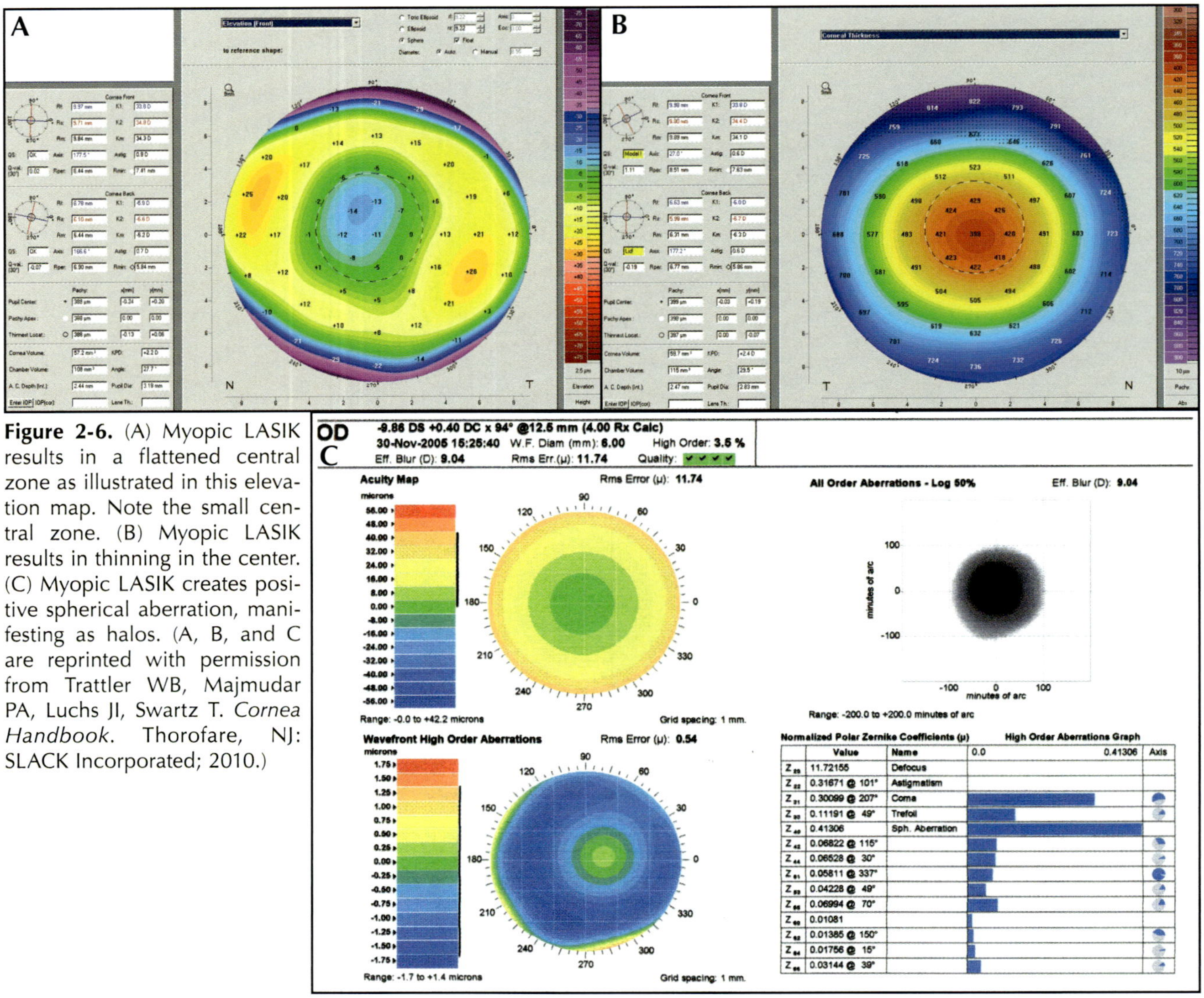

**Figure 2-6.** (A) Myopic LASIK results in a flattened central zone as illustrated in this elevation map. Note the small central zone. (B) Myopic LASIK results in thinning in the center. (C) Myopic LASIK creates positive spherical aberration, manifesting as halos. (A, B, and C are reprinted with permission from Trattler WB, Majmudar PA, Luchs JI, Swartz T. *Cornea Handbook*. Thorofare, NJ: SLACK Incorporated; 2010.)

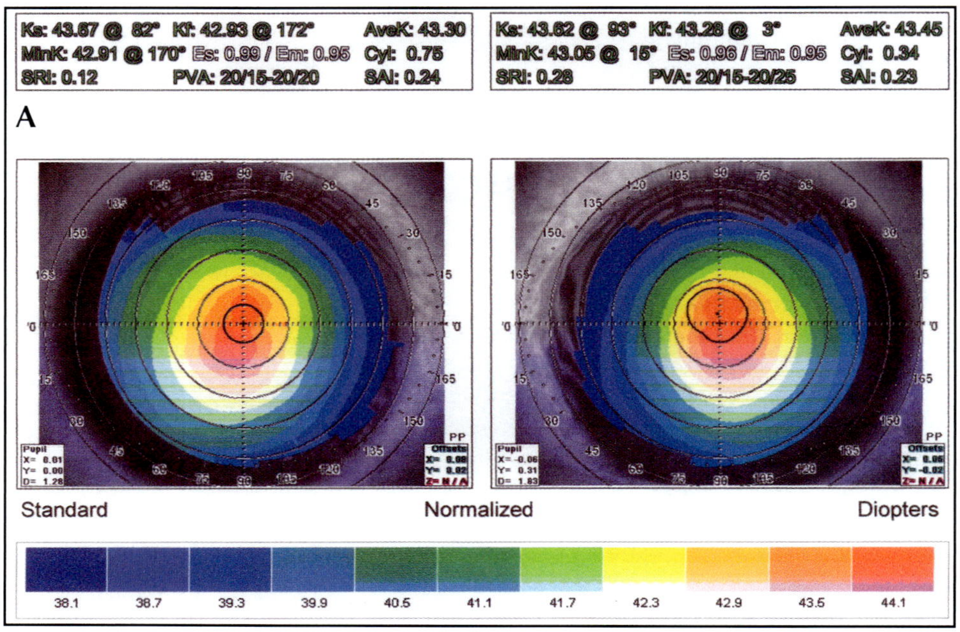


**Figure 2-7.** (A) Hyperopic LASIK results in a steepened central zone. (Reprinted with permission from Trattler WB, Majmudar PA, Luchs JI, Swartz T. *Cornea Handbook*. Thorofare, NJ: SLACK Incorporated; 2010.) *(continued)*

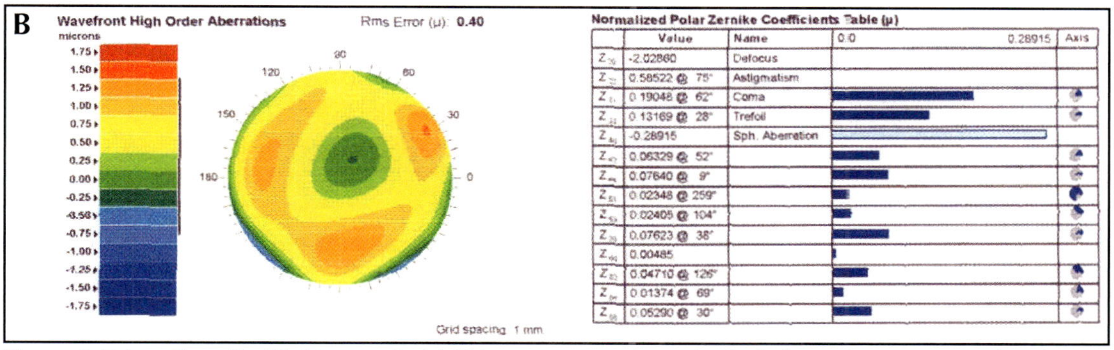


**Figure 2-7 (continued).** (B) Hyperopic LASIK creates negative spherical aberration. (Reprinted with permission from Trattler WB, Majmudar PA, Luchs JI, Swartz T. *Cornea Handbook*. Thorofare, NJ: SLACK Incorporated; 2010.)

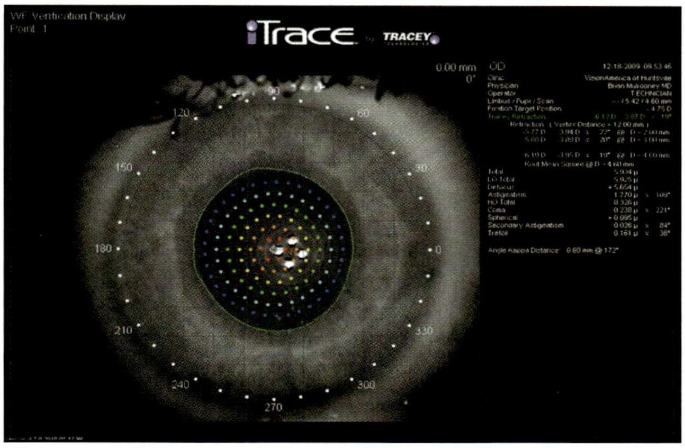


**Figure 2-8.** A large angle Kappa may complicate keratorefractive procedures.

Note the ratio of refractive change to keratometric change is not 1:1. The mismatch is thought to result from the change in posterior corneal curvature following keratorefractive surgery. In myopic ablative procedures, the posterior corneal surface is thought to become more negative at the same time the anterior corneal surface becomes less positive. The natural power ratio between the 2 surfaces is altered, and the assumptions used in keratometry create significant errors in power measurements.

## Intraocular Lens Calculations After Refractive Surgery

A considerable amount of research has been done to improve the ability to calculate intraocular lens (IOL) powers after a refractive procedure. Several methods are available to cataract surgeons to aid them in IOL power calculation. The clinical history method, sometimes referred to as the refraction-derived method, involves subtracting the change in refractive error induced by refractive surgery from the average corneal power measured prior to surgery. The equation to determine the change in the corneal power from the known pre- and postoperative refractive and keratometric values is

$$RE\Delta_{sp} = MR_{Preop} - MR_{Postop}$$

A sample calculation is shown below:

| | OD | OS |
|---|---|---|
| Ks Preop | 45.00 (Average) | 45.50 (Average) |
| MR Preop | -6.00 | -4.50 |
| MR Postop | -0.25 | -0.50 |
| Ks Postop | 40.75 | 41.25 |

| | OD | OS |
|---|---|---|
| $RE\Delta_{sp} = MR_{postop} + MR_{preop}$ | $RE\Delta_{sp}$ = -0.25 – (-6.00) = +5.75 D | $RE\Delta_{sp}$ = (-0.50) – (-4.50) = +4.00 |
| $K_{sp} = K_{preop} - RE\Delta_{sp}$ | 45.00 – 5.75 = 39.25 D | 45.50 – 4.00 = 41.50 D |

To determine the change in corneal power based on the refraction in the corneal plane, the change in refraction must be converted using the following equation:

$$RE\Delta_{cp} = \frac{RE\Delta_{sp}}{1-(0.014*RE\Delta_{sp})}$$

This value can then be subtracted from the preoperative keratometry value to determine the keratometry value for the corneal plane ($K_{cp}$).

The contact lens method uses the known values of power and base curve combined with over-refraction to determine the power of the cornea.[26]

| | OD | OS |
|---|---|---|
| $OR_{sp}$ = MR with CL+CL power | ORsp = -3.00 + (-3.00) = -6.00 | ORsp = -1.50 + (-1.50) = -3.00 |
| BC of CL = 337.5/BC (mm) | 337.5/7.4 = 45.61 | 337.5/7.5 = 45.00 |
| $OR_{cp} = OR_{sp}/1+(0.014*OR_{sp})$ | -6.00/1+(0.014* -6.00) = -5.55 | -3.00/1+(0.014* -3) = -2.13 |
| $K_{CL}$ = BC of CL + $OR_{cp}$ | 45.61 + (-5.55) = 40.06 D | 45.00 + (-2.13) = 42.87 D |

Videokeratography measures the central corneal power inside the approximately 3-mm zone measured by keratometry and may give a more accurate power to use in IOL calculation formulas. For eyes that have had refractive surgery, the corneal power derived from clinical history, contact lens refraction, or videokeratography should be used in a third-generation theoretic formula, such as the Hoffer Q, Holladay, or SRK/T, to calculate the IOL power used during cataract surgery.[27]

Cheng and Lam[28] investigated the K-value obtained from the Gaussian optics formula (CalK) based on postoperative corneal topography by Orbscan II (Bausch & Lomb, Rochester, NY) and ultrasound pachymetry, comparing them to those obtained from the clinical history method (estK). A high correlation was noted between the K-value obtained by the clinical history method and the Gaussian optics formula ($R = 0.97$, $P < 0.001$). The mean difference between the 2 methods was 0.13 D. However, Preussner and colleagues found that ray tracing is superior to Gaussian optics in calculating corneal power, the purpose of IOL calculation.[29]

Aramberri recommends adjusting the SRK/T formula using the double K method. He found using the preoperative K value from keratometry or topography for the effective lens position calculation and using the clinical history method with the vergence formula improved the accuracy of IOL calculation S/P keratorefractive surgery.[30] Gimbel and Sun[31] evaluated target refractions based on measured and refraction-derived keratometric values by comparing them with postoperative achieved refractions. Differences between target refractions were calculated using 5 IOL formulas and 2 A-constants. Refraction-derived keratometric values led to more accurate IOL power calculations, along with using the Holladay 2 or Binkhorst 2 formula.

Chen and colleagues[32] suggested using the flattest keratometry value by calculation and aiming for -150 rather than plano in lens calculation to reduce the likelihood of hyperopia after cataract surgery following keratorefractive surgery. Gimbel and colleagues[33] also recommended using the smaller of the actual or refraction-derived keratometric values for calculating IOL power. As increasing numbers of baby boomers who are S/P keratorefractive surgery qualify for cataract surgery, it is likely that specific parameters will develop to avoid hyperopic postoperative results.

## Conclusion

The understanding of natural corneal optics and how they are changed with keratorefractive surgery is required for all corneal surgeons. Surgical planning must incorporate the knowledge to safeguard the patient from visual quality issues arising from drastic changes in corneal architecture. While night vision issues, glare, and distortion are minimized by increased ablation zones and improved ablation profiles, significant treatments in less-than-ideal patients may result in undesirable topographical abnormalities.

## References


1. Duke-Elder S, Wybar KC. Cornea. In: Duke-Elder S, ed. *System of Ophthalmology, Vol. 2: The Anatomy of the Visual System.* London, UK: Henry Kimpton Publishers; 1961:95-131.
2. Gipson IK, Joyce NC, Zieske JD. The anatomy and cell biology of the human cornea, limbus, conjunctiva, and adnexa. In: Smolin G, Foster CS, Thoft RA, Azar DT, Dohlman CH, eds. *Smolin and Thoft's the Cornea: Scientific Foundations & Clinical Practice.* Philadelphia, PA: Lippincott Williams & Wilkins; 2005:1-17.
3. McMenamin PG, Steele C, McGhee CNJ. Cornea: anatomy, physiology, and healing. In: McGhee CNJ, Taylor HR, Gartry DS, Trokel SL, eds. *Excimer Lasers in Ophthalmology: Principles and Practice.* London, UK: Martin Dunitz; 1997:41-45.
4. Davson H. *Physiology of the Eye.* 5th ed. New York, NY: Pergamon Press; 1990.
5. Maurice DM. *The Cornea and the Sclera.* London, UK: Academic Press; 1985.
6. Warwick R. *Eugene Wolff's Anatomy of the Eye and Orbit.* 8th ed. London, UK: Chapman & Hall Medical; 1997:235.
7. Vracko R, Benditt EP. Basal lamina: the scaffold for orderly cell replacement. Observations on regeneration of injured skeletal muscle fibers and capillaries. *J Cell Biol.* 1972;55(2):406-419.
8. Hogan MJ, Alvarado JA, Wedell JE. *Histology of the Human Eye.* Philadelphia, PA: WB Saunders; 1971.
9. Krachmer JH, Mannis MJ, Holland EJ. *Cornea, Vol I: Fundamentals, Diagnosis and Management.* 2nd ed. London, UK: Elsevier-Mosby; 2005.
10 Farrell RA, McCally RL. Corneal transparency. In: Albert DM, Jakobiec FA, eds. *Principles and Practice of Ophthalmology.* Philadelphia, PA: WB Saunders; 2000:629-643.
11. Arffa R. *Grayson's Diseases of the Cornea.* 4th ed. St Louis, MO: Mosby; 1997.
12. Meek KM, Boote C. The organization of collagen in the corneal stroma. *Exp Eye Res.* 2004;78:503-512.
13. Daxer A, Fratzel P. Collagen fibril orientation in the human corneal stroma and its implications in keratoconus. *Inv Ophthal Vis Sci.* 1997;38:121-129.
14. Meek KM, Tuft SJ, Huang Y, et al. Changes in collagen orientation and distribution in keratoconus corneas. *Inv Ophthal Vis Sci.* 2005;46:1948-1956.
15. Hayes S, Boote C, Tift SL, Quantock AJ, Meek KM. A study of corneal thickness, shape and collagen organization in keratoconus using videokeratography and X-ray scattering techniques. *Exp Eye Res.* 2007;84:423-434.
16. Joyce NC, Meklir B, Joyce SJ, Zieske JD. Cell cycle protein expression and proliferative status in human corneal cells. *Invest Ophthalmol Vis Sci.* 1996;37:645-655.
17. Holly FJ, Lemp MA. Tear physiology and dry eyes. *Surv Ophthalmol.* 1977;22:69-87.
18. Stein HA, Slatt BJ, Stein RM, Freeman MI. *Fitting Guide for Rigid and Soft Contact Lenses: A Practical Approach.* Philadelphia, PA: Mosby; 2002:3-12.
19. Müller LJ, Marfurt CF, Kruse F, Tervo TM. Corneal nerves: structure, contents, and function. *Exp Eye Res.* 2003;76:521-542.
20. Robin JB, Rich LF, Elander RE. *Principles and Practice of Refractive Surgery.* Philadelphia, PA: WB Saunders Co; 1997.
21. Fannin TE, Grosvenor T. *Clinical Optics.* 2nd ed. Boston, MA; Butterworth-Heinemann; 1996.
22. Klyce S. Night vision after LASIK. *Ophthalmology.* 2004;111(1):1,2.

23. Munnerlyn C, Koons S, Marshall J. Photorefractive keratectomy: a technique for laser refractive surgery. *J Cataract Refract Surg.* 1988;14:46.
24. Baikoff G, Lutun E, Ferraz C, Wei J. Analysis of the eye's anterior segment with optical coherence tomography: static and dynamic Study. *J Fr Ophtalmol.* 2005;28(4):343-352.
25. Freedman KA, Brown SM, Mathews SM, Young RS. Pupil size and the ablation zone in laser refractive surgery: considerations based on geometric optics. *J Cataract Refract Surg.* 2003;29(10):1924-1931.
26. Haigis W. Corneal power after refractive surgery for myopia: contact lens method. *J Cataract Refract Surg.* 2003;29:1397-1411.
27. Hoffer KJ. Intraocular lens power calculation for eyes after refractive keratotomy. *J Refract Surg.* 2004;20(6):783-789.
28. Cheng CK, Lam DS. Keratometry for intraocular lens power calculation using Orbscan II in eyes with laser in situ keratomileusis. *J Refract Surg.* 2005;21(4):365-368.
29. Preussner PR, Wahl J, Lahdo H, Dick B, Findl O. Ray tracing for intraocular lens calculation. *J Cataract Refract Surg.* 2002;28:1412-1419.
30. Aramberri J. Intraocular lens power calculation after corneal refractive surgery: double-K method. *J Cataract Refract Surg.* 2003;29:203-206.
31. Gimbel HV, Sun R. Accuracy and predictability of intraocular lens power calculation after laser in situ keratomileusis. *J Cataract Refract Surg.* 2001;27:571-576.
32. Chen L, Mannis MJ, Salz JJ, Garcia-Ferrer FJ, Ge J. Analysis of intraocular lens power calculation in post-radial keratotomy eyes. *J Cataract Refract Surg.* 2003;29:65-70.
33. Gimbel HV, Sun R, Furlong MT, van Westenbrugge JA, Kassab J. Accuracy and predictability of intraocular lens power calculation after photorefractive keratectomy. *J Cataract Refract Surg.* 2000;26:1147-1151.

Chapter 3

# Maps and Scales

Tracy Schroeder Swartz, OD, MS, FAAO; Ilan Cohen, MD; Ray-Ann Lin, MD; Megan Buliano, OD; and Y. Ralph Chu, MD

Corneal topography depicts the variations on the surface of the cornea. Because the cornea is not perfectly spherical, nor does it perfectly coincide with any other geometrical abstraction, we need to consider the characteristics on each point along its surface in order to understand its properties.

The cornea has 2 surfaces responsible for the refraction of light: the anterior and the posterior. The anterior surface is more important because approximately 90% of refraction occurs there. The posterior surface contributes roughly 10% of the total corneal power in a virgin eye. This assumption could lead to significant errors in eyes with keratoconus or postkeratorefractive surgery.

Numerous topographers enable measurement of the surface characteristics of the cornea. Each one uses slightly different formulas or techniques to derive the topographical map. To complicate matters, each topographer offers a wide range of plots to display the information obtained using similar but not identical scales, based on user preferences. When evaluating a topographical map, one must note the scale used and the type of map displayed to avoid misinterpretation.

## Scales

To view a topographical map correctly, it is important to understand the general shape of the curvature patterns and how it relates to scaling. The same map may appear differently depending on the scale used. Thus, determining which scale to use in a particular situation is the key to success.[1]

Initially, a standardized absolute scale was proposed,[2] ranging from 9.0 to 101.5 D. The central portion of the range was measured with 1.5-D step intervals and the extreme limits of the range in 5.0-D step intervals. Although this range covered the entire power spectrum seen in corneal practice, salient topographic features were occasionally lost within the 5.0-D intervals, particularly at the low end of the scale. Hence, this was modified by the Klyce/Wilson Scale,[3] which ranged from 28.0 to 65.5 D in equal 1.5-D step intervals. It has still been argued that the 1.5-D interval is so wide that irregularities in corneal topography may be masked. An example of changes in topographic patterns associated with increased step size is shown in Figure 3-1. Figure 3-1A shows more detailed irregularity compared to its counterpart (Figure 3-1B) due to smaller step size.

However, it has been demonstrated that the 1.5-D scale can detect all the topographic characteristics identified by a more sensitive 1.0-D scale in a consecutive series of patients that included contact lens-wearing corneas, early to moderate and advanced keratoconus, penetrating keratoplasties, extracapsular cataract extraction, excimer laser photorefractive keratotomy, radial keratotomy, aphakic epikeratophakia, and myopic epikeratophakia.[4] In 1999, the American National Standards Institute (ANSI) issued a report titled, *Corneal Topography Systems—Standard Terminology, Requirements* (ANSI Z-80.23-1999).[5,6]



Wang M. *Corneal Topography: A Guide for Clinical Application in the Wavefront Era, Second Edition (pp. 21-32)*

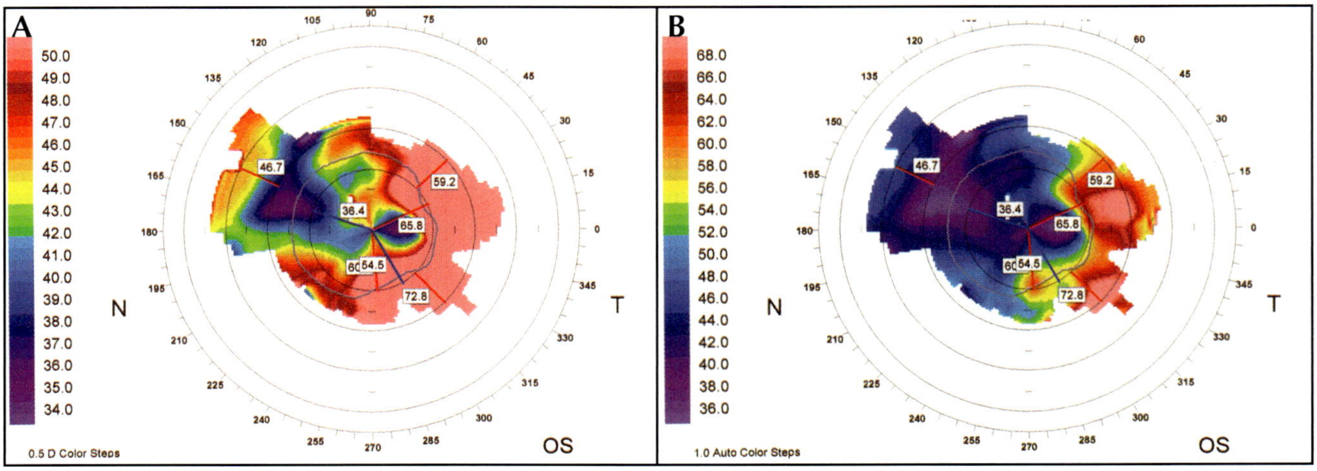


**Figure 3-1.** (A) An axial curvature map using a step size of 0.5 D. (B) The same axial curvature map using a step size of 1.0 D. Note the detail changes as the step size changes.

TABLE 3-1.

**Differences Between the American National Standards Institute and Universal Standard Scale**

| SCALE NAME | INTERVAL SIZE (D) | RANGE OF POWERS (D) | DISPLAYED POWERS (% OF 388 TOPOGRAPHIC MAPS OF 12 CORNEAL CONDITIONS) |
|---|---|---|---|
| ANSI | 1.5 | 29 to 59 | 99.2 |
| ANSI | 1.0 | 34 to 54 | 96.6 |
| ANSI | 0.5 | 39 to 49 | 86.2 |
| USS | 1.5 | 30 to 67.5 | 99.9 |

This standard was anticipated to encompass the presentation of information, the standardized scale, scale interval, and the representative color palette used for curvature and elevation maps. It would allow users of corneal topographers to directly compare the topography maps produced by different manufacturers. However, Annex B of the ANSI standard, which defines scale intervals, the scale center, and a color convention, does not specify a single, well-defined color palette but rather suggests a variety of numeric and color scale combinations.[5]

In an effort to overcome this potential point of confusion, an alternative color scale was proposed—the Universal Standard Scale (USS). The USS was able to overcome the problems encountered with the ANSI standard by associating a single, well-defined numerical scale with a single, well-defined color palette. Table 3-1 highlights the differences between the ANSI and USS scales. This method has been shown to produce maps that were consistent and could be rapidly and correctly interpreted. The USS displays a range of powers that encompass 99.9% of both naturally occurring and surgically induced corneal shapes. The USS is based on 1.5-D intervals and a well-defined color scale that would be most relevant for average clinical uses.[7] The 1.5-D interval gives the best sensitivity, specificity, and range.[7]

Table 3-2 describes the ability of topography scales to display corneal powers by relating interval size to dioptric range. There is no standardization of topographic scales between commercial companies. This makes it more difficult to compare examinations performed using different systems. For example, in the absolute/standardized scale default mode, the Humphrey Atlas (Carl Zeiss Meditec, Jena, Germany) ranges from 38.5 to 50.0 D in 0.50-D intervals, while the out-of-the-box absolute default scale for the Tomey TMS-4 (Tomey Corporation, Nagoya, Japan) ranges from 9 to 101.5 D.

## INTERPRETATION

When evaluating a topographic display either through a printed report or on the instrument's screen, one should study maps in a structured way to avoid mistakes in interpretation. The guidelines that follow will aid in successful interpretation of the maps.[8] Once a topographic

TABLE 3-2.

**Topographical Maps Use Colors to Denote Curvature**

| COLOR | POWER (D) | |
|---|---|---|
| Red | 48.0 | Steep |
| Orange/yellow | 45.0 | |
| Yellow/green | 43.5 | Average |
| Green/light blue | 42.0 | |
| Blue | 39.0 | Flat |

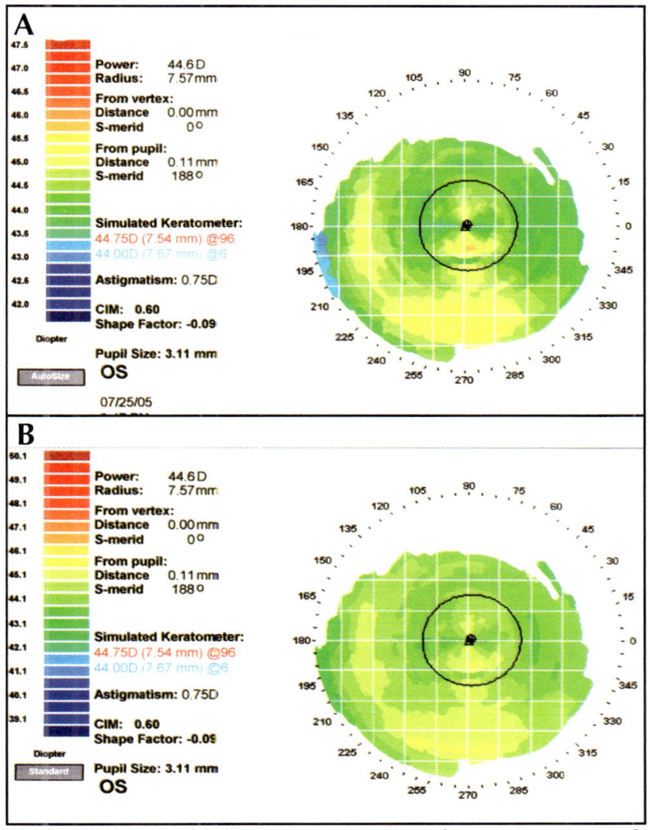


**Figure 3-2.** (A) Mild dry eye causing irregular astigmatism with the autoscale. (B) Mild dry eye appears less irregular when using the standard scale.

image has been captured, it is scaled and graphically represented in a color-coded contour map. Depending on the scale used for color conversion, identical maps may, in fact, appear to be different. Scale ranges and color representation vary among topographers, which makes direct comparisons between topographers open to interpretation. Color-coded contour maps of corneal surface power have been adopted as a standard presentation scheme in corneal topography. They markedly facilitate the viewer's interpretation through the association of power with color and recognition of pathologic features with the patterns formed by the map contours. Color-coded contour maps were initially developed for videokeratoscopy, and with the introduction of projection-based topography systems, a similar color-coded system was applied to elevation maps. Warm colors, red and orange, are used to represent relatively higher powers (steeper curvatures); green and yellow are used for powers associated with normal corneas; and cool color hues of blue are used to denote relatively lower powers (flatter curvatures). For elevation maps, high areas were depicted by warm colors, and low areas were depicted by cool colors. This concept, along with standard scale, provides an intuitive basis for the interpretation of corneal topography.[4] For example, in a case of keratoconus, the red area on a height map corresponds to the highest point, which is the apex of the cone. In the same case, the red area on a curvature or power map is the steepest area, which is usually located adjacent to the cone inferiorly.

As you can see in Figure 3-2, the absolute/standardized scale significantly expands the dioptric range used. Clinically significant irregularities may be masked when comparing eyes with widely disparate curvature readings. When the range is standardized, the steepest curvatures appear red, while the flattest curvatures appear blue. General patterns remain the same, but intricate curvature changes disappear because the interval of measurement also increases from 0.25 to 0.50 D.[1]

The use of a standardized and fixed color scale for routine clinical examination is important for consistent and correct evaluation of corneal topography (Table 3-3).

TABLE 3-3.

**Comparison of Absolute and Relative Scales**

| COLOR STANDARDIZED/ ABSOLUTE SCALES | NORMALIZED/ RELATIVE/AUTOSIZE |
|---|---|
| Standardized | Nonstandardized |
| Good for comparison | Comparison of maps is more difficult |
| Large step sizes | Small steps |
| Low resolution | High resolution |
| Large range of powers | Narrow range of powers |
| Good for screening | Subtle features present |
| Good for gross pathology | Good for detail |

Autosizing or normalized scales lend confusion. Because the range of powers for the cornea varies, physiologic asymmetry or astigmatism may be amplified by an adaptable scale and may lead to misdiagnosis of pathology. An example of this is shown in Figure 3-2, a patient with mild dry eye. The irregular astigmatism is more evident using the auto scale. Alternatively, a cornea with substantial irregular astigmatism can be made to look less abnormal with an adjustable scale.[4]

The allocation of colors on an absolute/standardized scale is related to the distribution of corneal powers in the normal population. Central corneal power has an approximate Gaussian distribution (represented by a bell-shaped curve). The mean central corneal power is 43.50 D, which is depicted by a color from the middle of the spectrum. Approximately 66% of the population has a central corneal power within one standard deviation of the mean (42 to 45 D), and this is represented by the adjacent colors on the scale. Less than 3% of the population has a central corneal power beyond ±3 SD, represented by red and dark blue. If these colors are present on an absolute scale map, the cornea is unlikely to be normal.[7]

## Autosize/Normalized Scale

The normalized scale (relative, adaptive) or autoscale automatically adjusts and subdivides a specific cornea into several dioptric intervals based on the actual dioptric range of the cornea measured. Based on color representation, maps may appear to represent similar dioptric curvatures when using this scale, but depending on a patient's specific corneal curvature, these intervals may vary in range and dioptric value. This may falsely give the appearance that all maps represent equal curvatures.

A normalized scale uses a set number of colors that are automatically adjusted to fill the range of dioptric values for that single map. The mean power for that cornea is positioned in the center of the scale. The normalized scale has the advantage over the absolute scale by fusing narrower steps between the contours, which provides more detail. Some systems limit how small the steps can be so that the information generated is still clinically relevant. However, as the scale may be different for almost every examination, it should be checked carefully before studying the map.

The automatic scale is a useful tool for examining a single eye in greater detail, as the smaller range will highlight variation and subtle changes with the caveat that normal variations may seem accentuated to the point of being questionable surgical candidates. For example, the use of a normalized scale can produce a pair of maps of similar appearance for a patient with advanced keratoconus in one eye (using a large step interval) and a subclinical cone in the other eye (using a small step interval).[7] The automatic scale may also be beneficial in patients having undergone laser-assisted in situ keratomileusis (LASIK) with visual complaints where small irregularities may cause problems with visual acuity.

## Standard/Absolute Scale

The standard or absolute scale assigns the same color to a specific dioptric interval of curvature and forces that cornea's parameters to fit within that range. Although the range varies by instrument, each individual instrument's range is consistent. Therefore, for each map viewed, a direct comparison of images from different eyes or from curvature changes of one eye (preoperative and postoperative refractive surgery patients) can be made quickly and accurately. Because there has been no standardization of scales between commercial companies to date, this makes it more difficult to directly compare examinations performed using different systems.

A potential limitation of the standard scale is its inability to highlight subtle corneal changes that are important to evaluate when considering refractive surgery. Misinterpretation can exist due to the large range in intervals and loss of detail. Because the ranges and parameters are standard, 2 different maps can be compared—unlike with the autosize scale. This scale is most useful when comparing maps over time and with varying interpreters. It gives the best results for gross evaluations of the cornea.

## Map Displays

Topographers capture data from points on the corneal surface using various technologies. Placido imaging is the most commonly used system, but Scheimpflug imaging and slit scanning are also employed. From these primary data points, a wide range of maps can be displayed by the computer. The maps are usually color coded for easier interpretation by the clinician.

### Curvature Maps

Curvature or power maps include axial, tangential, and refractive maps. The most commonly used curvature map is the axial map. This map depicts the anterior curvature of the cornea at each point along its surface, usually up to a diameter of 7 mm. To know the curvature of a point on a spherical surface, we need to find the circle that best fits the plane curve at the surface point of interest and determine the local radius of curvature (K), where K = 1/R. The radius of curvature (R) is measured in millimeters. Curvature is the inverse of the radius, measured in D The optical power of the cornea at any given point is a function of the curvature at that point but is not the same as the curvature. The smaller the radius of curvature, the more curved the surface. Curvature may be displayed using several types of maps: axial and tangential or meridional.

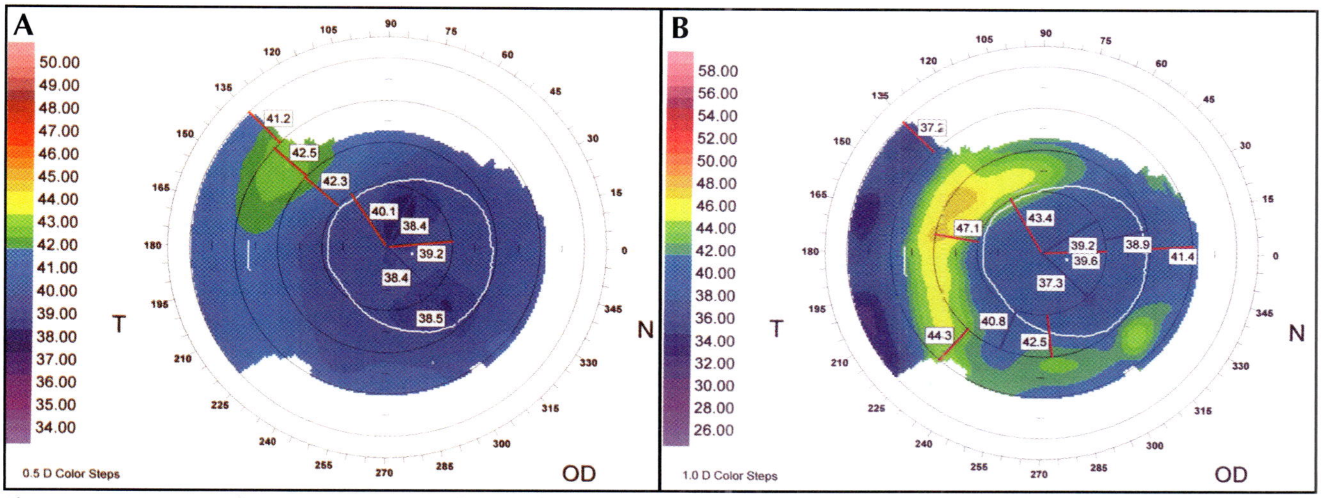


**Figure 3-3.** (A) An axial map. (B) A tangential map of the same eye. Note the focal changes seen with this map are more detailed than those of the axial map.

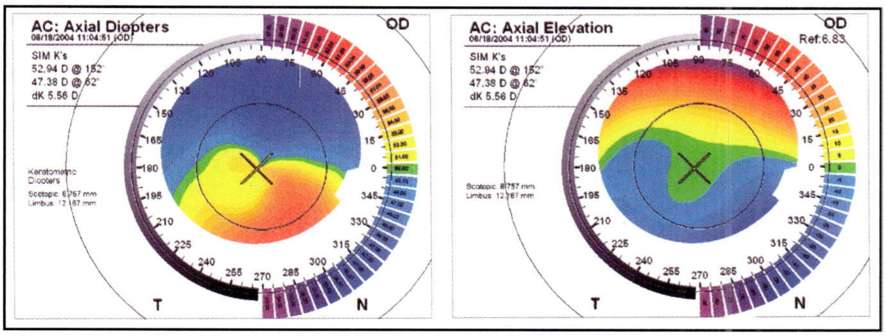


**Figure 3-4.** Elevation and axial maps of the same eye show that the inferior portion is not actually elevated, but rather depressed below that of the reference sphere due to the sharp curve of the cornea inferiorly.

Axial curvature maps are obtained by measuring the curvature of the cornea at each point relative to a specified axis, usually the visual axis. The local radius for a corneal surface point can be measured as the distance from the point to the optic axis along the normal. Unfortunately, this requires the assumption that the center of curvature for the specific surface point is located along the optic axis. This radius is then called the axial radius of curvature. The center for all surface points is on the optic axis for spherical surfaces only, and the cornea is an aspheric surface. While this assumption was acceptable for keratometry, it introduces significant error in the corneal periphery. This effectively smooths small variations on the surface of the cornea and provides a less irregular map that is easier to read and understand.[8] The axial map gives a global view of the corneal curvature as a whole. However, axial maps tend to ignore minor variations in the local curvature. A comparison between an axial map and a tangential map for the same eye is shown in Figure 3-3. Figure 3-3A is an axial map, which is less irregular than Figure 3-3B, a tangential map.

The tangential map uses calculations based on a different mathematical approach to more accurately determine the peripheral corneal configuration. Tangential maps represent the local curvature of the cornea at each point in meridional direction relative to the other points on the particular ring. For this reason, they may be referred to as "meridional maps." Tangential maps are also sometimes referred to as "local curvature" or "instantaneous curvature." Because the axis of reference is different for each point, there is a higher degree of variability from point to point.[9] There is also a smaller number of mathematical assumptions (ie, the sphericity of the cornea) used in this formula. The tangential map can recognize sharp power transitions more readily than the axial map and eliminates the "smoothing" appearance that appears on the axial map for most topographers. Because tangential maps are more likely to illustrate focal irregularities, they are useful in contact lens fitting.

When reading a curvature map, it is important not to confuse "steepness" (typically pictured by hotter colors) with height. Curvature simply means that the shape of the cornea is changing, but it does not tell the direction of the change. For example, a curvature map of a keratoconic cornea characteristically shows red inferiorly, corresponding to the inferior distortion of the cornea inherent to the disease. The elevation map of the same eye in Figure 3-4 shows that the inferior portion is not actually elevated, but rather is depressed below that of the reference sphere, due to the sharp curve of the cornea inferiorly.

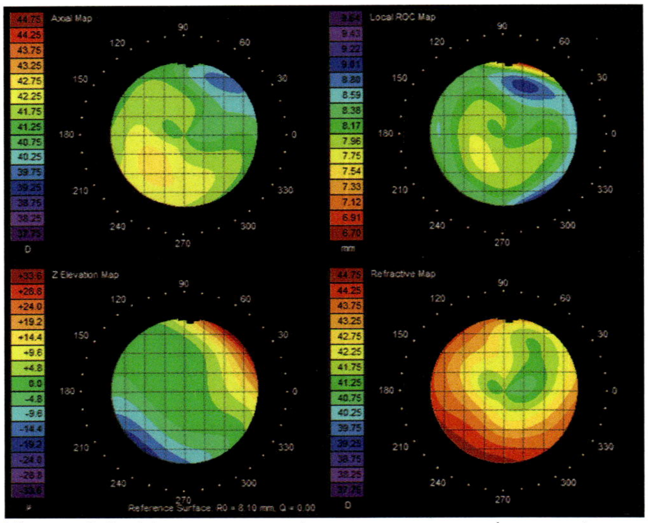


**Figure 3-5.** Many systems incorporate several maps into a single display. This patient reported visual distortion and glare, which was most easily explained by the refractive power map (lower right).

The refractive map displays the calculated refractive power of the cornea based on Snell's law of refraction. It correlates vision to corneal shape. It is not often used; however, it may identify distortion in vision related to focal irregularities in the cornea and explain vision loss not apparent upon slit-lamp examination (Figure 3-5).

## Elevation Maps

A topographical map of a landscape depicts each point on the map in relationship to sea level. In corneal topography, an elevation map needs to be depicted with relation to a reference plane. This plane is often a sphere with a diameter that most closely resembles the overall diameter of that specific cornea. Each point on the cornea that coincides with the reference sphere is represented by the color green. Warmer colors represent points that are higher than the reference plane, and cooler colors represent points lower than the reference plane. Remember that the refractive power of the cornea is not represented by the elevation itself but by changes in elevation.

In refractive surgery, elevation maps are extremely important. Because removing tissue most directly affects the elevation of the cornea, we have to understand elevation topography in order to grasp the effects that we are imparting on the cornea. The cornea is usually prolate, not perfectly spherical. Therefore, in order for a topographical map to have a quantitative and qualitative meaning, we need to know how the reference sphere correlates to the corneal surface. This attribute may be fixed in some topographers and can be chosen by the user in others.

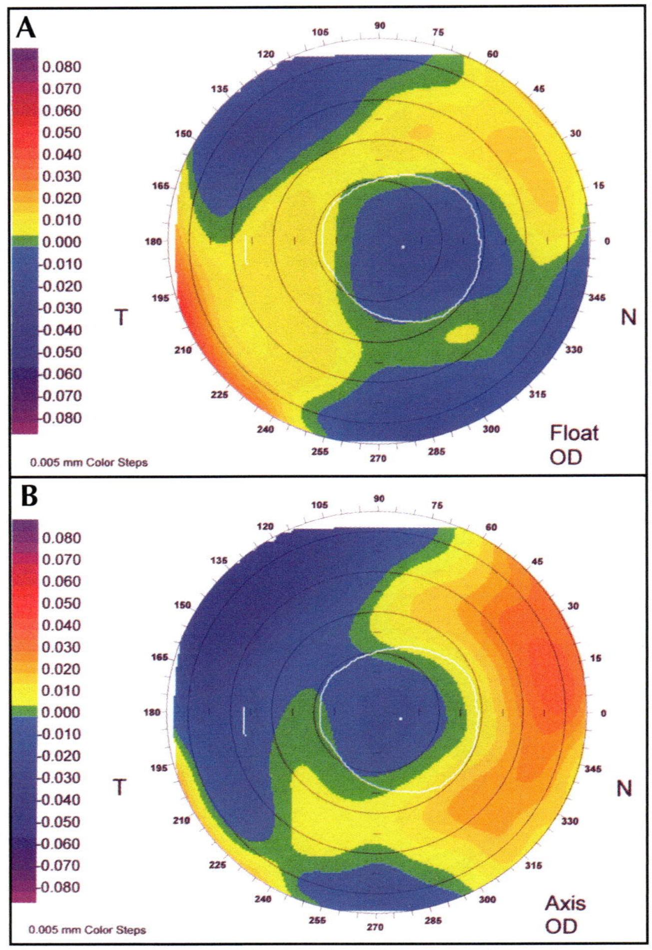


**Figure 3-6.** Operator choices for alignment of anterior elevation map displays include (A) float alignment, where there are no constraints assigned to the reference sphere and (B) centered alignment, where the center of the sphere is constrained to the viewing axis. *(continued)*

Changing the size, shape, or alignment of the reference sphere will have an impact on the topography map, just as changing the sea level would impact the heights of structures on the land surface. For practical applications, the reference plane is usually set to a sphere. The size of the sphere is chosen such that it best fits the cornea in question.

Choices for alignment vary, but often include float, centered, pinned, or apex. In Figure 3-6, the same eye has been mapped using the 4 choices. When using float alignment, there are no constraints assigned to the reference sphere. The diameter and the location of the sphere are chosen to maximize the area of contact between the reference sphere and the cornea. This is the default alignment for most topographers. When using centered alignment, the center of the sphere is constrained to the viewing axis with the ability to move along that axis. Pinned alignment imposes the pin (P) constraint, which forces the reference sphere and the data surface to intersect on the viewing axis. The sphere

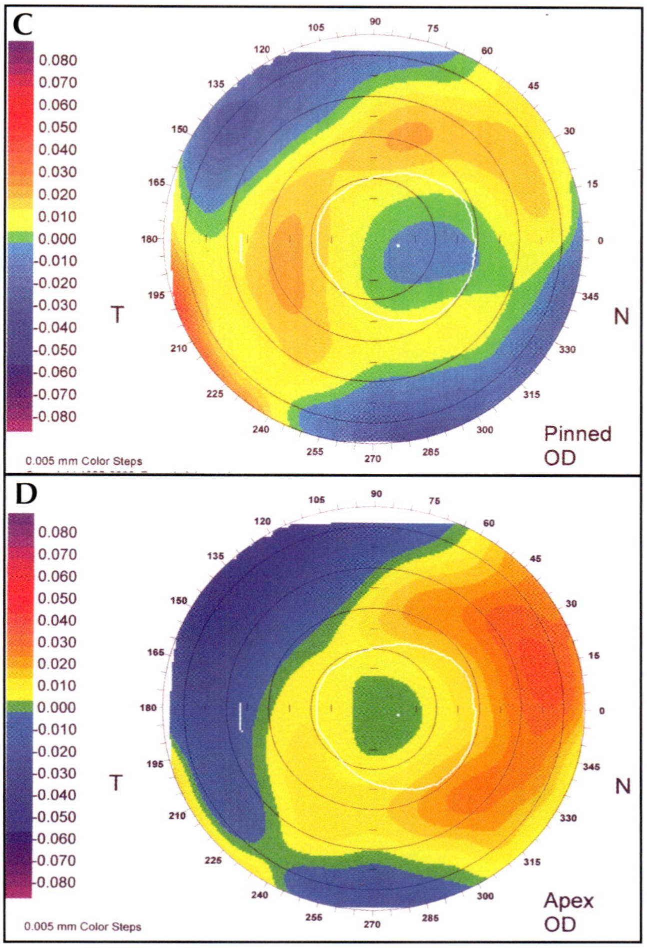


**Figure 3-6 (continued).** Operator choices for alignment of anterior elevation map displays include (C) pinned alignment, which forces the reference sphere and the data surface to intersect on the viewing axis and (D) apex alignment, which imposes both the center and pinned constraints.

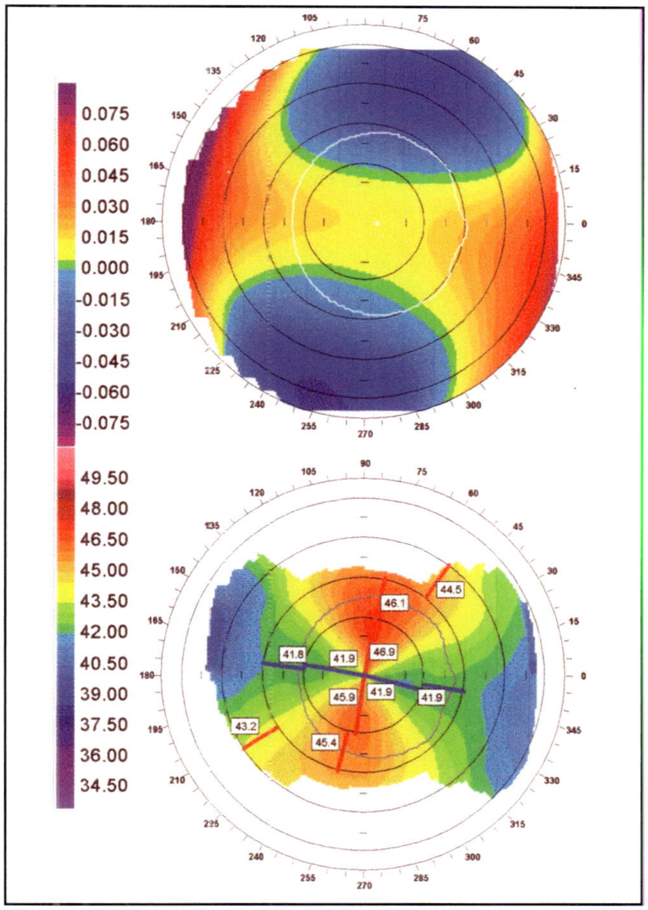


**Figure 3-7.** An elevation and axial power map in an eye showing with-the-rule astigmat sm.

center may be off-axis in this scenario. Apex alignment imposes both center and pin (C + P) constraints. The sphere surface intersects the data surface on the viewing axis, and the center of the sphere lies on the viewing axis.

It is important to realize that the axial curvature map and anterior elevation map are related, but do not directly correspond. Figure 3-7 shows an elevation map and an axial power map in an eye that has with-the-rule astigmatism. When we follow the vertical axis from a point superiorly toward the center, we see that elevation increases as we approach the center and decreases as we move inferiorly. This means that the curvature is steep along this meridian, as shown in the axial map. The steep meridian here is represented by the vertical bow-tie pattern. Note that the warm and cold colors are somewhat reversed when you compare an elevation map to a curvature map because a change in elevation causes a change in curvature.

In refractive surgery, we often need to compare pre- and postoperative topographical maps. The goal is to determine where tissue was removed and how much tissue was removed. We can then correlate this to the refractive effect that was achieved with the keratorefractive surgery. Elevation mapping directly illustrates tissue removal. Some programs perform a pre- and postoperative analysis based on the anterior elevation and pachymetry maps to calculate the exact amount of tissue that was removed at each point. This is useful in detecting postsurgical irregularities such as decentered ablation or central islands. Curvature maps should not be used to identify decentered ablations because they may exaggerate the decentration, exemplified in Figure 3-8.

General understanding of the anterior elevation topographical map can be applied to the posterior elevation topography. The posterior elevation map is created much like the anterior elevation map in design, with the exception that it represents the posterior surface of the cornea. The choices for alignment of the posterior surface elevation maps are the same as those for the anterior surface: float, centered, pinned, or apex. These are shown in Figure 3-9.

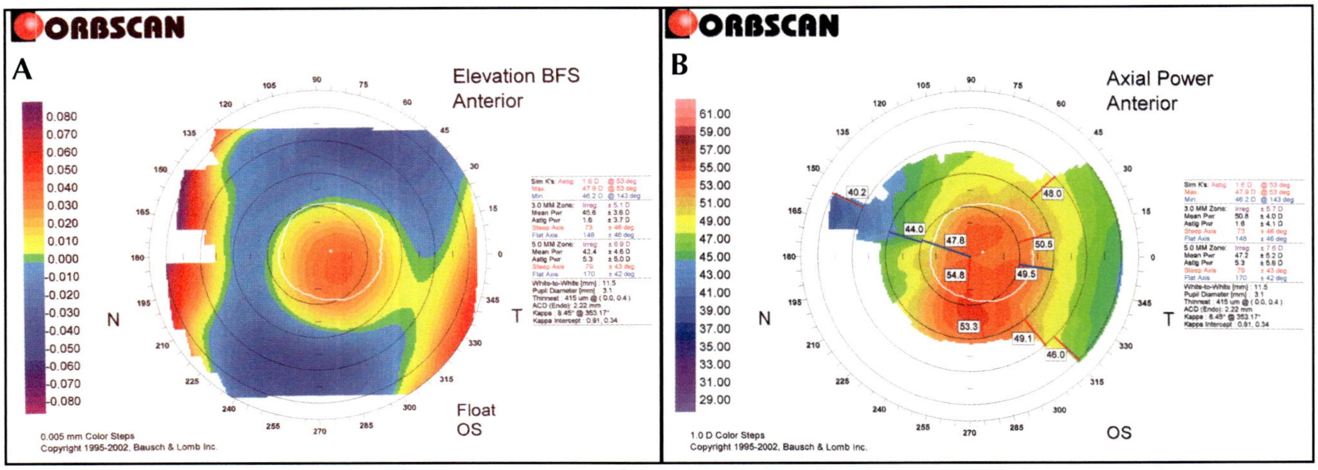


**Figure 3-8.** (A) Elevation maps rather than curvature maps should be used to identify decentered ablations. (B) Curvature maps tend to exaggerate the decentered area and should not be used to identify decentered ablations.

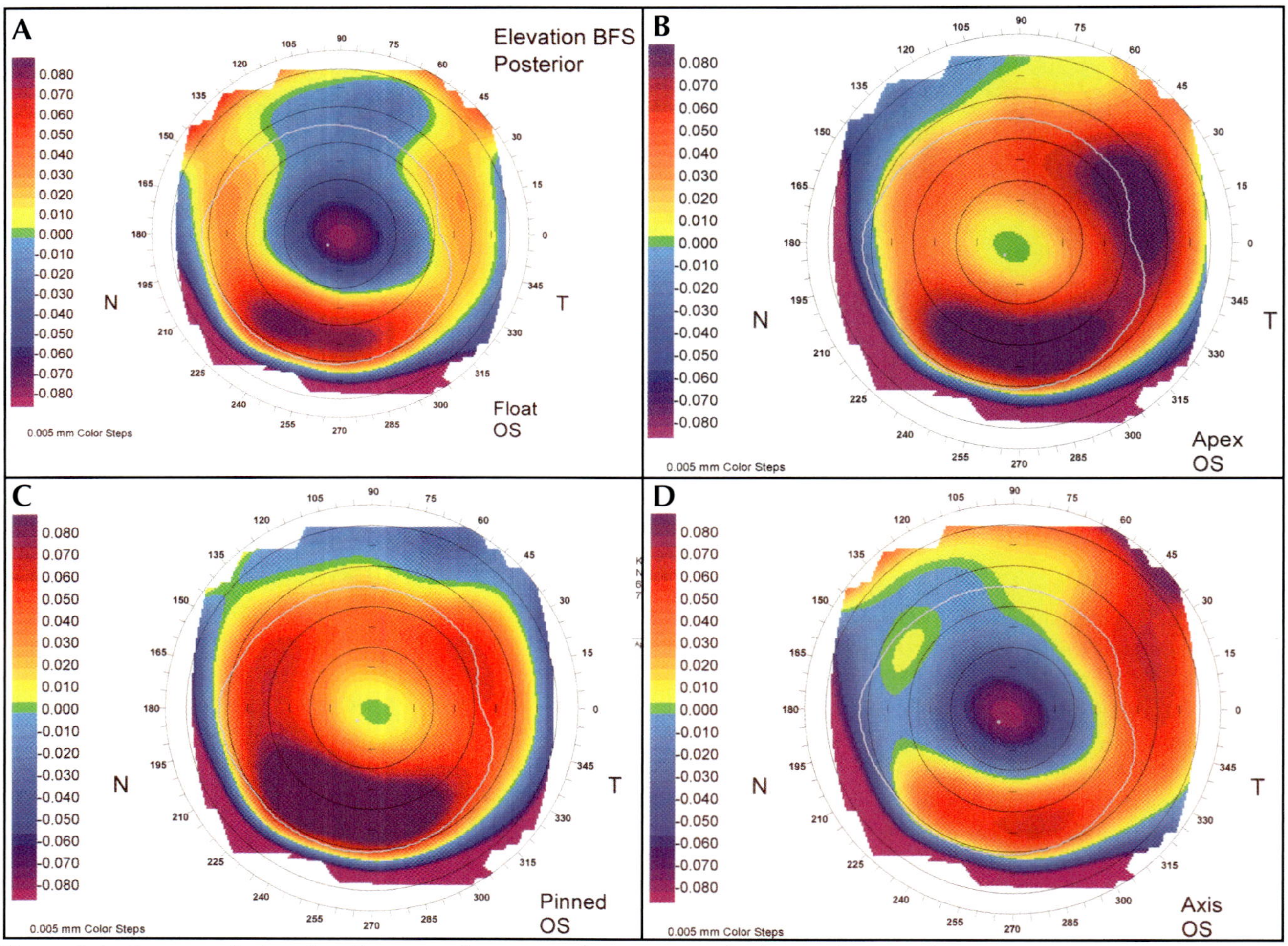


**Figure 3-9.** Operator choices for alignment of posterior elevation map displays include (A) float alignment, where there are no constraints assigned to the reference sphere; (B) centered alignment, where the center of the sphere is constrained to the viewing axis; (C) pinned alignment, which forces the reference sphere and the data surface to intersect on the viewing axis; and (D) apex alignment, which imposes both the center and pinned constraints.

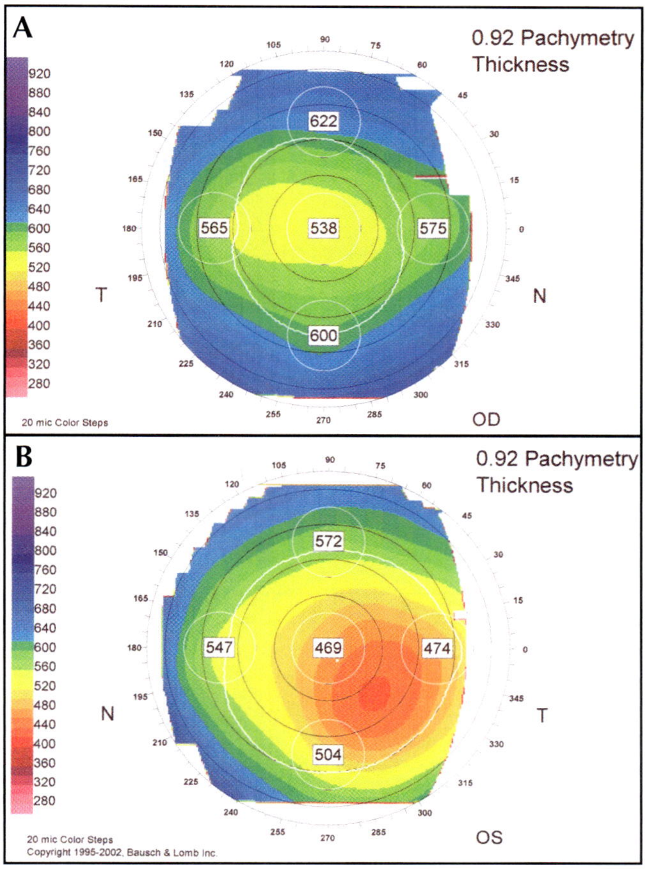


**Figure 3-10.** (A) Pachymetry map from a healthy patient. (B) Pachymetry map from a patient with keratoconus.

# Pachymetry Maps

Slit scanning, Scheimpflug, and anterior segment optical coherence tomography imaging technology yield pachymetry data. It gives us information not only about the central or paracentral points of the cornea customarily obtained by ultrasound pachymetry, but also about the distribution of the thickness along the surface. Figure 3-10 shows a pachymetric map from a healthy patient (Figure 3-10A) and a patient with keratoconus (Figure 3-10B).

Pachymetry information is useful in glaucoma assessment, as well as in screening refractive surgery candidates and estimating residual corneal bed thickness postoperatively. These data are invaluable when combined with the other maps to rule out keratoconus or forme fruste keratoconus. Figures 3-11 and 3-12 illustrate the subtle differences between the forme fruste keratoconus, true keratoconus, and pellucid marginal degeneration. Corneal thinning corresponds to the apex of the cone in keratoconus (Figure 3-12A) and inferior to it in cases of PMD (Figure 3-12B). Early topographical signs may only be found on the posterior surface using tomography.

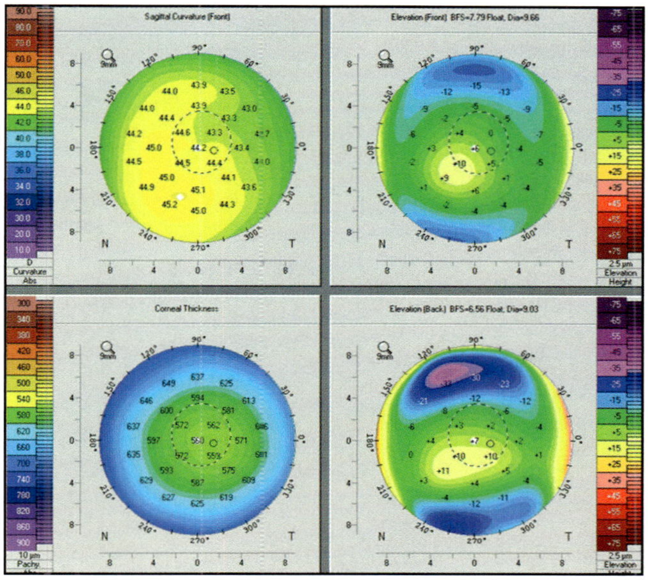


**Figure 3-11.** Subtle topographic abnormalities in forme fruste keratoconus. Note the slightly decentered posterior elevation, and displacement of the thinnest point. There is mild asymmetry on the curvature map.

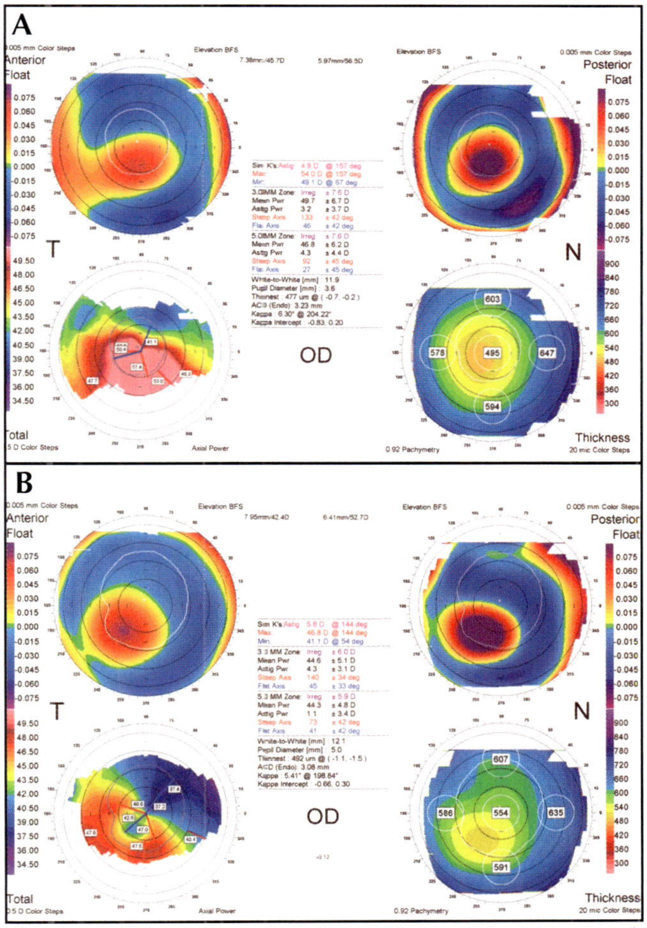


**Figure 3-12.** (A) The ectasia in keratoconus tends to be central. (B) The ectasia in PMD tends to be inferior.

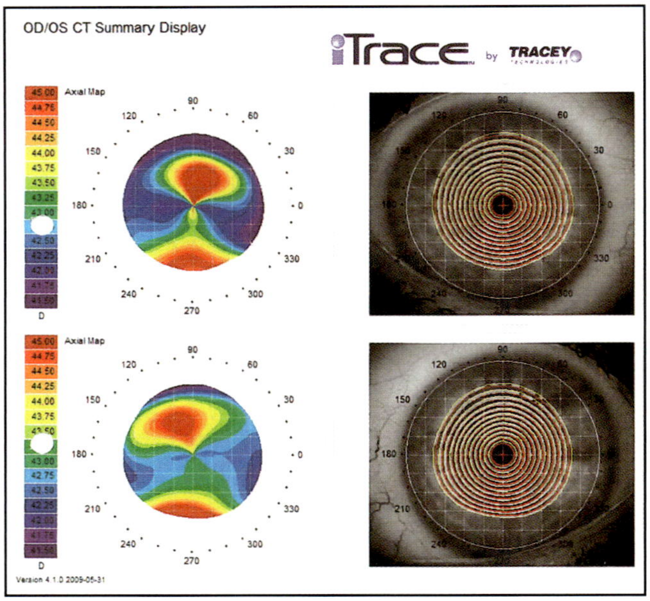


**Figure 3-13.** When topography maps appear nonsensical, dry eye may be the etiology, as in this case. With treatment, the topography should become more regular.

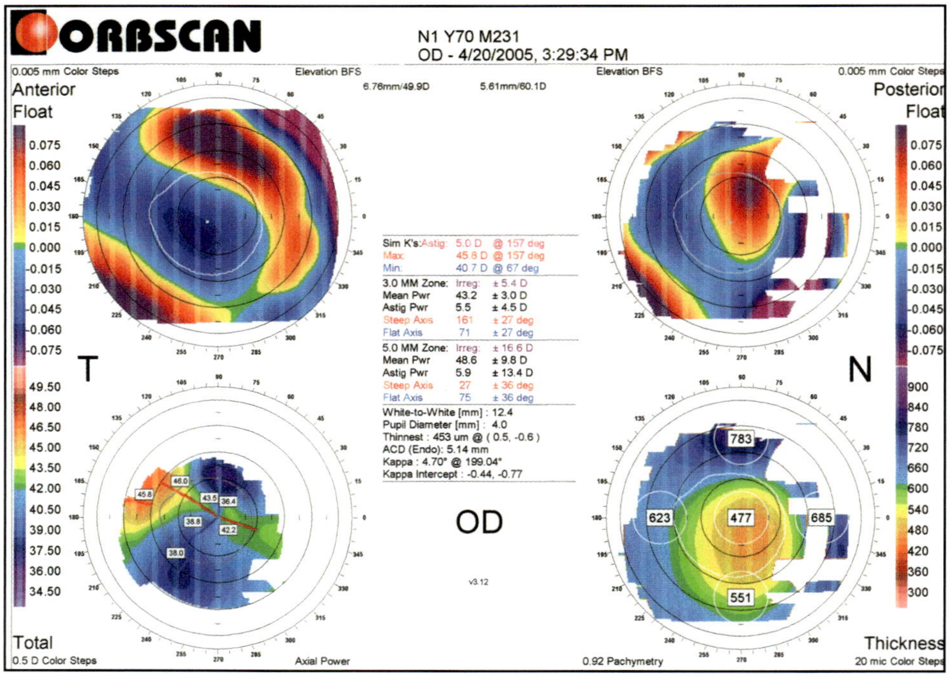


**Figure 3-14.** Data loss resulting from INTACS segments.

# Topographic Map Interpretation

When looking at a topography map, you need to consider the clinical picture and interpret the map in that perspective. Correct identification of the type of map is crucial—is it a curvature map or elevation map? When comparing maps over time, it is necessary to examine the scale. Some clinical entities that commonly interfere with the accuracy of topographic maps include corneal opacities, dry eye and insufficient tear film, eye movements, and contact lens wear.

A corneal scar can interfere with the data acquisition by a slit-scan topographer. The slit-scanning unit may misinterpret the opacity as a corneal surface, resulting in errors in both pachymetry and posterior elevation maps. A disrupted tear film can interfere with the reflection of light from the cornea, create artificially steepened areas, or lead to miscalculations based on missing data points. Irregularities resulting from a dry eye can be seen in Figure 3-13. INTACS corneal ring segments (Valley Eye Associates, Appleton, WI) can also result in loss of data in certain systems, as seen in Figure 3-14.

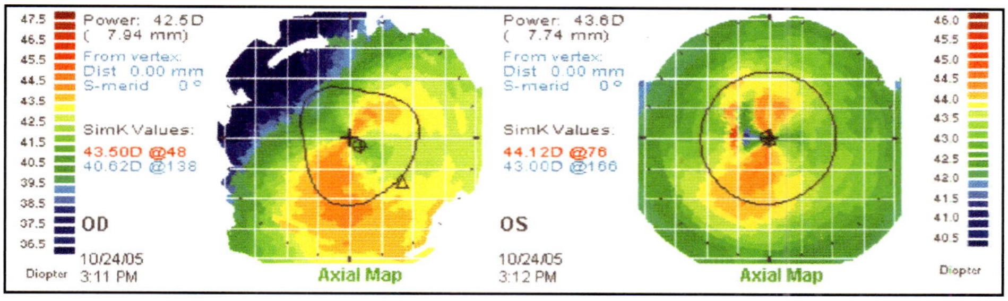


**Figure 3-15.** Contact lens warpage can result from overwear of both soft and gas permeable lenses, and lenses must be discontinued before final diagnosis or IOL selection in the case of patients pursuing cataract surgery. It is easy to mistake warpage for ectatic disease, and pachymetry facilitates the differential diagnosis.

Minimal eye movements are required for data collection, especially for the slit-scanning systems where data capture requires more time. Some topographers may accomplish this process faster than others, and this may be helpful in patients who have difficulty opening their eyes or who cannot maintain fixation for long.

Contact lens wear may distort the shape of the cornea. An example of contact lens warpage in a gas-permeable lens wearer is shown in Figure 3-15. This is not uncommon in hard contact lens wearers and in prolonged soft contact lens wearers. These eyes may resemble early keratoconus on topography. For this reason, it is recommended that contact lens wear be discontinued for a sufficient duration to allow the cornea to return to its natural shape. A common rule of thumb is 1 week plus 1 week for each decade of gas-permeable lens wear. Tomographers facilitate this differential diagnosis, but careful ultrasound in all 4 quadrants can be used as well.

Epithelial surface irregularities such as superficial punctate keratitis, recurrent corneal erosions, and abrasions can also interfere with topography. They typically cause focal irregularities or loss of data (seen as white spots on maps). It is important to let such irregularities heal before important topography-based decisions are made.

## Conclusion

Topography has become an indispensable tool for the clinician in assessing the qualities of the corneal surface. The ability to interpret and understand various topographical maps can be complex given the variety of technology available. It is especially important for the refractive surgeon who assesses the eligibility of a candidate for elective surgery to understand the characteristics of the different types of maps for proper interpretation and clinical utility.

## References

1. Lebow KA, Grohe RM. Differentiating contact lens induced warpage from true keratoconus using corneal topography. *CLAO J.* 1999;25(2):114-122.
2. Maguire LJ, Singer DE, Klyce SD. Graphic presentation of computer-analyzed keratoscope photographs. *Arch Ophthalmol.* 1987;105:223-230.
3. Wilson SE, Klyce SD, Husseini ZM. Standardized color-coded maps for corneal topography. *Ophthalmology.* 1993;100:1723-1727.
4. Oshike T, Klyce SD. Corneal topography: basic concepts. In: Brightbill FS, ed. *Corneal Surgery—Theory, Technique, and Tissue.* 3rd ed. St. Louis, MO: CV Mosby; 1999.
5. Smolek M, Klyce SD, Hovis JK. The universal standard scale: proposed improvements to the American National Standards Institute (ANSI) scale for corneal topography. *Ophthalmology.* 2002;109:361-369.
6. Secretariat, Optical Laboratories Association. *American National Standard for Ophthalmics—Corneal Topography Systems: Standard Terminology, Requirements.* Merrifield, VA: Optical Laboratories Association. American National Standards Institute; 1999:ANSI Z80.23-1000.
7. Corbett MC, Rosen ES, O'Brart DPS. Presentation of topographic information. In: Corbett M, O'Brart D, Rosen E. *Corneal Topography: Principles and Applications.* London, UK: BMJ Books; 1999:31-59.
8. Applegate RA. Comment on characterization of the inherent error in a spherically-biased corneal topography system in mapping a radially aspheric surface. *Refract Corneal Surg.* 1994;10:113-114.
9. Roberts C. Characterization of the inherent error in a spherically-biased corneal topography system in mapping a radially aspheric surface. *Refract Corneal Surg.* 1994;10:103-116.

# Section II

# Topographic Technologies

Chapter 4

# Topographic Technologies

Tracy Schroeder Swartz, OD, MS, FAAO; Zuguo Liu, MD, PhD; Xiao Yang, MD; and Mei Zhang, MD

The principles of topography are based on the reflections of a concentric ring of light upon the cornea. Variations in curvature and astigmatism are represented as an asymmetry of the keratographic patterns. Modern keratoscopes incorporate complex images in the analysis of topographic anomalies. Refractive surgery and the quest for better understanding of corneal shape (versus curvature) resulted in new technologies with increased precision in evaluating complex corneal shapes. Technologies include Placido disk imaging, PAR, slit scanning, Scheimpflug imaging, ultrasound, interferometric, and optical coherence tomography (OCT) systems. This chapter contains a brief overview of each technology.

## Placido Disk Imaging

Placido imaging is based on the overlay of concentric mires on the cornea. Keratoscopes permitting the direct observation of illuminated mires upon the cornea demonstrate the Placido ring. The closer the mires, the steeper the axis. The wider the rings, the flatter the axis. It was the first technology to be used to evaluate the shape of the cornea in conjunction with computer analysis. While systems may differ somewhat, all contain a transilluminated Placido target in the shape of a cone or disk, an imaging system containing an objective lens and camera, a video frame grabber, and a computer for image analysis. The number, position, color, and thickness of the rings vary between systems.

Placido systems are typically divided into 2 types: near (also called small targets) or distance (called large targets). Near target systems typically allow for imaging with lower illumination and enjoy greater corneal coverage. However, they are sensitive to focusing adjustments, and facial anatomy may hinder measurement. Large target systems require more illumination and are less sensitive to focusing error but cover less of the cornea.[1]

Most systems project images of illuminated keratoscope rings onto the corneal surface to produce a virtual image of the Placido disk about 4 mm behind the corneal vertex.[2] An example is shown in Figure 4-1. They directly measure the curvature of the cornea and calculate the elevation map using a coordinate system from the curvature data. This requires assumptions about the corneal geometry, however. Elevation is generated by fitting slope data to a predefined mathematical model, which may be spheric, aspheric, or a conical section. While this practice is reasonable in normal corneas, it may result in serious error in diseased eyes or in eyes having undergone keratorefractive surgery.[3]

Studies regarding the accuracy of early Placido disk systems found acceptable levels of accuracy and reproducibility. However, most test objects were spheres.[4] Systems tend to be more accurate centrally than peripherally, and defocus increases errors. Clear surfaces are required for clear mires. Reported accuracy of dioptric power varies from 0.1 to



Wang M. *Corneal Topography: A Guide for Clinical Application in the Wavefront Era, Second Edition (pp. 35-42)*

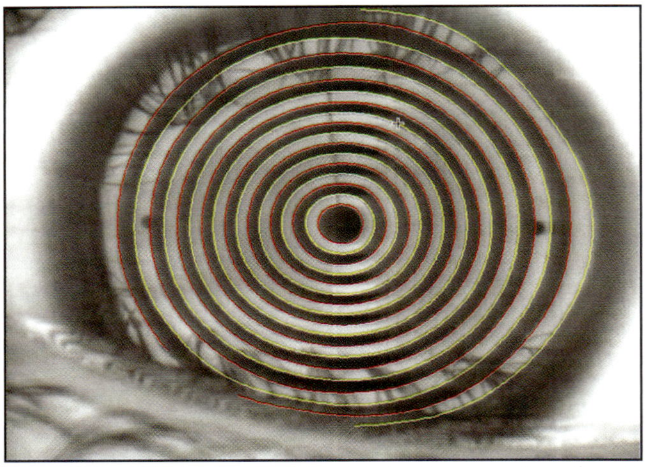

**Figure 4-1.** A placido image. (Reprinted with permission of Joe S. Wakil, MD.)

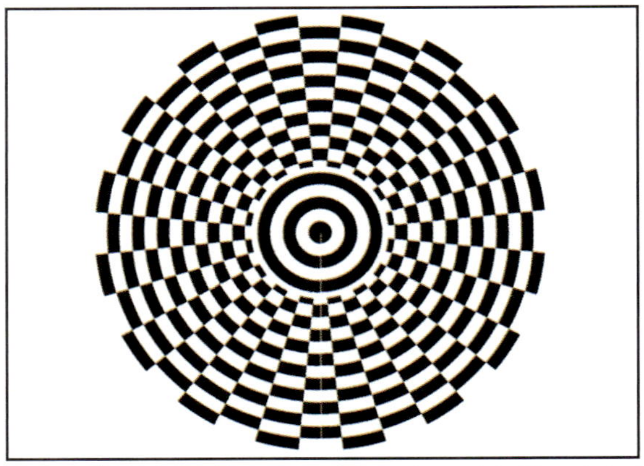

**Figure 4-2.** AstraMax system's polar grid. (Reprinted with permission of Aleksandar Stojanovic, MD.)

0.25 D and from approximately 0.018 to 0.045 mm in the radius of curvature.[5]

Variants on Placido disk technology include a 3-dimensional grid system, such as the AstraMax system (Lasersight Technologies, Inc, Winter Park, FL) shown in Figure 4-2. Rather than using a Placido disk, a polar grid provides both radial and concentric data points, enabling measurement of radial distance and rotational concentric changes in the cornea. The AstraMax uses 3 cameras to obtain multi-angled shots, measuring each data point independently of an adjacent point. A raw image is shown in Figure 4-3.

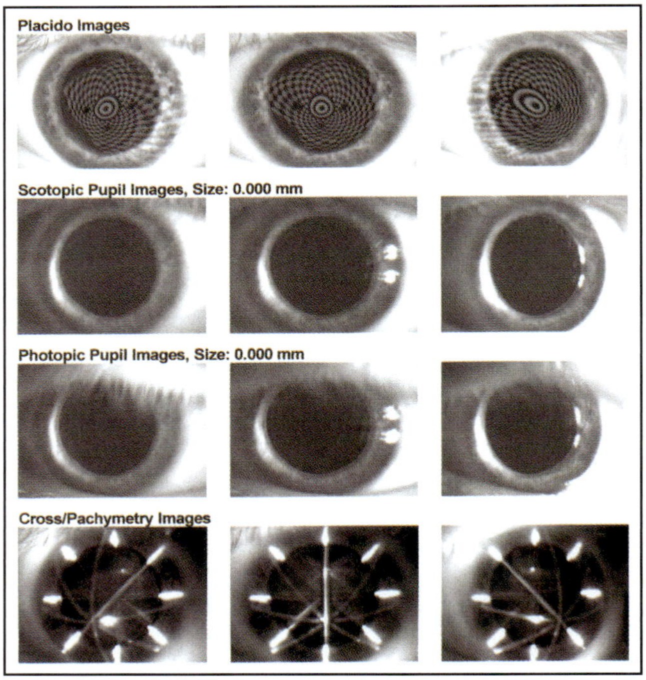


**Figure 4-3.** AstraMax raw image of a keratoconic cornea.

# ELEVATION-BASED SYSTEMS

Several systems measure elevation directly: the PAR Corneal Topography System (CTS; ParTech, Inc, New Hartford, NY), Orbscan (Bausch & Lomb, Rochester, NY), Scheimpflug imaging, and OCT. The first systems were the PAR and the Orbscan slit-scanning systems, which use a triangulation method to measure the elevation, and curvature data were calculated without the error of geometrical assumption.[6]

## Rasterstereography and the PAR Corneal Topography System

Rasterstereography is a method of topographical evaluation that creates an elevation map. Unlike Placido disk systems, it does not depend on the reflectivity of the corneal surface and can provide information about the entire corneal, limbal, and interpalpebral conjunctival surfaces.[7] Because a smooth reflective surface is not required, images can be obtained with epithelial irregularity or defects, sutures, or stromal ulceration.

The PAR CTS was the first topography system to produce an elevation map of the corneal surface using rasterstereography.[8] It projected a grid onto the corneal surface and computed elevation data based on the distortion of the grid. The PAR system requires that a small amount of fluorescein be placed in the tear film, and the images are collected using standard fluorescence-based photography. Image acquisition is rapid and relatively insensitive to focusing. From the known geometry of the grid projection and imaging system paths, rays can be intersected into 3-dimensional space to compute the X, Y, and Z coordinates of the surface.[9]

The PAR CTS can provide elevation, curvature, and keratometry maps. Unlike Placido disk-based videokeratoscopes, the PAR CTS produces a true elevation map and requires neither a smooth reflective surface nor precise spatial alignment for accurate imaging.[10] Based upon the fact that the cornea is an asymmetric refractive surface, the PAR corneal elevation map can be obtained by comparing corneal height with a spherical reference surface, which is the average cornea elevation or a certain preset standard height. The actual corneal surface is either above or below this reference surface measured at individual points.

Unlike Placido disk-based videokeratoscopes, the PAR System requires neither a smooth reflective surface nor precise spatial alignment for accurate imaging.[11] The system demonstrated the ability to image irregular, de-epithelialized, and keratectomized corneas. The PAR CTS can be installed on slit-lamp microscopes, surgical microscopes, or automatic optometry instruments, allowing topographical examination intraoperatively.

Currently, there is limited information on the normal corneal topography with the PAR CTS, and it is rarely used in clinical practice. Naufal and colleagues[12,13] investigated corneal elevation maps in 100 normal eyes of 50 subjects using the PAR system. Five categories were identified in their study: unclassified, regular ridge, irregular ridge, incomplete ridge, and island. They found the surface of the normal cornea was not smooth and spherical, and surface irregularities ranged from small central islands of elevation to complete, elevated bands crossing the cornea. Priest and colleagues[13] investigated the accuracy and precision of the elevation topography from the Tomey Topographic Modeling System (TMS-1) and the PAR CTS. Based on quantitative analysis of elevation measurements, they concluded that the CTS represented surface topography more accurately than the TMS-1.[13]

# TOMOGRAPHY

Tomography is the creation of a 3-dimensional model from 2-dimensional images and is accomplished using slit scanning, Scheimpflug imaging, OCT, and ultrasound systems.

## Slit-Scanning

Slit-scanning technology is currently used by a single system, the Orbscan. The Orbscan uses a scanning slit-beam similar to the parallel pipes used in biomicroscopy and direct stereotriangulation to measure the anterior corneal surface. During the 1.5-second examination, 2 scanning slit lamps project a series of 40 slit beams angled at 45 degrees to the right and left of the video axis. Twenty slits are projected from the left and 20 from the right. Proprietary software image registration attempts to minimize the influence of involuntary eye movements during data acquisition.

The typical display used by the Orbscan incorporates 4 images: the anterior and posterior elevation maps, the curvature (axial) map, and the pachymetry map. An example is shown in Figure 4-4. When used for screening, Tanabe and colleagues recommended using 10- or 20-µm scales for elevation maps, which best identified abnormal corneas.[14]

Modis and colleagues investigated the anterior and posterior corneal shape, curvature, and thickness of normal human corneas using the Orbscan. Scanning slit topography seems to be a reliable technique for the evaluation of normal corneas not only for anterior shape and curvature, but also for a real pachymetry gradient recording.[15] This was the first system to yield pachymetry data. However, the accuracy of these measurements remains controversial. It is generally accepted that Orbscan measurements of central corneal thickness are greater than ultrasonic pachymeter measurements in virgin eyes.[16] The role of the Orbscan pachymetry is limited by lack of repeatability for peripheral measurements, however, and is recommended for central CT measurements only.[17]

Kawana and colleagues compared central corneal thickness measurements of 3 pachymetry devices in eyes after laser in situ keratomileusis (LASIK). They found in post-LASIK eyes, Orbscan II scanning slit topography significantly underestimated corneal thickness. Noncontact specular microscopy gave smaller thickness readings than ultrasonic pachymetry, but these 2 units showed an excellent linear correlation.[18]

## Scheimpflug Imaging

Scheimpflug imaging is based on a principle named after and patented by Austrian Theodor Scheimpflug in Vienna in 1904. To best appreciate the advantages of this modality for ophthalmologic imaging, let us review basic principles and limitations of an ordinary camera.

A typical camera uses 3 imaginary surfaces, referred to as planes: the film plane, the lens plane, and the plane of sharp focus. A camera's film is fixed upon the film plane. The lens plane passes through the optical center of the lens and is perpendicular to the lens axis. The lens will depict any object that is positioned on the plane of sharp focus crisply onto the film plane. For an ordinary camera, these 3 planes are all parallel to each other, and, therefore, all 3 planes are perpendicular to the lens axis. As long as a given application only calls for limited depth of focus, this setup works well. The depth of focus is the range over which the film plane can be moved while maintaining an image of acceptable sharpness.

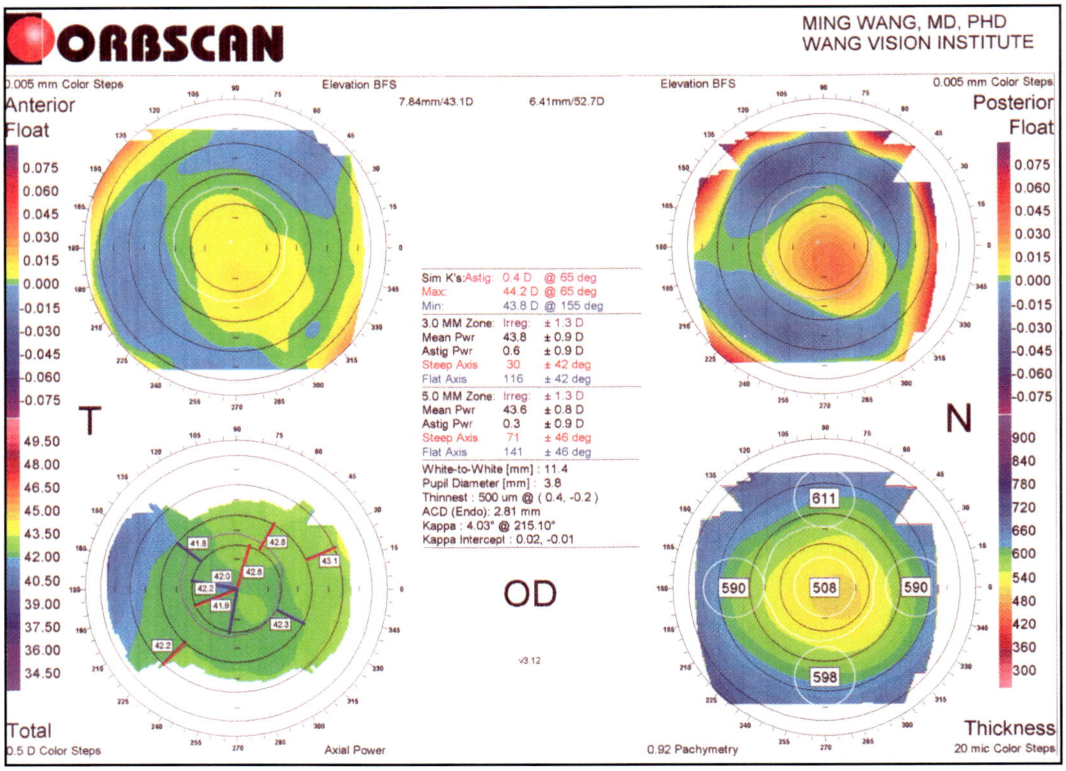


**Figure 4-4.** Typical Orbscan quad map of a normal eye.

Ophthalmologic applications require an extended depth of focus to effectively image the entire anterior segment. In Scheimpflug imaging, the 3 planes are not parallel but slanted so they intersect in a line or, simplified, in a point of intersection. Put more elaborately, the Scheimpflug principle states that if the lens is tilted in a way that the resulting lens plane intersects the film plane, the plane of sharp focus, due to its dependence upon the lens plane, must also pass through that same line of intersection. This line is sometimes referred to as the "Scheimpflug line." The benefit this setup brings is extended depth of focus. Extended depth of focus has a trade-off: distortion of the image. The Pentacam (OCULUS, Wetzlar, Germany) computes the acquired picture to compensate for the distortion.

Scheimpflug imaging gives a complete picture from the anterior surface of the cornea to the posterior surface of the lens as viewed through the pupil, as shown in Figure 4-5. Three-dimensional models of the front surface (Figure 4-6) and back surface (Figure 4-7), as well as pachymetry (Figure 4-8), are created.

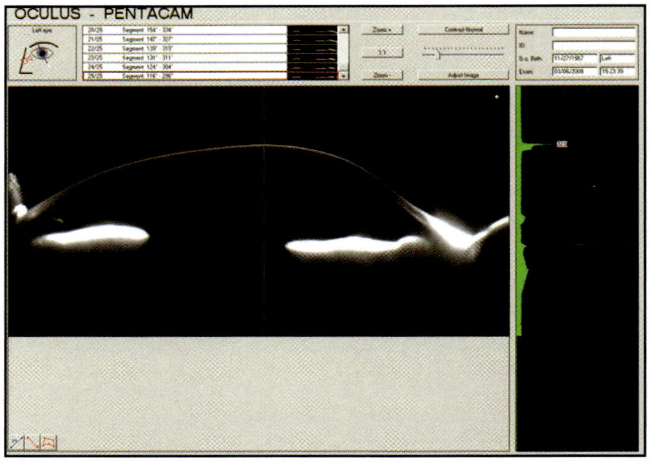


**Figure 4-5.** Clinical Scheimpflug image in a patient with keratoconus.

## Ultrasound Digital Topography

The Artemis system (ArcScan, Inc, Morrison, CO) uses high-frequency ultrasound scanning enhanced by digital signal processing. Ultrasonic echo data from consecutive parallel B-scans of the cornea spaced at 250-μm intervals are digitized and stored. Using the I-scan obtained by computing the analytic signal magnitude of the deconvolved ultrasound signal, layer thickness measurements are made with a precision of 2-μm standard deviation at 120-μm intervals along each scan plane. The data are stored as an array, z (x,y), mapping thickness (z) onto horizontal and vertical (x,y) spatial coordinates. Pachymetric maps are then constructed by plotting local thickness against measurement point position. This technique provides the corneal surgeon with a new tool for the topographic evaluation of the thickness of anterior corneal layers in normal and

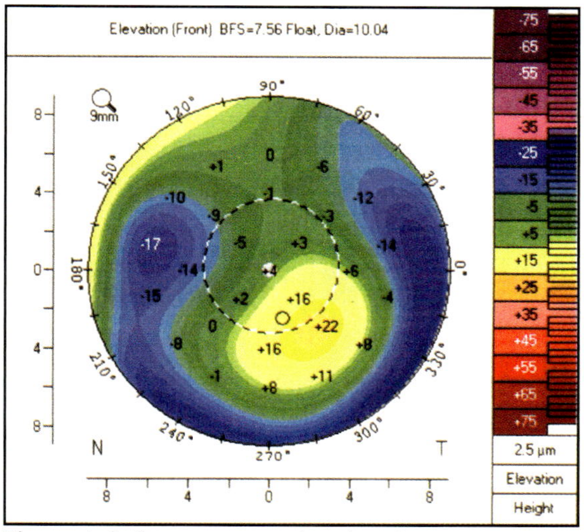


**Figure 4-6.** Pentacam anterior elevation map.

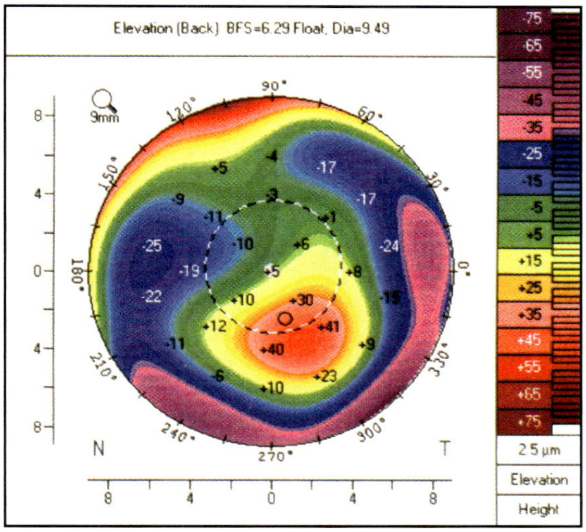


**Figure 4-7.** Pentacam posterior elevation map.

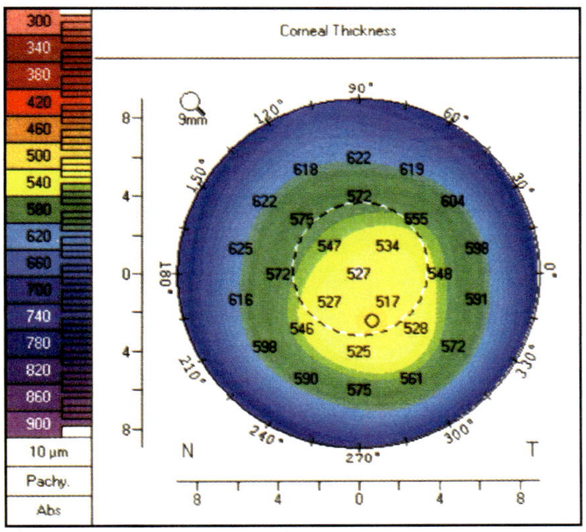


**Figure 4-8.** Pentacam pachymetry map.

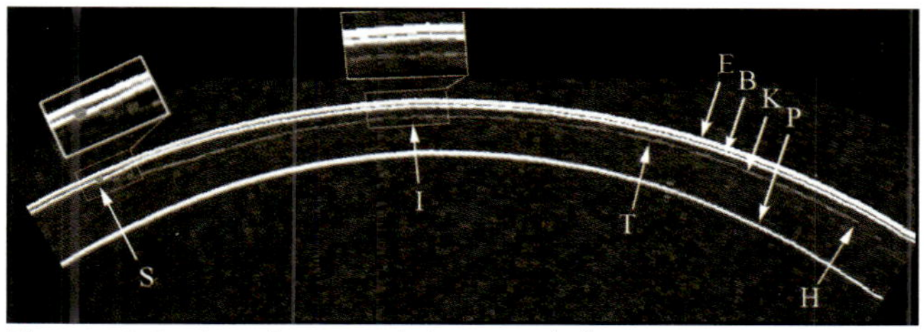


**Figure 4-9.** An ultrasound image of the cornea S/P LASIK. S = Break in Bruch's membrane. I = Interface. T = Flap demarcation. E = Epithelium. B = Bowman's membrane, K = Flap. P = Endothelium. H = Outer edge of flap. (Reprinted with permission of Dan Z. Reinstein, MD.)

pathologic corneas with high precision. The resolution of the Artemis is sufficient to distinguish individual corneal layers such as the epithelium, stromal component of the flap, and residual stromal bed. In addition, the technique is not limited to optically transparent tissue.[19] An example of the images obtained with this technology is shown in Figure 4-9. The common display used is the C12 array, illustrated in Figure 4-10. This array was created from scans of the right cornea of a patient scanned prior to LASIK and 6 months postoperatively.

Reinstein and colleagues investigated precision, imaging resolution, 3-dimensional thickness mapping, and clinical utility of a new prototype—3-dimensional very high-frequency (VHF; 50 MHz) digital ultrasound scanning system for corneal epithelium, flap, and residual stromal thickness after LASIK. They found VHF digital ultrasound arc-B scanning provides high-resolution imaging and high-precision 3-dimensional thickness mapping of corneal layers, enabling accurate anatomical evaluation of the changes induced in the cornea by LASIK.[20]

## Interferometric System

This technique uses laser holographic interferometry fringe patterns to depict deviations of the corneal surface. Interferometry is based on the principles of light wave interference. It records the interference pattern generated on the corneal surface by 2 coherent wavefronts. High accuracy is theoretically possible.[1] Fringe patterns can be interpreted as contour maps of surface elevations where the difference between the 2 consecutive fringes is equal to an elevation difference of half the light wavelength (about 0.5 μm). The shape of the cornea can be calculated by adding this amount to the reference sphere elevation. Unfortunately, interferometric methods are sensitive to eye movements, and a system is required to maintain head position. Despite reported sensitivity of less than 0.1 D of curvature within the 5-mm vertex[5], the system is too complicated to gain a foothold in the field.

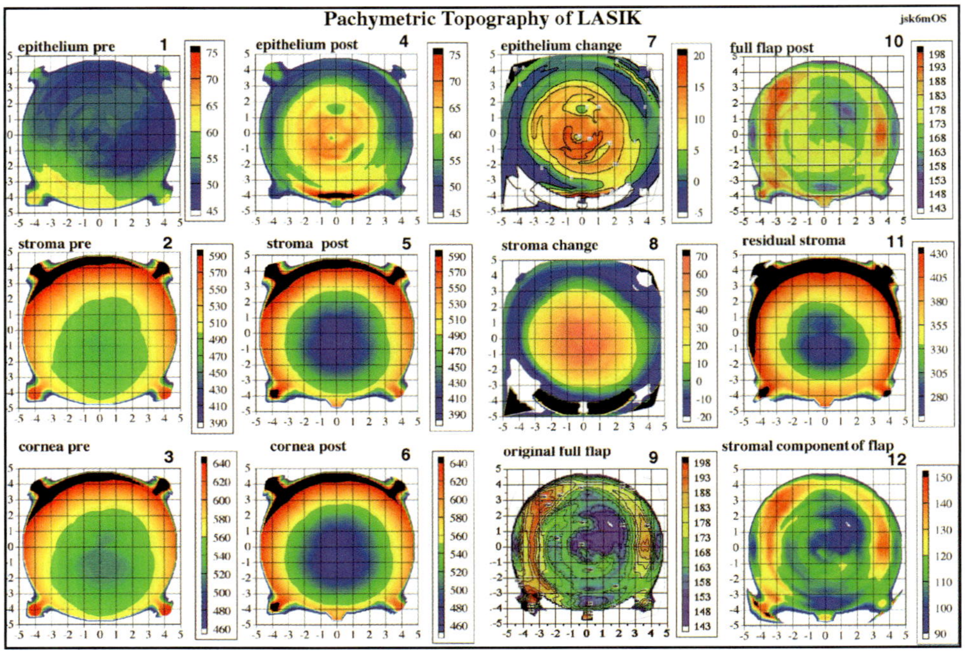


Figure 4-10. The C12 Artemis display. (Reprinted with permission of Dan Z. Reinstein, MD.)

# Optical Coherence Tomography

This technology, which originally was used to evaluate the posterior pole and retina, has been adapted for use on the anterior segment. OCT uses cross-sectional scanning based on reflection and scattering of light from the structures within the anterior segment. The light source is split into measurement and reference beams. Ocular structures reflect the measurement beam and interrelate with the reference light reflected from the reference mirror, creating interference. The coherent or positive interference, an increased resulting signal, is measured by the interferometer and allows determination of the reflecting structure's position.

A cross-sectional image of the anterior segment structures anterior to the lens is produced (Figure 4-11). It is also more functional than confocal microscopy because it can provide images of the entire anterior portion of the eye quickly, including pachymetry maps (Figure 4-12). Additional advantages include it being a noncontact test and that it uses no coupling medium.

The use of light as an analysis medium also has disadvantages. The depth of penetration is limited to the anterior segment, and image quality may be greatly reduced in cases of scarring or pannus. Initial clinical use of anterior segment OCT was mainly focused on measurement of phakic IOL placement, angle analysis in glaucoma, and flap detection after LASIK.[21,22]

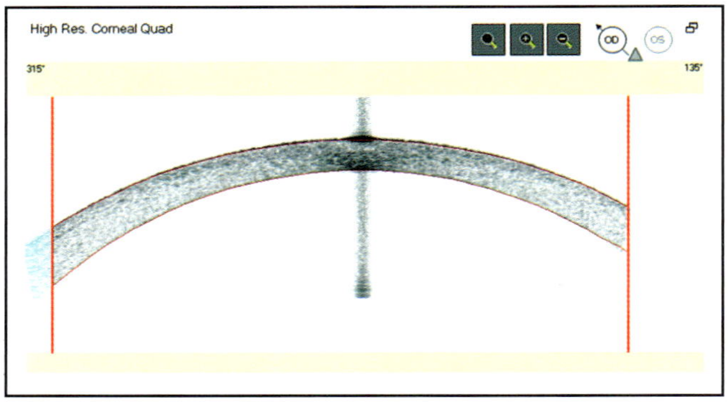


Figure 4-11. OCT yields a cross sectional image of the cornea.

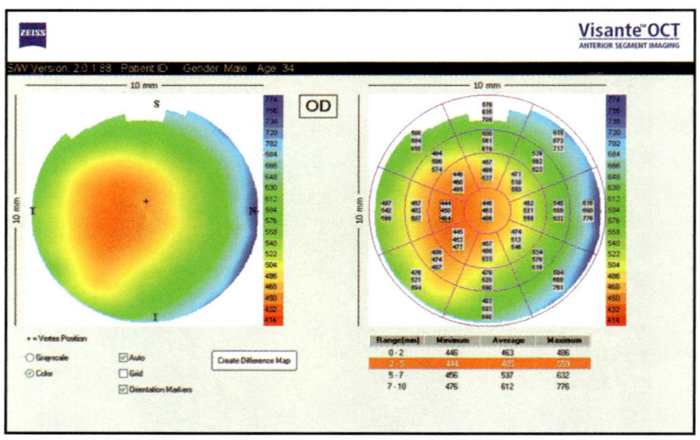


Figure 4-12. OCT pachymetry mapping.

# Conclusion

Understanding topographic technology and how each system derives the maps is important for clinical interpretation. Placido disk is the most widely used and understood by clinicians. Tomographers are gaining popularity and offer views of both surfaces as well as optical pachymetry, attributes appreciated by both refractive and cataract surgeons.

# References


1. Corneal topography. *Ophthalmology*. 1999;106(8):1628-1638.
2. Binder PS. Videokeratography. *CLAO J*. 1995;21(2):133-144.
3. Mandell RB. The enigma of the corneal contour. *CLAO J*. 1992;18:267-273.
4. Koch DD, Foulks GN, Moran CT, Wakil JS. The Corneal EyeSys System: accuracy analysis and reproducibility of the first generation prototype. *Refract Corneal Surg*. 1989;5:424-429.
5. Mejia-Barbosa Y, Malacara-Hernandez D. A review of methods for measuring corneal topography. *Opt Vis Sci*. 2001;78:240-253.
6. Litoff D, Belin MW, Wynn SS, Smith RS. PAR technology corneal topography system. *Invest Ophthalmol Vis Sci*. 1991;32(4 suppl):922S.
7. Arffa RC, Warnicki JW, Rehkopf PG. Corneal topography using rasterstereography. *Refract Corneal Surg*. 1989;5(6):414-417.
8. Nemeth J, Erdelyi B, Csakany B. Corneal topography changes after a 15 second pause in blinking. *J Cataract Refract Surg*. 2001;27:589-592.
9. Belin MW, Litoff D, Strods SJ, Winn SS, Smith RS. The PAR Technology Corneal Topography System. *Refract Corneal Surg*. 1992;8(1):88-96.
10. Belin MW, Cambier JL, Nabors JR, Ratliff CD. PAR Corneal Topography System (PAR CTS): the clinical application of close-range photogrammetry. *Optom Vis Sci*. 1995;72(11):828-837.
11. Belin MW, Zloty P. Accuracy of the PAR corneal topography system with spatial misalignment. *CLAO J*. 1993;19(1):64-68.
12. Naufal SC, Hess JS, Freidlander MH, Granet NS. Rasterstereography-based classification of normal corneas. *J Cataract Refract Surg*. 1997;23:222-230.
13. Priest D, Munger R. Comparative study of the elevation topography of complex shapes. *J Cataract Refract Surg*. 1998;24(6):741-750.
14. Tanabe T, Oshika T, Yomidokor A, et al. Standardized color-coded scales for anterior and posterior elevation mapping of scanning slit corneal topography. *Ophthalmology*. 2002;107(7):1298-1302.
15. Modis L Jr, Langenbucher A, Seitz B. Evaluation of normal corneas using the scanning-slit topography/pachymetry system. *Cornea*. 2004;23(7):689-694.
16. Giraldez Fernandez MJ, Diaz Rey A, Cervino A, Yebra-Pimentel E. A comparison of two pachymetric systems: slit-scanning and ultrasonic. *CLAO J*. 2002;28(4):221-223.
17. Cho P, Cheung SW. Repeatability of corneal thickness measurements made by a scanning slit topography system. *Ophthalmic Physiol Opt*. 2002;22(6):505-510.
18. Kawana K, Tokunaga T, Miyata K, Okamoto F, Kiuchi T, Oshika T. Comparison of corneal thickness measurements using Orbscan II, non-contact specular microscopy, and ultrasonic pachymetry in eyes after laser in situ keratomileusis. *Br J Ophthalmol*. 2004;88(4):466-468.
19. Reinstein DZ, Silverman RH, Trokel SL, Coleman DJ. Corneal pachymetric topography. *Ophthalmology*. 1994;101(3):432-438.
20. Reinstein DZ, Silverman RH, Raevsky T, et al. Arc-scanning very high-frequency digital ultrasound for 3D pachymetric mapping of the corneal epithelium and stroma in laser in situ keratomileusis. *J Refract Surg*. 2000;16(4):414-430.
21. Hirano K, Ito Y, Suzuki T, Kojima T, Kachi S, Miyake Y. Optical coherence tomography for the noninvasive evaluation of the cornea. *Cornea*. 2001;20(3) 281-289.
22. Belin M, Holladay J, Michelson M, Woodhams JT, Ahmed I. The Pentacam: precision, confidence, results and accurate "Ks." Insert to *Cataract & Refractive Surgery Today*. 2007;55:341-347.

Chapter 5

# Placido Disk-Based Topographic Systems

## ATLAS 9000 Corneal Topographer

Dianne Anderson, OD, FAAO

The ATLAS 9000 Model (Carl Zeiss Meditec, Jena, Germany) corneal topographer (CT) is a large cone Placido disk system designed to measure corneal curvature and produce color-coded maps for the detection of corneal conditions and pathologies. This system also aids in the screening and postoperative management of refractive procedures such as laser-assisted in situ keratomileusis (LASIK), photorefractive keratectomy (PRK), and multifocal and toric intraocular lenses (IOLs) and in the selection and fitting of rigid gas-permeable (RGP) contact lenses. The field of view of the camera system is large enough to capture the limbus boundaries of the eye, thus allowing white-to-white (limbus-to-limbus) measurements, as well as the determination of the geometric center of the eye for better contact lens fitting and eye registration.

The ATLAS 9000 Placido disk-based system projects a series of 22 concentric infrared (950 nm) light rings onto the cornea of the eye. An image of the reflected rings is captured with a digital camera. The ATLAS system analyzes thousands of data points in the image to measure the distances between rings and their relationships with each other in order to reconstruct the corneal surface into a color-coded topography map. The ATLAS system can display the image of the cornea in a variety of ways, including curvature, elevation, and aberrations. The ATLAS system also has the ability to capture both scotopic (without light) and photopic (with light) pupil images. With the exception of the keyboard and printer, the ATLAS system integrates all hardware components in a single unit, including the image acquisition optics, the system computer, and a flat panel display screen.

### Image Acquisition

The patented Cone-of-Focus technology used by the ATLAS system is the most critical part of the system's alignment and focusing mechanism.[1] The 22 rings of the large cone are separated by a smaller Cone-of-Focus at the location of the 9th ring. This smaller cone protrudes outward and reflects on the eye at a fixed, known distance from the camera. This reflection appears on the live video image as a larger separation between the rings surrounding the small cone. As the cone is brought closer to the cornea, the cone ring moves closer to the inner ring. As the cone is brought further from the cornea, the cone ring moves closer to the outer ring. The properly focused image results in even separation between the rings surrounding the cone. ATLAS' Cone-of-Focus uses a triangulation method to find the exact location and distance of the rings. A "triangle" is formed between the cone, the corneal surface, and the Placido rings.



Wang M. *Corneal Topography: A Guide for Clinical Application in the Wavefront Era, Second Edition* (pp. 43-102).

During an examination, the patient's chin is positioned in the chin rest assembly in front of the projection head. The clinician administering the exam aligns the projection head and, using a joystick, focuses on the patient's eye and activates the system. The user presses the joystick or spacebar to stop data acquisition. The ATLAS SmartCapture Image Analysis technology captures images at a rate of 15 per second before the joystick button/spacebar is pressed,[2] which stops the collection of images. When using this option, SmartCapture analyzes these images and chooses the 4 best images for processing on the "exam preview screen," or the best acceptable single image on the "exam results screen."

After you capture an image, the "exam preview screen" is the default display setting for the ATLAS 9000. Both the "exam preview screen" and the "exam results screen" allow you to evaluate image quality, recapture or save images, acquire additional images, edit pupil and limbus contours, select the doctor and operator for the exam, and add remarks. While the "exam preview screen" displays the last 4 images (displayed in chronological order, left to right) in the image frame buffer (or 4 best images if the SmartCapture option is used), the "exam results screen" displays only the last image (or best image if the SmartCapture option is on).

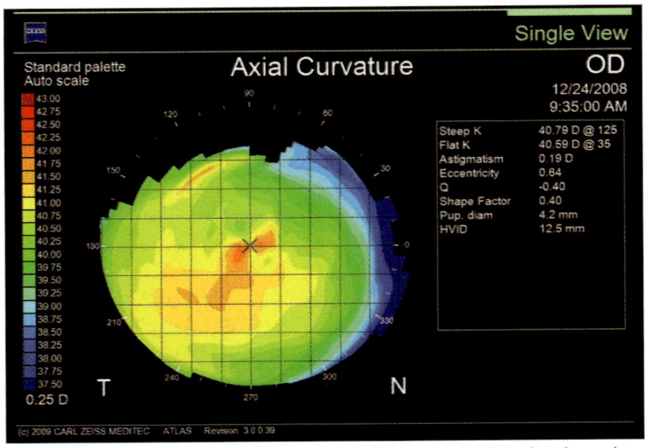


**Figure 5-1.** ATLAS Axial Curvature View may be displayed in mm or D.

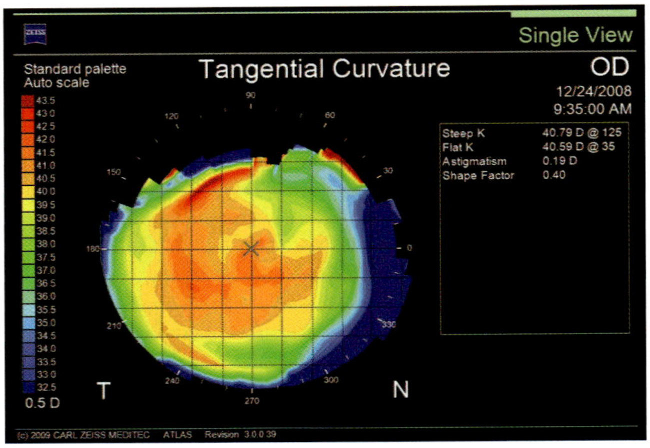


**Figure 5-2.** The Tangential View gives more detail about the topographical characteristics of the cornea compared to the axial map.

# Image Analysis: Views

ATLAS supports 13 different types of views of the exam image: Axial Curvature, Tangential Curvature, Elevation, Irregularity, Rings Image, Keratometry, Refractive Power, Mean Curvature, Corneal Wavefront, Image Simulation, Point Spread Function (PSF), Modulation Transfer Function (MTF), and PathFinder II Corneal Analysis. Masterfit II Contact Lens Software is an optional program for RGP designing.

## Axial Curvature View

The Axial Curvature View displays the axial curvature of the cornea using 23 colors to represent dioptric power or radius of curvature in mm (Figure 5-1). The Axial View is actually a calculation of curvature rather than "true" refractive power when displayed as keratometric diopters (D). The color-coded display visually corresponds to the "flat" and "steep" axes, well-known to keratometry users.

The Axial View treats every single data point as if the whole cornea would be a sphere that matches the local slope and position of every data point. The distance from the point of interest on the corneal surface to the optical axis defines the axial radius of curvature. The Axial View has been established in the field, but it does not represent the true local curvature. Axial Views naturally incur more smoothing when measuring the corneal surface toward the periphery and may not reflect subtle changes. Because it shows a "perfect sphere" as flat, the Axial View is unable to take into account corneal spherical aberration (SA).

## Tangential Curvature View

The Tangential Curvature View (Figure 5-2) displays the cornea as a topographical view but bases the calculation on the local curvature of a given meridian, resulting in more detail than the Axial View. The Tangential View bases its calculation on a different mathematical approach and is also known as instantaneous or local curvature. This algorithm is more accurate at calculating the periphery of the cornea. This view may also recognize sharp transitions in power more easily and eliminates the "smoothing" appearance of the topographical view as seen in the axial or sagittal view. This is often useful in following healing trends after surgery or in viewing pathologic eyes. The Tangential View is helpful for locating the size and position of specific features on the corneal surface, such as the apex of corneal steepening in keratoconus, boundaries of a treatment zone after corneal refractive surgery, pterygia, and corneal scarring.[3]

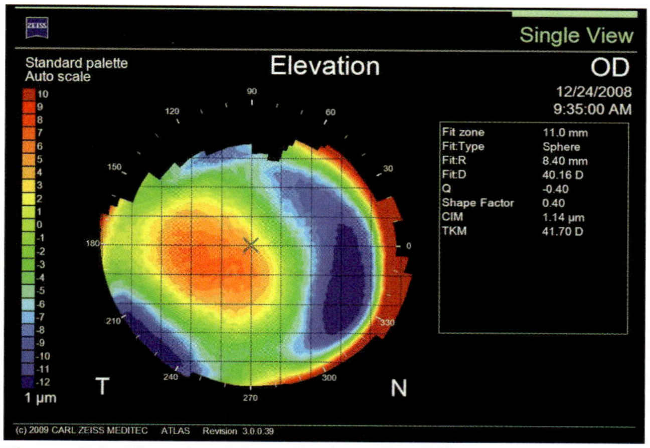


**Figure 5-3.** Elevation View displays the difference in height of the cornea in micrometers (µm) from a reference sphere.

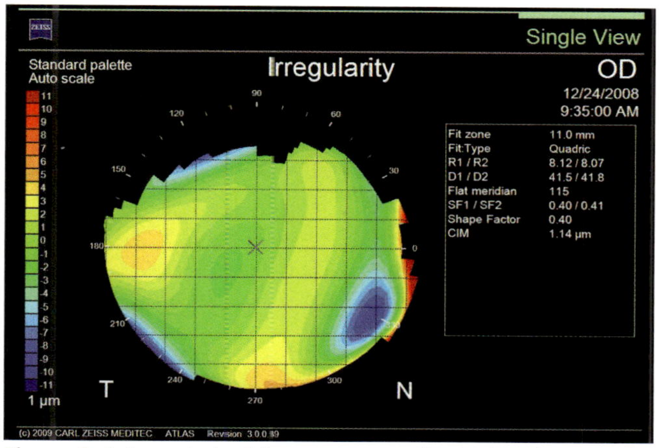


**Figure 5-4.** Irregularity View uses nonspherical surfaces as the reference object rather than the reference sphere used in the elevation map.

The Tangential View does not force the center of curvature of the best-fit sphere to lie along the optical axis. The location of the center of curvature for each point is calculated by a best-fit sphere to the local neighborhood at the point of interest on the corneal surface. The distance from the point of interest to the center of the locally best-fit sphere represents the tangential (or instantaneous) curvature. The Tangential View may be a better representation of true local curvature.

## Elevation View

The Elevation View displays the difference in height of the cornea in microns (µm) from a reference sphere (Figure 5-3). ATLAS superimposes a reference sphere onto the corneal surface, measuring the difference between the reference and the real corneal surface. Elevation is measured as differences in height from the reference sphere as positive and negative µm. The corneal surface may be above the reference sphere, resulting in a positive difference and appear red in the Standard Colors, or below the reference sphere, resulting in a negative difference and appear blue in the Standard Colors.[4]

The reference sphere may be automatically computed or created using parameters entered by the user. It is important to keep in mind that the elevation is measured in µm, not D, and that Axial and Elevation Views cannot be directly compared. The value of measuring the corneal surface in µm is that small elevations or depressions on the corneal surface created by surgery or pathology can be carefully documented, giving a level of detail not possible using the curvature views. Because the shape of the normal cornea is aspheric (ellipsoidal) rather than spherical, it is challenging to locate subtle deviations in elevation maps even in normal eyes, as well as those with nonpathologic corneal shape changes, such as astigmatism.

## Irregularity View

The Irregularity View takes the best-fit surface methodology of the Elevation View one step further by using nonspherical surfaces as the reference object (Figure 5-4). A best-fit toric ellipsoid surface is subtracted from the corneal elevation data to yield the irregularity that cannot be described by a reference ellipsoid that accounts for both the asphericity and toricity of the cornea. The Irregularity View shows how different the cornea is from a normal eye, representing the elevation difference between the "normal" best-fit ellipsoid surface and the actual measured corneal surface.[5]

## Rings Image View

The Rings Image View or *photokeratoscopic image* displays the actual captured image of the eye with the reflected rings (Figure 5-5). In addition to the Rings Image, Scotopic (no light, large pupil) and Photopic (with light, small pupil) images may also be displayed if captured at image acquisition. Overlay options include Zoom Rings Image to display a zoomed-in rings image to 10 mm; Limbus Contour to display green markings at the location of the limbus contour and to measure the horizontal visible iris diameter (HVID); Geometric Center to display a crosshair enclosed by a circle designating the point on the cornea corresponding to the center of the limbus contour; and Rings to outline ring edges. Data options in the display include pupil diameter, HVID, and photopic and scotopic pupil diameter.

## Keratometry View

The Keratometry View simulates the data obtained using a standard keratometer (Figure 5-6). This view provides readings for each semi-meridian in 3 zones: central (0 to 3 mm), midperiphery (3 to 6 mm), and periphery (6 to 9 mm). The steepest semi-meridians in each zone are displayed in red D values, and the flattest meridians are

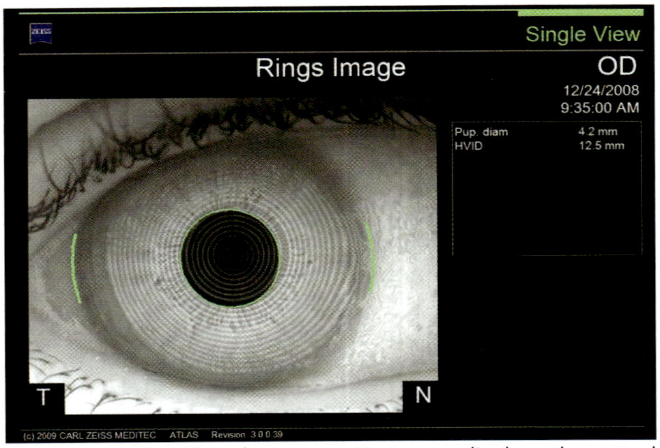


**Figure 5-5.** The Photokeratoscoptic Image displays the actual captured image of the eye with its reflected rings. Scotopic (no light, large pupil) and Photopic (with light, small pupil) images may also be displayed. Overlays such as limbus contour may be used to determine the horizonatal visible iris diameter.

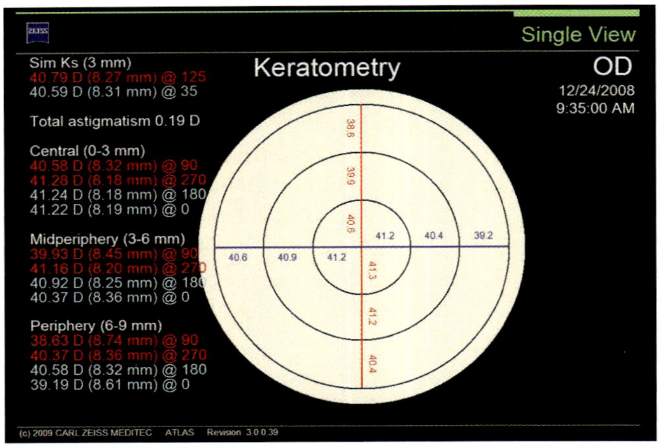


**Figure 5-6.** Keratometry View simulates the data obtained using a standard keratometer. Values for the 3 zones are displayed as well.

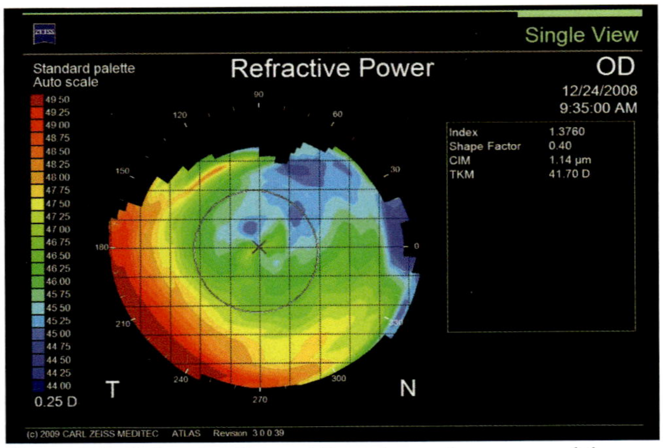


**Figure 5-7.** Refractive Power View shows the power of the eye in its refractive state, measured only in D.

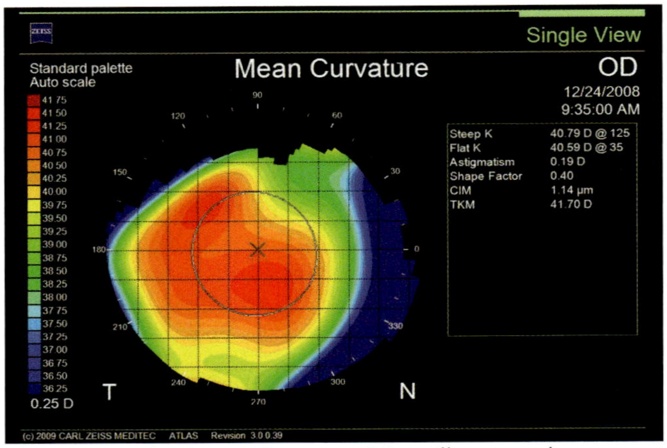


**Figure 5-8.** The Mean Curvature View illustrates the average curvature of the 2 principal curvatures for any given point on the cornea, and contains curvature information along 3 dimensions of every single data point.

displayed in blue D values. The data are listed by semi-meridian and zone on the left of the screen. The simulated keratometer values at the top left of the display are computed in a similar way to the computations performed by keratometers commonly used to measure the central 3 mm, assuming the principal axes have a 90-degree shift. Eccentricity values are also displayed for meridians at 0, 10, 15, 20, 25, and 30 degrees.

## Refractive Power View

The Refractive Power View shows the power of the eye in its refractive state, measured only in D (Figure 5-7). Sometimes called a *Snell's Law Map*, this view measures the refraction of light rays using Snell's Law as they pass through the corneal surface. Taking into account SA, the Refractive Power View more closely illustrates how light rays behave as they strike the cornea. Refractive Power Views may differ from Axial Views in their readings of power and radius for the same exam. Significant differences can be seen in the periphery and in eyes with unusual or abnormal shapes due to the effect of the SA.

## Mean Curvature View

The Mean Curvature View is the average curvature of the 2 principal curvatures for any given point on the cornea (Figure 5-8). As the Axial and Tangential Views are defined along individual meridians (or slices of the cornea), the Mean View contains curvature information along 3 dimensions of every single data point. The mean curvature is the average curvature in all directions around the data point, while axial and tangential curvature is limited to the semi-meridian. As a result, the Mean View suppresses corneal astigmatism and is insensitive to patient fixation. The advantage of the Mean View is that it may better detect subtle abnormalities because it has the ability to suppress nonpathological features, such as corneal astigmatism, while preserving pathological features such as keratoconus.

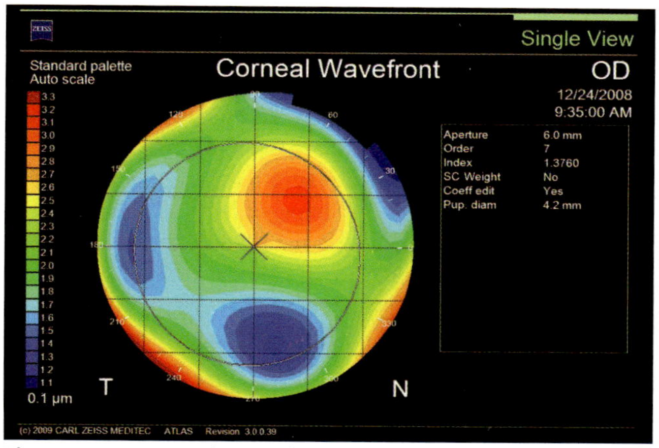


**Figure 5-9.** Corneal wavefront represents aberrations based upon topography, and described using Zernike Polynomials like total eye aberrometry.

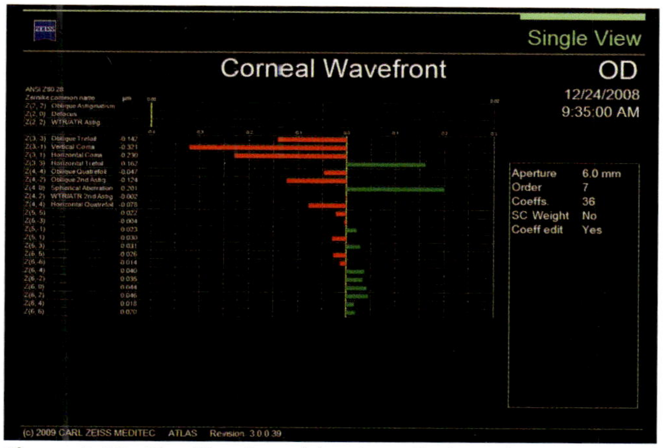


**Figure 5-10.** The Zernike table view displays the names and values of the Zernike coefficients (up to order 4), along with horizontal bar graphs of the Zernike coefficients values.

## Corneal Wavefront View

The Corneal Wavefront View displays corneal wavefront aberrations (Figure 5-9). The corneal wavefront is calculated from corneal topography using an algorithm that incorporates the shape of the cornea using ray tracing, technology that traces light rays from the fovea out of the eye. Wavefront aberration is measured as the optical path difference, the difference between the corneal wavefront and an ideal wavefront at the entrance pupil.

Total aberration of the eye as measured by wavefront aberrometers depends on pupil size and accommodation and generates the refractive error of the eye. Corneal wavefront aberrations are relatively stable over time, are not affected by pupil size or accommodation, and do not provide information about the refractive error of the eye. Using the Wavefront View Editor, corneal wavefront can be displayed in color, number, profile, surface, or Zernike table format. The Zernike table view displays the names and values of the Zernike coefficients (up to order 4), along with horizontal bar graphs of the Zernike coefficient values (Figure 5-10). Various coefficients can be selected or removed. You can also enable or disable compensation of Stiles-Crawford weighting (directional sensitivity of the photoreceptors) in the calculation of the aberrations.

## Image Simulation View

The Image Simulation View displays a corneal focal plane image simulation based upon the corneal PSF (Figure 5-11). Images available for use in the simulation include a 20/100 "E" image, an eye chart (20/50 to 20/10), and a beach scene image.

## Point Spread Function View

The PSF View is a monochrome display representing the PSF arising from the Corneal Wavefront (Figure 5-12).

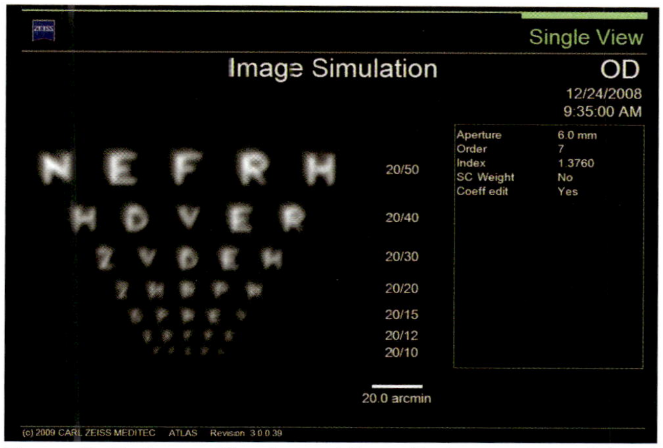


**Figure 5-11.** Image Simulation View displays a corneal focal plane image simulation based upon the corneal PSF.

The PSF shows the distribution of light on the focal plane of the anterior cornea, not including the effects of diffraction. The PSF View can be displayed as an Image (default view), Surface, or Profile view.

## Modulation Transfer Function View

The MTF View is a monochrome display representing the MTF arising from the Corneal Wavefront (Figure 5-13). The MTF View can be displayed as a Profile (default view), Surface, or Image view.

## PathFinder II Corneal Analysis

PathFinder II is a unique software feature for the ATLAS 9000 System, designed to assist in identifying abnormal and pathologic corneas based solely on anterior corneal topography.[6] It uses statistical parameters derived from anterior corneal topography for its analysis (Figure 5-14). Clinical data make it possible to compare findings in an individual

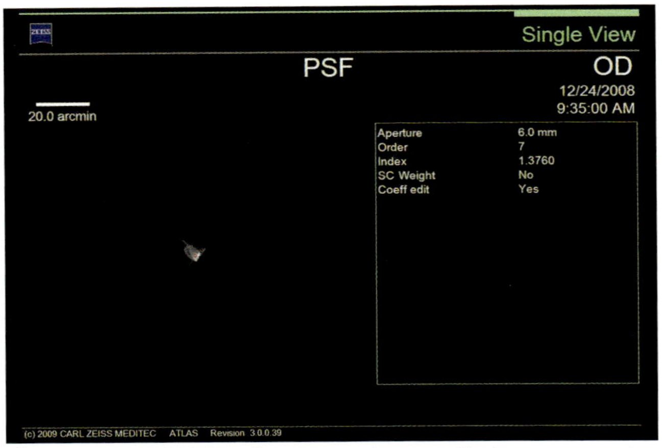


**Figure 5-12.** PSF View is a monochrome display representing the PSF arising from the Corneal Wavefront.

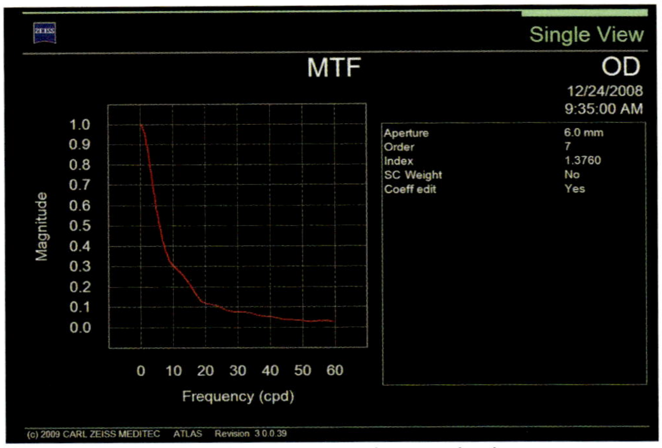


**Figure 5-13.** MTF View is a monochrome display representing the MTF based on the Corneal Wavefront.

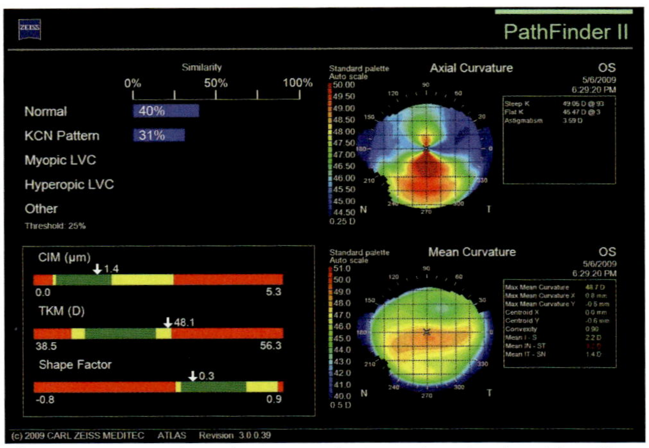


**Figure 5-14.** PathFinder II Analysis assists in the identification of abnormal and pathologic corneas based on statistical parameters derived from anterior corneal topography.

patient to expected findings from different populations of individuals with eyes that have various known conditions or pathologies. Using a trained Support Vector Machine (SVM) algorithm, PathFinder II displays the probability (from 0% to 99%) that the corneal topography matches each of the categories established in the PathFinder II clinical study database.[7] Of the 12 corneal parameters analyzed, 3 evaluate the corneal irregularity measurement (CIM), or mean apical curvature/toric keratometric mean (TKM), and shape of the cornea (Shape Factor). The remaining 9 parameters are derived from the Mean Curvature View.

An SVM algorithm performs classification by constructing multidimensional hyperplanes that optimally separate the clinical (or training) data into specific categories using the analyzed parameters. SVMs are considered to be one of the most successful classification algorithms in the data processing field.[8] For each topography exam, the PathFinder II SVM algorithm assigns a percent probability of the exam to match the trained categories.

Each corneal parameter used by PathFinder II is color-coded (green = normal, yellow = borderline, red = abnormal) to indicate the degree to which it matches the values established for the normal population, based on a multicenter clinical study. The multiclinical sample data set covers 95% of the normal eye population with a 95% confidence. The statistical parameters (CIM, TKM, and Shape Factor) are displayed in bar plot format with color-coding shown in the bar plot itself. The 9 other parameters, based on the Mean Curvature View, are displayed in the Mean Curvature View Data Box, and the values themselves are color coded.

PathFinder II analyzes 12 different corneal parameters for a particular exam and compares them to a comprehensive clinical database that contains parameter reference values for 5 categories of conditions and pathologies: normal, keratoconus pattern, myopic laser vision correction (LVC), hyperopic LVC, and other.

The normal cornea is typically aspherical in shape with TKM, CIM, and Shape Factor in the normal range. No abnormal or asymmetric topography patterns, such as inferior steepening, abnormal elevation, or curvature, can be seen in the Mean Curvature View. PathFinder II's clinical database for the normal category includes normal corneas with no corneal pathology and no history of refractive surgery or other ocular surgery. These corneas were screened with other modalities, such as corneal pachymetry, and were determined to be good candidates for LVC.

PathFinder II clinical database for the keratoconus pattern category includes established keratoconus, suspect keratoconus (subclinical/forme fruste keratoconus), and pellucid marginal degeneration. Keratoconus is defined as the true pathological condition, which causes thinning and wrinkling of the cornea, along with a cone-like protrusion of the cornea in its later stages. Keratoconus can also produce high regular astigmatism, irregular astigmatism, and topographical patterns with inferior steepening.

PathFinder II's clinical database for the myopic LVC category includes corneas that have undergone myopic LVC (LASIK, PRK, or laser-assisted subepithelial keratectomy [LASEK]).

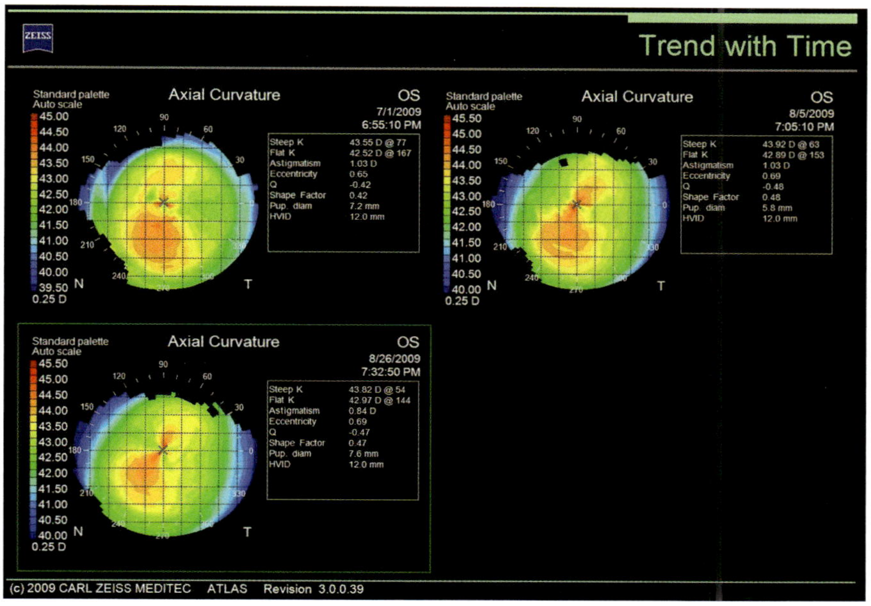


**Figure 5-15.** The Trend with Time Display shows the currently active exam and up to 3 previous exams for the same eye in chronological order.

PathFinder II's clinical database for the hyperopic LVC category include corneas that have undergone hyperopic LVC (LASIK, PRK, or LASEK).

PathFinder II's clinical database for the "other" category include corneal diseases, pathologies, or surgeries that can potentially affect the corneal surface, such as postoperative corneal transplant, intracorneal ring segments, radial keratotomy, post-LASIK ectasia, corneal scars, etc.

The PathFinder II display incorporates 4 views. The Probability View displays the previous 5 categories with blue color bars representing the 2 highest probabilities. The Parameters View consists of bar graphs of the 3 statistical data parameters: CIM, TKM, and Shape Factor. The User-Selectable View default is the Axial Curvature View and is customizable. The Mean Curvature View, a special mean curvature view with 9 additional parameters, cannot be customized.

## Image Analysis: Displays

The ATLAS software lets you select 8 different display types for the exam data:

- The Single View Display shows a single view of a single exam for the selected patient.
- The Overview Display shows 4 different views of the same exam for the selected patient.
- The OD/OS Compare Display shows 2 different views of left and right eye exams for the same patient on the same display. Two views on the left side of the display are for the right eye (OD) exam, and the same views for the left eye (OS) are on the right side. ATLAS automatically selects the exam of the other eye based on the date of exam, but manipulation of the exam is easily performed.
- The 2-Difference Display shows 2 exams for the same eye and illustrates their difference. The top exam (Exam 1) is subtracted from the bottom exam (Exam 2).
- The 3-Difference 5-Map Display provides information regarding changes between multiple exams, helpful in monitoring healing following corneal surgery. It is also useful to follow contact lens-induced change over time to determine the effect that the lens is having on the cornea. Three exams for the same eye are selected, and 2 differences are calculated. Exams 1, 2, and 3 are shown, respectively, left to right on the top of the display. Exam 1 will be subtracted from Exam 2, and a difference map will be calculated and displayed on the lower left. Exam 2 will be subtracted from Exam 3, and a difference map will be calculated and displayed on the lower right.
- The Trend with Time Display shows the currently active exam and up to 3 previous exams for the same eye (Figure 5-15). The exams are always displayed in chronological order (left to right, top to bottom).
- The Trend Analysis Display shows up to 4 exams for the same eye, along with a table of data analysis parameters (Figure 5-16). By default, only the current day's exams for the same eye are displayed, if possible. However, you can select any 4 exams to include in the Trend Analysis Display. The exams are always displayed in chronological order (left to right). The Trend Analysis Data Parameters Table displays apical radius (Ro), sagittal height (for a specified chord length); eccentricity along either the flat, steep, or custom meridian; flat and steep Sim Ks; HVID; and pupil diameter values for each image. The mean and standard deviation values for these parameters are also displayed for the images.

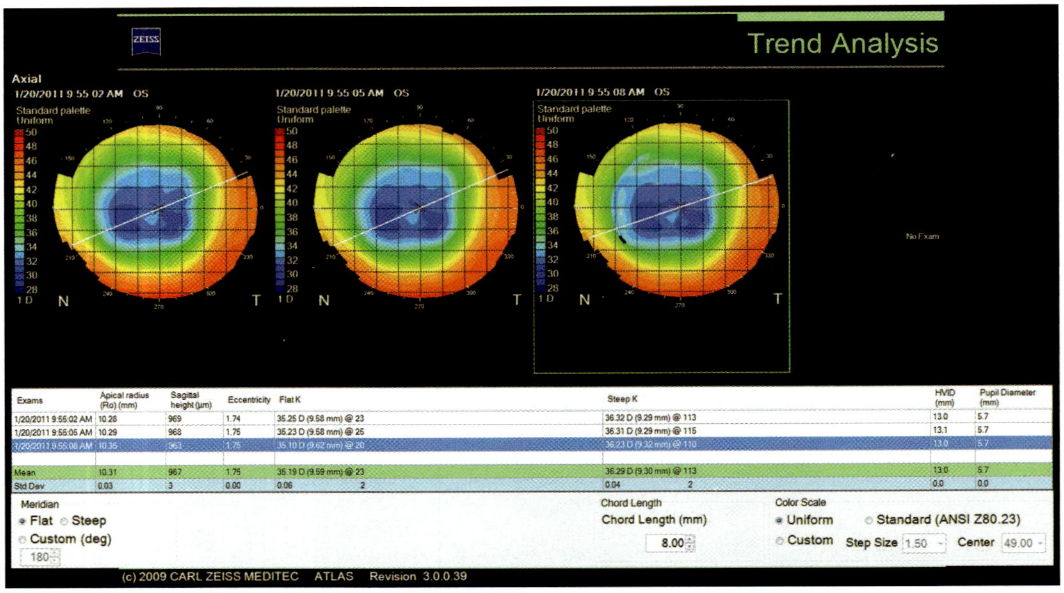


**Figure 5-16.** The Trend Analysis Display shows up to 4 exams for the same eye, along with descriptive parameters.

- The Custom Display can show 4 different views for the selected patient. Any combination of exams and views can be selected. This differs from the Overview Display, where all views are for the same exam. You can select the exams and views for the Custom Display. ATLAS has 6 default parameter sets: Pathology, Cataracts, Contact Lens Fitting, Refractive Surgery, Screening, and Screening (Expanded). Default displays can be customized within each of these parameter sets.

## MasterFit II Contact Lens Software

The optional MasterFit II Contact Lens Software enables the user to design RGP contact lenses and to simulate the resulting fluorescein pattern on the cornea. MasterFit II features both topographic- and keratometric-based lens fitting methods.[9] Based on customizable fitting preferences, MasterFit II will recommend the most appropriate lens type, including spherical, aspheric, front toric, back toric, and bitoric designs, and designs a custom lens that best achieves the desired fitting preferences (Figure 5-17).

MasterFit II also features region-specific databases of stock (finished) lenses that may be used as an alternative to creating custom lens designs.

The Fluorescein Map is a green color map of simulated fluorescein tear film layer thickness (between the back surface of the contact lens and the cornea) for the current selected lens design shown over the ring image of the eye (Figure 5-18). The shades of green correspond to the values (μm) shown on the scale at the left of the screen—darker green areas have small tear film thicknesses, while brighter greens areas have larger tear film thicknesses. The software will initially place the lens at the geometric center of the

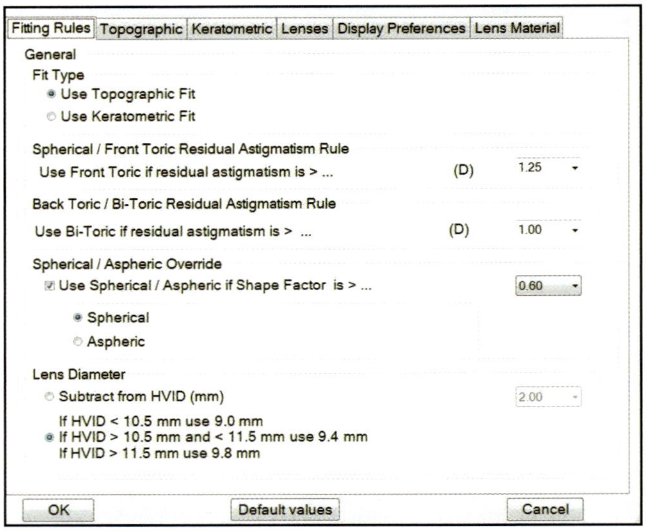


**Figure 5-17.** MasterFit II Fitting Rules are set to these default values. Users can reset these values to personal preferences.

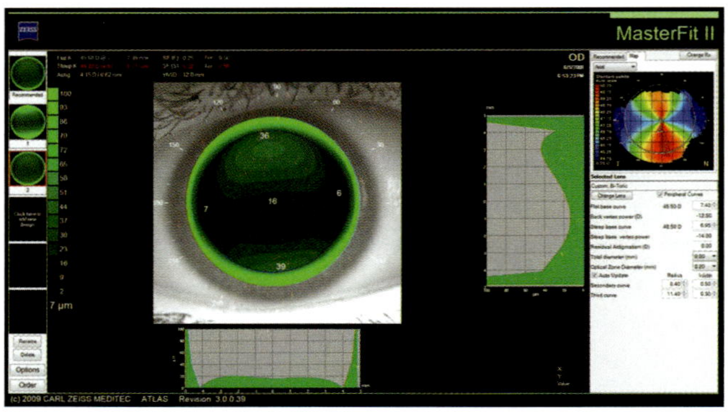


**Figure 5-18.** MasterFit II Simulated NaFl Pattern Display shows the recommended RGP lens based on the chosen fitting rules. Lens design thumbnails on the left allow the user to add and edit up to 5 lens designs to the recommended design. Horizontal and vertical tear film thickness graphs appear below and to the right of the simulated image, respectively.

cornea. You can manually move the lens by clicking inside it and dragging up-down and/or left-right.

MasterFit II's topography-based fitting optimizes the tear film clearance. The topographic fitting algorithm attempts to create a contact lens design that will provide the selected tear lens thickness using the methodology described in Figure 5-17:

- The center of the lens should clear the central cornea by approximately 20 µm.
- There should be a midperipheral clearance of approximately 8 µm along the horizontal meridian (Sim K axis closest to 180 degrees).
- There should be midperipheral clearance of approximately 40 µm, allowing for unobstructed movement along the vertical meridian (Sim K axis closest to 90 degrees).

The user may create multiple lens designs per topography exam to simulate the effect of adjusting the available lens parameters on the fluorescein pattern. After finalizing the lens design, the user may print the lens design using the order form templates provided, or the order form may be saved as a PDF and sent by e-mail to the preferred laboratory.

# The Tomey TMS Corneal Topographer

Stephen D. Klyce, PhD and Bradford L. Tannen, MD

The analysis of corneal topography is now the standard of care in anterior segment practices. The first CT commercially available was the Computed Anatomy, Inc (New York, NY) Corneal Modeling System (CMS) in 1987.[10,11] It incorporated many of the Louisiana State University Eye Center research laboratory findings in its implementation.[12] Of greatest impact was the incorporation of the color-coded display of corneal surface curvature.[13] This device had limited commercial success owing to its cost but was remarkable in that it measured both anterior corneal curvature as well as corneal thickness profiles, capabilities subsequently available in the Bausch & Lomb (Rochester, NY) model Orbscan II. Computed Anatomy was acquired by the Tomey Corporation (Nagoya, Japan) in the early 1990s following the introduction of the Computed Anatomy Topography Modeling System (TMS-1). This model became the earliest "work horse" CT, supplanted eventually by subsequent Tomey models. At this writing, the Tomey TMS-4a ("TMS-4") is commercially available with software version 5.2D. This section will review the features of the TMS-4 as well as the capabilities of the software. It should be noted that not every capability of the TMS-4 software can be covered here; priority is given to those of most frequent clinical use.

## General Characteristics

Several methodologies have been used to measure corneal curvature, including interferometry, profilometry, and Placido disk reflective methods. While interferometry has the greatest potential sensitivity of measurement, interference produces fringes according to the deviation of a measured surface from a reference surface. If the distortions in the measured surface become much greater than a few wavelengths of the measuring light wavelength, the fringes produced will merge and become indistinguishable. In essence, interferometry is too sensitive a measurement technique to apply to the imperfect optics of the eye. Profilometry is the technique used by slit-based topographers and fluorescein-stained tear film techniques (rasterstereography). The early version Orbscan I used anterior corneal surface data obtained with a scanning slit to estimate corneal topography, while the Pentacam (OCULUS, Wetzlar, DE) uses a rotating slit to obtain these data. However, direct measurement of the corneal profile does not provide sufficient resolution for accurate depiction of corneal topography. The Placido reflective technology appears to have the requisite sensitivity of measurement and is employed by all of the commercially successful CTs, including the upgraded Orbscan IIz. Developing technologies like high-frequency ultrasound and high-speed anterior segment optical coherence tomography continue to evolve, but at present have limited utility in clinical practice in measuring corneal topography.[14,15]

There are 2 basic approaches used with the Placido disks. Some use a large faceplate with a large working distance to project images of mires onto the corneal surface. This approach has the advantage of less critical focus and the disadvantage of corneal shadows created by the brow and the nose of the patient, which can obscure portions of the peripheral mire images. Other CTs use a small cone-shaped Placido disk target with a short working distance. The advantage of this arrangement is a greater potential coverage of the corneal surface, with the disadvantage of being more sensitive to error in focus. Both types have seen commercial success. All of the Tomey models have used the small cone-type Placido disk.

# Topographic Displays

CTs project a Placido pattern onto the corneal surface, capture this with a digital camera, determine the precise location of each of the mires, and convert these positions into curvature at each measurement point. The curvature data are expressed in a number of ways; mm are often used for contact lens applications, while the units of D are most often used for clinical diagnostics. The curvature data available from CTs are generally conditioned with the keratometric index (1.3375), such that the values presented include the dioptric power of the tear film/air interface (about 48 D) and the dioptric power of the endothelial/aqueous humor interface (about -5 D). This makes dioptric power values equivalent to total corneal power and conveniently correspondent to keratometry.

The scales available on the TMS-4 include the absolute scale, the Klyce/Wilson scale, the Maguire/Waring scale, a user-adjustable scale, and a normalized scale. Normal clinical use of the TMS-4 involves use of one of the 1.5-D contour interval scales (absolute or Klyce/Wilson), which show the relevant topographic features without overemphasizing details.[16] The scales are implemented with a color palette that consists of contrasting colors that make the contour boundaries obvious so that corneal topographic irregularities are not masked. This strategy of a combination of a fixed range, a fixed interval, and a well-selected color palette is essential for proper interpretation of corneal topography. Further emphasis on the importance of proper topographic scale choice is presented elsewhere in this book.

Curvature data are commonly calculated with 3 different approaches. The standard map with the TMS-4 displays corneal surface dioptric power with a spherical approximation method commonly referred to as axial power (Figures 5-19 and 5-20A). This is the baseline map that is ordinarily used in routine clinical screening. The strength of this method for calculating and displaying corneal topography is that it removes the corneal positive SA component from the power calculation. The remaining curvature displayed retains more of the shape characteristics seen in the normal cornea: steeper (higher power) in the central region and flatter (lower power) in the periphery.

A second display of corneal curvature available on the TMS-4 is the refractive power map (Figure 5-20B). This method for calculating corneal power uses Snell's law, which is necessary for accurate ray tracing in order to evaluate the corneal contribution to the aberrations measured with wavefront sensors. Note that the negative SA of the natural lens (as well as the modern aspheric IOLs) compensates to some extent for the positive SA of the cornea.

A third display of corneal curvature available on the TMS-4 is the instantaneous map (Figure 5-20C). This label is shortened from *instantaneous radius of curvature*, which offers the most detailed look at local changes in the corneal curvature. Because of the method of calculation, the instantaneous map contains significant noise artifact that may mislead the user to assume that a cornea has an abnormally high amount of higher-order aberrations (HOAs). However, the instantaneous map increases the detail of curvature changes, particularly in the corneal periphery, and may be the only means to evaluate the peripheral

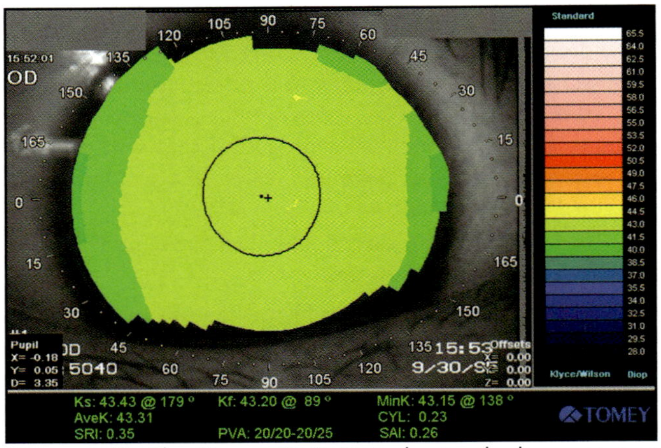


**Figure 5-19.** The Tomey TMS-4 single standard power map using the Klyce/Wilson scale. This is a cornea from a normal eye. This map conveys all the characteristics of a normal cornea: uniform central powers tapering toward the limbus, relatively smooth contours, and K readings near 43 D. An outline of the pupil is shown with its location and diameter noted in the lower left-hand corner. The central cross indicates the position of the vertex normal at the alignment axis of the TMS-4. The central small square represents the position of the pupil center. Corneal statistics are displayed in the lower panel. Sim K1 is labeled Ks and Sim K2 is labeled Kf in this version of the software.

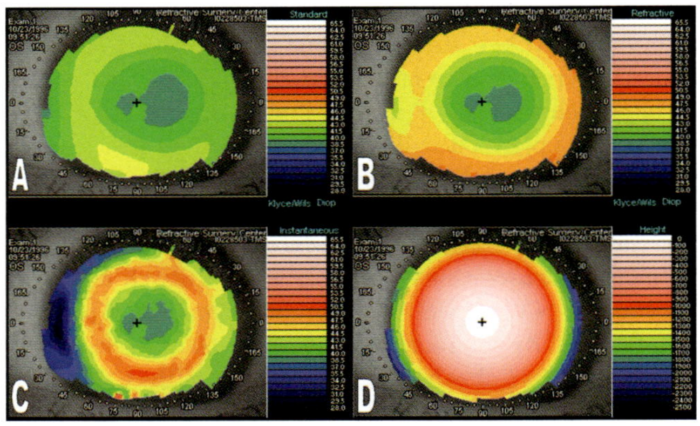


**Figure 5-20.** The TMS-4 multimap display is used here to illustrate the appearance of a single exam (cornea after PRK) with the 3 different power maps and the height map. (A) The standard power display. (B) The refractive power map. Note the central powers are the same as A, but allowing for SA steepens the peripheral powers. (C) The instantaneous map shows the "red ring" in the transition zone, which modern algorithms have overcome for the most part. Note the additional noise compared to A. (D) Without amplification, the true height map is unable to show useful detail of the shape changes responsible for the power maps.

optics of the cornea after myopic refractive surgery (MRS). Generally, amplifying corneal power distribution beyond that shown with the standard axial power map shows details that are not of consequence to vision or to diagnostics. However, the instantaneous map clearly shows the transition zone characteristics after refractive surgery, and these may be responsible for night vision complaints after refractive surgery (Figure 5-20C).

The final map type available on the TMS-4 is the height map (Figure 5-20D). The raw height map is of itself not useful diagnostically except in extremely aberrated corneas. The main component of the height data is a sphere, and this masks the small curvature changes that are clearly shown with the power maps. However, the TMS-4 offers 2 additional displays that allow inspection of distortions in true cornea shape. The enhanced height map is created by subtracting an average sphere that fits the raw height data. The enhanced height map produces an aberration structure, which bears a similarity to wavefront displays as both are in units of µm. A second routine, the height difference map, displays the difference in height data between 2 corneal examinations. This allows the change in shape induced by refractive surgery to be displayed, which can be useful to compare planned versus achieved shape changes.

A difference map is also available to show changes in corneal power with time or condition. As with the height change map, the power difference map permits the evaluation of changes in corneal power induced by refractive surgery, contact lens wear, or other condition (Figure 5-21).

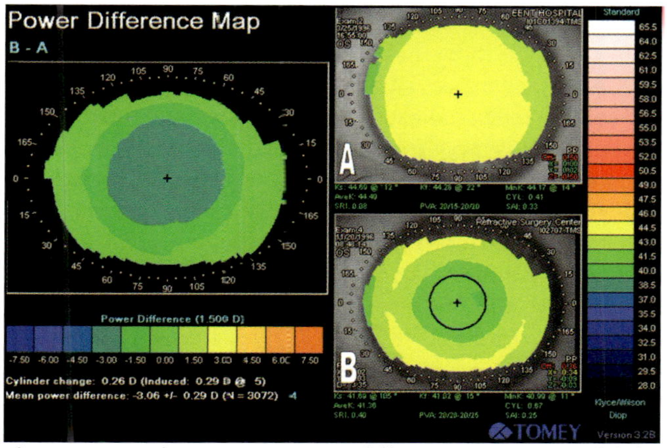


**Figure 5-21.** The TMS-4 power difference map is useful for examining the actual effect of a refractive surgical procedure on the corneal topography. (A) The preoperative cornea. (B) Postoperative result. (C) The difference between pre- and postoperative examinations

Each of the maps available on the TMS-4 embodies a number of user-selectable features. The cursor can be moved around on a map to view the radius and power at any measured point. The same routine can be used to estimate the distance and difference in power between any 2 points. This same ruler function can be used to obtain a calibrated "white-to-white" measurement. The TMS-4 measures the margins of the pupil in the video image it captures, and the pupil outline can be superimposed on any of the maps, as noted in Figure 5-22. Astigmatism is calculated in a number of ways: orthogonal, instantaneous, and zonal. Orthogonal astigmatism is similar to standard keratometry. Instantaneous astigmatism gives an indication of corneal irregularity, while zonal astigmatism is useful for planning astigmatic surgery and for contact lens applications. Other features that are user selectable include the presence or absence of the eye image, a routine for verifying the accuracy of the mire tracking, a slide-making utility, exam backup, import and export, and several grid overlays for measurement.

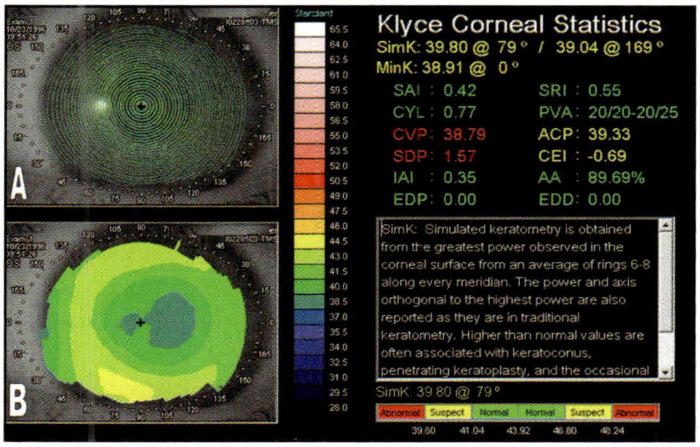


**Figure 5-22.** TMS-4 statistics display. (A) Raw image of the eye with the mires overlaid with the green rings found by the computer is useful for verifying the accuracy of the processing. (B) The standard map display of corneal topography. The right half of the figure displays the statistics calculated for the examination. Indices that are green in color indicate values within ±2 standard deviations of the value found in normals. Those yellow in color indicate suspect values that lie between 2 and 3 standard deviations from the normal. Those red in color represent abnormal values more than 3 standard deviations from the normal. The cutoff values are indicted for every statistic in the scale at the bottom of the panel. These change appropriately for each statistic by moving the mouse cursor over one of the statistics. The definition for each statistic is obtained in the same manner.

By itself, the color-coded contour map is useful for classifying corneal topography, but it does not lend itself directly to quantitative evaluation of specific values of clinical interest. A number of corneal topographic indices are available on the TMS-4; some, such as the simulated keratometry data, were designed for direct clinical use. Other indices were designed primarily for use in the automatic discrimination software described below. Each of the indices was evaluated for a group of normal corneal topographies to determine the mean and standard deviation for the normal population. To assist the user in distinguishing among normal, potentially abnormal (suspect), and clearly abnormal corneal topography, each index is color coded. A green-colored index indicates a value that is within 2 standard deviations from the normal average. A yellow-colored index indicates a caution (ie, that an index is 2 to 3 standard deviations from the normal average). A red-colored index indicates a value that is more than 3 standard deviations away from the normal average. Some of the statistical indices can be displayed on the standard maps as in Figure 5-19. More extensive statistics are found on the statistics display (see Figures 5-20 through 5-22).

The first indices enumerated for the TMS-4 and now standard on all CTs are those associated with simulated keratometry (SimK).[17,18] SimK1 gives the dioptric power and associated angle of the principal meridian, SimK2 gives the dioptric power and associated angle of the meridian orthogonal to the principal meridian, and MinK gives the dioptric power and associated angle of the meridian with the lowest overall dioptric power. The simulated keratometric cylinder of the corneal surface (Cyl) is obtained from the SimK readings.

The surface asymmetry index (SAI) measures the difference in corneal powers at every ring (180 degrees apart) over the entire corneal surface.[19,20] The SAI is often higher than normal in keratoconus, PKP, decentered MRS procedures, trauma, and contact lens warpage. Adequate spectacle correction is often not achieved when SAI is high. The surface regularity index (SRI) is a correlate to potential visual acuity (PVA) and is a measure of local fluctuations in central corneal power.[17,18] When SRI is elevated, the corneal surface ahead of the entrance pupil will be irregular, leading to a reduction in best spectacle-corrected visual acuity. High SRI values are found with dry eyes, contact lens wear, trauma, and PKP.

The PVA is derived from a clinical correlation[18] of SRI versus the best spectacle-corrected visual acuity. The PVA is given as the range of best spectacle-corrected Snellen visual acuity that might be expected from a functionally normal eye with the topographical characteristics of the analyzed cornea. Diagnostic evaluation should consider the fact that tear film breakup can greatly influence PVA (and SRI). Prolonged gazing at a fixation target by a patient without blinking can produce tear film breakup, transiently reduced vision, and abnormal values of PVA and SRI. With proper blinking, abnormal values of PVA are associated with true irregular corneal astigmatism as is often observed with keratoconjunctivitis sicca, contact lens warpage, lamellar keratoplasty, and herpes keratitis. SRI and PVA are extremely valuable diagnostically to differentiate visual deficit; if an eye exhibits good corneal potential but suffers visual loss when best-corrected, the deficit will be associated with compromised internal optics, retinal disease, or neural deficit.

The average corneal power (ACP) is an area-corrected average of the corneal power ahead of the entrance pupil.[19,20] This value is generally a more accurate measurement to use for IOL calculations than keratometry values, particularly in postsurgical corneas. The corneal eccentricity index is a measure of corneal eccentricity, an overall global shape factor. The newest software version also permits the user to obtain eccentricity values for each meridian on the corneal surface. A positive (normal) value is obtained for a prolate surface, a nil value for a sphere, and a negative value is used to indicate an oblate surface. Higher-than-normal values are found with keratoconus, and negative values are often found with symptomatic contact lens wear and MRS corrections.

The standard deviation of corneal power (SDP) is calculated from the distribution of all corneal powers in an examination.[21] The coefficient of variation of corneal power (CVP) is calculated from SDP divided by the grand average of corneal powers. This fundamental statistic is high when there is a broad range of powers in the corneal surface and has been found to be a good measure of corneal multifocality. High values of CVP are found in moderate to severe keratoconus corneas, as well as during corneal transplants in the early postoperative period. Manifest refraction of an eye with high CVP will be difficult to achieve, but attention to refraction is important in such a patient to attain spectacle tolerance. The CVP value given has been scaled up by a factor of 1000.

The irregular astigmatism index (IAI) is an area-compensated average summation of inter-ring power variations along every meridian for the entire corneal surface analyzed.[22] The IAI increases as local irregular astigmatism in the corneal surface increases. IAI is high in corneal transplants shortly after surgery; persistence often heralds suboptimal best spectacle-corrected vision. The analyzed area (AA) gives the fraction of the corneal area covered by the mires that could be processed by the TMS-4 software. AA is lower than normal for corneas with gross, irregular astigmatism, which causes the mires to break up and not be resolved. A lower-than-normal AA is found with early postoperative corneal transplants, advanced keratoconus, and trauma. AA can also be artificially low during a squint or when the eyes are not opened wide.

The elevation/depression diameter (EDD) is the equivalent diameter of the area found to contain powers within the pupil 1 D or more from the mode. It is calculated from twice the square root of this area divided by pi. The units are millimeters. The elevation/depression power (EDP) calculates the average power of apparent islands (or peninsulas) and valleys for those areas of the cornea that are within the demarcated pupil. If the pupil is not available for a given exam, EDP is calculated from an area 4 mm in diameter centered on the CT axis. Together with EDD, EDP can be used to estimate the size of so-called central islands after excimer laser sculpting. Any power within the pupil that is 1 D or more beyond the mode (most frequently occurring power) is multiplied by the cornea local area it represents (area compensation); this total is then divided by the total area of the summed powers. The units are D. Normal corneas with high cylinder, corneal grafts, and clinical keratoconus will also exhibit degrees of abnormal EDP and EDD.

Modern corneal topography algorithms and devices offer reliable and repeatable measurements of surface curvature. In addition to the basic features described above, the TMS-4 offers several advanced features that take advantage of the consistent examinations that can be obtained.

## Screening Software

The presence of keratoconus or suspect keratoconus pattern in corneal topography is a contraindication for standard refractive surgery as it puts the cornea at risk for developing keratectasia. This is a particular concern for LASIK, where keratectasia can occur 6 to 18 months or more after surgery in corneas exhibiting suspect keratoconus topography[23] as well as for PRK, where keratectasia can occur 4 to 5 years after surgery in such corneas (personal communication, R. Zaldivar, 2005). Corneal topography is the most sensitive method for detecting suspect keratoconus[24,25] and, because of this, often there are no other signs, although careful retinoscopy may reveal a slight scissoring of the light reflex in these cases. Suspect keratoconus topographic patterns often present as a subtle asymmetry in corneal power. Because all corneas exhibit some degree of asymmetry, in order to differentiate between these normal variations and changes consistent with suspect keratoconus, a quantitative analysis is indicated.[24,25] The TMS-4 has 2 keratoconus screening programs (Figure 5-23). The Klyce/Maeda method[22] uses discriminant analysis and a decision tree to report the similarity in percent of a corneal topography to clinical keratoconus. The Smolek/Klyce[26] method extends this approach using neural networks to assign a similarity value to corneas with clinical keratoconus and gives a severity index of the pathology. In addition, the latter method was also trained on suspect keratoconus topographies (Figure 5-24). A number of complementary corneal topographic indices were developed to aid in the discrimination of keratoconus from other corneal pathologies in order to increase the specificity of the tests.[22] The opposite sector index represents the maximum difference between average corneal powers between any 2 opposite sectors. The differential sector index represents the maximum difference between average corneal powers between any 2 sectors. The center/surround index is the difference in average corneal power between the central 3-mm diameter of an analyzed area and an annulus surrounding this central area from an inner radius of 1.5 mm to an outer radius of 3 mm. This index is used to capture central keratoconus. These and other indices already described are used in the calculation of the keratoconus index (KCI) and the keratoconus severity index.

Here is one caveat in the use of these screening utilities: although the training sets of topography examinations contained a number of different types of corneal topographic anomalies in addition to normal corneas and those with keratoconus, they were trained to detect only keratoconus. Hence, presented with a clear example of topographic pellucid marginal degeneration, the screening utilities will each

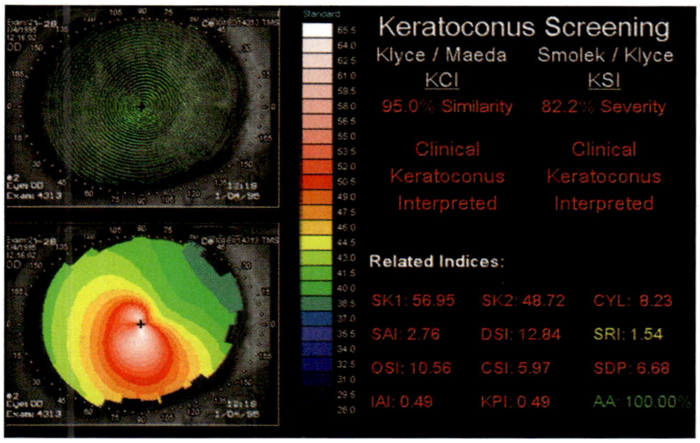


**Figure 5-23.** The TMS-4 keratoconus screening tool analyzing a cornea with moderate keratoconus. The statistical indices presented are fully described in the text.

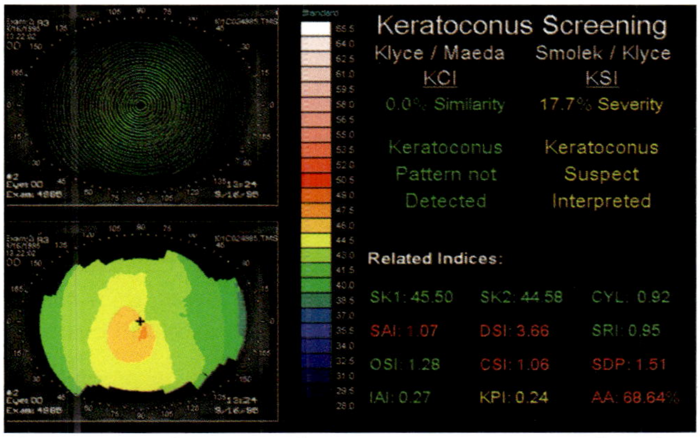


**Figure 5-24.** The TMS-4 keratoconus screening tool analyzing a cornea that is suspect keratoconus. Note that the Klyce/Maeda method reports the absence of clinical keratoconus, while the Smolek/Klyce method reports the presence of suspect keratoconus. This is not a contradiction: the Klyce/Maeda method only recognizes clinical keratoconus; suspect keratoconus was not part of its training.

report the absence of keratoconus, with keratoconus indices colored green. Therefore, it is important that these utilities not be used as general screening programs for refractive surgery because abnormal corneal conditions other than keratoconus are also contraindications for conventional refractive surgical techniques.

Hjortdal and co-workers[27] were the first to show the utility of Fourier decomposition in corneal topography analysis. They demonstrated that the average power, cylinder, and irregular astigmatism could be extracted from each mire. The TMS-4 implements a Fourier decomposition display (Figure 5-25) along the lines suggested by these authors. With this implementation, the power values along each of the mires are fit sequentially with a 1-dimensional Fourier Series analysis, which provides a radial micro-zonal analysis. This routine decomposes corneal power data into zonal spherical equivalent, zonal cylinder, zonal asymmetry, and zonal higher-order irregularity. In addition, each of these variables is also given for 3- and 6-mm zones. These data

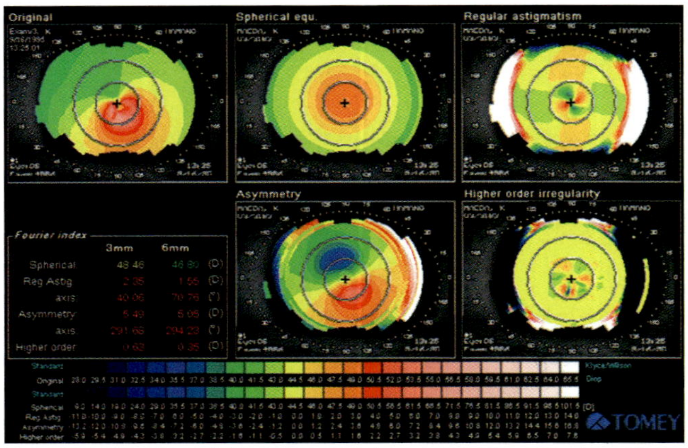


**Figure 5-25.** The TMS-4 Fourier decomposition display. Here, a keratoconus cornea is decomposed into spherical, cylindrical, asymmetrical, and higher-order irregularity components. Because the analysis is done on a ring-by-ring basis, the cylinder component is not radially linear.

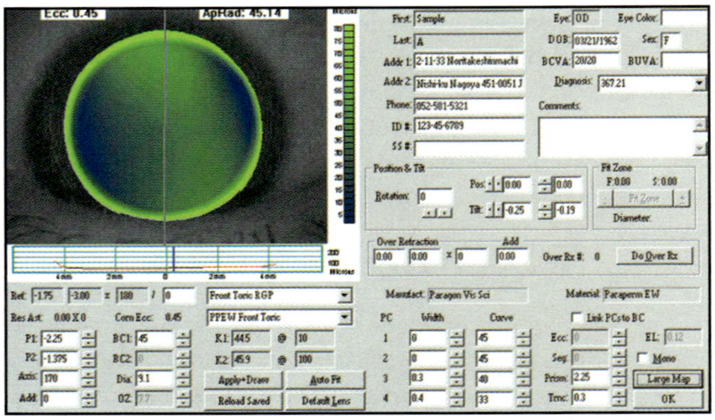


**Figure 5-26.** The TMS-4 has an extensive contact lens program with a large built-in library of commercial contact lenses as well as customizable one-off routines. The map simulates the clinical fluorescein test and is useful for inspecting the lens clearance. It updates if base curve or other parameters are adjusted.

can be useful for the analysis of the quality of refractive outcomes for different approaches. The approach has been used to evaluate corneal topographic effects of cataract surgery,[28] irregular astigmatism and contrast sensitivity after PRK,[29] and keratoconus progression[30]; to establish normative data for normal corneas versus those with pathology or surgery[31]; to examine the effects of overnight wear of contact lenses worn for orthokeratology[32]; and to evaluate visual acuity after PKP.[33]

The TMS-4 has contact lens fitting software that has evolved from the TMS-1 program, one of the first such utilities available on a CT. Using elevation and position data allows a 3-dimensional representation of the cornea to be analyzed for a contact lens fit using several rules similar to those used by contact lens fitters. Eccentricity and K readings are available from the corneal statistics, and these are used to select an initial contact lens fitted to the corneal surface from those lens characteristics that are stored on the TMS-4. The contact lens is then mathematically lowered onto the corneal surface by properly controlling the lens tip and tilt. This allows the clearance between the contact lens and the corneal surface to be calculated, and the amount of clearance is indicated using a simulated fluorescein exam (Figure 5-26). If necessary or desired, the operator can then make adjustments to the lens design, such as base curve and diameter while observing the effect on the fit. This program has been used successfully to obtain good fits with RGP contact lenses for both normal and irregular corneas.[34,35]

# Conclusion

The TMS-4 is the latest Placido disk-based Tomey CT, whose predecessors included the very first clinical device capable of producing a data-rich map of corneal shape, the Computed Anatomy CMS. Nearly all of the advances in corneal topography were made with the CMS topographer and its descendants, including scales and color palettes that promote rapid and accurate interpretation, display types that allow the clinician to examine topography in greater detail and to appreciate changes over time, topographic statistical indices that provide quantitative assessment of corneal shape factors and corneal optical quality, and screening programs that differentiate suspect keratoconus and clinical keratoconus from normal individual variations in corneal shape. Corneal topography analysis has made huge strides from the early 1980s, when keratometry and keratoscopy were state of the art. Without this essential tool, which has become the standard of care in anterior segment practice, there is no doubt that refractive surgery would have remained underdeveloped and would not have achieved the enormous success it has today. It was the CT that taught us that small functional optical zones, central islands and peninsulas, and decentrations are clear detractors of visual quality. It was the CT that detected suspect and early keratoconus to classify these patients as ineligible for standard refractive surgical procedures. These are just a few of the many advancements that define the critical role the TMS CT has played in the development of corneal shape analysis, a science that has provided both the clinician and the refractive surgery patient with better information, safer surgery, and ultimately clearer vision for the past 20 years and will continue to do so in the years to come.

# Acknowledgments

This work was supported in part by an unrestricted grant to the Department of Ophthalmology, Mount Sinai School of Medicine from Research to Prevent Blindness Inc, New York, NY. The authors are indebted to Marguerite B. McDonald, MD, Ophthalmic Consultants of Long Island, New York, for providing the patient examinations used to illustrate this chapter.

# The Magellan Mapper

Michael J. Endl, MD and Claus M. Fichte, MD

Over the past decade, the number of corneal refractive procedures has reached an all-time high. Increasingly, eye-care providers have become aware of potential postoperative complications. One of the most feared outcomes following subtle laser procedures is the development of progressive corneal ectasia. If the physician is to fulfill his or her primary goal of "do no harm," then prevention is the key.

Although various authors have published risk criteria as a guide to practitioners,[36] preoperative screening for corneal ectasia presently has no standardized detection methods.

Clinicians currently rely on keratometric, slit lamp, and standard topographic "red flags" when evaluating the candidacy of a keratorefractive patient. Some CTs—like the Magellan Mapper from Nidek (Fremont, CA)—provide refractive surgeons with a helpful tool to avoid unwanted complications.

The Magellan features new software that includes a neural network application capable of predicting various corneal diseases and postsurgical outcomes. Based on corneal statistics derived from topographic data, the software classifies and predicts the probability of several categories in an easy-to-read bar graph below the traditional axial map. This is the first application of an artificial intelligence system that uses a previously trained set of logic rules "learned" from sets of ectatic and normal patient topographies.[36]

Unlike previous keratoconus screening programs, the Magellan is able to differentiate between astigmatism, keratoconus suspects (KCS), true keratoconus, and pellucid marginal degeneration. In addition, the mapper's neural network is able to assign a percentage of probability, or grade, to these disease states. This will potentially allow users to better document and follow their patients for progression over time. Lastly, the software can also detect the probability of previous myopic and hyperopic refractive surgery, as well as PKP.

Another feature of the Magellan software is the high resolution of the map displays, made possible through improvements in the dual-edge ring-finding algorithms. As a cone-based Placido system, the mapper enjoys a smaller working distance than traditional Placido disk systems; this improves corneal coverage. The cone features a streamlined 30-ring projector. However, the system can locate both edges of each ring, which allows the Magellan's new algorithm to detect 60 rings of data. This provides an astounding 21,600 data points. As these are evenly distributed across the cornea, that translates to twice the resolution of traditional topographers.

Figure 5-27 illustrates a typical Magellan printout with the traditional axial map, a grouping of indices, and their

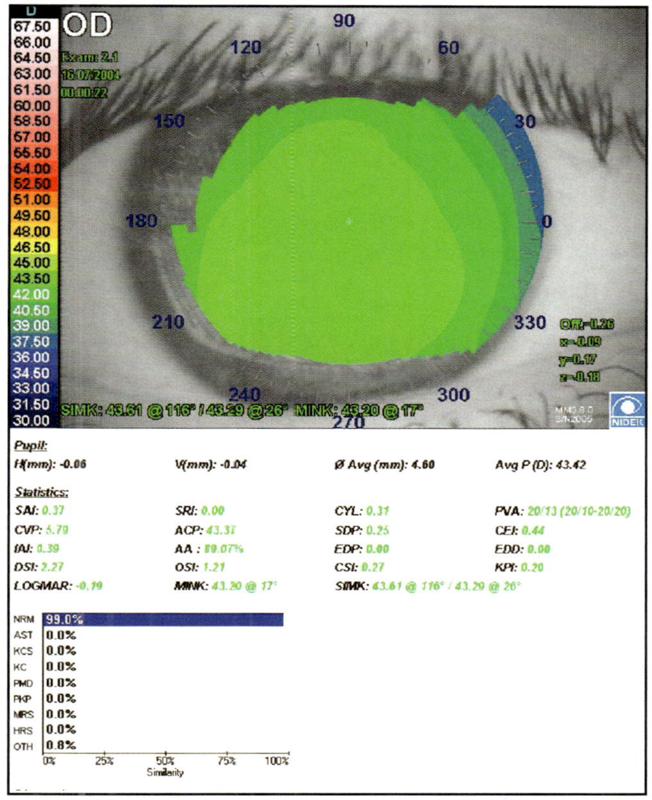


**Figure 5-27.** This topographical map has the characteristics of a normal cornea (99.0%).

values. In addition, an easy-to-interpret bar graph with classification categories is displayed that includes a percentage of that category's probability. Placing the computer mouse over any of the abbreviated indices or classifications reveals a full explanation of the title and its significance.

Refractive surgery is no longer just in the realm of the LASIK surgeon, as cataract/IOL surgery now requires the same precise results. The dramatic technology advances in small-incision phacoemulsification, aspheric multifocal IOLs, and diagnostic instrumentation have led our patients to demand the same "freedom from glasses" that our LASIK patients have come to expect. The new paradigms require results that are within ±0.25 D sphere with ≤0.50 D cylinder as well as good contrast sensitivity and functional reading vision. Expectations often exceed what current IOLs can provide unless we are "right on the money." To this end, the authors have found a second application of the Magellan Mapper extremely useful.

Aspheric IOLs have been shown to effectively reduce SA in implanted eyes, with improved optical quality over previous spherical lenses.[37] Studies have shown that customized selection of aspheric IOLs based on corneal wavefront measurements is possible and produces better visual outcomes compared to unselected patients implanted with aspheric IOLs.

As opposed to wavefront aberrometers that provide the sum total HOAs of the entire visual system, the Magellan provides corneal HOA calculations that can be used in everyday IOL selection by the cataract surgeon. This is something the authors have been routinely doing since 2005 by attempting the "best match" selection from "aberration-free" (eg, Bausch & Lomb AO platforms) or negative SA IOLs in the marketplace (such as Tecnis [Abbott Medical Optics [AMO], Santa Ana, CA] and Wavefront [Alcon, Fort Worth, TX] platforms).[38,39]

# Clinical Applications

## Corneal Refractive Surgery

Any information that can help the refractive surgeon avoid the dreaded postoperative complication of progressive corneal thinning is beneficial. Keratoconus prevalence has been reported in the range of 50 per 100,000.[40] However, as these patients are many times dissatisfied with their glasses or contact lenses, the incidence is significantly higher for the refractive surgeon.

There remains no substitute for a complete medical history and full slit-lamp examination to best evaluate a preoperative patient's potential risk for ectasia following excimer laser surgery. Although pachymetry and preoperative keratometry readings are an essential part of every refractive surgery evaluation, corneal topography has become the "standard of care" when it comes to identifying irregular corneal astigmatism and disease states.

Despite advances in instrumentation and graphics, most modern kerato-mapping systems lack the ability or programming to help identify early progressive disorders, such as keratoconus or pellucid marginal degeneration. Most practitioners are comfortable recognizing advanced thinning and irregular or asymmetric maps. However, detecting early changes or possible forme fruste keratoconus remains a clinical dilemma.

The advanced resolution and user-friendly bar graphs of the Magellan Mapper provide a much needed screening tool for the identification of abnormal corneal shape preoperatively. Using this statistical information may help prevent undesirable postoperative outcomes by recommending against surgery for patients with evidence of progressive ectatic disease. Figure 5-28 shows a Magellan printout of a patient having properties consistent with keratoconus. Also note that the indices listed in red are abnormal.

Alternatively, patients classified with mild characteristics that are consistent with KCS on the bar graph may be best treated by surface ablation or PRK (if at all).

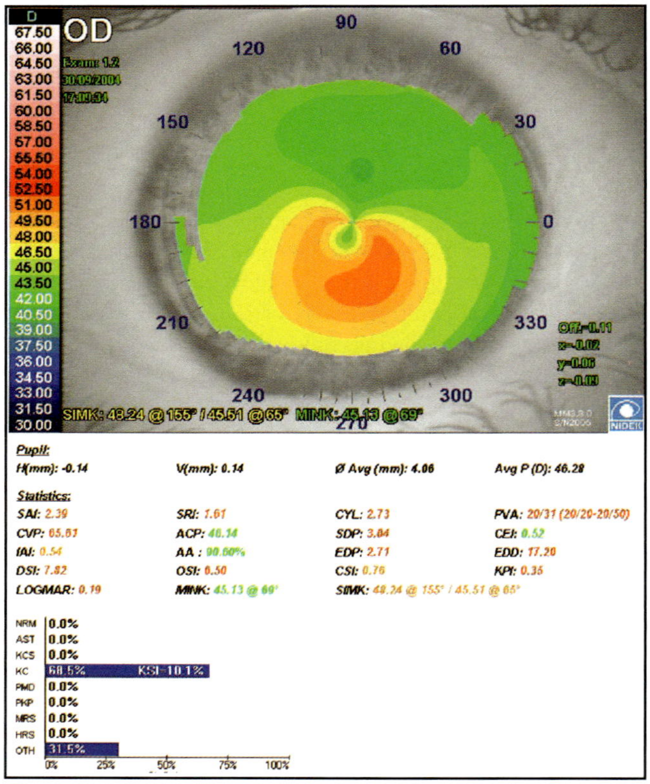


**Figure 5-28.** This topographical map has the characteristics associated with clinical keratoconus (68.5%) with a severity index of 10.7%. This map also contains features characterized as unclassified variations (31.5%).

It should be noted that any removal of corneal tissue could theoretically accelerate the progression of early ectatic disease. Most experts agree that surface ablation poses a lower risk than the creation of a corneal flap (whether 90 or 160 µm) plus ablation depth. Moreover, recent studies of up to 12 years have demonstrated the long-term safety and refractive stability of PRK.[41]

Figure 5-29 shows a preoperative map that registers properties associated with KCS in a patient who underwent uncomplicated surface ablation. The same patient's preoperative Orbscan, shown in Figure 5-30, did not display any of the classic "red flags" associated with early ectasia. Such red flags include pachymetry readings with a thinnest point less than 470 µm or more than a 100-µm difference from the thinnest point to the 7-mm zone; posterior elevation (compared to best fitting sphere) greater than 40 µm; high irregularity indices at 3- and 5-mm zones; and (perhaps most important) the overall correlation of the highest/thinnest point coinciding on the anterior, posterior, and pachymetry maps.[42]

Figure 5-31 shows the postoperative stable Magellan classification graph consistent with characteristics of MRS. This case may represent a patient who was spared the increased risk of postoperative progressive irregular thinning brought on by the creation of a microkeratome cut.

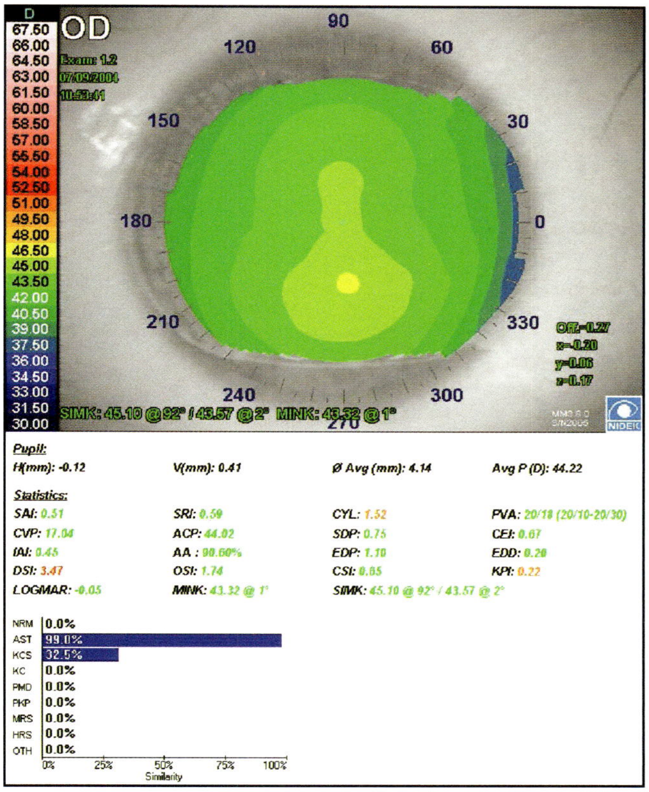


Figure 5-29. The topographical image shows characteristics associated with a cornea with 1.52 D of cylinder (99.0%) and KCS (32.5%).

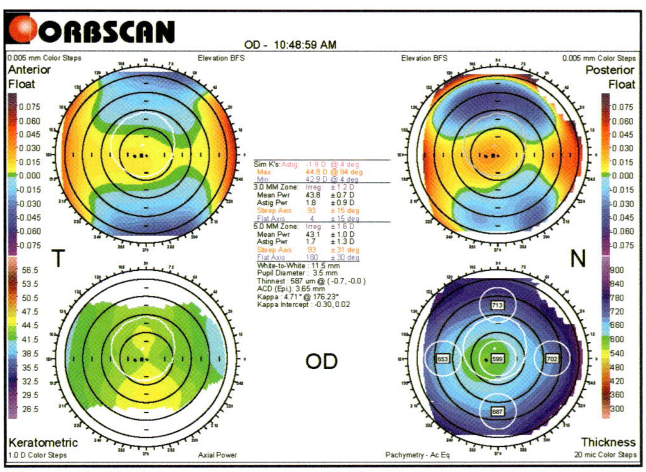


Figure 5-30. The preoperative Orbscan map of the same eye shown in Figure 5-29. Note there is no indication of ectasia.

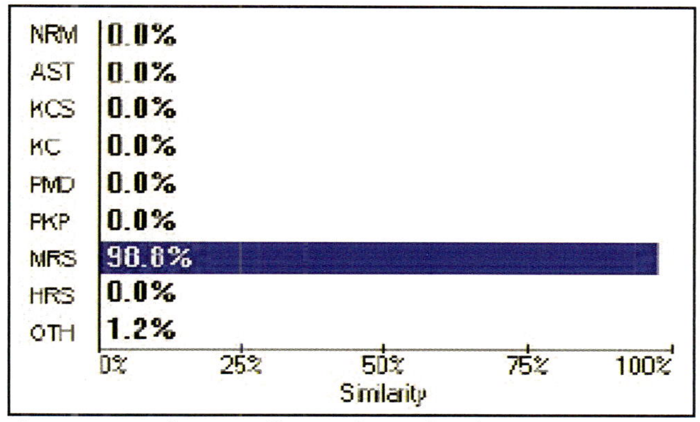


Figure 5-31. The Magellan analyzes the characteristics of the cornea and determines if the characteristics are associated with various conditions. In this case, the map is characteristic of MRS (98.8%).

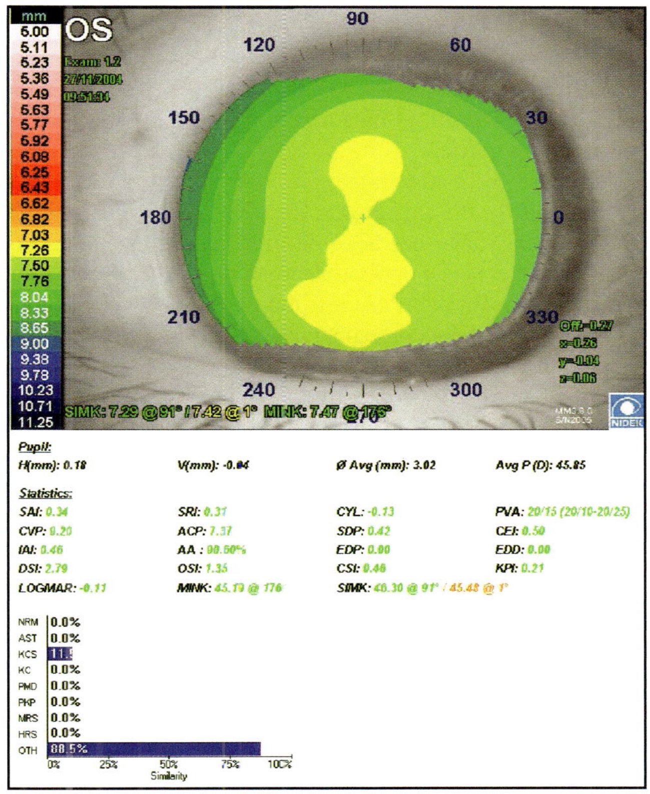


Figure 5-32. This map shows characteristics associated with unclassified variations (88.5% likelihood) and keratoconus suspect (11.5%).

It should be noted that the previously mentioned characteristics for Orbscan screening compliment the outlined Magellan statistical classification. This is illustrated in Figures 5-32 and 5-33. Both show cases where the Magellan topographical maps are consistent with mild KCS, while the Orbscan maps appear unassuming at first glance. Upon further review, the "hottest" region on the Orbscan posterior float (upper right of quad map) is greater than 40 μm from the best-fitting sphere, and the difference between the thinnest region and the 7-mm zone on corneal pachymetry is more than 100 μm. Again, these characteristics are consistent with early keratoconus-like changes, and this is a patient who perhaps should be followed without any refractive surgery until further information is gathered.

As refractive technology continues to evolve, wavefront-based excimer ablations are emerging as the procedure of

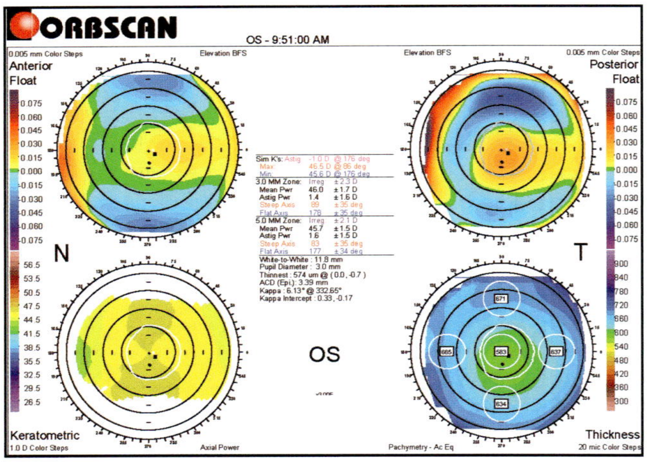


**Figure 5-33.** Orbscan map of the eye shown in Figure 5-32. Note the elevation on the posterior float (upper right of quad map).

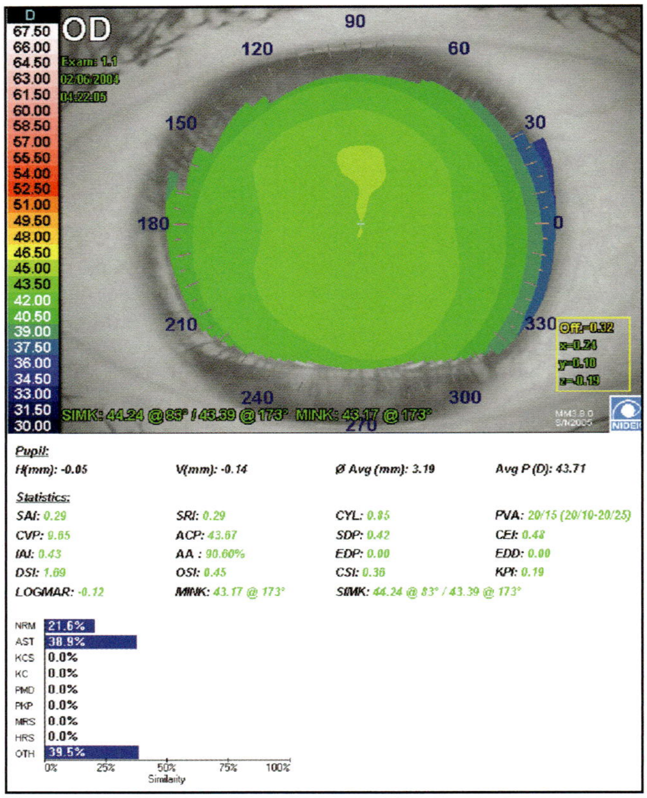


**Figure 5-34.** This axial map has the characteristics associated with unclassified variations (OTH = 39.5% likelihood), 0.85 D of cylinder (AST = 38.9%), and normal topography (21.6%).

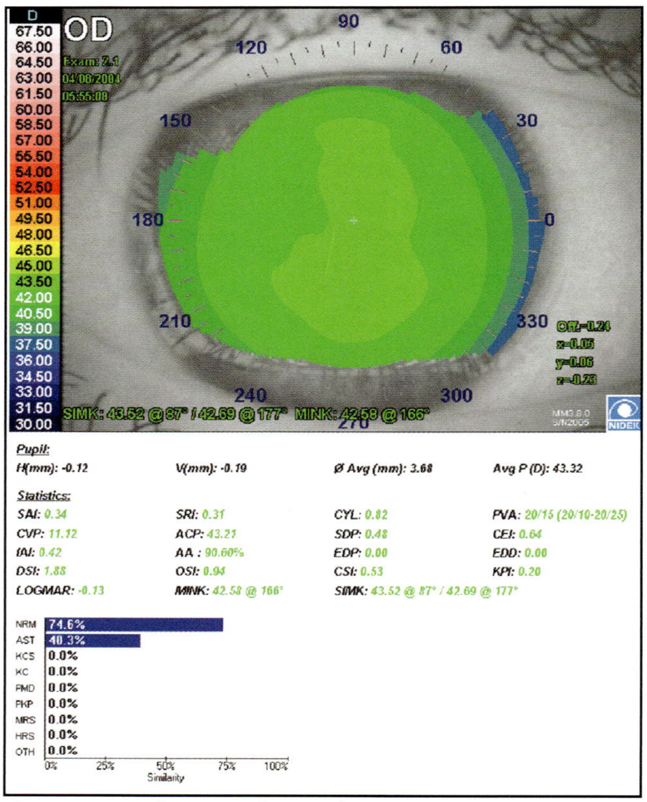


**Figure 5-35.** This map shows characteristics associated with a normal cornea (75.6%), as well as features of a cornea with 0.82 D of cylinder (AST 10.3%).

choice for optimum visual quality. In order for these types of customized treatments to work, a match must be made between the wavefront data and the pattern to be traced on the patient's cornea.

Because the preoperative wavefront information is the entire basis for the ablation profile, the capture of a patient's true corneal shape has become more important than ever. One cannot expect a perfect outcome if the data used to create the treatment plans are less than optimal. The Magellan Mapper's statistical corneal analysis is designed to differentiate between classic early ectasia signs and other abnormal shapes that may be more likely to appear with extended contact lens wear and corneal warpage (personal communication, Drs. S. Klyce and M. Smolek, November 5, 2004).

Most refractive surgeons recommend discontinuation of soft lenses at least 2 weeks prior to wavefront measurement and hard lenses or RGP lenses a minimum of 1 month before refractive evaluation. As contact lens warpage from RGP lens use has been noted to produce an irregular corneal shape for up to 6 months,[43] any axial maps that appear asymmetrical on preoperative evaluation should be followed and correlated with clinical history before surgery is considered.

Figure 5-34 shows an axial map of a refractive surgery candidate that on initial exam displayed some mild irregular astigmatism. The Magellan classifier registers in the "other" category. Note that no ectatic characteristics were triggered. Upon further history, this patient had been out of her extended-wear soft contact lenses for just 1 week.

Figure 5-35 shows her follow-up exam after being out of lenses for over 1 month. We now see a more regular axial map with the reclassification of only "normal" and "astigmatism."

The previous case is a perfect example of subtle contact lens warpage detected by the Magellan that might otherwise be overlooked. These findings allow the refractive surgeon to collect more accurate wavefront information and thus produce better postoperative results.

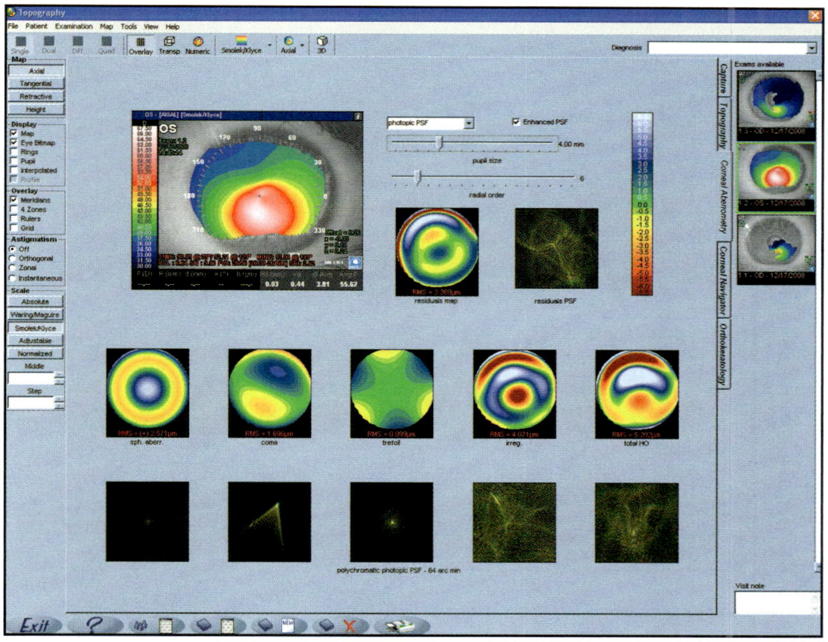


**Figure 5-36.** The aberrometry display includes the selected topographical map and wavefront maps related to typical aberrations (SA, coma, trefoil, 2-degree astigmatism, irregularities, and other HOAs) with corresponding PSFs.

## Lens-Based Refractive Surgery

The bouquet of IOL choices are ever expanding so that the concept of "one size fits all" has become a historical artifact. At the present time, IOL surgeons must choose from lenses that are aberration neutral or correct for negative or positive SA.

In general, HOAs degrade optical quality. Although there may be some benefits, such as a natural defense against ocular chromatic aberrations[44] or a decrease of image deterioration by myopic defocus,[45] most clinicians agree that, for HOAs, "the lower the better."

The cornea, with its high refractive power, is a primary contributor to HOAs. Based on a typical 6-mm papillary diameter, the cornea produces about + 0.28 µm of SA.[46]

The AMO Tecnis family of lenses (ie, ZA00 multifocal; ZB00 monofocal) induces -0.275 µm of SA to attempt to neutralize the "average" positive SA produced by the cornea. Dr. Holladay has suggested that a small amount of residual negative SA may be beneficial in presbyopes as it can increase the cornea's central power at near with pupillary constriction.[47]

The Alcon family of lenses uses different negative SA factors based on research attempting to approximate the residual SA measured in the emmetropic youthful eye. The ReStor (3.0) SN6AD1 corrects -0.10 µm of SA and the aspheric wavefront IQ monofocal and toric (SN6 series) lenses adjust for -0.20 µm. The intent here is to produce a small residual amount of positive SA as seen in young adult eyes of athletes and US Navy pilots at their peak visual performance.[48,49]

The Bausch & Lomb AO platforms (Crystalens, Akreos) are aberration "neutral" or without any positive or negative aberration induced. Thus, these lenses are less sensitive to minor decentration or tilt in the capsular bag. The previous generation of IOLs from all manufacturers induces various amounts of positive SA.

Patients with previous MRS (including radial keratotomy, lamellar procedures, and excimer laser ablations) typically have a significantly increased value to their positive corneal SA above +0.28 µm. Conversely, those patients with a prior history of hyperopic refractive surgery tend to present with corneas measuring overall negative SA.

As each patient's corneal shape and wavefront profile is unique, our practice has found the corneal-HOA calculation feature of the Magellan Mapper extremely valuable in choosing the best IOL to match the patient's anatomy. Figure 5-36 is an example of the corneal aberrometry page available for the surgeon's review. The corneal aberrometers module adopts a model based on the Zernike decomposition to derive aberrometric terms from corneal surface wavefront analysis. All of the aberrometry work was part of a larger software program created with Dr. Stephen Klyce during his long-term scientific consultancy for Nidek Technologies (personal communication, Cesare Tanassi, April 10, 2010).

Starting from the topographic map, the software computes the most significant Zernike terms (up to the 30th order). Thanks to a technique of wavefront approximation with Zernike polynomials, typical wavefront aberrations (such as SA, coma, trefoil, 2-degree astigmatism, and other HOAs) can be expressed as weighted sums of Zernike terms. Wavefront deformation maps are built and plotted in coded colors. For each aberration, the chromatic PSF and the simulated eye-chart are calculated and plotted.

As illustrated in Figure 5-36, the aberrometry page displays several components: the selected topography, wavefront deformation maps related to typical aberrations (SA, coma, trefoil, 2-degree astigmatism, irregularities,

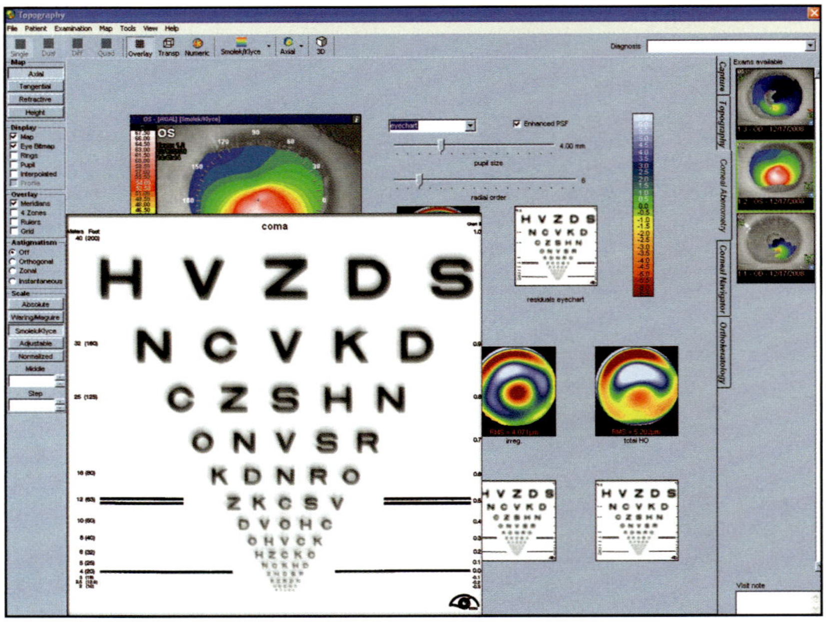


**Figure 5-37.** Simulated Snellen eye chart. This can be a very useful tool when attempting to explain the effects of corneal shape and previous refractive surgeries on visual function to patients.

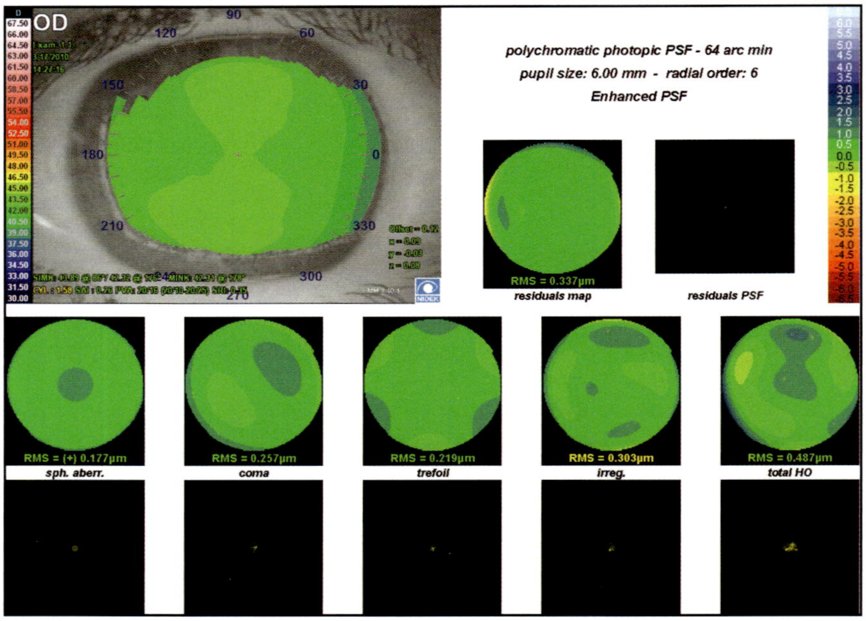


**Figure 5-38.** Measurement of SA can be beneficial when considering implantation of an aspheric IOL with a lower amount of asphericity. This value can be found beneath the spherical aberrometry map (second row, left).

and other HOAs), the residuals map, PSF, and simulated eye charts. For each aberrometric term, the following are illustrated: wavefront deformation map, color-coded RMS value (bad, suspect, normal depicted as red/yellow/green), PSF, and simulated eye chart.

The surgeon can review the PSFs and simulated eye charts (Figure 5-37) in either photopic or scotopic mode. For each aberration term, the simulated eye chart will be calculated and displayed below the corresponding wavefront deformation.

The effect of pupil size can be varied from 3 to 9 mm. It is important to measure and correctly set the patient pupil parameters as HOAs become significant (>4 mm) and large (increase ≥6 mm). Moreover, as the negatively aberrated IOLs available were calculated based on the cornea's positive SA at a 6-mm pupil, we recommend that the maps also be set at 6 mm to attempt to best use the wavefront data collected.

Following are examples of how we have used our Magellan in deciding what IOLs to implant in our cataract patients. Figure 5-38 of patient PR shows the right eye has RMS = +0.177 µm corneal SA and very low other HOAs, a "good match" for one of the Alcon platforms. The OS (Figure 5-39) has RMS = + 0.30 µm and low other HOAs, a "good match" for one of the Tecnis platforms. The surgeon can now decide whether to "mix and match" or just choose one of these platforms.

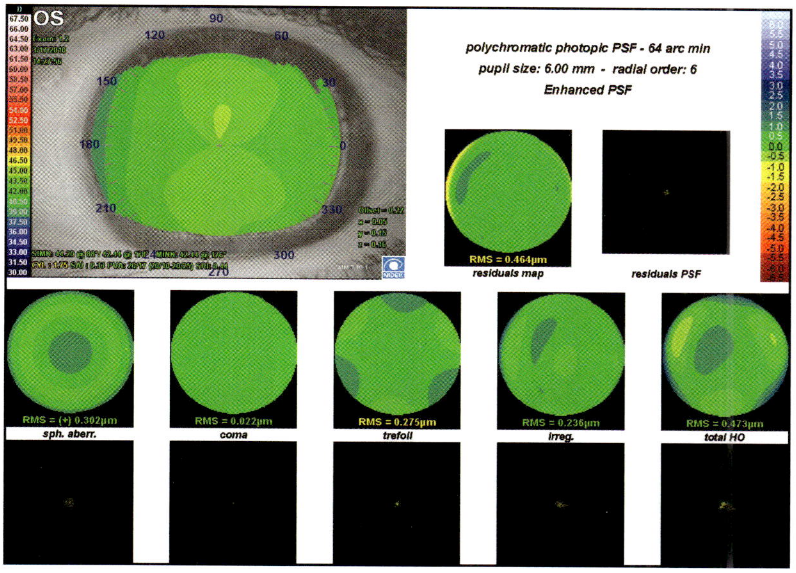


**Figure 5-39.** Higher amounts of SA are better addressed with an IOL with a larger amount of asphericity.

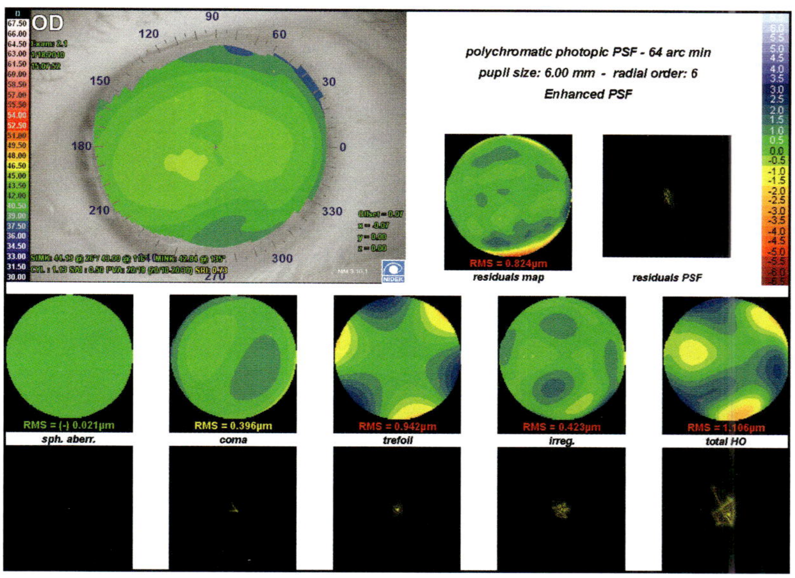


**Figure 5-40.** Negative SA found in this eye combined with an IOL with negative SA correction would suffer increased HOAs. An aberration-free IOL is a better choice.

Figure 5-40 of patient VK's OD shows negative SA RMS of -0.021 and high amounts of other HOAs. This patient had no previous eye surgery, and if an "average" positive corneal SA had been assumed, the surgeon may have actually induced more HOAs by implanting a negative SA lens. An aberration-free (Akreos) platform was chosen here to attempt to avoid further changes to the low measured SA and not exacerbate the higher degrees of coma if the lens were to tilt or decenter.

Figures 5-41 and 5-42 are of patient JH who had "old" LASIK in her OD and left her OS untreated for monovision. Her OD shows high rms of +0.85 SA and very high rms for other HOAs. A decision now has to be made. Does one want to go SA neutral with an aberration-free platform or choose a negatively aberrated lens (such as Tecnis set at -0.275 SA), reducing the +SA somewhat but risking an increase in the other factors? Her OS "virgin" cornea shows rms of only +0.185 SA with medium other HOAs. The OS is theoretically a candidate for one of the Alcon wavefront platforms (set for -0.20 SA). Having this HOA information and evaluating the effects of SA as well as of the other HOAs can be helpful to making a better IOL decision and makes it less likely that you will be surprised by an unanticipated outcome in vision quality.

Figure 5-43 of patient JW's OD shows the classical topographical pattern post-RK surgery. Observe the 4 flatter regions over the old corresponding RK cuts. Note the extremely high HOAs in all categories. The patient adamantly wanted multifocal visual rehabilitation. After extensive counseling, the best option for him was the aberration-free Crystalens AO.

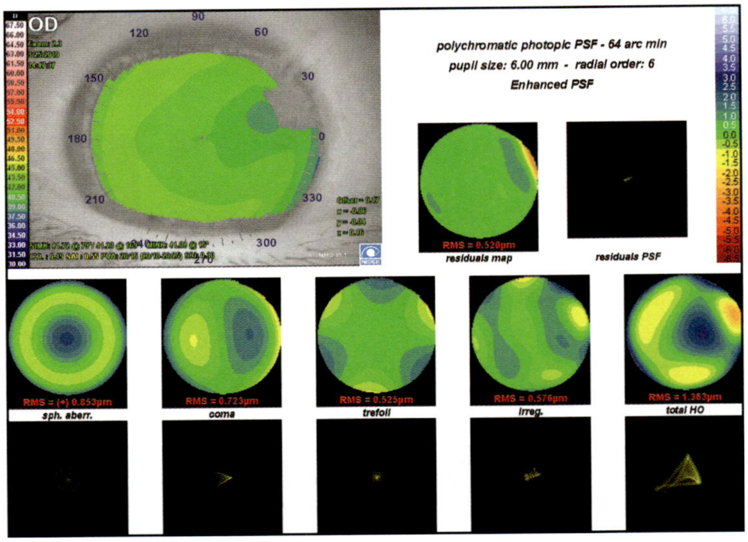


**Figure 5-41.** A map from an eye S/P LASIK with increased SA (+0.853 µm). This patient may benefit from a stronger aberration-correcting IOL.

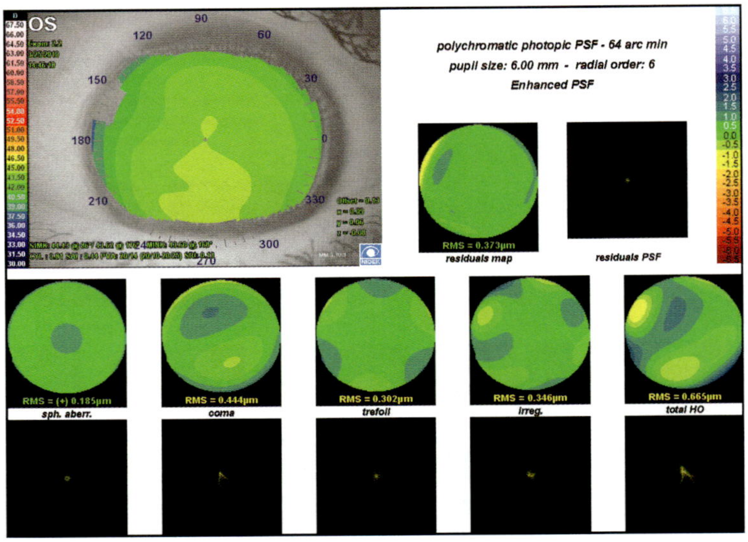


**Figure 5-42.** The fellow eye of the patient in Figure 5-41 was left untouched for monovision and thus had far less SA.

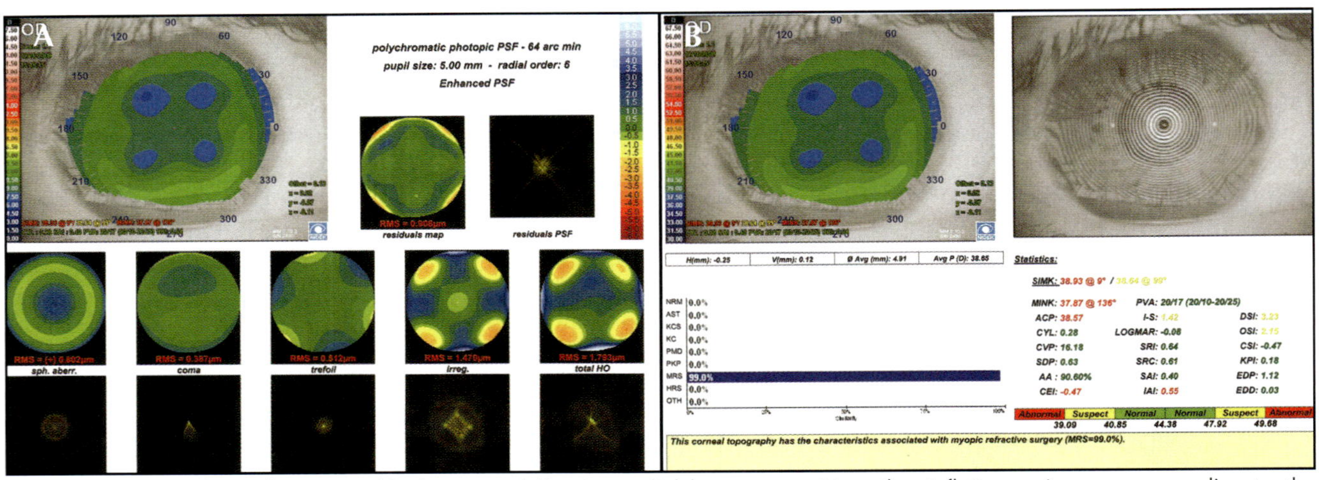


**Figure 5-43.** (A) Classical topographical pattern following radial keratotomy. Note the 4 flatter regions corresponding to the RK incisions and extremely high HOAs in all categories. The patient adamantly wanted multifocal visual rehabilitation. (B) The Magellan uses the indices to categorize the patient and correctly identified this as an eye with a history of MRS. The patient wanted to undergo implantation of a presbyopia-correcting lens, but multifocal I classical topographical pattern post-RK surgery. Observe the 4 flatter regions over the old corresponding RK cuts. Note the extremely high HOAs in all categories. The patient adamantly wanted multifocal visual rehabilitation. IOLs are contraindicated in eyes with this amount of irregular astigmatism.

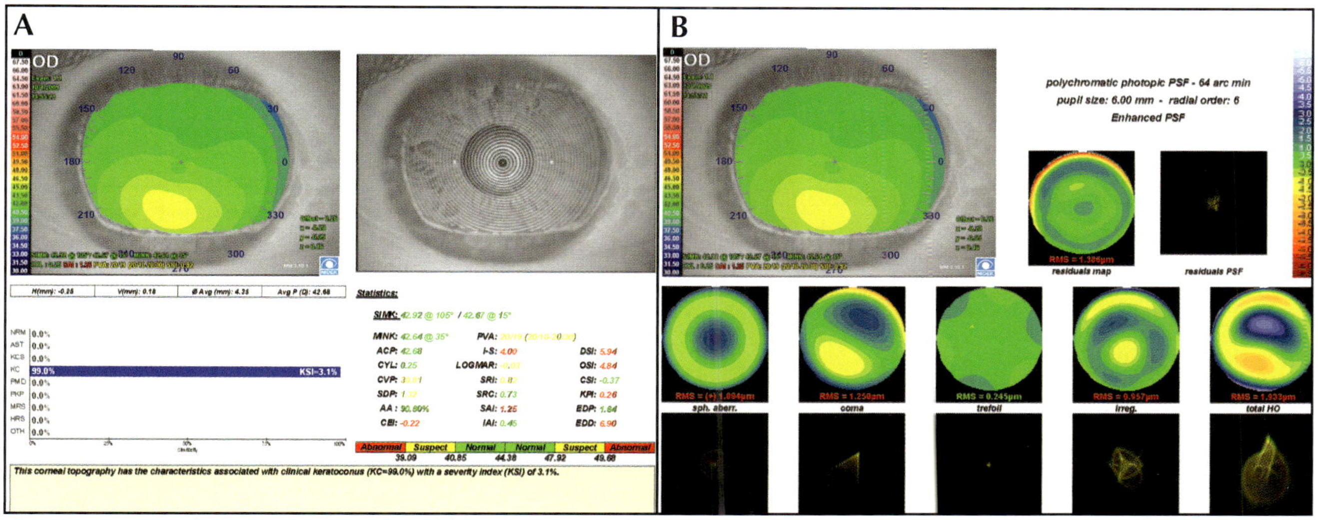


**Figure 5-44.** (A) This patient was referred for surgery OD due to a PSC cataract. Refraction and manual Ks were "spherical," but the Magellan found topography with 99% artificial intelligence-based association with keratoconus with a severity index of 2.9%. Note the inferior steepening, but the central mires are quite regular, consistent with his refraction and Ks (both manual and IOL Master, Carl Zeiss, Jena, Germany). (B) The navigator view shows very high HOA RMS in almost all categories. An aberration-free IOL platform was the most reasonable choice. Multifocal IOL implantation should be avoided.

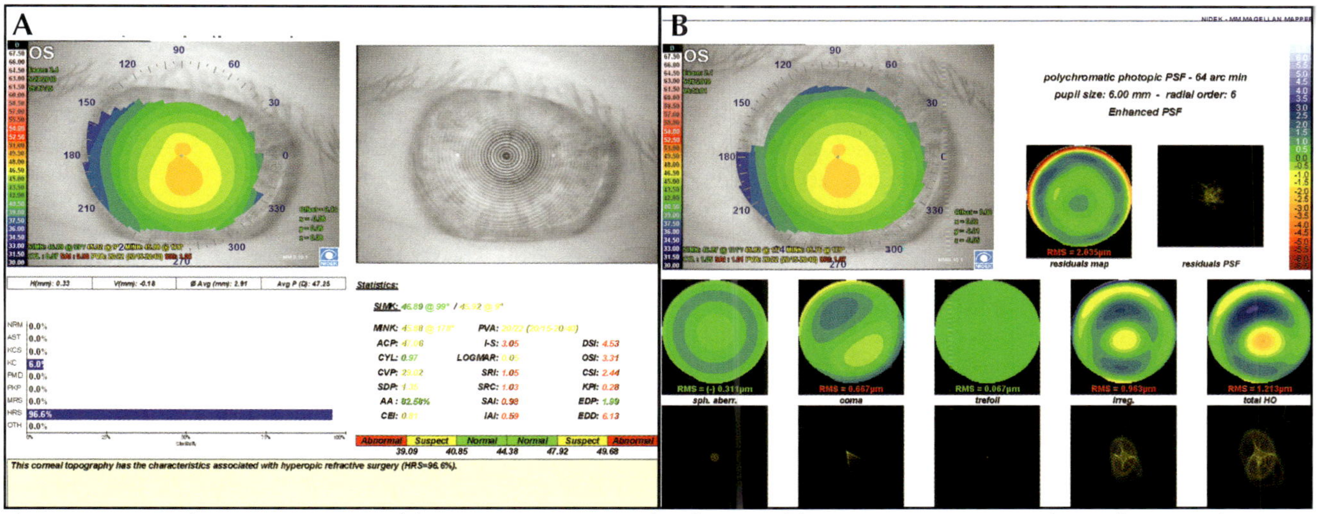


**Figure 5-45.** (A) This patient presented for cataract surgery with a history of hyperopic LASIK. Note the well-centered excimer ablation on the axial map with the neural network indices correctly identifying the previous hyperopic refractive surgery (96.6% HRS). (B) The aberration map shows a high degree of negative corneal SA (-0.311). An aberration-free IOL or perhaps an earlier-generation spherical IOL that will induce some positive SA would be beneficial.

Figure 5-44 is of patient MK, a 54-year-old man referred for OD surgery for a PSC cataract. His refraction and manual Ks were close to "spherical." His past ocular history was not contributory. The Magellan aberrometer view shows topography with 99% artificial intelligence-based association with keratoconus with a severity index of 2.9%. Note the inferior steepening, but the central mires are quite regular, consistent with his refraction and Ks (both manual and IOL Master, Carl Zeiss Meditec). The navigator view shows very high HOA RMS in almost all categories. In our view, the aberration-free Akreos AO platform was the most reasonable choice.

Figure 5-45 illustrates patient CB presenting for cataract surgery with a history of hyperopic LASIK. Note the well-centered excimer ablation on the axial map with the neural network indices correctly identifying the previous hyperopic refractive surgery (96.6% HRS). Here, the aberration map (Figure 5-45B) shows a high degree of negative corneal SA (-0.311). The surgeon can consider an aberration-free IOL or perhaps in this case an earlier-generation spherical IOL that will induce some positive SA to best match this wavefront.

## Other Refractive Applications

In addition to the Magellan's advanced screening features and corneal wavefront profiles, the mapper has advanced contact lens-fitting software with simulated fluorescein test images and a library of available contact lens parameters. Last, the topographer has an available orthokeratology module. Detailed axial scans, dual and quad multimaps, and difference mapping provide the clinician with precise fitting and therapeutic diagnostics.

## Conclusion

The Magellan Mapper and its novel classification system can provide clinicians with accurate, easy-to-read topographies as well as color-coded corneal wavefront aberration maps that complement any refractive evaluation. The high-resolution images and expanded range of indices make this topographer an invaluable tool for pathology detection and management.

# THE KERATRON CORNEAL TOPOGRAPHERS

Renzo Mattioli, PhD and Nancy K. Tripoli, MA

The Keratron family of CTs are Placido-based, non-spherically-biased, and computer-assisted (Figure 5-46). The original Keratron, introduced in 1993 by Optikon 2000 (Rome, Italy) was designed to satisfy the demand for more precise and intuitive corneal measurement by overcoming limitations in an earlier generation of CTs. In 1999, Optikon recognized the need for a portable, modular topographer and introduced the Keratron Scout, a CT that can be handheld, fitted on a generic slit lamp with a slide adaptor, or positioned intraoperatively with a weight-balanced arm and sterile disposable covers. In 2002, an external unit, the Keratron Bridge, was added to update the Keratron providing image grabbing, power supply, and USB interface with any standard PC, either desktop or laptop. The Keratron Piccolo was introduced in 2006 to take advantage of USB2 general-purpose computer technology. A version of the Keratron Scout, the Keratron Piccolo, fits on a slit-lamp carriage and uses the display of a PC rather than an integral display of its own. The Keratron Onda is a new-generation instrument that acquires corneal topography and the ocular wavefront (OW) contemporarily and at various accommodation states of the eye. Its PC is embedded, and it can be connected via LAN cable to an external PC. All currently available Keratrons are equipped with corneal wavefront analysis, IR pupillometry (except the Piccolo), and a number of new accessories.

Scout is a full 32-bit software package that is compatible with the Windows XP, Windows Vista, and Windows 7 (Microsoft Corporation, Redmond, WA) operating systems. It operates all Keratron topographers, even those dating back to 1993-1994, and can be upgraded from Optikon's Web site at www.optikon.com.

Before describing these and other Keratron family software features and clinical applications, it is important to understand the Keratron's unique method of corneal reconstruction that reveals corneal shape details that are not commonly evident with most other topographers.

## The Quest for Accurate Corneal Topography

In the past 25 years, the color-coded corneal maps produced by CTs have become an indispensable tool for clinical understanding of corneal shape. The challenge of videokeratoscopy has been to present clinically relevant corneal shape information in pictorials that are well understood to discourage overinterpretation. In addition to maps of corneal power, CTs have also mapped corneal height and used the height unit to fit contact lenses and predict or evaluate refractive surgical techniques, such as PRK, LASIK, LASEK, and intrastromal rings.

Since the early 1990s, a new generation of lathes has allowed fabrication of custom contact lenses with far more complex shapes that can conform to the large variety of keratoconic corneas. In the same period, ophthalmic excimer laser technology has been greatly improved by the introduction of flying spot technology and high-speed eye-trackers, which allow custom modelling and custom retreatments. Both of these applications could be linked to CTs and guided by corneal topography measurements. However, the applications needed data with higher accuracy and local spatial resolution than could be achieved by spherically-biased methods.

In the past, Placido-based CTs were criticized as theoretically incapable of producing accurate corneal height information.[50-52] It was argued that the corneal surface description could not be recovered from Placido images without irrevocable limits on accuracy. The Keratron was designed to overcome such criticism. The problems to be solved were (1) accurately measuring the cornea so that the maps and other applications are trustworthy; (2) providing a color-coded map unit that shows corneal shape detail; (3) supporting software processing with precision hardware; (4) rigorously testing the accuracy produced by the

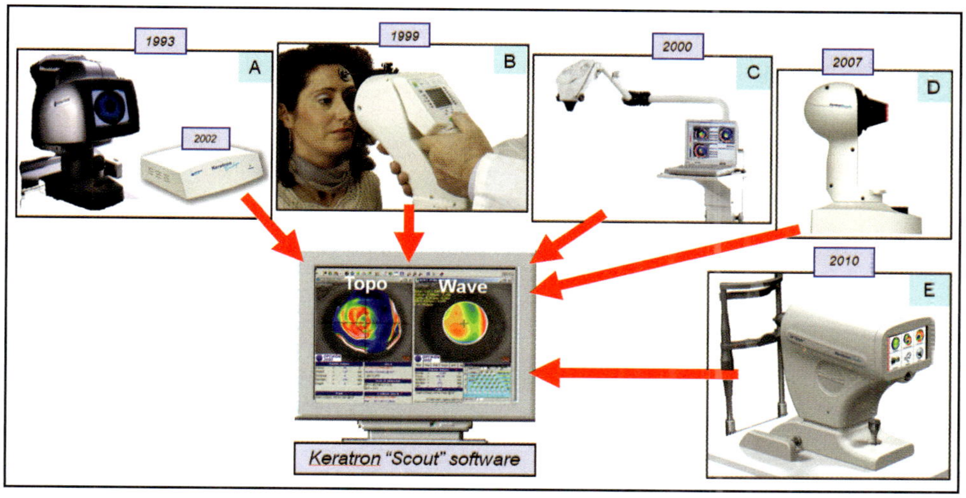


**Figure 5-46.** Scout software processes corneal topography and wavefront maps from all the Keratrons. (A) Keratron with Keratron Bridge. (B) Keratron Scout, handheld. (C) Keratron Scout, intraoperative. (D) Keratron Piccolo. (E) Keratron Onda.

hardware/software configuration; and (5) using the configuration to demonstrate as much information as possible to the clinician. This section describes the challenges of Placido-based CTs and the Keratron's design implementations to meet those challenges.

## Clinical Information in a Corneal Topography Color-Coded Map

Prior to the introduction of the Keratron, the leading commercial CTs showed maps of "corneal power" as measured along a number of radials. The unit shown was axial power whose mathematical definition is the power of a sphere, centered on the CT axis that has the same tangent as the cornea at each measurement position on a corneal profile. Axial power is inversely proportional to the radius of the sphere, using the "thin lens law" ($D = \frac{337.5}{Ra}$), and that radius is the distance from the surface position to the CT's axis measured along a surface normal. Mathematically, it is defined as

$$Ra = \frac{x\,(1 + (dz/dx)^2)^{1/2}}{(dz/dx)}$$

where z is sagittal height and x is the distance from the axis. Axial power represents the "tilting" of the surface downward from apex to periphery. Its historical relevance lies in its use in the ophthalmometer, and its scientific relevance is derived from the fact that the tangent to a surface determines refraction.

Because the corneal surface is smooth, its height changes gradually from position to position. The surface's rate of change, the tangent, reveals more detail about corneal shape than does height. However, the "bending" of the cornea reveals even more details. The geometric unit that describes the bending of the cornea in a given direction through a given point is the local, also called *tangential*, *meridional* or *instantaneous* curvature, which is the inverse of the radius of a circle whose profile matches the profile of the corneal surface at each measurement position. The radius of the sphere (Ri) is defined as

$$Ri = \frac{(1 + (dz/dx)^2)^{3/2}}{(d^2x/dx^2)}$$

where z is sagittal height and x is the distance from the axis. The sphere used to measure axial power does not have the same instantaneous curvature as the cornea at the same reflective position unless the cornea is spherical. Unlike the sphere, the center of curvature does not necessarily lie on the CT axis. Axial power at any point has been shown to be the average of the instantaneous curvature from the center to that point.[53]

## Traditional "Spherically Biased" Methods to Deduct Axial Power From Placido Reflections

Prior to the Keratron, the leading commercial CTs derived axial power by (1) measuring the power of the cornea to magnify the image of a mire[54] or (2) matching the size of a reflected mire to the sizes of mires reflected from a series of spheres.[55,56] Figure 5-47, left, shows the problems of these methods. The diagram shows rays from a mire reflecting from a cornea (solid line) and a sphere (dotted line). A point on the sphere (A) and a point on the cornea (B) will reflect the same ray to the lens and form the same image in the reflected mire pattern. However, the sphere and the cornea have different axial radii, heights, and instantaneous curvatures. Traditional axial power measurement records the radius of the sphere as the radius of curvature of the cornea. This results in mild error for axial radii and more extreme error for height and instantaneous curvature.

The false assumption that a sphere and a cornea, which reflect the same ray to the lens, have the same powers and heights is called "spherical equivalency" or "spherical bias."[55] When axial power is measured by mire magnification or mire size, corneal height cannot be determined because, for a selected reflection position, an infinite family of combinations of tangents and heights can produce the same axial power. It has been definitively demonstrated

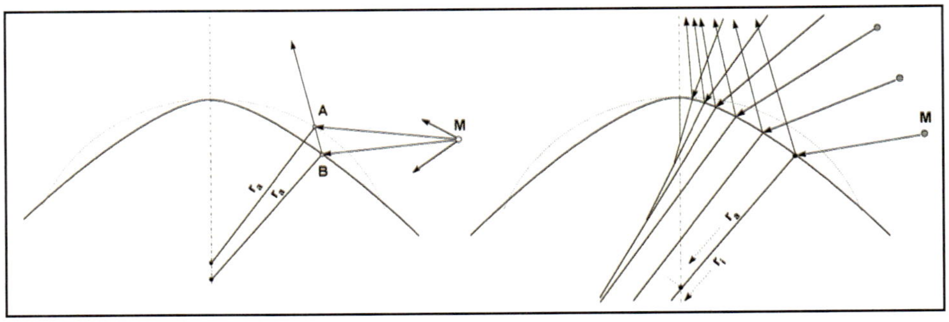


**Figure 5-47.** (Left) Spherically biased algorithms identify the ray reflected from the cornea as equivalent to a ray from the same mire (M) reflected on a sphere. (Right) The Keratron arc-step instead reconstructs the whole corneal profile as a continuous sequence of arcs, from vertex to periphery, resulting in higher accuracy of both heights and curvatures.

that this assumption leads to incorrect height measurement.[54,55] The reliance of early CTs on spherically biased measurement techniques resulted in the false assertion that all reflective CTs must be inaccurate for measuring height and instantaneous curvature.[50,51]

## Corneal Surface Reconstruction Using the Keratron Arc-Step Algorithm

An arc-step algorithm such as that used by the Keratron is a surface reconstruction method that is not spherically biased and is not completely new. It was introduced by Allvar Gullstrand in 1896[57] and resurrected in different formats by Doss in 1981[58] and by other authors between 1989 and 1992.[59-61] Nevertheless, the arc-step was usually assumed to be difficult to implement in a commercial CT without smoothing data with polynomial fitting or the like.[62]

The Keratron identifies a continuous sequence of arcs, starting at the vertex, that accurately reconstruct a corneal profile along each of 256 radials, as shown in the right image of Figure 5-47. A cornea reflects rays from each mire through the lens to produce a unique reflected mire pattern for that cornea. The radii of the arcs in the Keratron's reconstructed profile are adjusted until they reflect rays from the appropriate mires to the lens and produce the reflected pattern. The generic arc-step reconstruction method can describe aspheric corneal profiles because the second and more peripheral arcs need not be centered on the CT axis. There is one and only one sequence of arcs that can satisfy a unique sequence of mire reflections along a radial.

An unsmoothed arc-step algorithm was implemented on the Keratron to provide accurate height measurements and to produce meaningful maps of instantaneous curvature.[63] When the profile is reconstructed, it yields the instantaneous curvature, height, tangent, and axial power at each intersection of 2 arcs. This obviates the need for calculating one corneal descriptor from another because curve-fitting and mathematical derivations necessarily erode measurement accuracy and/or spatial resolution.[64,65]

## Keratron Maps of Axial and Curvature Units

Maps that depict unbiased units demonstrate the clinical utility of axial power for traditional reference to optics and instantaneous curvature for shape visualization. The detail that is missing from an axial power map, but is depicted by an instantaneous curvature map, is clinically significant.[66,67] For example, on an axial map of a normal astigmatic cornea such as that in Figure 5-48 (top, left), the toricity of regular astigmatism seems to extend to the periphery. When the same cornea is depicted using instantaneous curvature as shown in the same figure, middle left, it now appears that the astigmatism is confined within an approximately circular region of curvature above 37 D, the "corneal cap" (green and yellow). That region is surrounded by a flat peripheral region (blue), which becomes even flatter toward the periphery, reaching a maximum flatness of 15 D (23 mm) or more. The existence of the corneal cap, which appears on most normal corneas, has implications for contact lens fitting and also may prove valuable in early diagnosis of disease. The diagram in Figure 5-48 (bottom,

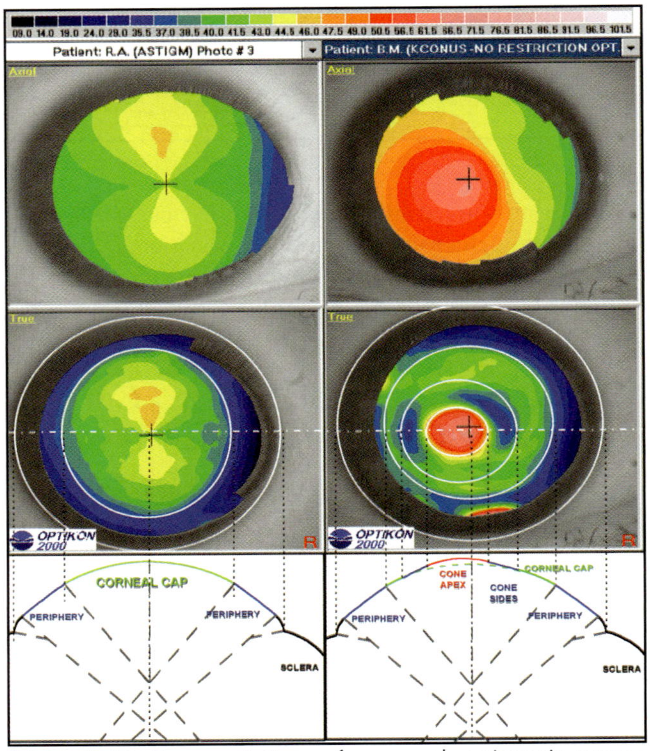


**Figure 5-48.** Representations of a normal, astigmatic cornea (left) and a keratoconic cornea (right) include the axial power (top) and curvature maps (middle) and color-coded local curvature along the 9 o'clock corneal profile (bottom).

left) represents a corneal profile from 9 o'clock to 3 o'clock. The relatively uniform curvature across the corneal cap in this direction, shown in green and corresponding to the green in the curvature map, changes in the periphery, which is relatively flat, shown in blue corresponding to the blue in the map.

Viewing an axial power map of keratoconus, as shown in Figure 5-48 (top, right), can lead to a misinterpretation of shape because a large corneal region seems to be affected by the cone. The instantaneous curvature map (Figure 5-48, middle, right) shows that the most highly curved region of the cone is only 2 mm in diameter, and curvature decreases rapidly to a large corneal region that is unaffected by the cone. The diagram (Figure 5-48, bottom, right) shows that the cone is characterized by a highly curved central region that involves the corneal vertex, surrounded by a somewhat flatter annular region. Much of the corneal cap is unaffected by the cone.

The importance of depicting corneal shape details is well illustrated by maps of a cornea after PRK, such as that in Figure 5-49. On this axial map (left), the steepness of the edge appears to involve a large annular region surrounding a generally flat center. On the curvature map (right), the steep bending of the cornea over the ablation's edge can be appreciated. More importantly, some central island anomalies, which are critical to vision following PRK, are not visible on the axial map but are seen on the curvature map.

Detecting and understanding corneal warpage caused by contact lenses is also aided by an instantaneous curvature map, as shown in Figure 5-50. On the curvature map (left), the distinctive pattern includes a flat annular region (blue) surrounded by alternating steep (red) and flat (blue) regions. The map on the right side is obtained by subtracting corneal height from the height of a sphere. Although the map contains less detail than either axial or curvature maps, it shows that a highly curved corneal region, indicated by the large cross, differs from the surrounding region by only 5 μm. To reveal this detail requires an operator's option for positioning the reference sphere and also precise height measurement so that small color steps describe localized corneal shape features.

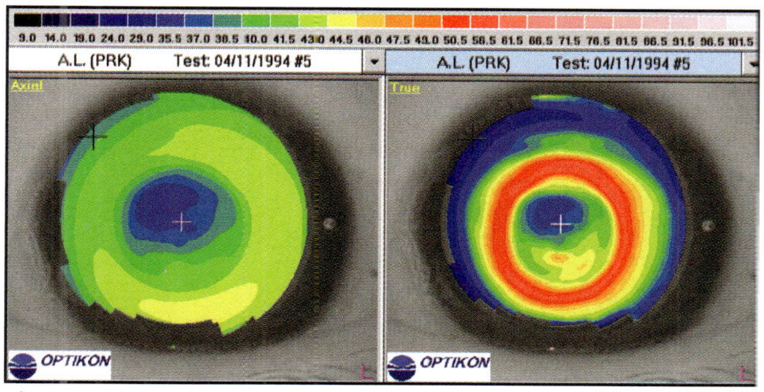


**Figure 5-49.** The instantaneous curvature map (right) of a post-PRK cornea clearly shows shape features, like the steep bending over the edge of the ablation and central islands, that are not clearly visible in the axial power map (left) of the same cornea.

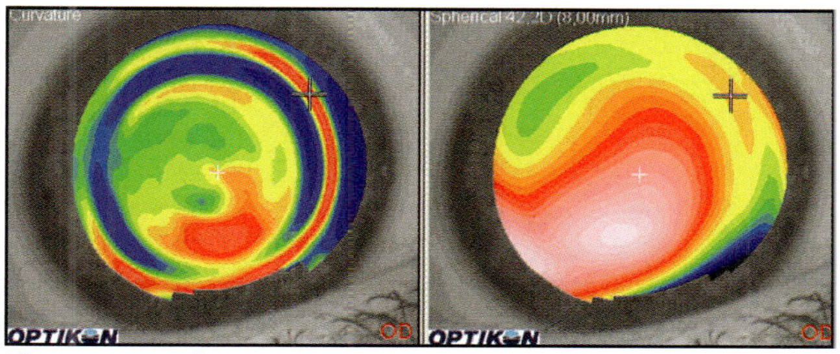

**Figure 5-50.** The instantaneous curvature map (left) and height or "spherical offset" map (right) depict the same cornea with contact lens warpage.

## The Spherical Offset Map

A map of absolute sagittal height (ie, depth with respect to the corneal plane) would always appear as a series of concentric colored doughnuts because the decreases in height from center to periphery are much greater than any circumferential variations in height. Therefore, another surface similar to the cornea's must be subtracted and the differences in heights mapped. Simulations of normal corneas have been proposed as the basis for subtraction, but the normative shape of the cornea is disputed, complex, and highly variable, making the use of a single "normal" reference of little value. Therefore, the Keratron subtracts a sphere, a shape that can be easily visualized by users. Difference values near zero are colored yellow and represent positions where the sphere's surface and the cornea's surface coincide. This is illustrated in Figure 5-50, right. Positions where the cornea rises above the sphere are colored in shades of red, and positions where the cornea dips below the sphere are in shades of green-blue. With this convention, the map is analogous to a topographic map of the earth.

The positioning of the sphere radically alters the appearance of the map, and users must understand and become accustomed to the alternative views of height. When we first introduced "spherical offset" height maps, users were frequently disappointed by the smooth, general appearance of this kind of map and the lack of detail, even on diseased corneas. To allow them to enhance heights in the region of interest (eg, the apex of a keratoconus, the optical zone of a postrefractive treatment), the Keratron allows the sphere to be fit tangent to the apex (as in Figure 5-51) or to any position selected by the user, either tangent to a given point or passing through 3 reference points, which is especially useful to align pre-post ablation height differences as in Figure 5-52.

# Keratron Basic Features

The accuracy and cost-effectiveness of a measuring instrument depend on the appropriateness of each of its components to the overall objective. To implement the

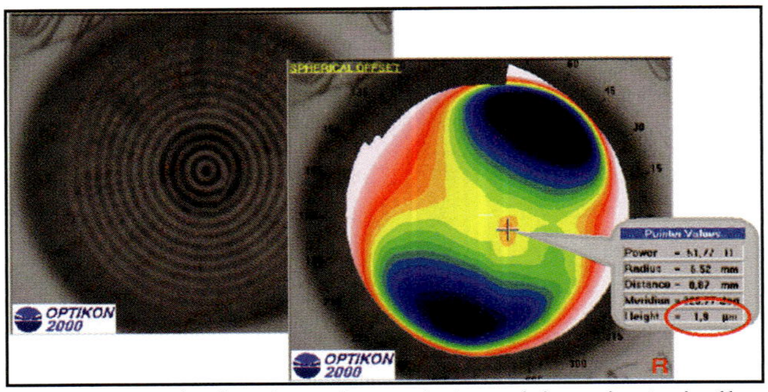


**Figure 5-51.** The height scale resolution of the spherical offset map can be adjusted to measure detail like this 1.9-μm ectatic scar.

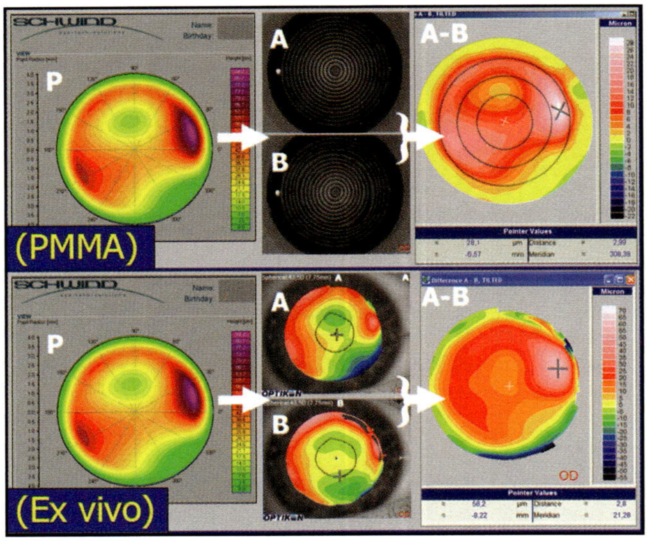


**Figure 5-52.** The pre-post height difference (A minus B) after an application of the Schwind ESIRIS laser treatment to an aspheric PMMA surface (top row) and to a living eye (bottom row), which shows the accuracy of the Keratron Scout for measuring corneal heights.

arc-step algorithm on a commercial instrument required special attention to inherent problems, for example numerical instability and extremely sensitive ring tracing.[51,59] The subpixeling and other proprietary numerical methods and design solutions adopted for the Keratron are described in more detail elsewhere.[68] The following is a list of the Keratron's main features and the resulting unique benefits.

## Height Accuracy

Earlier CTs had proven successful in measuring spheres,[56,69-71] but were highly inaccurate for measuring aspheres.[54,55] Since 1993-1994, the Keratron has been tested by several independent researchers on nonspherical profiles.[72] Tripoli and colleagues[73] measured, on a set of normal prolate, rotationally symmetric surfaces, an error within 0.25 μm within the central 3-mm zone and an error within 1 μm for entire surfaces. Under similar conditions, a TMS-1 (Computed Anatomy) height error was within

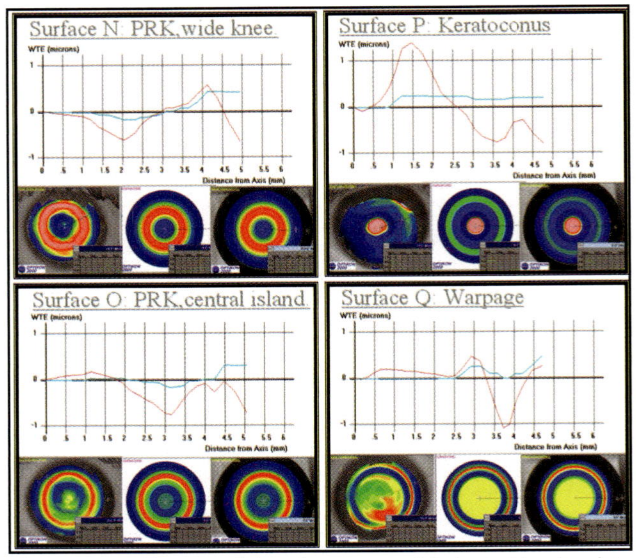


**Figure 5-53.** Four model surfaces were fabricated to simulate the 4 clinical conditions shown on the left. Accuracy was always within ±1.5 μm.

85 μm.[54,74] Another frequent criticism of CTs is their disregard for the circumferential rise and fall of an astigmatic surface, which theoretically deflects mire reflections. Evidence that this real optical effect produces inconsequential errors in the reconstruction on surfaces with up to 12 D of regular astigmatism has been published elsewhere.[75,76]

Attempting to measure more complex surfaces encountered in clinical and surgical practice can lead to even larger height and curvature errors with spherically biased methods.[72,73] The multiple transitions from flat to steep to flat areas present a real challenge for topographic algorithms. Optikon conducted in-house testing on 4 surfaces that mimicked clinical cases and presented the results at the 1996 Association of Research in Vision and Ophthalmology annual meeting (Figure 5-53).[77] In spite of the greater complexity of such shapes, the error remained within less than 1.5 μm. The testing has been repeated on the Keratron Scout with results similar to the Keratron. The examples in Figures 5-48 through 5-53 demonstrate the flexibility of the arc-step for tracking complex profiles without smoothing details.

In addition to other applications like custom contact lenses and laser links, the Keratron's height accuracy is very useful for verifying the specified custom laser ablation pattern as implemented, including file transfer, ablation design algorithm, and "fluence." Figure 5-52 shows an example of such a custom ablation pattern (on the left) and the post-minus pretreatment height measurement by a Keratron Scout (on the right). In the top row, the ablation was applied on curved plastic surfaces, and the yellow annular zone (difference = 0 μm) corresponds to the untreated zone. The bottom row shows the effect of the same specified ablation on a living eye. This example depicts a case by Dr. Camellin, treated with the ESIRIS laser by Schwind Eye-Tech solutions (Kleinhostheim, Germany) and the

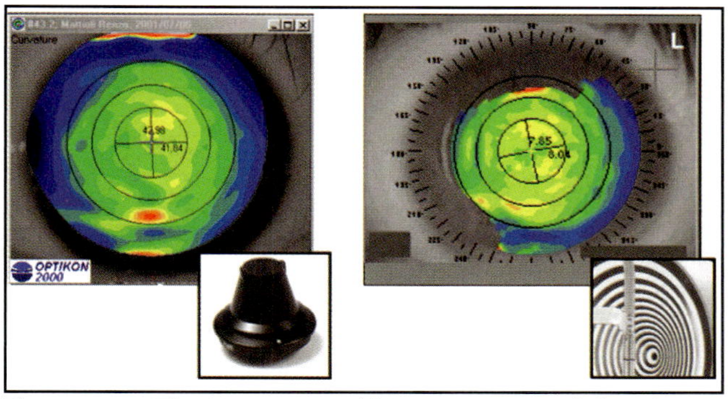

**Figure 5-54.** The Keratron "Dekking" type cone (left) achieves greater corneal coverage than large "Placido disk" topographers (right) when imaging the same cornea.

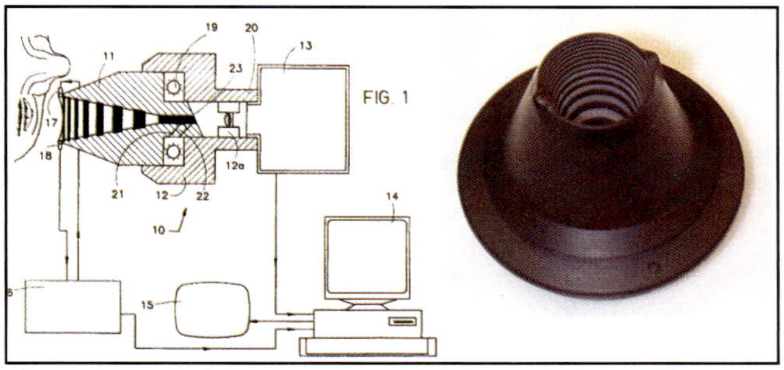

**Figure 5-55.** The Keratrons' Eye Position Control System (EPCS) includes an infrared beam that intercepts the corneal vertex and permits image acquisition only when the cornea is within a narrow range of Z distance.

Scout-ORKw (Optimized Refractive Keratectomy—wavefront) corneal wavefront link.[78]

## Corneal Coverage, Focusing, and Positioning

The use of a cone containing lighted mires is not new. It was introduced by Dekking in 1930 to place the mire arrangement close to the cornea in order to measure a larger area.[79] The Keratron mire reflections cover about 80% to 90% of a normal cornea in a well-opened eye, illustrated in Figure 5-54. However, the cone can be very sensitive to focal distance. To overcome this theoretical limitation, the Keratrons are equipped with a patented Eye Position Control System (EPCS), pictured in Figure 5-55, in which an infrared beam intercepts the corneal vertex. With this system, a picture can be taken only when the focusing, the "Z" positioning, is within a range as tight as 0.05 mm, which can guarantee a repeatability of ± 0.1 D or better (see next paragraph and Figure 5-56). Lateral (X, Y) decentering is not critical because of a software method called Eye Misplacement Control System (EMCS), which recalculates the spatial mire position in the measured direction.[68] Cantera and associates have verified that a misalignment in any direction, up to 1 mm, induces less than 0.1 D of change in the resulting curvature map.[80]

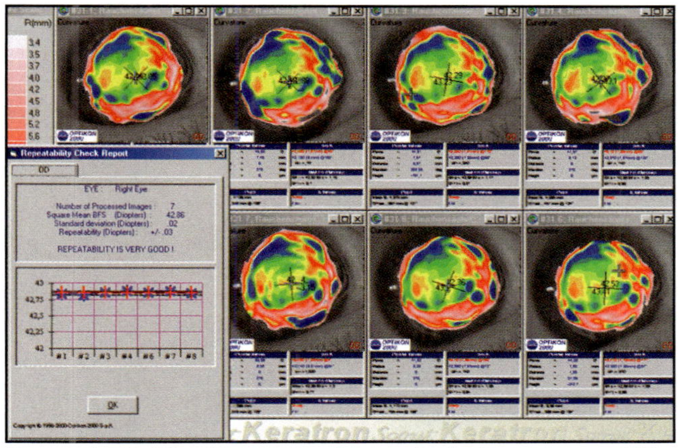

**Figure 5-56.** The Keratron software includes a repeatability check, shown here assessing the stability of acquisition by a surgeon through 7 intraoperative topographic images of the same eye.

## Repeatability Check

In spite of EPCS automated capture enabling, harsh movements and other occurrences (eg, blinking, tear film disruption) can still create artifacts that affect overall accuracy, especially in hand-held mode. To screen out unacceptable images, a repeatability check feedback function was introduced in the Scout software. The repeatability check window, seen in Figure 5-56, can be recalled at any time, or preset to automatic whenever 3 or more images of the same eye are acquired and processed. Normal eye repeatability is considered "good" with a deviation of the best fit sphere of processed maps within 0.24 D and "very good" if less than 0.12 D. Using this feature for self-training, it is not difficult to obtain repeatability well within 0.1 D, thus reducing the acquisition root mean square (RMS) height error to within less than 0.4 μm over a 6-mm zone.

## Range of Measurement

Even normal eyes frequently have an instantaneous curvature range between 20 and 50 D. In keratoconus, scars, and postsurgery, corneal curvature often shows a much greater range of power. To achieve their full potential, CTs must also be able to cover such extreme cases without losing too much local information or introducing artifacts. Figure 5-57 shows a case in which the local curvature ranges from less than 10 D (dark blue) in some areas to above 120 D (the measured point = 127.6 D) in others. Mires that are too close together limit an instrument's capability for measuring abrupt changes across the corneal surface. On the other hand, if the mires are too sparse, height reconstruction and detection of local distortion are impaired. With these opposite needs in mind, the Keratron's mire arrangement was optimized both in number and size of steps (28 mires uniformly spaced about 0.166 mm on a 43-D sphere), making use of both black-to-white and white-to-black mire borders.

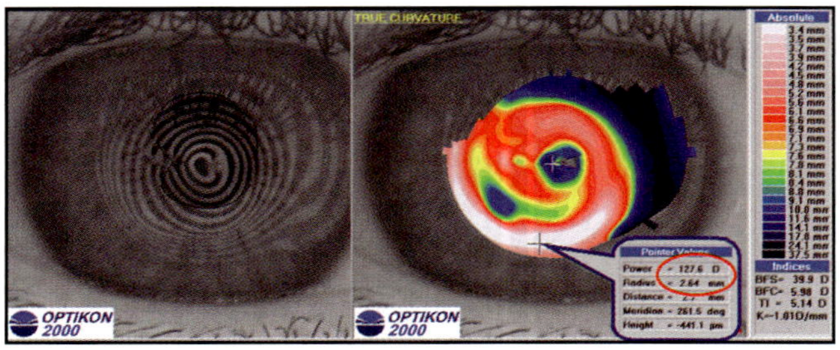


**Figure 5-57.** The Keratron's mire arrangement and subpixel edging algorithms allow the capture of detail in high resolution and over a large range of curvature. In this cornea, curvatures as steep as 2.64 mm (128 D) and as flat as 37.5 mm (9 D) are measured.

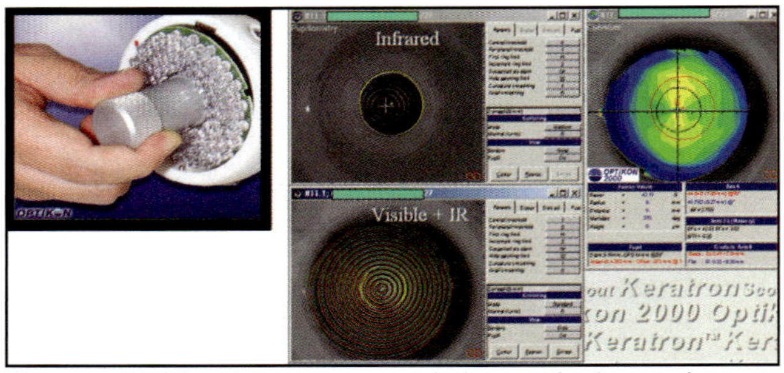


**Figure 5-58.** The Keratron can track the pupil edge in photopic and mesopic conditions and report it in topographic maps.

If mires were tracked at the middle of the rings as in most classic "cone type" videokeratoscopes, twice the number of rings would be needed for the same measurement distribution. This would limit the instrument's curvature measurement range to a maximum of 60 to 70 D.[68] Detecting the borders of alternating black and white mires instead ensures accurate tracking of mires even with complex, tangled patterns. In Figure 5-57, only some small edematous areas are unprocessed because the data were automatically discarded by tracking algorithms as unsuitable. Occasionally, special processing functions such as "dots editing" may be needed to recover mires that were automatically tracked incorrectly.

## Spatial Resolution

The Keratron's mire arrangement samples an average normal cornea at 166-μm spacing steps. This requires special edging techniques to prevent smoothing and losing important information about localized distortion such as scars. Precise mires tracking is accomplished by the Keratrons due to their subpixeling technique. Rather than just searching for black-to-white and white-to-black edges thresholds, the technique uses the entire gray scale information from all the pixels of each profile sector captured by the CCD camera. The resulting equivalent accuracy in detection of a ring position is less than 1/20 of a pixel.[68] The small ectasia in Figure 5-51, whose height is less than 2 μm, is detectable because of special tracking and arc-stepping algorithms that take full advantage of the crisp mire edge reflections. It could not be detected by nonreflective methods because the confusion in surface-scattered projected lines or slit light edges is typically much larger than the height of the feature. The mire reflections instead naturally describe even the smallest corneal scar (see Figure 5-51, left side).

## Pupil Tracking

The use of links between the corneal wavefront and the excimer laser in which a complex ablation pattern must be precisely aligned with pupil eye-trackers requires accurate measurement of the pupil center and edge, a feature that was less important when CTs were primarily diagnostic instruments. Furthermore, a measure of individual natural pupil dilation at night, or under mesopic-scotopic visual conditions, is often required in clinical preoperative practice. A dual infrared + visible illumination system has been implemented in both the Keratron Scout's (Figure 5-58, left side), and the Keratron's "lamp board." An assembly of software, firmware, and electronics allows acquisition of the eye image and tracking of the pupil edges in both mesopic and standard photopic light conditions.

The reconstruction of the pupil by the Keratron is performed on an internal reconstruction of a "clean picture" from the keratoscope image.[68] The mires must have been tracked correctly without induction of artifacts. In some cases, a "pupil editor" function can be used for hand correction. The pupil position at the 2 extreme illumination conditions is measured and represented with respect to corneal vertex. On average, in a normal population, the pupil center does not change significantly from photopic to mesopic condition.[81,82] Nevertheless, in some cases, the pupil center can be substantially displaced (0.25 mm in the case of Figure 5-58, right). In such a case, although the laser treatments are tracked on the photopic pupil, the ablated zone could be more properly centered on the largest naturally dilated area.

## The "Move Axis"

To measure curvature relative to the virtual pupil, surface measurements must be recalculated relative to a new axis. As with recalculating off-center images, a lateral translation will result in errors. Instead, the Keratron performs a 3-dimensional rotation of the corneal model. The "move axis" feature can also shift the corneal representation to any point desired by the user. This is useful to visualize the symmetry surrounding points of interest such as the keratoconic cone apex shown in Figure 5-59. This example also shows how the flat annular area surrounding the apex (A) creates a high astigmatism, typically against the rule in patients having an inferior keratoconus, because the meridional cut across the keratoconus and the apex is the local flattest meridian, and the steepest meridian is perpendicular. Moving the axis to the apex (B) shows the actual symmetry of the shape of keratoconus.

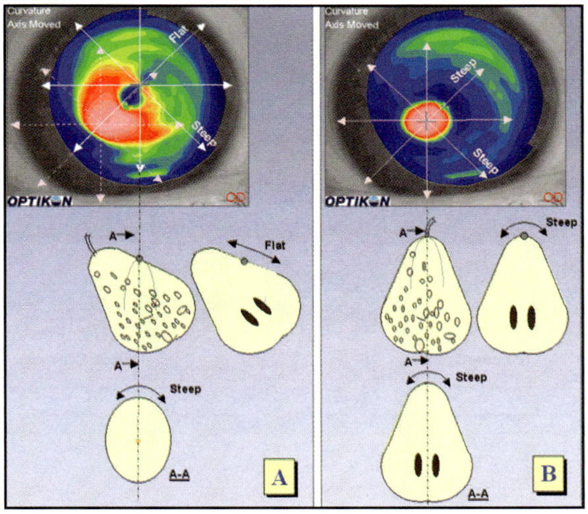


**Figure 5-59.** Keratron move-axis feature. Different views of the same keratoconus (A) before and (B) after moving the keratoscope axis to the cone center show that the keratoconus is symmetric.

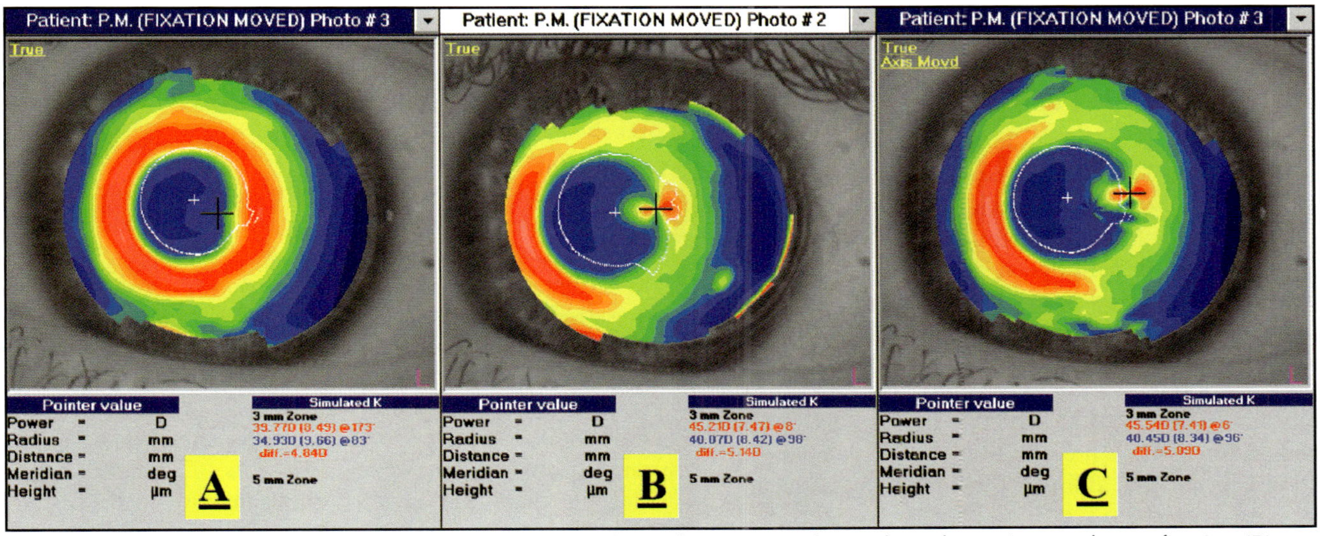


**Figure 5-60.** Using the Keratron move-axis feature (C) produces the same result as asking the patient to change fixation (B).

When an image is acquired while a subject gazes at the fixation light, as is shown in Figure 5-60, and the operator moves the axis, the resulting map looks remarkably similar to a map produced by requesting the subject to change his or her gaze. Thus, moving the axis produces a virtual rotation of the eye.[83] In Figure 5-60, normal fixation produces a typical postablation "knee," a red ring (A). If the patient is asked to fixate to the side, the vertex moves toward the periphery, and a small "hourglass" indicates the high astigmatism of the "knee zone" (B). The same image can be created using the Keratron's move-axis feature (C), showing that the feature mathematically rotates the cornea. The move-axis (C) preserves the entrance pupil position, whereas this important reference is lost when the patient changes fixation (B). This feature is particularly useful to measure the actual astigmatism when patients cannot keep fixation, such as during suture adjustment after PKP with the intraoperative Keratron Scout.[84]

## Process Editing and "Dots Editing"

When CT users acquire a corneal image and are shown only a colored map, they are unaware of the many choices that have been automatically made by the instrument. All measuring systems can occasionally produce artifacts or skip over regions. The ability to change the parameters that control Keratron processing can benefit the clinician who understands his or her objective. The Keratron offers the user the options to improve ring reconstruction in difficult cases, for example, by altering the sensitivity of borders, the incremental ring limit, the maximum number of meridians that can be interpolated, the sensitivity for finding the processing center, or the sensitivity for excluding suspected extraneous points. A versatile software feature called "Dots Editing" includes a number of tools to allow the user to reassign every black/white (green "dots") or white/black threshold (red "dots") to its proper ring. A complete removal of artifacts with this tool can be especially important before custom contact lens (CL) height-fitting or custom

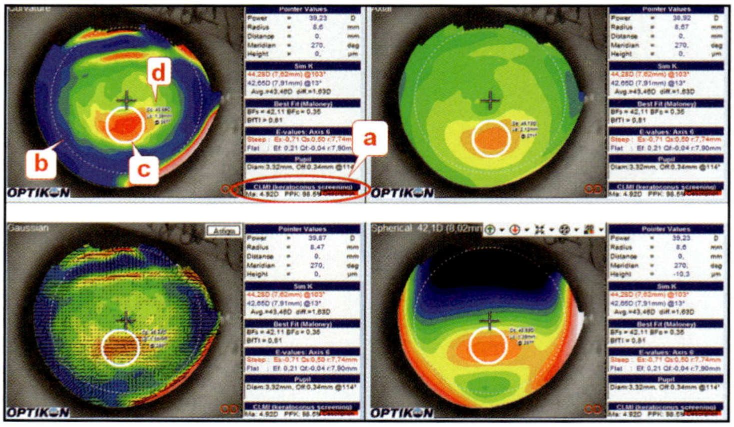


**Figure 5-61.** CLMI identifies a highly probable keratoconus (PPK = 98.5%) shown with 4 maps: curvature (top left), axial (top right), Gaussian (bottom left), and spherical offset with the sphere positioned tangent to the apex indicated by Cc (bottom right). The CLMI numerical values are shown in the screening panel (A). When PPK exceeds criterion by 20%, description data can be seen by clicking on yellow (>20%) or red (>45%) buttons. The description data include the 8-mm search area (B), the steepest 2-mm circle (C), as well as the average (Cc/Ca/Cg) in the circle and its location (D) from the vertex in polar coordinates.

laser link. The user is also permitted to clean a ring pattern by erasing artifactual areas but is not allowed to add rings or segments of rings arbitrarily.

## Intraoperative Functions

The Keratron Scout can be fit into an optional weight-balanced trolley (see Figure 5-46C), and sterile accessories allow the surgeon to take intraoperative corneal topography (ie, before and after a treatment). While the Keratron Scout is sterile sleeved, the surgeon can position and use upside-down buttons to start acquisition for either eye, capture an image, and even browse in the database and save the topography without needing to touch the PC keyboard. The intraoperative Keratron Scout has proved very useful in adjusting sutures after PKP and LKP,[84] during PTK treatments, and in measuring preoperative and/or de-epithelialized corneas before and after LASEK topo-link treatments.[85]

# Cone Location and Magnitude Indices, Gaussian Map, and Follow-Up Features

## The Cone Location and Magnitude Indices

The Cone Location and Magnitude Indices (CLMI), introduced by Drs. C. Roberts and A. Mahmoud in 2001,[86] were created to automatically distinguish keratoconic from normal corneas. CLMI is calculated by an algorithm that locates the steepest 2-mm diameter circular area of a dioptric map (axial, tangential, or Gaussian curvature). The central keratoconus index (KCI) is the difference between the average value within the steep circle and the average value of the remaining corneal area within 8 mm. The peripheral KCI measures the asymmetry of the cornea[87] as the difference between the average within the steep circle and the average within a circle on the opposite side of the cornea. A recently introduced calculation[88] allows continuous measurement from central to peripheral keratoconus.

CLMI was evaluated on 132 normal and 112 keratoconic eyes in 2005 by Twa[87] who applied a receiver operator characteristic curve analysis. He found that CLMI accuracy could be 90% at second place after his proposed C4.5 decision tree, with a specificity as high as 99% and a 79% sensitivity. This statistical analysis of screening had optimal results with axial maps.[87]

The CLMI were implemented in Scout software in 2005.[89] In scout.exe terminology, axial magnitude (Ma) is used for screening, and curvature (Cc) is used for description (Figure 5-61). The screening panel includes Ma and a statistic, percentage probability of keratoconus (PPK). If PPK is lower than a criterion, then a green circle indicates that the eye is not keratoconic. If PPK is higher than a criterion, either a yellow (for suspect) or red (for highly probable) button allows the user to get a description panel on the map. The description includes the "C1" circle (2-mm steepest zone), the circle's location relative to the vertex in polar coordinates, and the average D in that circle, Cc, Ca, Cg for tangential, axial, or Gaussian curvature maps, respectively (top left, top right, and bottom left in Figure 5-61). The main advantage of CLMI over other indices is that it locates the keratoconus and shows the clinician exactly where CLMI located the presumed cone apex, rather than using a hidden process. The clinician can look at the map to decide if the Ma or PPK could be due to an artifact or some clinical or surgical reason other than a keratoconus. Furthermore, the Cc parameter, which is the average dioptric power in the steepest circle C1 on curvature maps, is an especially valuable quantifier to follow the keratoconus, as described in a later section.

## The Gaussian Map

The Gaussian is the product of the steepest and flattest curvature in a plane perpendicular to a point of a surface. According to the Theorema Egregium by Carl Friderich Gauss (1828), this product is invariant for a flexible non-elastic surface. Gaussian curvature is therefore an intrinsic, invariant property of surfaces.[90] To illustrate the property, the Gaussian curvature of a flat sheet of paper is 0. When the paper is bent to any curvature in one direction,

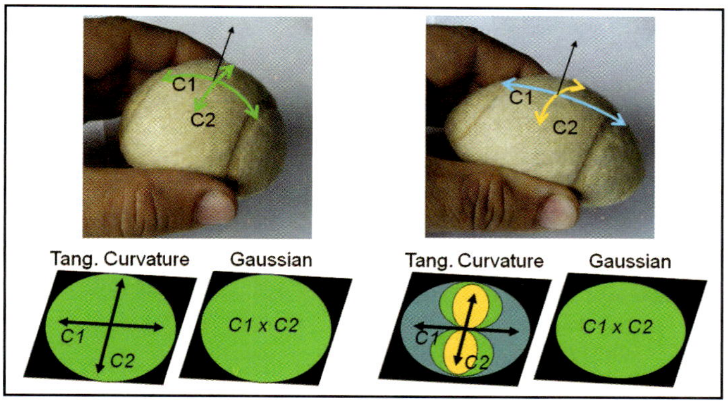


**Figure 5-62.** Gaussian curvature is an intrinsic property of any flexible, inelastic surface. Squeezing such a surface induces astigmatism on the (tangential) curvature map, but the product of the principal curvatures, C1 x C1, is invariant, and thus the Gaussian map is unchanged.

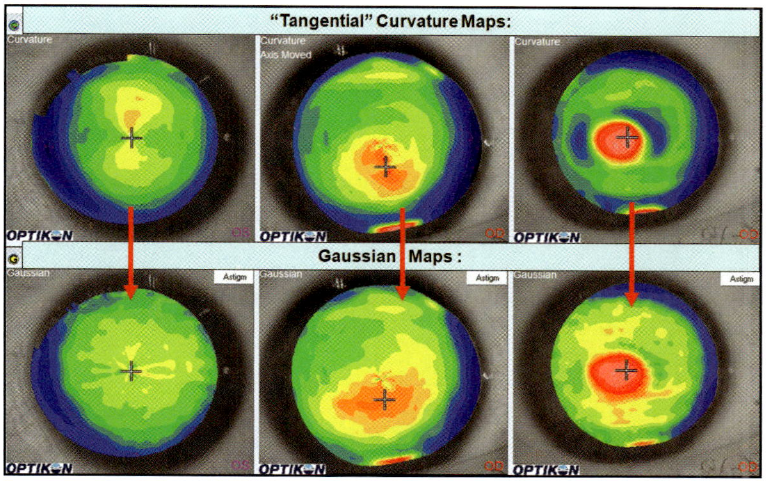


**Figure 5-63.** A comparison between curvature (upper row) and Gaussian maps (lower row) of 1 astigmatic (left) and 2 keratoconic (center and right) corneas shows that Gaussian maps do not depict astigmatism unless it is shown as a superimposed vector field. Gaussian maps do clearly reveal ectasia, whose locations are calculated independent from their distance from the corneal vertex.

it will remain straight (0 curvature) in the perpendicular direction. The steep times flat product will be 0, so the Gaussian curvature will remain 0. Squeezing a spherical surface, as shown in Figure 5-62, will make it steeper in one direction and proportionally flatter orthogonally. Surgeons who fit sutures on a donor cornea after PKP know that nonuniform tension will create astigmatism in the axial and (tangential) curvature maps. But, unless the wound is stretched to introduce cornea elasticity or permanent inelastic mechanical distortions, the Gaussian map will remain constant.

Unlike axial and tangential curvature calculations, the Gaussian curvature calculation is independent of the distance from the corneal vertex. Therefore, Gaussian maps can unequivocally show the apex of a keratoconus. This application was first proposed in 1997 by Barsky and colleagues.[91]

Gaussian curvature as implemented in the Scout software in 2007[90] is not actually the product, but the geometric average in D, the square root of the product C1 x C2:

$$G = (C1 \times C2)^{1/2}$$

where C1 and C2 are the 2 principal curvatures in that point.

Some authors have proposed a "Mean curvature" unit,[92] which is the arithmetic average of the same curvatures:

$$M = \frac{(C1 \times C2)}{2}$$

It can be easily demonstrated that the square of the 2 measures differs by the square of astigmatism:

$$G^2 = M^2 + (C1 - C2)^2$$

"Mean curvature" maps may appear quite similar to Gaussian if astigmatism is not high, but they are not invariant for the surface because they do not fulfill Gauss' Theorema Egregium.

Figure 5-63 shows differences between Gaussian maps (lower row) and curvature maps (upper row). Note the pair of maps of an astigmatic cornea on the left. On the Gaussian curvature map (bottom, left), the regular astigmatism cannot be seen, and the map appears no different from a rotationally symmetric cornea. Similarly, neither the blue sides nor the astigmatism in the apex of the keratoconus are visible in the middle and bottom right maps. Gaussian maps with vectors at points around the cornea allow visualization of astigmatism and its pattern (eg: Figure 5-61, bottom left). However, a curvature unit that hides astigmatism, as well as the flat sides that surround keratoconus apices, is not ideal for a complete clinical evaluation. Gaussian maps should always be viewed in conjunction with maps that depict other units and should never replace them.

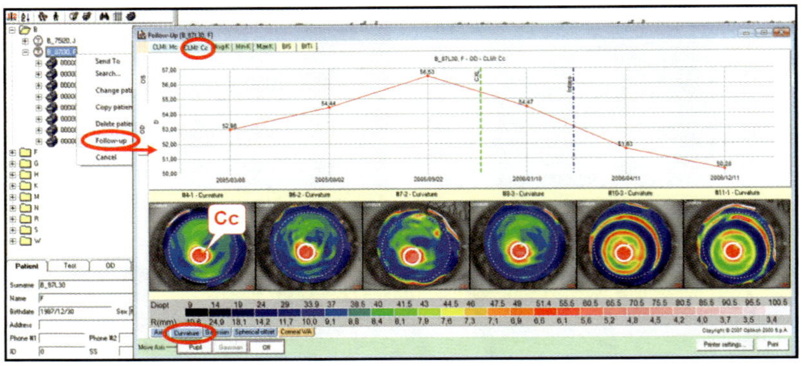


**Figure 5-64.** Follow-up of a case of keratoconus is shown in curvature maps and a plot of CLMI Cc from 6 tests over a period of almost 2 years. The first 3 tests were done before, and the fourth test after CXL treatment. The final 2 tests were done after an ICR implant. The parameter Cc proves to be ideal to show the natural progression of keratoconus and the stabilization after treatments.

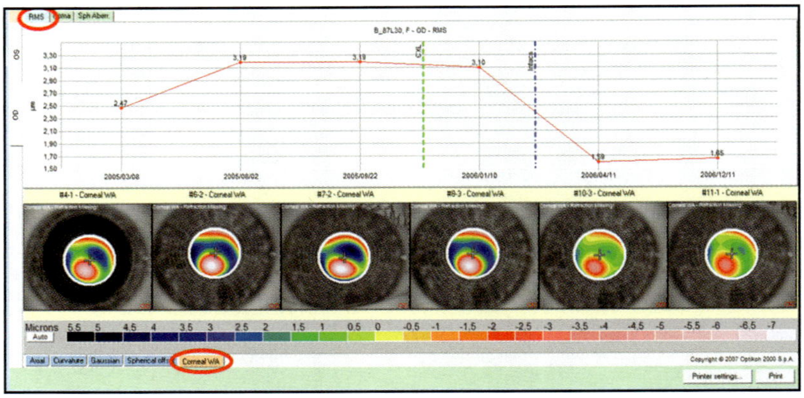

**Figure 5-65.** Follow-up of the same case as in Figure 5-64 is shown in a plot of HOAs of the corneal wavefront and corneal OPD maps. The higher-order RMS parameter quantifies visual improvement, rather than a shape factor, and is confirmed by patients' self-report.

In the new Scout software release, the CLMI applies Gaussian measurement to better locate the keratoconus apex as Cg, the CLMI circle C1 on the Gaussian map, and the unbiased location of the ectasia. There is a move axis to Gaussian apex option that places the map center of any type of map (curvature, axial, and spherical offset) on the center of circle C1. This option can be applied automatically to a number of maps, taken at different dates, in order to better evaluate Sim-K and other shape factors within the follow-up feature.

## The Scout Follow-Up Feature

When a patient has undergone a series of 3 or more tests, rather than comparing them in pairs (eg, with "pre-post" differences like those in Figure 5-52), the clinician can look at all the tests in a single window in order to evaluate over time the changes of the various maps and parameters including CLMI, Sim-K and other indices, or individual corneal and ocular aberrations.

Figures 5-64 through 5-67 show some examples of the Scout follow-up window. In this window, the clinician can choose 1) the patient's eye OD/OS (tabs on the left side); 2) the map type (circled in red, bottom left); and 3) the parameter (circled in red, top-left) to be plotted. The maps are updated in real-time and are shown in the middle of the window, just below the plot of the selected measurement unit. Their axes can be moved to the entrance pupil (button at the bottom left) or to the "Gaussian apex" (Cg), but only if a Gaussian map had been computed at least once. Moving the axis will affect all of the maps on the screen and the Sim-K readings but will not affect CLMI nor the aberrations. Corneal wavefront maps can also be shown with pupil size and aberrations chosen from the Zernike pyramid.

In Figure 5-64, we see the history of a keratoconic eye over almost 2 years and after 2 kinds of treatments. In the first 3 topographies, the progression of the cone steepness is evident by the increase of Cc (ie, the average curvature in D within the circle at the apex). After CXL treatment (test #8-3), Cc regressed by more than 2 D. After implantation of ICRs, the apical steepness dropped even more dramatically, by more than 6 D. Figure 5-65 shows the same patient's tests, for which the clinician has selected the Corneal WA (bottom tab, red circle, high orders maps) and to plot their RMS value (upper tab, red circle).

This figure gives us a different perspective than Figure 5-64. Rather than changes in the corneal shape, it shows the changes in the quality of vision. It explains why, in this particular case, the patient could not appreciate the regression of cone steepness after CXL, but recognized the greater improvement after ICR, which dramatically reduced HOAs, especially coma.

Critical to the decision of whether a keratoconic patient should have a CXL treatment or not, in addition to corneal thickness, is whether his or her ectasia is stable or progressing. This assessment is not an easy task when changes are slower or smaller than in the case shown in Figures 5-64

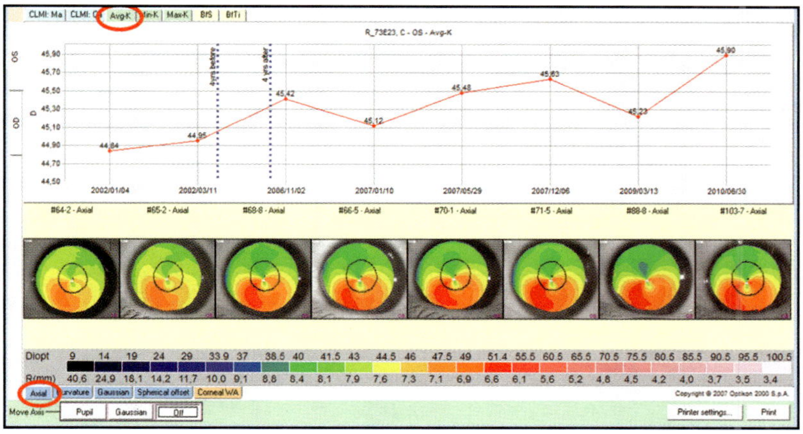

**Figure 5-66.** An unoperated keratoconic eye is followed over 8 years (2002 through 2010). Average Sim-K is plotted, and axial maps are shown.

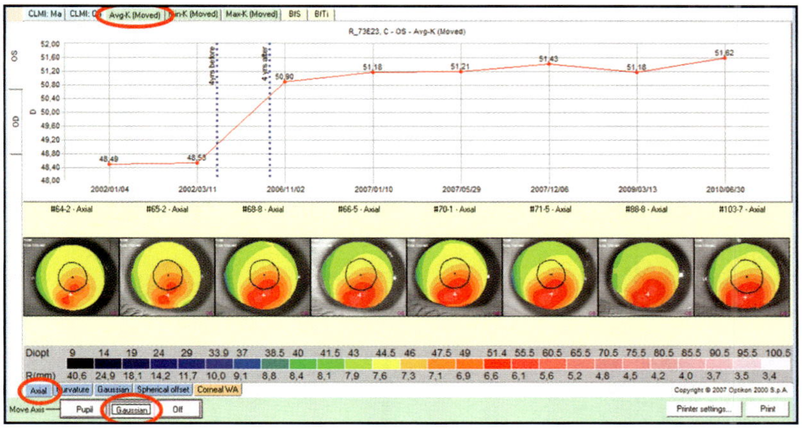

**Figure 5-67.** The same case as in Figure 5-66 is shown after (1) moving the axis of the axial maps to the "Gaussian apex," Cg, as calculated by CLMI, and (2) recalculating Sim K. The recalculated Sim K shows the likely progression during the 4-year gap between tests.

and 5-66. Most researchers who do not have a topographer with CLMI and the "move axis" feature determine whether the keratoconic ectasia is progressing by examining average Sim-K values, which are calculated on the corneal vertex of axial maps. This measurement can be reliable when the keratoconus apex is central. But in peripheral keratoconus, the disease progression can reduce the flat Sim-K reading rather than increasing the steep Sim-K reading, making Sim-K a very poor index as shown in Figure 5-66. Four years after the first 2 tests, even axial maps show an increase in the cone magnitude. Average Sim-K has increased by about 0.5 D, but in the subsequent maps, this value looks very fuzzy. If the axes of the same maps are moved to the Gaussian apex (see Figure 5-67), the etiology of average Sim-K is clearer and is consistent with CLMI Cc and Cg. After 4 years, the actual progression was almost 2.5 D, and in the following years, another 0.5 to 0.7 D. By referring to such a plot, the clinician can more objectively decide, and involve the patient in the decision, whether to do a CXL or perhaps wait for another 6 months of follow-up.

It has to be pointed out that plotting changes of only a few tenths of a D requires a well-calibrated Keratron and a good operator who makes use of the "repeatability check" (see Figure 5-56) to get precise measurements.

# Wavefront Analysis

Wavefront representations have been implemented in the Keratron Scout software since 2001.[93] These include measuring the Corneal Wavefront (CW)* from Keratron corneal topography, importing the OW from most commercial aberrometers through files containing Zernike terms and pupil data, and calculating the Internal Wavefront (IW) as the linear subtraction of Zernike terms (IW = OW – CW). Other wavefront representations include refraction maps from selected Zernike terms and simulating visual function (PSF, MTF) and performance (letter chart, visual acuity, night vision). A more detailed description of these functions,[94,95] as well as wavefront analysis[96] and Zernike polynomials can be found elsewhere,[97] and in the Scout "on-line-help." Here below, we summarize some basic topics of the new features that allow CTs to "talk the same language" as total wavefront analyzers.

*The terms *corneal* or *ocular wavefront* are used here as generic descriptions of either *wavefront error/wavefront aberration* or *optical path difference* (OPD). According to the OSA standard, both units can be used but the reader must be aware that they are opposite in sign. OPD maps appear similar in color convention to height maps, while wavefront error maps have opposite colors.

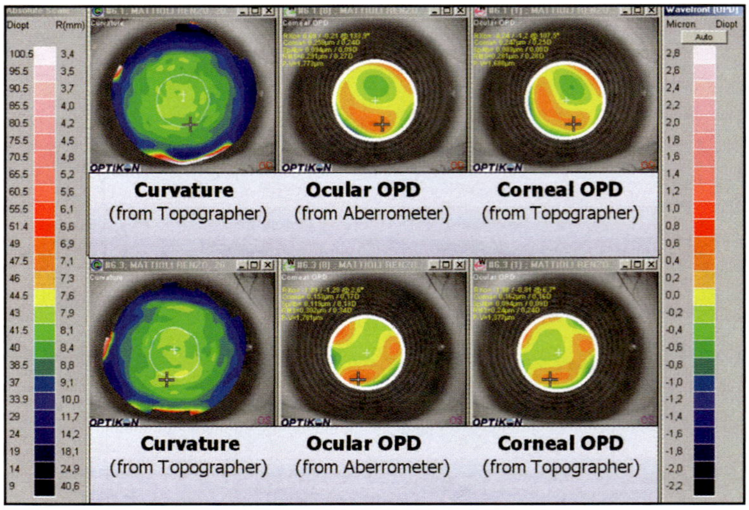


**Figure 5-68.** The right (top) and left eye (bottom) of one of the authors are shown as Keratron topography (left), ocular OPD (imported from a S/H aberrometer), and Keratron corneal OPD (right column).

## The Corneal Wavefront: A New Way to Represent Corneal Optics

The purpose of wavefront analysis (WA) is to measure wavefront aberrations, and the purpose of CT is to measure corneal shape. However, more than 70% of the eye's refraction is due to the corneal first surface. Corneal distortion always affects total OW aberration more significantly than any other interface. The CW, the component of the OW due to the cornea, can be calculated from CT height data and fit with a Zernike decomposition just as the OW can be measured by an aberrometer and fit with Zernikes. Placing the 2 Zernike representations side-by-side allows inspection of the OW and the contribution of the CW.

Figure 5-68 shows maps of the OW of one of the author's right and left eyes, measured with a Shack Hartmann aberrometer, and of the CW, derived from corneal topography. Only the high-order Zernike polynomials from 3rd to 5th radial order are shown. As usual, there is similarity between the OW and CW maps that shows how high-order aberrations of the cornea affect total ocular aberrations. However, when total ocular aberrations are very low, there is much less similarity between OW and CW representations of the same eye, and internal aberrations IW become the predominant component of the OW.

## From Corneal Geometry to Corneal Wavefront Maps

Since 1994, several authors have conducted studies of the CW from CT data, including Howland and colleagues[98]; Hemenger and colleagues[99]; and, in 1997, Schwiegerling and Greivenkamp.[100] A comprehensive collection of CW and IW studies under different patient conditions are among the work of Marcos and others[101,102] and Artal and colleagues.[103-106] Figure 5-69 illustrates a model of a simplified procedure based on the optical path difference (OPD; ie, the "least time" Fermat principle) in the "object space."[99,107] If a cornea had an ideal shape and minimal internal aberrations, then rays traced from the fovea would exit parallel from the cornea and form a flat wavefront (see Figure 5-69, green lines and yellow map on the top right) and the aberrations would be zero. If the cornea is distorted from this ideal shape (example Figure 5-69, orange lines), the rays in one section (the superior) enter the air first where they accelerate. Other rays (the inferior) remain in the cornea for a longer path and are retarded. In the time it takes for a ray to travel about 3 µm in the cornea, it would travel about 4 µm in the air (ie, rays travel [n-1] times faster in air than in cornea, where n is the assumed refractive index). For example, in Figure 5-69, a corneal distortion (b) of 3 µm will produce an OPD (a) 1 µm different from the ideal. As a result, we can adopt a simple "rule of 3" from corneal elevations:

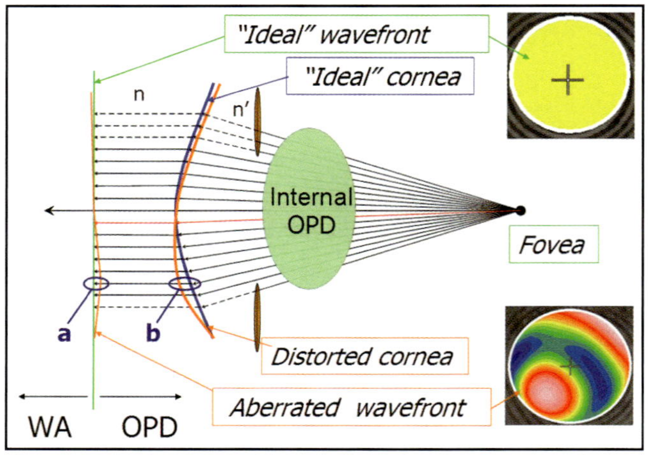


**Figure 5-69.** A cornea with an inferior keratoconus accelerates the rays in the superior and retards the rays in the inferior as compared with the ideal cornea. These physical distortions create a reversed aberrated wavefront whose height is scaled about 1:3 to the corneal distortion.

Every 3 µm of distortion from the ideal shape of the cornea will produce about a +1-µm difference in the OPD map and a -1-µm difference in the wavefront error map.

This simple rule can help estimate the thickness of a soft contact lens to add to the cornea or the amount of corneal tissue to remove from the cornea in order to produce a flat CW with no aberration, although some precautions should be followed for different refractive indices. The CW OPD maps (see Figure 5-68) closely resemble topographic height maps, but there are conceptual differences between the "spherical offset," which shows a cause, and OPD data, which show the effect. The "ideal cornea" is in fact an ellipsoid centered on the corneal vertex. Its definition depends on refractive indices and pupil position and requires matching the manifest patient refraction with the corneal curvature at a preset "refractive zone." In fact, the Zernike term, *defocus*, Z(2, 0), which depends on the axial length, is the only Zernike term that cannot be measured from the cornea alone and must be input from the manifest spherical equivalent refraction.

## Zernike Decomposition of Corneal Wavefront

In the wavefront module of the Scout software, the wavefront surface is calculated from corneal height, and Zernike polynomials up to the 7th order are least-squares best-fit.[108] For an accurate result, all corneal positions within the selected pupil, weighted for their subtended area, are involved in the fitting process. Piston and Tilt components (Zernike radial orders 0 and 1), although calculated, are not usually displayed.

## Zernike Selection and Graphical Representations of the Aberrations

The user can select the pupil size, from 3 to 9 mm, and any combination of Zernike terms to be represented by the wavefront map by clicking on specific buttons, arranged as suggested by the OSA standard pyramid.[109] For example, the user can select all orders from 2 to 7, the high orders only, the high orders and astigmatism, only radial orders from 3 to 5, or any combination of individual orders. When the selection is confirmed, the relevant weighted sum of Zernikes is calculated and reported in the map. The ray tracing, the PSF, MTF, or visual-simulation selected in the display panel at the top right in Figure 5-70 are updated to show the effect of using only the selected Zernike terms. Such a decomposition of the wavefront into selected Zernike "ingredients" can support the clinician's understanding of how individual or combined aberrations affect vision. In the "Zernike" display panel (Figure 5-71), a spectrum of the selected Zernike polynomials can be pictorially illustrated by selecting from the 5 different formats

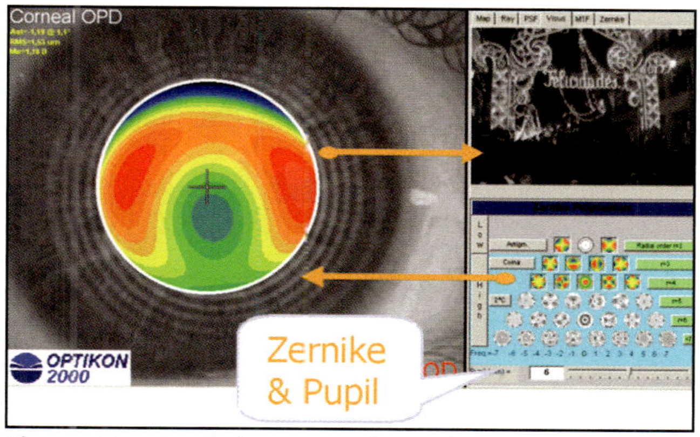


**Figure 5-70.** Pupil diameter and Zernike data selected in a Scout wavefront window will affect the corneal wavefront map, which further affects the simulation of the patient's vision.

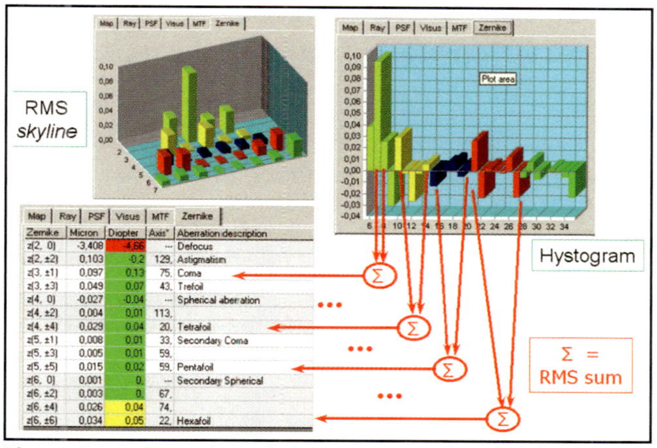


**Figure 5-71.** A number of alternative Zernike term formats are shown by the Keratron software.

("Histogram," "Color boxes," "RMS skyline," "Zernike list," or "Aberration summary").

A clinically relevant representation is the "Aberration summary." Here, the aberrations at the opposite sides of the OSA pyramid ("sine" + "cosine," or positive and negative F index) are presented not as individual Zernike terms, but as their RMS sum. This sum is expressed in µm as well as in "equivalent defocus" D and axis. For example, in the case in Figure 5-71, the amount of primary coma is 0.13 D at 75 degrees, or 0.097 µm RMS (or the combination of sine and cosine terms) at the selected pupil size. The equivalent defocus proposed by Dr. L. Thibos[110] expresses the wavefront variance in familiar dioptric terms. Reporting the Zernike terms in defocus equivalent D has the further advantage that D are fairly independent of pupil size, as shown in a study by Indiana University.[111] A green-yellow-red pattern in Figure 5-71 suggests a likely normality of individual aberrations.

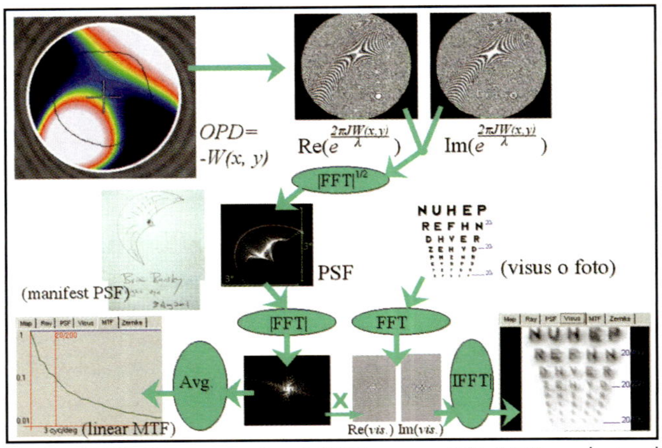


**Figure 5-72.** From wavefront OPD maps, PSF, MTF, and visual simulations are calculated using FFTs.

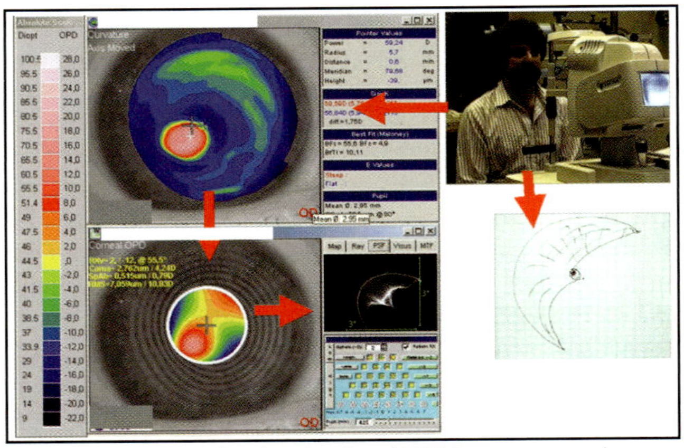

**Figure 5-73.** Example of a simulated PSF from a corneal wavefront map (OPD) compared with a drawing of the equivalent manifest PSF by the subject in scotopic conditions. (Reprinted with permission of Renzo Mattioli, PhD.)

### From the Wavefront to Point Spread Function, Modulation Transfer Function, and Visual Simulations

The calculation of the PSF, the MTF, the visual simulation of 2 different letter charts (from 20/500 to 20/100 and from 20/100 to 20/20), and pictures of night vision are not done by simple ray-tracing, but by complex mathematics using Fourier optics on the pupil size area and the Fast Fourier Transform (FFT), as summarized in Figure 5-72. Only this process produces faithful simulations[112] by including the effect of both the wave propagation and the diffraction created by the pupil edge. Simplified patterns or retinal spot-diagrams should not be confused with the real PSF.

### The Clinical Utility of Corneal Wavefront Measurement

CW measurement is not intended to replace WA. This new representation has special clinical utility because it evaluates corneal optics using the same "language" as wavefront analyzers and can be decomposed by Zernike fitting into representations analogous to WA, including simulated visual acuity, PSF, MTF, and other quantities that assess quality of vision. In this respect, the CW is a more sensible representation of corneal optics than either axial or refractive maps. Unlike WA, CT data allow investigators to assess the CW under varying conditions such as pupil size and position.

CW analysis can help clinicians understand patient comfort or discomfort despite apparently bad or good corneal conditions, may aid in the design of surgical interventions, and may predict the efficiency of strategies that concentrate on removing only extremely disturbing aberrations. Visual simulations of the CW are not to be regarded as a curiosity but as new, very powerful tools for clinicians. In addition to internal aberrations, light scattering, media opacity, and retinal problems may cause these simulations to differ from reality. However, in an example (Figure 5-73), we can appreciate how well the corneal PSF matches the patient's drawing of a small spot of light. Both the CW and the drawing were made under the same lighting, and therefore pupil, conditions. This example shows that the CW simulations, which directly derive from the corneal PSF, can be especially realistic in the presence of high corneal aberrations, which are difficult to measure directly with an aberrometer.

## Links With Excimer Lasers

Keratron height data can be output to files for any "third-party" software application. Specific links have been developed in agreement with Schwind Eye-Tech Solutions (Kleinostheim, Germany) and Nidek (Gamagori, Japan). These include a "topo-link" with Schwind, the Optimized Refractive Keratectomy—topography (ORK-t) software (now obsolete) and a versatile link with Nidek "FinalFit." Optikon pioneered with Schwind the adaptation of CW features to link a Keratron with an excimer laser system. The Scout software's CW was linked to the Optimized Refractive Keratectomy—wavefront (ORKw), software that had been previously developed by Schwind for OW links with ESIRIS and AMARIS. The first case of a photoablative treatment using a corneal wavefront link was made by Dr. M. Camellin on February 2002.[78] Other medical researchers extended this experience in the next few years, including Bonci,[113] Barraquer (Bogotà, Colombia), Arbelaez,[114] Rummelt,[115] Siganos,[116] and others. (For more complete and updated documentation, contact Schwind's APM department and the Web site at www.eye-tech-solutions.com.)

In principle, the following are advantages of a CW link with respect to topography, OW, or both:

- Optimization of the ablation pattern volume

- Simpler comparison of results with the target
- Overcoming some limits of Munnerlyn formulas[117,118]
- The possibility of aberration management
- The possibility of interaction with aberrometers

A more detailed description of these arguments can be found in quoted papers and in a book on LASEK and ASA edited by Camellin.[119]

## Fitting Contact Lenses With the Keratron's Software

The Keratron's accuracy in tracking both small local and peripheral corneal distortion produces sensitive height-difference fluorescein pattern algorithms to guide a user through easy design and simulation of contact lenses fitting. The user interface is ergonomic for easy familiarization, even for old-fashioned practitioners. Classic methods allow users to select or fit lenses according to central K-readings and corneal diameter. However, the Scout software's Contact Lens Editor (CLE) introduces a number of radically new height-fitting methods and protocols.

The CLE is a software module that is accessed by clicking any map or processed image from the database. Although maps usually cover 80% to 90% of the cornea, a preliminary extrapolation, placing 3 points around the limbal edge, is required to fill the gaps and to measure corneal diameter at the same time.

Some specially automated "lens-family protocols" are provided to guide the user through a large number of virtual trial-sets including the first, made for Horus (Verona, Italy) contact lenses[120] and similar sets including TS (Milano, Italy) and Soleko (Pontecorvo, Italy).

### The Scout Contact Lens Editor

The Keratron's CLE windows and menu offer several choices:

- Select a virtual trial set from among a wide number of CL manufacturers (registered users, see Scout CD-ROM or Optikon Web site) to simulate the fitting of a lens.
- Fit a custom multi-curve contact lens according to classical criteria "Contour" and "OC+2."
- Or, fit a custom lens using a "height-fitting" method that includes multi-curve (up to 5 zones), multi-conic (Figure 5-74), toric (up to 4 zones), or Ortho-K lenses (5 zones, inverse geometry, Figure 5-75).

A number of tools allow the user to evaluate and optimize fitting and design:

- A clearance panel (eg, bottom right in Figure 5-74B and C) plots the cross-sectional vertical distance between the lens and the cornea in µm. Clicking on the map is sufficient to select the meridian and see how the relevant clearance section changes.

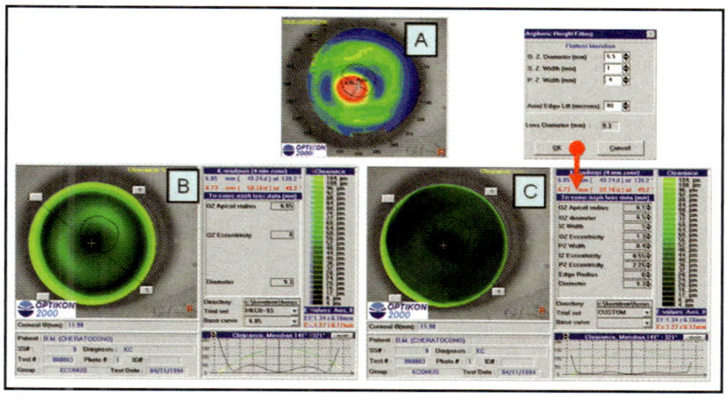

**Figure 5-74.** The Scout software module CLE is used to fit to a keratoconic cornea using a "virtual trial set" and a custom designed triconic lens.

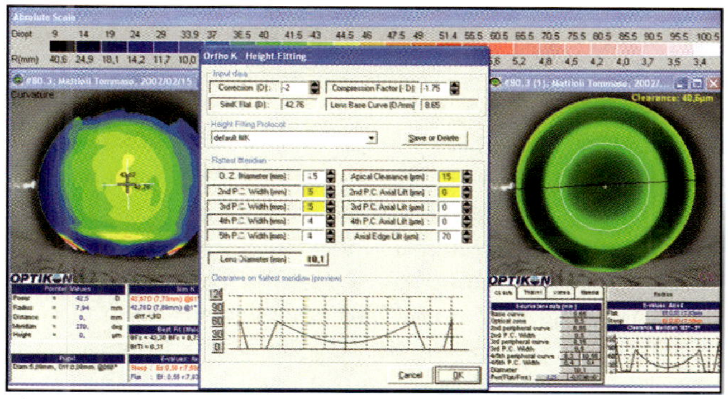

**Figure 5-75.** In this example of the CLE's use to fit a young patient with an ortho-K contact lens, the protocol projects a 10.1-mm lens to get 15 µm of clearance at the apex and a parallel fit in the midperiphery, with a "compression factor" of -1.75 D.

- Moving the lens by drag-and-drop to any point on the cornea simulates real lens movement on the eye and is used to find the point of maximum symmetry, a recommended first step.
- Tilting the lens along the flattest and steepest meridians, using 4 buttons on the map, simulates the effect of blinking, and gravity.
- Indenting the lens (ie, pushing in or pulling out) simulates the effect of indentation and compares this with the pattern of a tight lens.
- Programming the "lens selection protocol" (ie, the way the lens is first chosen within any trial-set). The protocol can be either classical curvature (ie, according to K-readings and toricity) or the default "height-fitting" protocol, which leaves an "apical clearance" of 10 µm.
- Evaluating the residual cylinder of a front spherical lens or designing the ideal front toric with a lens power input and calculator panel.

Figure 5-74 shows contact lens fitting to a keratoconic cornea (A) using the Scout CLE and 2 methods: B) a lens selected from a "virtual trial set" and C) a custom-designed triconic lens created automatically with the "height-fitting" (aspheric) feature. The "clearance panel" shows how well the contact lens conforms to the flat corneal meridian when the lens is properly placed on the cone's apex. Figure 5-75 shows an example of Ortho-K contact lens fitting. The user can create or select from among the available "height-fitting" protocols to modify the data. The protocol in this example projects a 10.1-mm lens to get 15 μm of clearance at the apex and a parallel fit in the midperiphery, with a "compression factor" of -1.75 D. The operator must then input only the desired correction in the panel (A), and the software will automatically calculate the parameters of a 5-curve CL reported in panel (C). Note the similarity between the desired (B) and achieved clearance plots (D), despite natural corneal asymmetries. It is unique to the Scout that all geometric components of the lens are not empirically extrapolated from Sim-K, Ro, and e values, but are calculated on actual corneal heights, measured by Keratron's along the flat meridian. This optimizes the design, even with complex and asymmetric corneas.

Lens designs can be saved and attached to the relevant corneal topography, up to 8 different designs per image.

The CLE fluorescein simulations have advantages over real fluorescein testing at the slit-lamp because the topographers' "virtual reality" fitting is static and does not stress the cornea. A physical test can hide how much the cornea is fitting itself to the lens as the lens shapes, possibly creating patient discomfort and warpages like those shown in Figure 5-50.

As a general result, many optometrists using a Keratron have improved their RGP first lens success fitting rate from the traditional 30% to 40% and up to 75% and above.[121]

## Calco Lenses and Other Third-Party Links

Not including Berkeley UC's OPTICAL research project,[122] Eikon's (Firenze, Italy) Calco was the first commercial third-party software provider to manufacture fully custom contact lenses based on Keratron data beginning in 1996.[123-125] In Latin, "Calco" means "cast." The basic idea of Calco Lens Designs is a strict integration between corneal topography and contact lens manufacture. The earliest contact lens manufacturing lathes were designed to cut sphere-based geometries. New-generation lathes (eg, the Rank-Pneumo Optoform, by Taylor Hobson, Leicester, UK, and later Precitech Keene, NH) overcame these limitations by designing complex aspherical profiles made of a large number of small steps with a resolution down to 10 nm. Such geometries can significantly improve comfort and global performance of an RGP lens. A natural evolution was to manufacture an optimized contact lens based on accurate elevation data from the Scout. This gives the fitter the capability of designing an aspheric lens according to fitting parameters rather than complex geometric ones. In fact, the first step in lens design is to define the desired tear layer shape (Figure 5-76). The "tear layer" screen contains data on how a lens fits a corneal semi-meridian. The lens design is controlled by the clearance between cornea and lens. Diameters and lifts are chosen in order to optimize the lens with respect to power, thickness, optical zone, correction of lens SAs, and multifocal optic options. This approach allows full control of the design because the parameter of clearance between the cornea and lens is much closer to fitting philosophy than the parameter of eccentricity. Moreover, working with clearance frees the fitter from the overhead of managing complex geometrical parameters. The use of Calco Lens Design has dramatically improved first fit success rate and patient comfort in a number of complex situations.

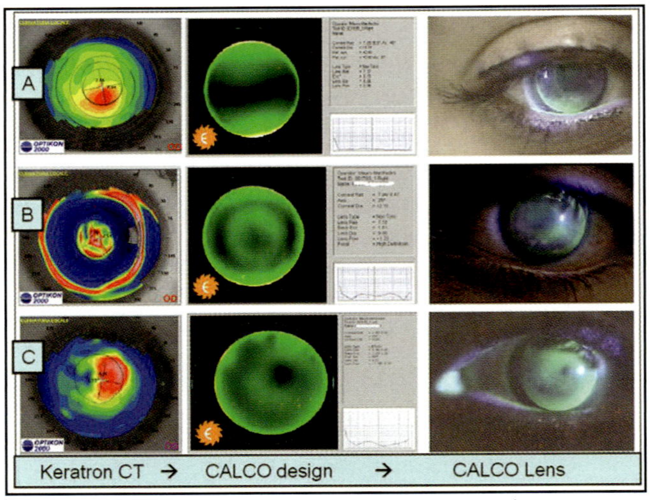


**Figure 5-76.** CALCO windows include the tear-layer screen, which contains data on how a lens fits a corneal semi-meridian according to the parameter of clearance between the cornea and lens.

Figure 5-77 illustrates some examples:

- Early stage keratoconus: The design is chosen as a conform fit, moderately flat. The slit-lamp image confirms comfortable wear.
- Post-hyperopic PRK treatment: The design leaves a small central clearance; The slit-lamp image shows lens stability and good physiological response.
- A rare superior keratoconus: An axial symmetry design, confirmed by the patient and the slit-lamp image as having good positioning, high visual acuity, and comfort.

Following Eikon's Calco, other fully custom methods designed to link the Scout with third-party software have been developed by companies all over the world. Dr. Edward's WAVE[126,127] (Figure 5-78) is very popular, especially in the United States, as well as Europe's ProCornea's EyeLite and Ing. Liffredo's Focal Points.[128] These programs import complete data from the Keratron's Scout software to specialized labs (eg, Eikon, VerkerOptik [now

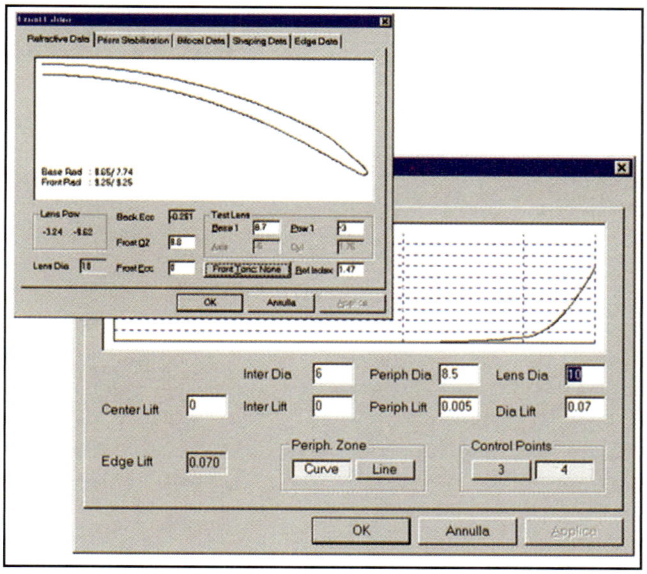

**Figure 5-77.** Examples of CALCO lens designs including early stage keratoconus, post-hyperopic PRK treatment, and a rare superior keratoconus.

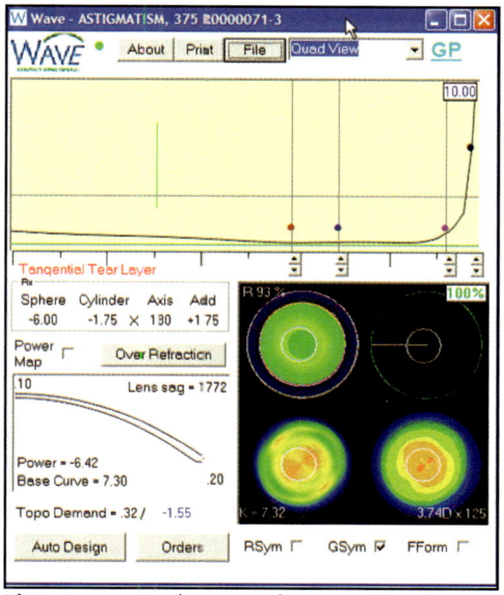

**Figure 5-78.** The popular WAVE program (www.wavecontactlenses.com) is shown in a screen shot. (Reprinted with permission from Renzo Mattioli, PhD.)

Optiek Verkerk, Amersfoort, The Netherlands], ProCornea [Eerbeek, The Netherlands], Essilor [Wiener Neudorf, Austria], No7 [East Sussex, UK], Eyequip [Jacksonville, FL], etc) to manufacture fully custom lenses.

## Conclusion

Thousands of users and researchers from around the world have been using the Keratron CTs since 1993 in their clinical practice and studies. Since then, the Optikon Keratron team has improved the software and hardware of this family of CTs. All Keratron owners are invited to register at www.optikon.com in order to download software updates and be notified by e-mail. We hope that all current and future Keratron users will continue to appreciate our commitment to maintain our state-of-the-art topographic systems. I invite them to continue to report to us their feedback and suggestions.

# AstraMax Comprehensive Diagnostic Workstation With Polar Grid Topography

David D. Liu, PhD; Jia Qu, MD; Shihao Chen, MD, OD;
Tracy Schroeder Swartz, OD, MS, FAAO; and Ming Wang, MD, PhD

Innovation and technology advancement has afforded ophthalmologists and optometrists with diagnostic equipment of unprecedented sophistication. As such, clinicians expect more measurements and diagnostic capabilities from modern-day topographers. LaserSight's AstraMax (Winter Park, FL) multi-camera topographer is designed for this purpose with hardware and software integration that gives the system a variety of corneal and pupil diagnostic functions.[129] One of AstraMax's most critical measurements for custom ablation is the anterior and posterior corneal elevation with a range from 0.00 to 2.60 mm and accuracy to ±1 μm. AstraMax acquires images in less than 0.2 seconds, eliminating the need for software or straps to compensate for eye movements. AstraMax also generates anterior and posterior axial, instantaneous curvature maps and different comparative options of the displays, processing data within 10 to 15 seconds. Information can also be displayed as point spread and modulation transfer functions (PSF and MTF), Zernike coefficients, plus a variety of physician-adjusted preferences to customize the software.

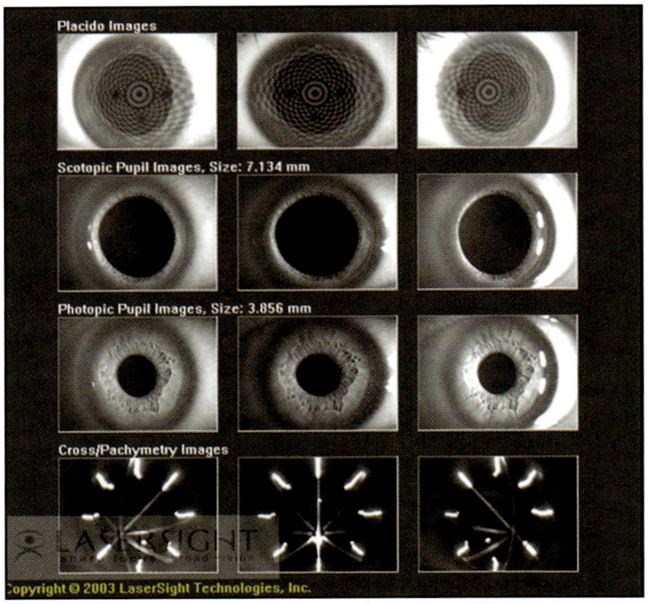


**Figure 5-79.** A quick sequence of exposure to targets using controlled illumination is captured within 0.2 seconds.

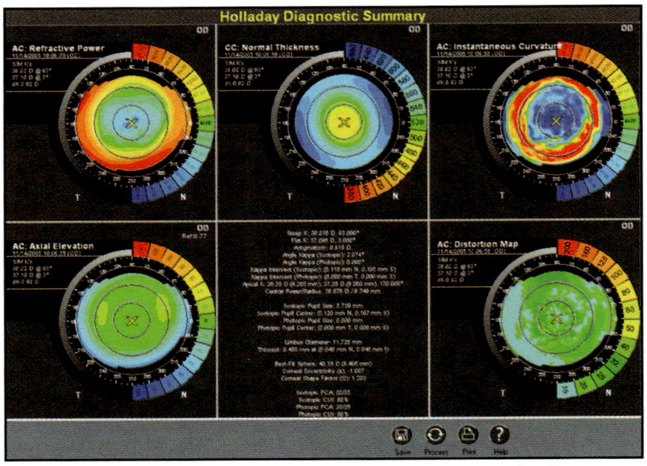


**Figure 5-80.** The Holladay Diagnostic Summary displays critical clinical information.

# Multiple Parameter Measurements in a Single Acquisition

AstraMax uses synchronized, multi-camera imaging systems to capture multiple images for various measurement purposes without the mechanical scanning of the acquisition head. This eliminates the source of error associated with the movement and the extended discomfort associated with scanning technologies. Anterior topography, whole corneal pachymetry, and posterior topography can be acquired in a single measurement. Dynamic pupil size and location relative to the visual axis center under various illumination conditions, cornea limbus diameter, and geometric center can be acquired as well. All of these parameters are particularly critical for a custom ablation algorithm when using laser refractive surgery.

As shown in Figure 5-79, a quick sequence of exposure to targets using controlled illumination is captured within 0.2 seconds. This simultaneous acquisition eliminates the error caused by mechanical movement of scanning measurement techniques.

## Comprehensive Diagnostics Displayed in a Single Screen

AstraMax offers standard data displays, including anterior and posterior elevation and curvature, pupil and limbus measurement, pachymetry, and optical analysis. Elevation, axial curvature, instantaneous curvature, and refractive power maps are available for both anterior and posterior corneas. Single map, dual maps, difference maps, and quad maps are also available for one or more corneal exams displays. Both 2- and 3-dimensional color maps and 3-dimensional contour displays are available. The Holladay Diagnostic Summary displays critical clinical information (Figure 5-80).

## Corneal Optical Analysis Tools

AstraMax offers advanced optical analysis capabilities using Zernike analysis, ray-tracing modeling, and image simulation. It incorporates corneal wavefront analysis, corneal MTF, and corneal PSF. All optical analysis functions are displayed 3-dimensionally. These analysis tools can help the clinicians understand the optical property of the cornea and communicate the diagnosis to the patient. For example, the corneal PSF illustrates the superior resolving capability of a prolate-shaped cornea compared to the oblate shape (Figure 5-81).

AstraMax also provides corneal Zernike analysis capabilities to analyze the corneal aberration. Figure 5-82 analyzes SA with respect to the asphericity (Q value) of the corneal models, including spherical, prolate and oblate ellipsoid, toroid, and astigmatic oblate and prolate models.

## Polar Grid and Concentric Ring Patterns

The pattern used in AstraMax is a combined concentric ring and polar grid pattern[130] as illustrated in Figure 5-83. Standard corneal topography uses a set of concentric rings as a reflective target to measure the axial aberration of the corneal surface. The radius of each ring at each angular direction (the radial direction) represents the surface aberration of the point along the radial direction only. Along each ring, there is no information along the circumferential direction. With a polar grid pattern as represented in Figure 5-83, information along radial and circumferential

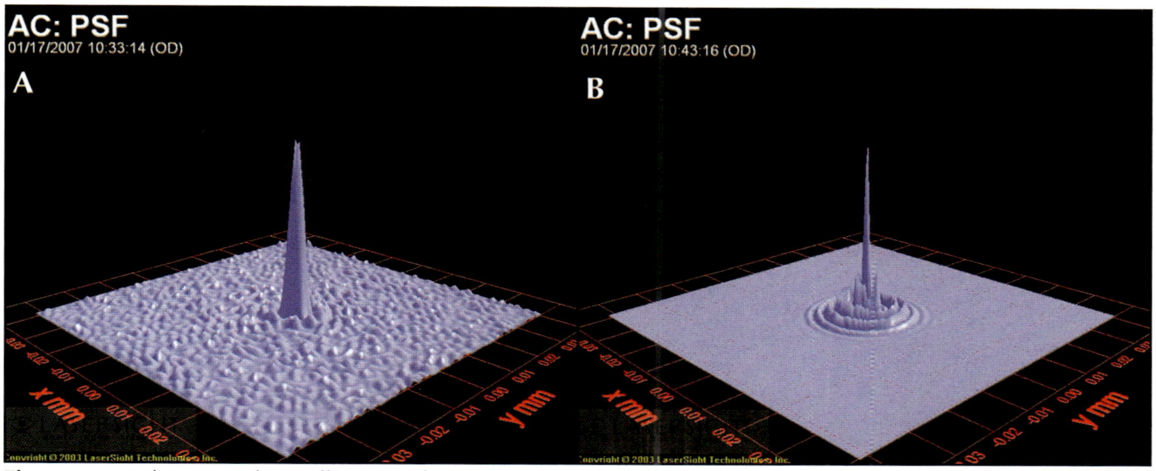


**Figure 5-81.** The corneal PSF illustrates the superior resolving capability of a prolate-shaped cornea.

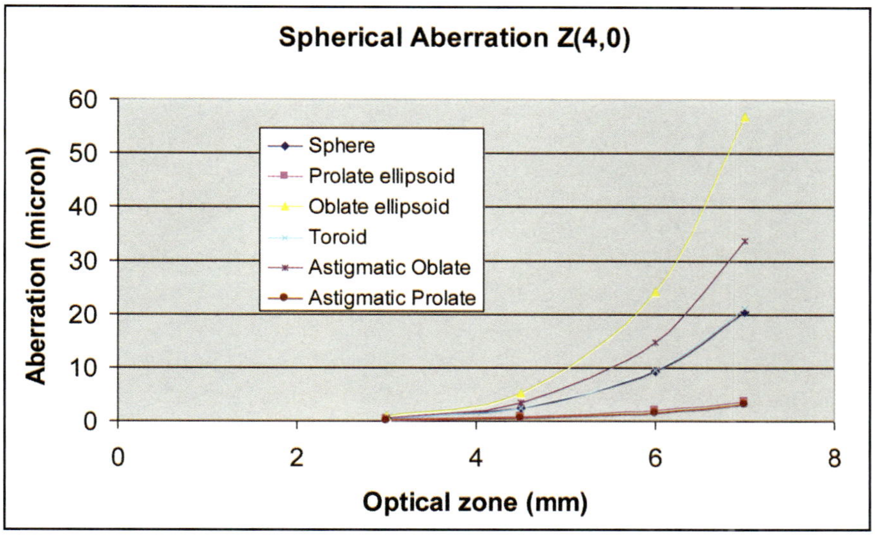


**Figure 5-82.** The corneal PSF illustrates the reduced resolving capability associated with oblate shape.

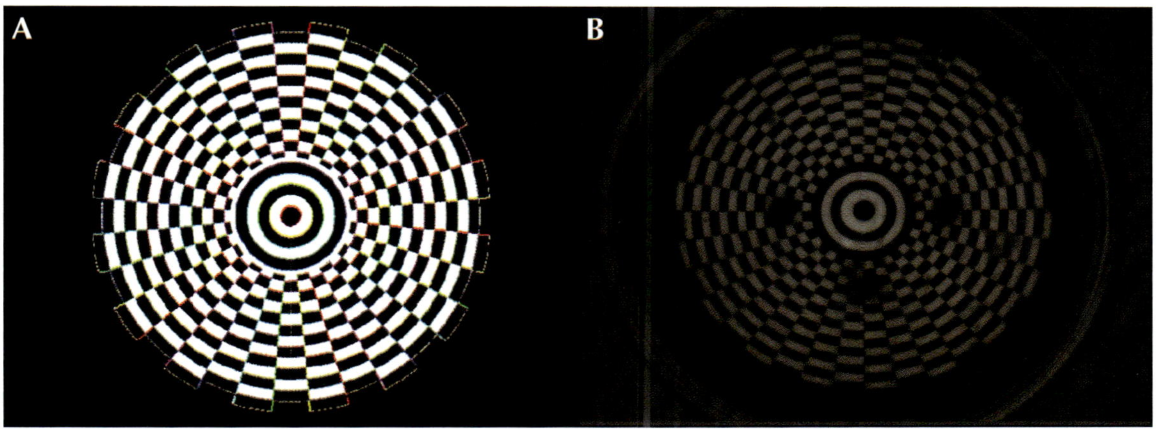


**Figure 5-83.** SA analysis with respect to the asphericity (Q value) of the corneal models, including spherical, prolate and oblate ellipsoid, toroid, and astigmatic oblate and prolate models.

directions are captured and processed. For concentric rings and axial symmetrical objects, measurement and analysis are performed only along radial directions. For asymmetrical objects, critical information is missing along the circumferential direction with concentric ring-only Placido.

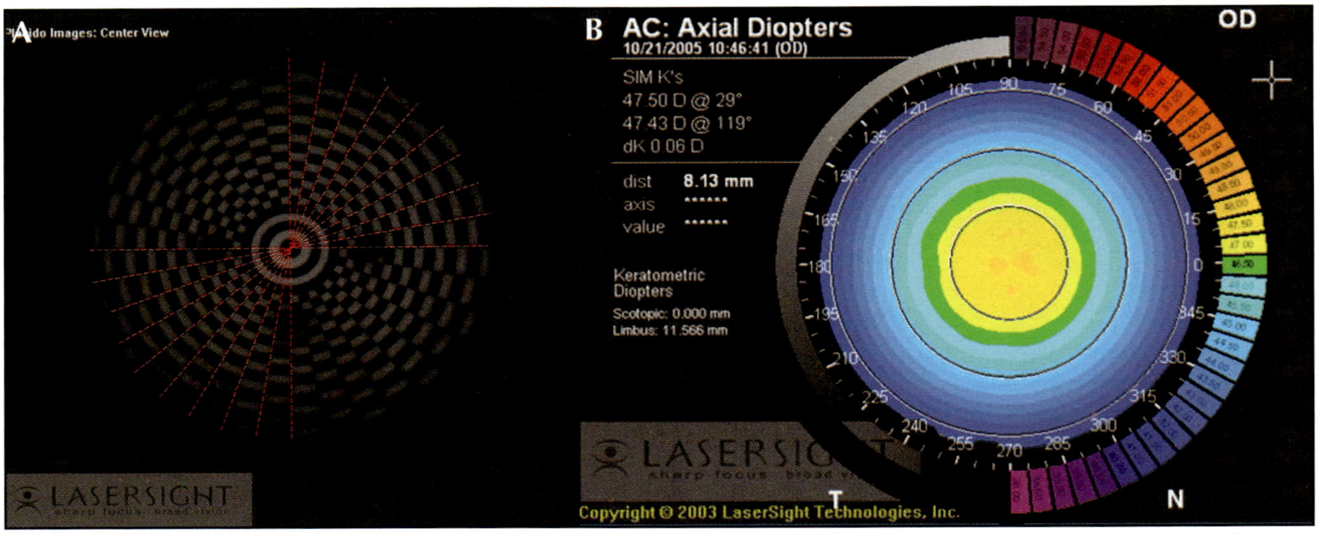


**Figure 5-84.** (A) The pattern used in AstraMax is a combined concentric ring and polar grid pattern. (B) The target used to create reflections on the cornea.

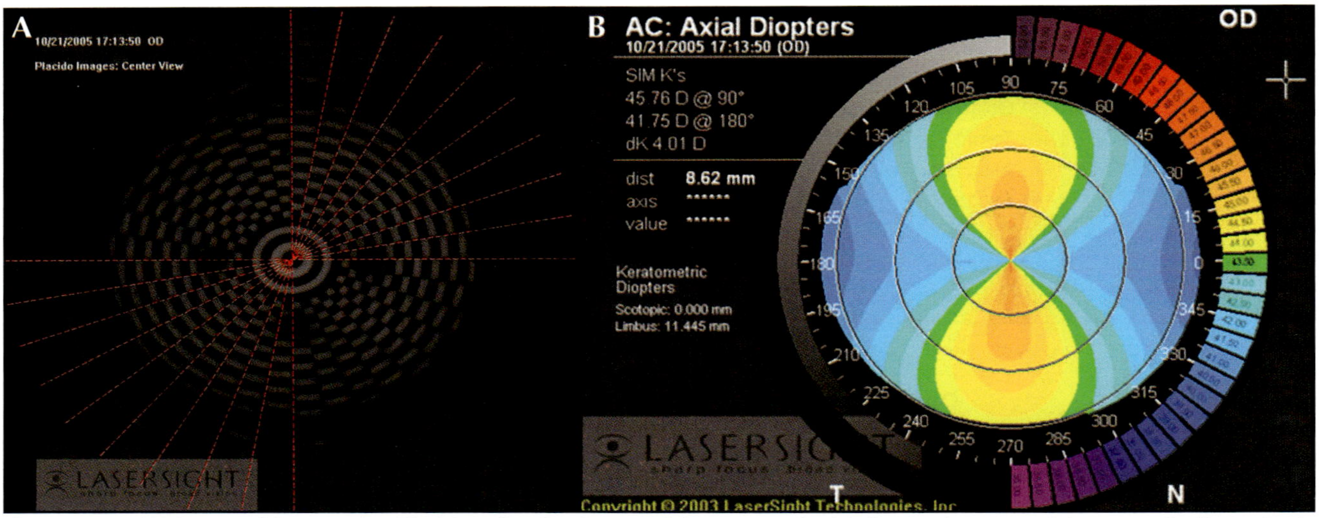


**Figure 5-85.** (A) Image of the anterior Placido reflection image of the patented grids for a sphere or axial symmetrically aspheric surface. Reflected image of a cornea with 4 D of corneal astigmatism. (B) Axial image of a cornea with 4 D of corneal astigmatism.

## Orthogonal Polar Grid and Axial Asymmetrical Objects

For axial asymmetrical objects, AstraMax performs analysis using concentric rings as well as spokes. For radial direction, concentric rings are used. For circumferential direction, a new measurement parameter, the twist angle map, is obtained to further illustrate the complex nature of optically axial asymmetrical objects. Measurement and analysis are performed along both axial and circumferential directions. Image is stretched differently in all directions, and image is twisted according to the twist angle. AstraMax captures the reflective twist, and, likewise, refractive twist measurement can be obtained using optical ray tracing of the anterior twist measurements.

A sphere is an axial symmetrical surface where concentric rings alone are adequate to measure the anterior surface. An astigmatic surface, however, best illustrates the effectiveness of the polar grid to address torsional twist. Figure 5-84 is the image of the anterior Placido reflection image of the patented grids for a sphere or an axial symmetrical aspheric surface. The spokes are roughly 10 degrees apart. Figures 5-85 and 5-86 are the reflected images of 4 D astigmatic and 8 D astigmatic surfaces of the polar grid patterns. The 10-degree spokes are "twisted" toward the flat axis (horizontal axis). The amount of twist varies according to the magnitude of the astigmatism and the angular region of the surface. Figure 5-87 is a summary of the twist angle for various astigmatic surfaces with respect to a no-twist spherical or axial symmetrical aspheric surface. It can be

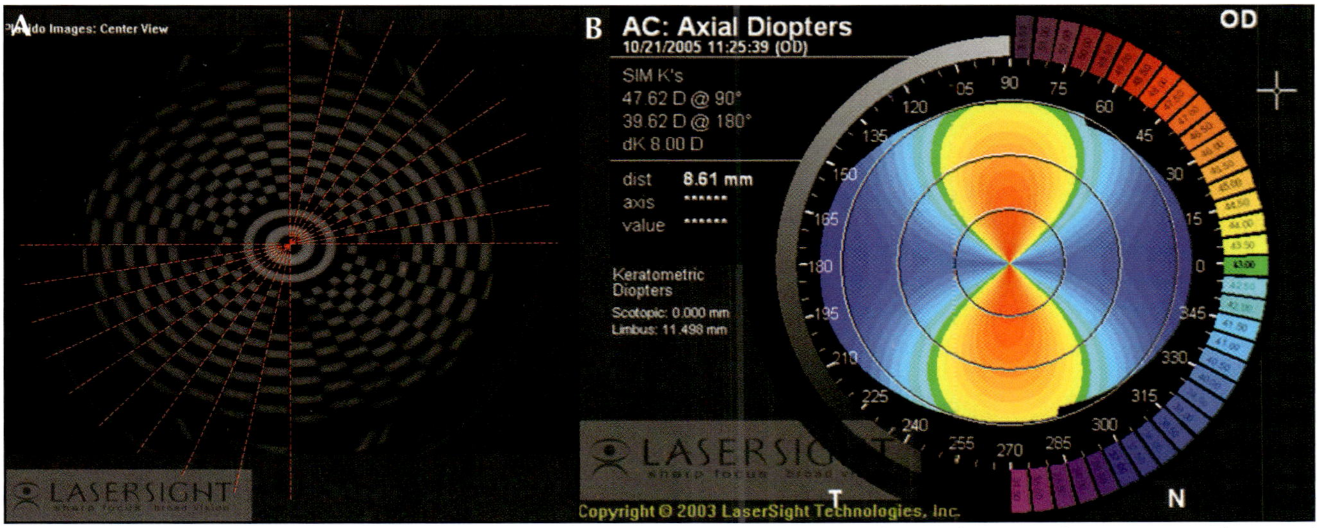


**Figure 5-86.** (A) Reflected image of a cornea with 8 D of corneal astigmatism. Note the 10-degree spokes are "twisted" toward the flat axis (horizontal axis). The amount of twist varies according to the magnitude of the astigmatism and the angular region of the surface. (B) Axial image of a cornea with 8 D of corneal astigmatism.

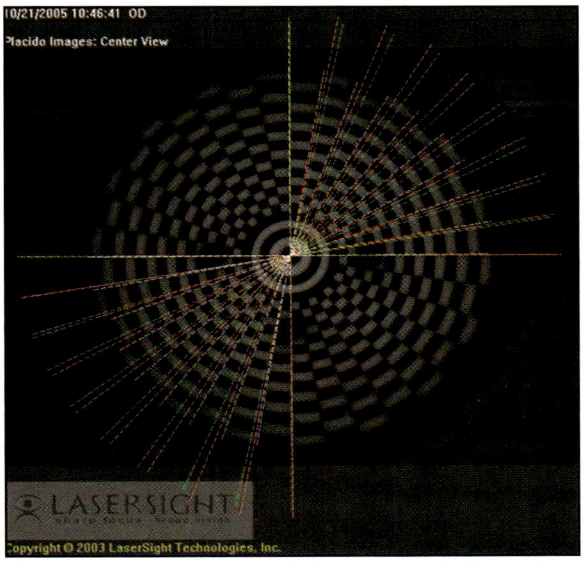


**Figure 5-87.** A summary of the twist angle for various astigmatic surfaces with respect to a no-twist spherical or axial symmetrical aspheric surface.

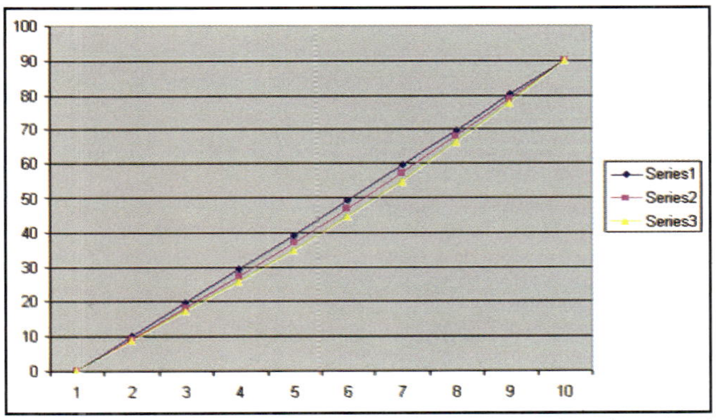


**Figure 5-88.** Image twist occurs where the twist bends toward the flat axis. The minimum twist occurs at the steep and flat axis, while the maximum twist occurs in the middle of the steep and flat axis.

observed that the twist has several characteristics with regard to the optical property of the cornea:

- The object no longer reflects rays in the same plane as the incident rays. Instead, it may reflect rays in a different plane, causing the object image to twist.
- By applying Snell's law, this twist ray characteristic will also be in the refractive domain, causing the image formed to be twisted.
- The twist also causes objects to reflect in a way that may enhance (compress) or weaken (stretch) the images of different parts of the object, causing additional image-forming complexity to the imaging optical system (in this case, the astigmatic reflective or refractive surfaces).

## Accumulated Twist Angle and Twist Change Rate

Image twist occurs according to Figure 5-88, where the twist is bending toward the flat axis. The minimum twist occurs at the steep and flat axis, while the maximum twist occurs in the middle of them. In this figure, between 0 and 10 degrees, the image is compressed along the circumferential direction. Likewise, between 80 and 90 degrees, the image is stretched. In the middle between 40 and 50 degrees, there was very little compression, or stretching, even though the maximum accumulated twist occurs in this middle region.

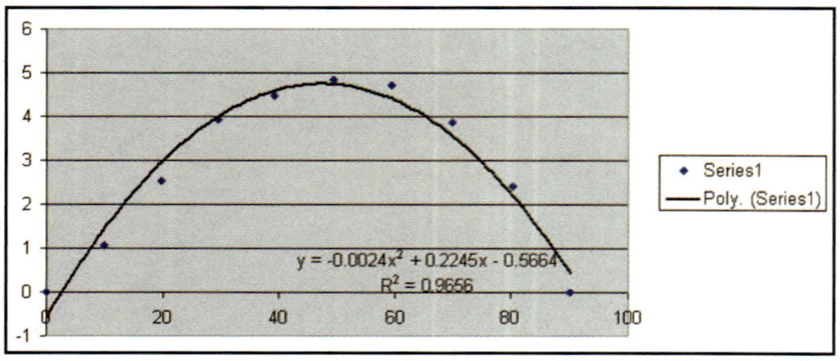


**Figure 5-89.** The accumulated twist angle within 0- and 90-degree region where the horizontal axis is angular direction theta and the vertical axis is the accumulated twist angle. For this 8 D astigmatic surface, the maximum twist angle is 4.8 degrees at 45-degree location. Note that the accumulated twist angle fits a second-order polynomial quite well, and its coefficients are proportional to the magnitude of the astigmatism as can be seen from this figure, in this case, a factor of 2.

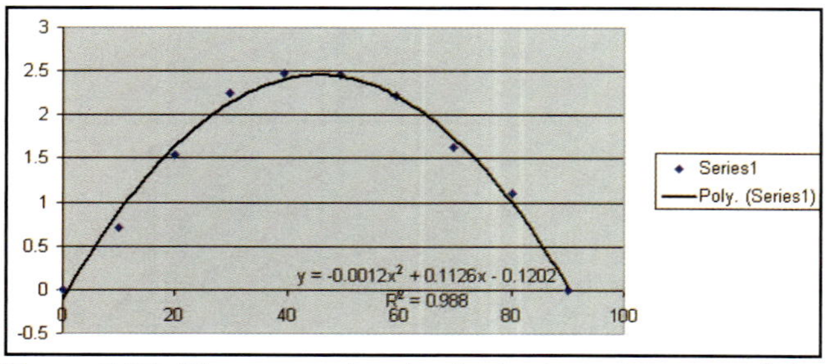


**Figure 5-90.** The accumulated twist is clockwise, toward the flat axis. There were no twists at 0 and 90 degrees. For this 4 D astigmatic surface, the maximum twist angle is 2.4 degrees at 45-degree location.

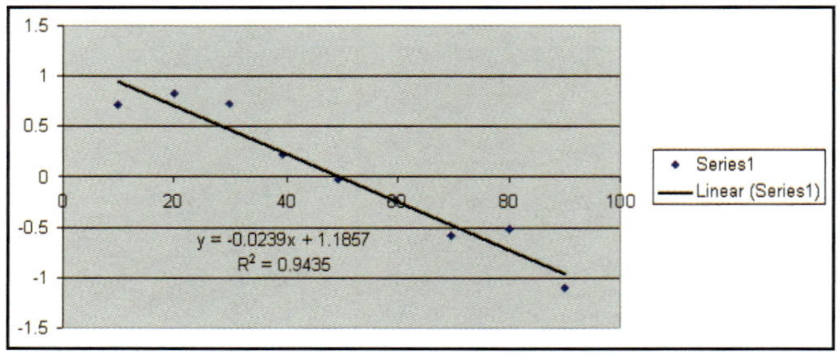


**Figure 5-91.** By taking the derivative of the accumulated twist angle, we can get the twist rate of change of this 4-D astigmatic surface, where the range of the twist rate is between approximately 1 to -1 degree for the angular range of 0 and 90 degrees.

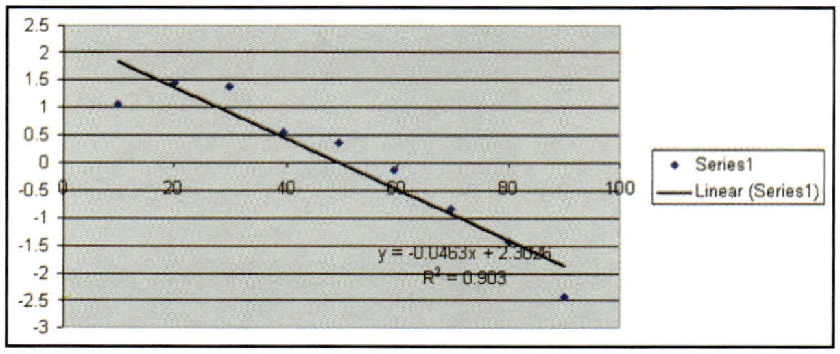


**Figure 5-92.** By taking the derivative of the accumulated twist angle, we can get the twist rate of change of this 8-D astigmatic surface, where the range of the twist rate is between approximately 2 to -2 degrees for the angular range of 0 and 90 degrees. Note that a linear relationship fits the data quite well, and slope and offset are proportional to the magnitude of the astigmatism, in this case a factor of 2 compared to Figure 5-92.

The accumulated twist angle within the 0- and 90-degree region is documented in Figures 5-89 and 5-90, where the horizontal axis is angular direction theta and the vertical axis is the accumulated twist angle. The accumulated twist is clockwise, toward the flat axis. There was no twist at 0 and 90 degrees. The maximum twist happens at about 45 degrees. Please note that the accumulated (whole body) twist is bending toward the flat axis (0 degrees), and the maximum bending occurs at about 45 degrees and slowly returns to zero twist at 90 degrees. Therefore, the rate of twist (twist angle per angular section) has to change sign where the maximum twist occurs (see Figures 5-89 and 5-90). By taking the derivative of the accumulated twist angle, we can get the twist rate of change as shown in Figures 5-91 and 5-92.

## Dynamic Pupil Measurement and Iris Recognition

AstraMax uses programmable infrared illumination to allow the image capture and measurement of the pupil parameter of diameter and location. The unique design of the illumination angle allows for detailed capture of the pupil and iris and iris recognition. This important information, when combined with the simultaneously acquired topography data, is crucial to the alignment and registration of the eye during laser refractive surgery.[131-133]

AstraMax is capable of using controlled illumination light sources and capturing the pupil size and location with respect to the visual axis under various conditions. Figure 5-93 is the captured scotopic pupil data. In Figure 5-94, the same eye captured the pupil data under photopic conditions. Both the pupil size and location are dynamic, changing with time and illumination condition. Proper assessment is important to determine the nominal pupil offset under the proper conditions when data are to be used in laser refractive surgery.

Due to AstraMax's unique design of illumination and imaging optics, iris patterns are distinctively revealed, recorded, and analyzed under programmable illumination intensity as shown in Figure 5-95. Iris registration and alignment capabilities are important, particularly when treating patients with significant astigmatism.[133,134]

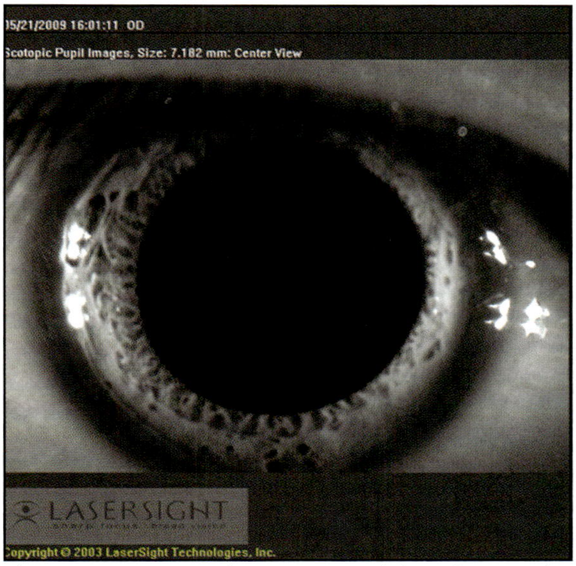


**Figure 5-93.** Captured scotopic pupil data showing the pupil size (7.18 mm).

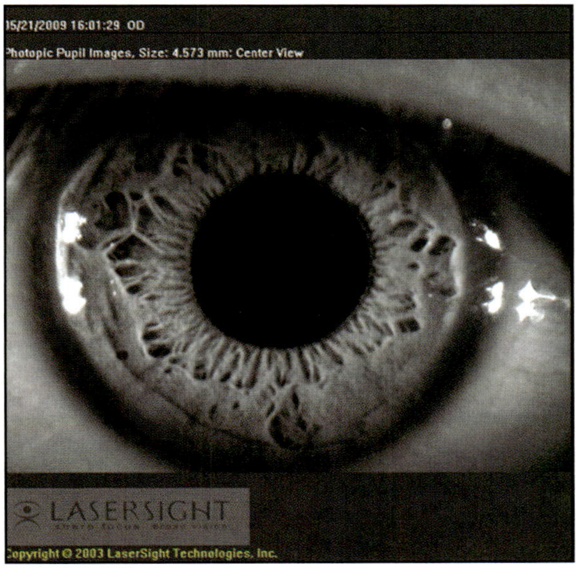


**Figure 5-94.** The same eye as in Figure 5-93 is captured under photopic condition, showing pupil size of 4.57 mm.

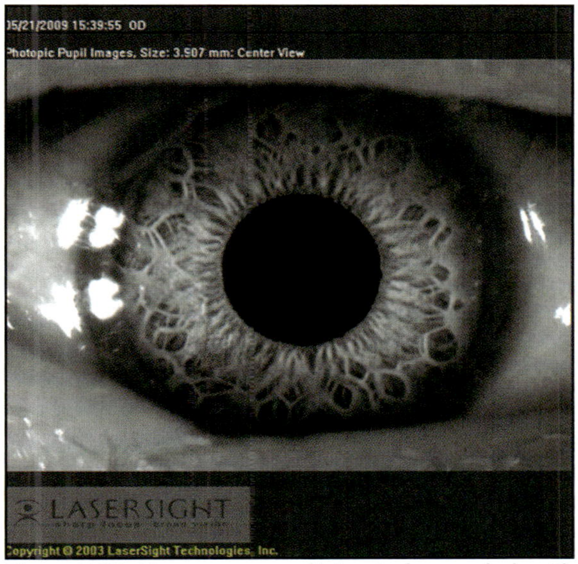


**Figure 5-95.** Iris patterns are distinctively revealed, with pupil diameter, which is used to align the patient eye during surgery.

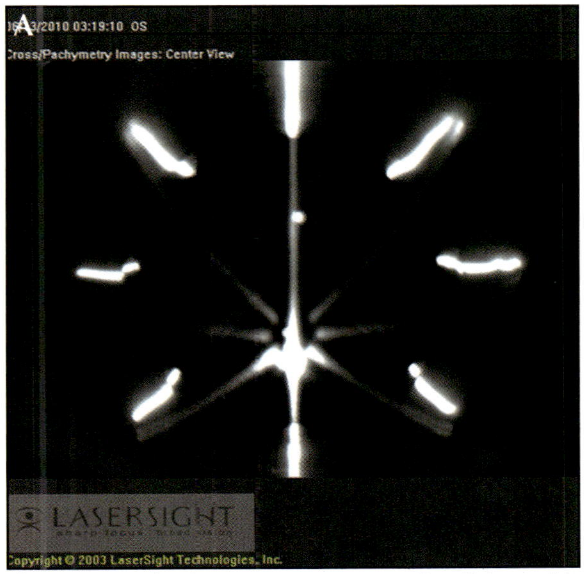


**Figure 5-96.** The 3-camera system uses 8 radial acquisition meridians to optically measure the corneal thickness along normal direction. (A) This is the view from the middle camera. *(continued)*

## Whole Eye Instantaneous and Simultaneous Optical Pachymetry

AstraMax uses 3 gen-locked cameras arranged at the proper angle to capture an optically bent focal plane that matches the contour of the cornea through an optical projector of a starburst pattern onto the cornea. Three stereo cameras capture the starburst pattern, and advanced image-processing algorithms digitally measure the whole eye corneal thickness. As can be seen in Figure 5-96, the current design offers 8 radial acquisition meridians to optically measure the corneal thickness along the normal direction. The advantage of the technique is the instantaneous and simultaneous acquisition of the whole data points by all 3 cameras at the same time. The disadvantage is the somewhat loose data density. Future improvement includes additional meridians with dense data points and more advanced image processing to obtain higher spatial resolution.

Other than whole-eye pachymetry, additional anterior segment information such as anterior chamber depth and IOL thickness and lens opacity can also be obtained (see Figure 5-96). Posterior topography is obtained by the

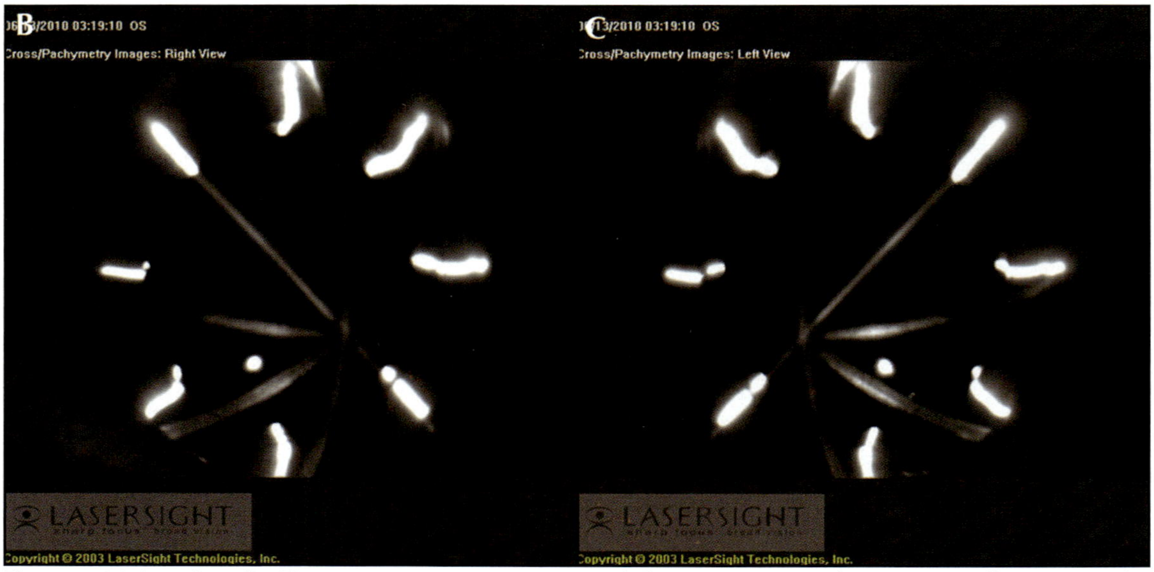


**Figure 5-96 (continued).** The 3-camera system uses 8 radial acquisition meridians to optically measure the corneal thickness along normal direction. (B) This is the view from the side camera. (C) This is the view from the other side camera.

combination of anterior topography and whole-eye optical pachymetry.

## Conclusion

An instantaneous and simultaneous comprehensive diagnostic instrument is clinically important, particularly in laser refractive surgery. Polar grid, combined with concentric rings, offers additional information not available from a concentric ring-only Placido system. Twist angle is a function of astigmatism, and the distribution is highly correlated to the optical transfer function of the cornea. Simultaneous and dynamic pupillometry, iris recognition, and corneal topography are critical to the overall assessment of the patient's eye and, in particular, to the clinicians involved with laser surgery when alignment of the eye and visual axis is of significance. A comprehensive diagnostic workstation with instantaneous and simultaneous measurement capabilities provides effective tools in topo-guided laser refractive ablation for particularly problematic and complex corneas.[131]

# TOPOLYZER

Mirko R. Jankov II, MD, PhD; Renato Ambrósio Jr, MD, PhD; Diogo L. Caldas, MD; Ana Laura C. Canedo, MD; Leonardo N. Pimentel, MD; Bruno F. Valbon, MD; and Sissimos Lemonis

The Allegretto Topolyzer (Alcon, Fort Worth, TX; Figure 5-97) is a Placido disk corneal topography system with an integrated autokeratometer, which facilitates best focusing on the reflected mires on the cornea and allows for an automatic acquisition of the Placido's image. This provides quick, precise, and very repeatable data with excellent image centration. The instrument has a software link with the Alcon WaveLight excimer laser platform for custom topographic-guided treatments.[135-137]

The Topolyzer has 11 rings of the Placido disks that are projected on the cornea (Figure 5-98), so that up to 22 reflection edges are recorded by a CCD camera and up to 22,000 measuring points are detected by the software (Figure 5-99). Basically, the reflected image of the Placido's disk is captured, and the slope (distance) of the rings is computed for calculating the topographical maps. The distance between the reflected rings will be smaller in steeper corneas and larger in flatter surfaces. The integrated

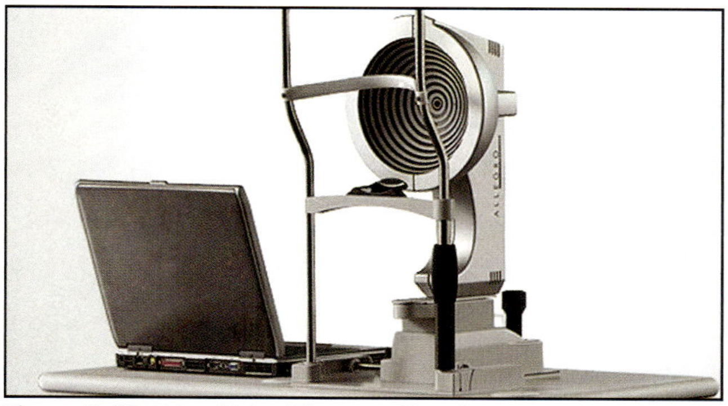

**Figure 5-97.** WaveLight Allegretto Topolyzer system.

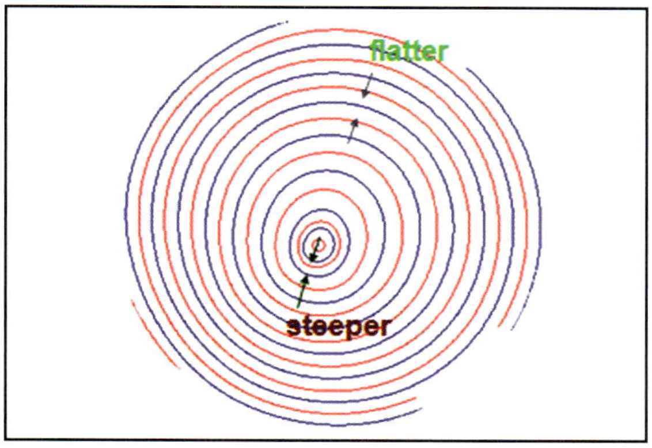


**Figure 5-98.** Red and blue lines represent the edges of the rings as detected by software. Smaller distance between the lines represents steeper areas of the cornea, while larger distance represents flatter surfaces.

keratometer enables the Topolyzer to have an accuracy of 0.1 D for keratometric readings (15 µm). The range of measurements is between 9 and 99 D (3- to 38-mm radius). There is a calibration routine using a model eye with a radius of 8.00 mm, which should be repeated periodically according to the manufacturer's recommendations.

## Measurement Technique

During the examination, the patient should be comfortably positioned at the chin and forehead support, with eyes aligned in the direction of the side marking line. The patient is asked to blink normally, open his or her eyes, and look at the fixation target in the center of the rings. The alignment and focusing are facilitated by the integrated autokeratometry, which guides for perfect positioning, so that it automatically takes the image (Figure 5-100). In cases of poor quality of the measured surface where automatic imaging is not possible, one can take the measurement with the manual activation arbitrary to the examiner. As with any Placido disk-based topographer, Topolyzer measurements are sensitive to tear film deficiency and irregularities; therefore, a strict measurement protocol and regular blinking is important for correct measurements.

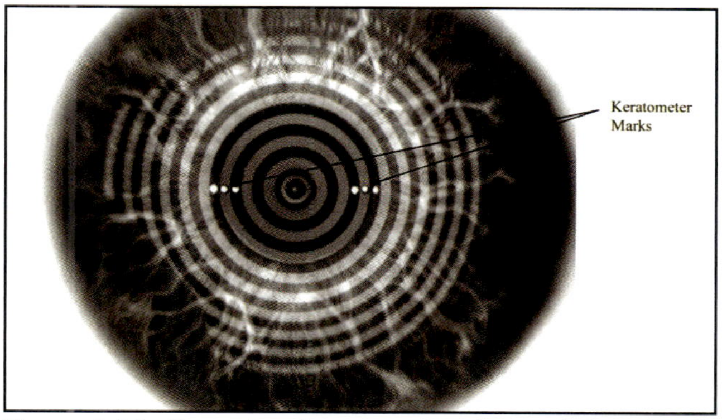


**Figure 5-99.** Raw photokeratoscopic photo of the Placido disk's reflection from the cornea, together with the keratometer marks. Note how the nose (lower left) and the eyelashes together with the eyebrows (superiorly) form a shadow, decreasing the number of detected ring edges, thus the amount of measured data.

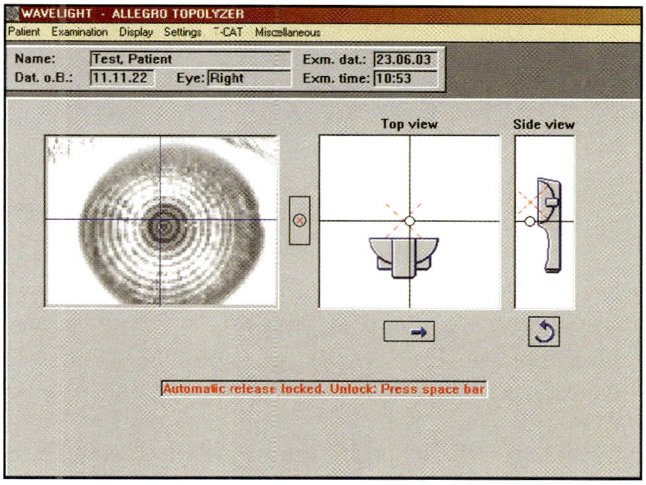


**Figure 5-100.** Automatic release comprises 3 view windows: left window for rough x, y, and z centration and middle and right window for automatic release, together with the alignment instructions in the form of an arrow for correct focusing.

If the case is considered for customized topography-guided ablation treatment (T-CAT), at least 4 (and up to 8) measurements should be taken sequentially (Figure 5-101). In this case, only the measurements taken automatically would be eligible for export and further analysis for the topography-guided customized treatments on the treatment planner portal software of the WaveLight Allegretto Wave excimer laser.

It is important to note some important parameters of quality to proceed with T-CAT. The pupil should be identified by a black and white circle, ensuring that the software did not erroneously recognize the real edge of the pupil as one of the inner circles (switch off the visualization of the corneal rings and only check for the pupil margin detection).

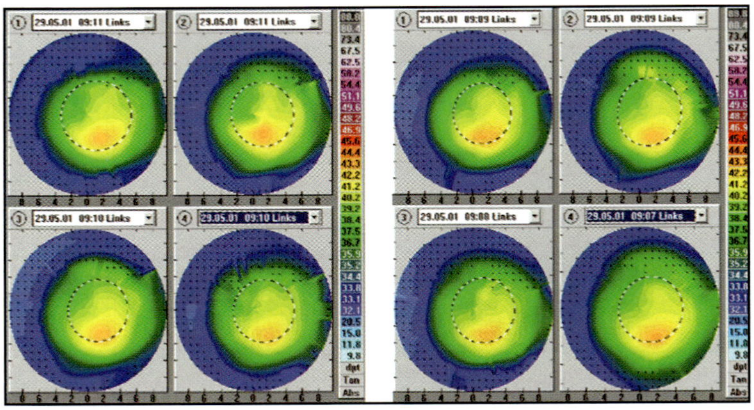

**Figure 5-101.** Repeatability demonstration "in vivo."

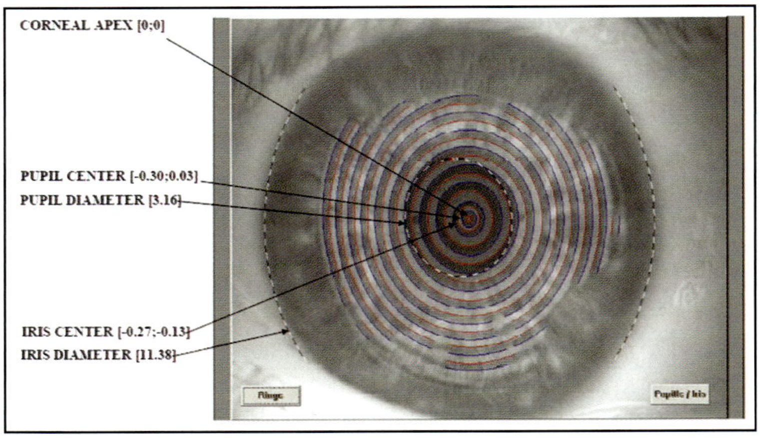


**Figure 5-102.** Photokeratoscopic photo of the Placido disks' reflection from the cornea, together with the software edge detection analysis: pupil (center and diameter), limbus (iris center and diameter), and ring edges of the Placido disks' reflections.

Another parameter is the percentage of the imaged or measured area compared to the full available image (abbreviation used by the software is analyzed area [AA]). Depending on the settings, the software either extrapolates the area that is not really measured, based on the surrounding measured ones, marking that area with black points, or it will simply be omitted and left as a white area without any information.

Only the area with uninterrupted Placido rings (Figure 5-102) and without the black dots will be considered for T-CAT. The measured area should be at least 60%. As this figure strongly depends on preoperative Ks, as well as the surface quality, one should aim to have at least enough data to cover the area of the intended ablation optical zone, typically 6.0, or 0.5-mm smaller in cases of the patients with smaller pupils. As an additional safety measure, the treatment planner portal software will automatically exclude measurements not providing adequate amounts of data for the desired optical zone.

## Display Modes

The Topolyzer exam provides relevant clinical information, starting from the evaluation of the photokeratoscopic image. The corneal apex is defined in cartesian polar coordinates as x = 0 and y = 0. This is the center of the Placido's reflex, and it is very important to have the patient adequately fixating to the fixation light inside the central inner ring. The pupil is identified, and its center is positioned accordingly to the apex. The limbus edge (or iris edge, as defined by the software) is also identified, and the best circle is fit such that its center is also characterized (see Figure 5-102).

The overview display provides most of the relevant clinical information (Figure 5-103). This display contains the photokeratoscopic image with the edge detection layer (upper left) along with the sagittal or tangential curvature map (upper right). The real (not simulated) central keratometric readings from a built-in keratometer for horizontal and vertical axis (or steeper and flatter, depending on the software settings), together with the astigmatism and its axis, are also displayed (lower left) and color coded: any data related to the flatter axis are displayed in blue, while data showing the steeper axis are marked in red. Next is the white-to-white measurement of the limbus (or corneal diameter, as defined by the software), and finally the corneal eccentricity (ecc), another conic constant to describe asphericity (Q). The formula for converting ecc to Q is as follows:

$$Q = -ecc^2$$

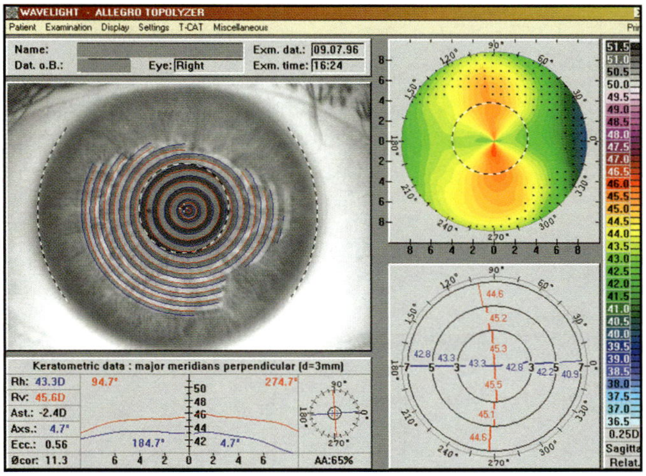


**Figure 5-103.** Overview display—an example of pure myopic astigmatism, sagittal map with relative OCULUS color scale and 0.25-D interval.

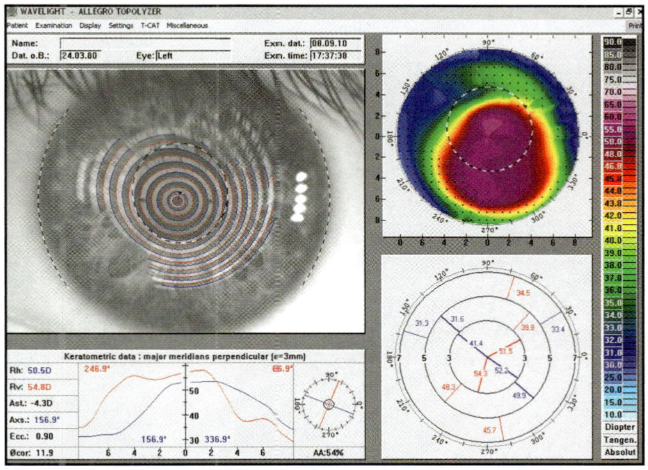


**Figure 5-105.** Overview display—an example of the patient in Figure 5-104 3 days after the implantation of 2 intracorneal ring segments of 200 and 250 μm (nasally and temporally, respectively). Tangential map shows absolute OCULUS color scale and 0.50-D interval. Note the remarkable decrease of the corneal curvatures and astigmatism, as well as formation of a relatively regular optical zone of approximately 4.5 mm on the keratometric profile map (lower left).

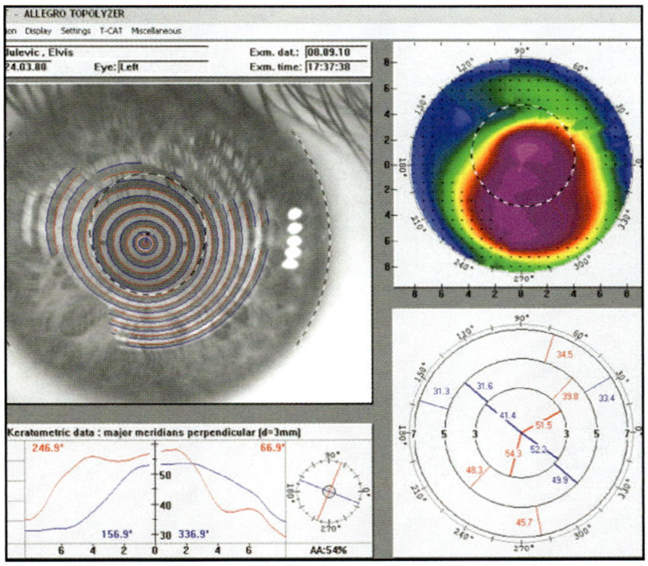


**Figure 5-104.** Overview display—an example of keratoconus, tangential map with absolute OCULUS color scale, and 0.50-D interval. Note the distortion of the rings on the raw image (upper left).

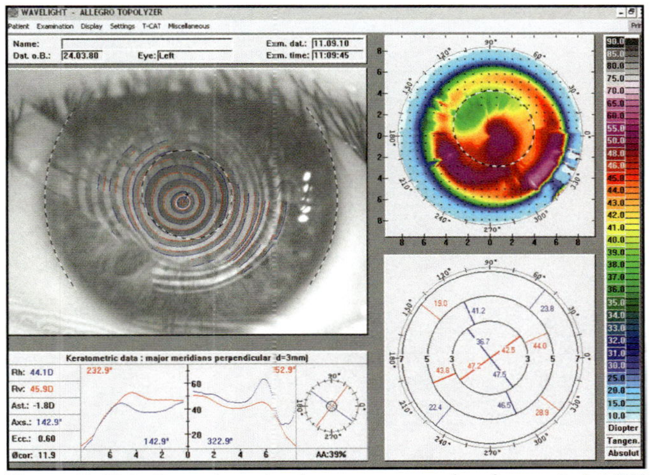


**Figure 5-106.** Overview display—an example of myopic LASIK of -5.00 D. The tangential map shows absolute OCULUS color scale and 0.50-D interval. Note a regular optical zone of approximately 5.5 mm represented as a straight line on the keratometric profile map (lower left).

The keratometric profiles along the major orthogonal axis calculated along all of the measured corneal diameter are also provided (lower left corner), together with keratometric readings at 3-, 5-, and 7-mm zones (lower right corner).

Topolyzer is capable of recognizing quite complex corneal shapes, such as keratoconus (Figure 5-104), cornea with intracorneal ring implanted for KC of the same patient (Figure 5-105), cornea after myopic LASIK (Figure 5-106), and cornea after hyperopic LASIK (Figure 5-107). Cases of elevated hyperopic astigmatism with a very high kappa angle are adequately detected (Figure 5-108) and can be used for correct ablation zone centration planning in case of excimer laser treatment.

The Topolyzer software performs a Fourier analysis, a mathematical process that decomposes a periodic function in a number of sine and cosine waves. The topographic map generated by the Topolyzer can be divided into individual components by Fourier analysis, allowing the study of spherical equivalent, decentralization, regular astigmatism, and irregularities from a single captured image (Figure 5-109).

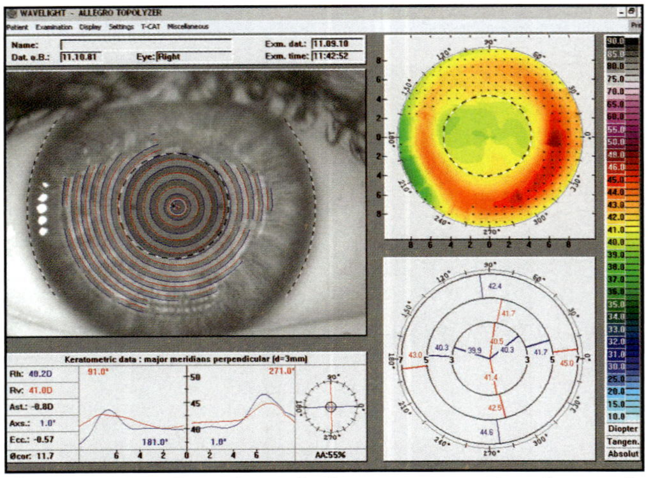


**Figure 5-107.** Overview display—an example of myopic LASIK of +4.0 D, tangential map shows absolute OCULUS color scale and 0.50-D interval. Note a regular optical zone of approximately 4.5 mm represented as a straight line on the keratometric profile map (lower left). Deflection circle of a hyperopic transition zone can be seen as a circular area of the missing rings on the raw image (upper left). That area is erroneously interpreted by the software as extremely flat and, therefore, color-coded with light blue on the curvature map (upper right).

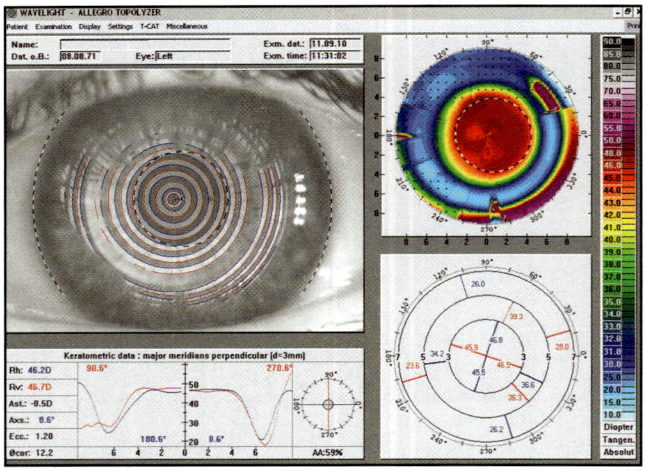


**Figure 5-108.** Overview display—an example of compound hyperopic astigmatism of Sph: +1.0 D and Cyl: +4.0 D @ 175. Tangential map shows absolute OCULUS color scale and 0.50-D interval. Note a significant kappa angle, represented by a line between the center of the pupil (cross) and the corneal apex (the central dot) on the raw image (upper left).

The Topolyzer exam also provides an analysis of corneal wavefront. Zernike polynomial decomposition of the anterior surface of the cornea provides lower-order aberrations and HOAs. The understanding of corneal SAs may be used for customizing aspheric IOLs in cataract surgery. Also, coma and other HOA terms may be useful for diagnosing keratoconus, irregular ablation, and other irregular conditions of the cornea (Figure 5-110).

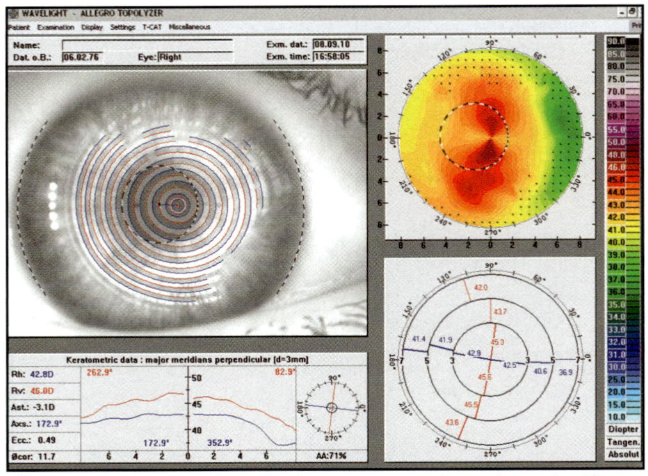


**Figure 5-109.** Fourier display—topography of a significant superior decentration of a myopic LASIK treatment. (Map on the left with the absolute OCULUS color scale and 0.50-D interval next to it.) The same curvature map is decomposed into 4 different components: spherical (upper middle), decentration (upper right), regular astigmatism (lower middle), and irregularities (lower right). Note a significant decentration component, while other components are quite low.

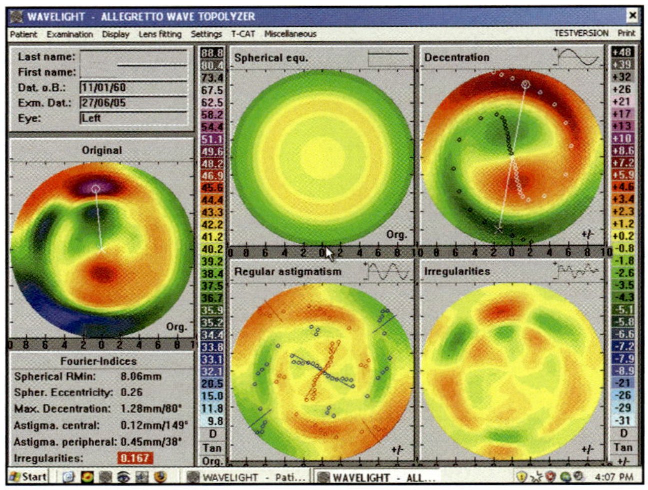


**Figure 5-110.** Zernike display—topography of a significant superior decentration of a myopic LASIK treatment (same patient seen in Figure 5-110). The curvature map is decomposed into Zernike coefficients expressed in mm (vector mode and 3-dimensional view chosen on this picture). Note a gross decentration described by significant tilt and coma coefficients of 8.22 and 1.99 μm, respectively, and some additional irregularities of 3-foil, 4-foil, and 5-foil, while other coefficients remained relatively low.

Keratometric indices are calculated to provide artificial intelligence to detect and stage keratoconus (Figure 5-111). A contact lens-fitting software module with a big database for different RGP and soft contact lenses is also available (Figure 5-112).

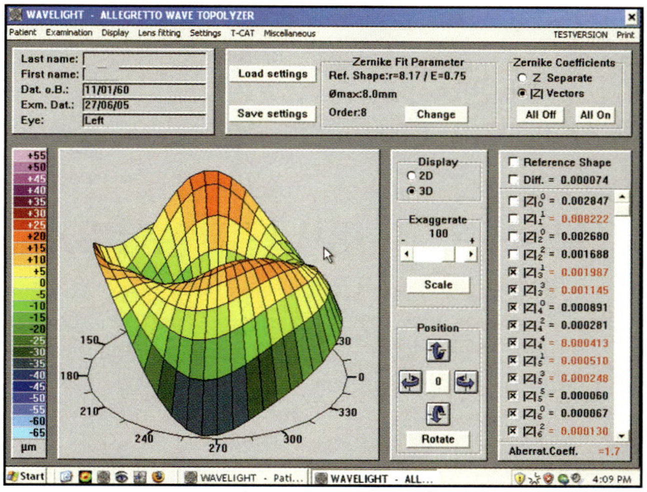


Figure 5-111. Keratoconus indices display—topography of a mild case; together with the curvature map (upper right with the absolute OCULUS color scale and 0.50-D interval next to it), a map of the decentration component from the Fourier analysis is displayed (upper left). In the upper middle, between the maps, a series of indices with their respective values is displayed (red being outside normal limits), as well as the classification of the keratoconus level (KC stage 1-2 in this case).

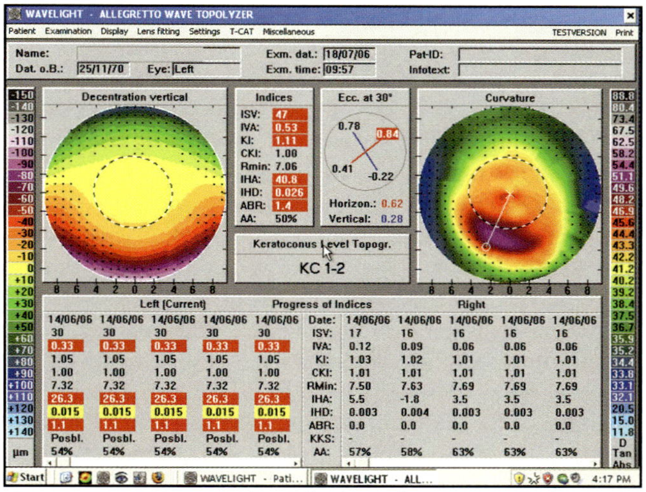


Figure 5-112. Contact lens display—fluorescein trial simulation of a fit for a mild keratoconus (the same as in Figure 5-111) with a RGP CL (r = 7.70, eccentricity of 0.45 and the outer diameter of 9.80 mm).

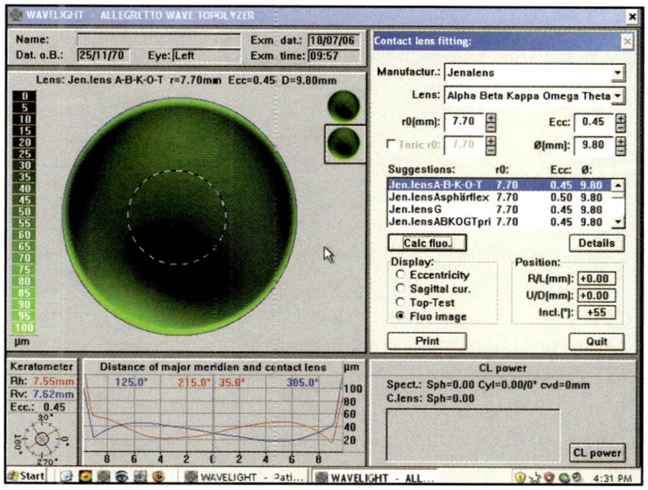


Figure 5-113. Height map display—topography (upper right) of a significant superior decentration of a myopic LASIK treatment (the same as in Figure 5-109); software automatically chooses the best-fit reference toric ellipsoid for a "pinned" fit, where the reference shape touches the corneal map in its center (an asphere with a radius of 0.27 mm and eccentricity of 0.26 in this example).

The Topolyzer is a topography system efficient in generating data and useful maps for diagnosis of corneal diseases, but one of the most important applications of this equipment is the ability to plan and export data to the Alcon WaveLight laser systems.[135,138,139] For this reason, expression of data as height maps with the pupil center data is essential (Figure 5-113). The main indications for customized topography-guided ablations using the Topolyzer are primary cases of high astigmatism, especially those with high kappa angle, irregular astigmatism due to corneal scars and retreatment of a small optical zone, decentered ablation and postradial keratotomy, and penetrating or lamellar keratoplasty. Data validation for quality, repeatability, and proper centration prior to exporting, as described earlier (measurement technique), is essential for predictable outcomes.

The Topolyzer is a topography system that is a powerful diagnostic tool, with good accuracy and repeatability, which are very important for correct and successful measurement of various natural and iatrogenic corneal shapes. Moreover, one of the most important applications of the Topolyzer is planning customized ablations for LVCs with the Alcon WaveLight laser systems and T-CAT treatment planner portal software.

# EyeSys 3000 and EyeSys Vista

Sonya M. Dakin, COT and Joe S. Wakil, MD

The EyeSys 3000 system manufactured by EyeSys Vision Inc (Houston, TX) is a patented multiresolution Placido technology along with high-resolution 4-camera optics that provides unparalleled corneal measurement reliability and precision.[140] The multiple-resolution corneal reflection pattern encodes reflection features in such a way as to automatically adjust the measurement resolution depending upon the curvature of the surface. The downfall of most CTs on the market today is the fact that they use a standard number of rings to identify and quantify all corneal abnormalities. In certain cases, subtle changes are overlooked because they are lost in the "red sea" due to extremely steep keratometric readings.[141] In high curvature areas, high-frequency patterns can merge together so that they cannot be reliably resolved while low-frequency patterns stay far enough apart so that a measurement can be made. In low curvature areas, patterns spread out so that high-resolution patterns are required to maintain high spatial sampling.

The EyeSys 3000's technology offers the customization based on the overall keratometric condition of the cornea. For instance, for a relatively high curvature corneal area (keratoconus), the EyeSys needs only 14 rings to accurately identify and display the keratometric characteristics. When evaluating a moderate-curvature cornea (normal eyes), the EyeSys increases the number of rings to 79, and, lastly, the very low-curvature corneas increase the rings to the maximum number, which are 131 rings. By adapting the resolution of these areas, the EyeSys 3000 can increase measurement reliability and precision using techniques that are not possible with single-resolution reflection patterns.[142] The EyeSys 3000 also has the ability to locate the pupil's centroid and measures its size by using a dedicated IR pupil camera.

Along with the EyeSys 3000, EyeSys Vision also produces an EyeSys Vista unit, which brings new freedom to corneal topography while retaining the quality and excellence that are the hallmark of EyeSys products. The Vista offers eye-care practitioners a simple affordable and dependable tool for precise corneal topography. The portability and unparalleled versatility of the EyeSys Vista enables it to perform topography in all clinical environments. Patients confined to a bed or wheelchair can easily be examined, and supine patients can be mapped in the operating room under a surgical microscope.

## EyeSys Design Philosophy

The EyeSys 3000 uses a multiresolution Placido technology to ensure the most reliable and reproducible information possible. The Vista CT is designed to be detached and used with a laptop computer as a stand-alone, portable, hand-held corneal topography unit with full software benefits. The EyeSys system was developed in 1986 as an industry leader, and with its most recent release of the EyeSys 3000 and Vista, it is still an industry leader. The EyeSys Vista CT is designed for convenient handheld use and has special electronic features such as auto-capture and tilt sensing along with auto-correction to ensure accurate and precise corneal topography and keratometric data on par with any tabletop unit. This includes using the system in a vertical mode on supine patients, such as during surgery (ie, to document flap orientation and condition at the end of standard LASIK procedures).

The EyeSys Placido is noted for using edge detection of the Placido mires to provide precise determination of ring location for highly accurate corneal topography measurements. The Placido design of the Vista is the same as that of the larger EyeSys 3000 system, covering the central cornea at around 0.9 mm to over 10 mm in the normal peripheral cornea. This larger Placido design provides for a longer working distance than smaller cylindrical Placido cones. The longer 12.5-mm working distance has the advantage of being less sensitive to positional errors in focusing and alignment that significantly improves the reproducibility and accuracy of the system. The EyeSys Vista hardware has this advantage working in its favor under both conditions—mounted on the slit-lamp base and when used in a handheld manner. The reproducibility results are impressive at less than ±0.10 D in the hands of an experienced user.

It is important to always remember that, with corneal topography measurements, one is measuring the anterior tear film surface of the cornea—truly the "lens of the eye." This is the refractive surface that provides the vast majority (>75%) of the eye's refractive power. Please note that although some topography systems emphasize that the cornea has anterior and posterior surfaces, this can be misleading because, optically, with tear film on the living cornea, there are actually 3 refractive interfaces: air/tear film, tear film/corneal stroma, and corneal stroma/aqueous humor. Effectively, nature has provided for these last 2 refractive interfaces of the cornea to practically cancel each other out, leaving the anterior tear film as the effective refractive power interface of the cornea.

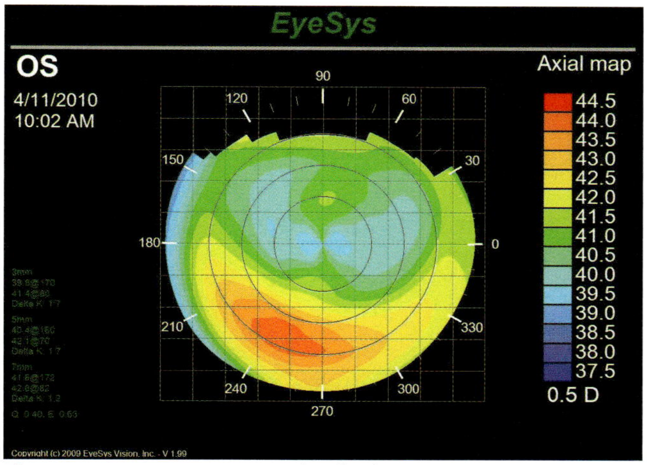


**Figure 5-114.** Main topography display.

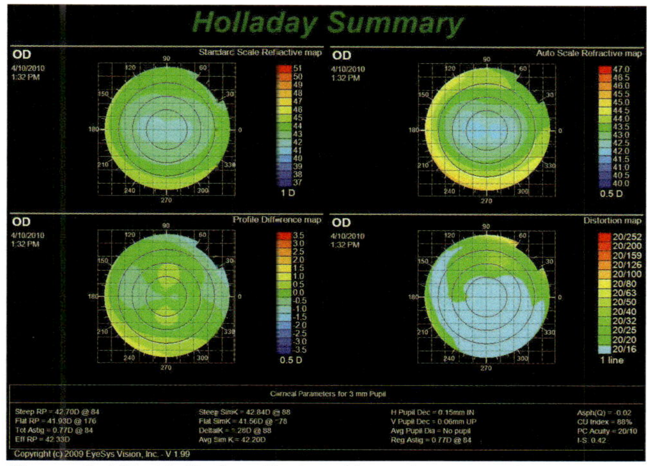


**Figure 5-115.** Holladay display. Note the corneal parameters listed at the bottom: Sim Ks, radial power values, pupil measurements, asphericity, CU index, I-S value, and PC acuity.

To ensure ideal vision correction, matching the available surgical procedures or corrective lens choices in addressing each patient's visual deficits depends heavily upon performing the correct diagnosis of the aberration sources in each patient's eyes. The EyeSys is designed to meet this goal for every patient in an easy-to-use and comprehensive format, creating a new standard of visual function analysis well beyond the antiquated Snellen refraction.

# Displays

The corneal topography calculations and displays are generated from the EyeSys 3000 and Vista Placido image of the cornea and are fully customizable within the software. Using advanced edge detection software, the Placido image of the cornea is analyzed across all of the ring edges from center to periphery. Along with patient name and identification number, OD/OS label, and time of exam, standard keratometric readings are generated at the 3-mm zone of the cornea to accurately measure its central curvature and simulate keratometer measurements for routine use. These K readings are provided with every corneal topography display, as shown in Figure 5-114.

Additionally, a refractive power reading of the cornea is calculated for the 3-mm zone in similar fashion to the K readings, but based on Snell's law of refraction to more accurately describe the refractive power of the central cornea. A single effective refractive power reading is given for the entire central 3-mm zone of the cornea to be used primarily for IOL calculations. This number has been popularized by Jack Holladay, MD, as an improvement in understanding central corneal refractive power contribution in more accurately calculating the necessary IOL power for eyes postrefractive surgery. The Holladay Diagnostic Summary available with the compatible EyeSys software package to the Vista hardware has become an industry standard—a single-page display that provides additional corneal indices to comprehensively analyze the cornea and simplify corneal diagnosis (Figure 5-115). These indices include the inferior-superior (I-S) index, a corneal uniformity index (CUI), an aspheric Q factor of the cornea, and the unique potential corneal acuity (PCA) measurement that provides a direct objective measure of mire quality related to the tear film of the eye, in effect helping measure potential dry eye problems.

Beyond the numeric data of K readings, refractive power readings, and other corneal indices, color maps are provided to depict the unique features of each cornea. With the 2-dimensional images, there are a number of algorithms available, providing complete corneal analysis. These include the Axial Map, Local Radius of Curvature Map (Tangential), Refractive Map, Z Elevation Map, High-Order Aberration, Contact Lens Map, and Wavefront Map (Figures 5-116 and 5-117).

The Vista hardware is used to capture the Placido image automatically upon centering and focusing of the video image as the patient fixates upon a coaxial fixation point. This automatic capture occurs through triangulation of a low-power laser beam reflected off of the corneal vertex at a calibrated distance from the Placido. Once captured, the Placido image is displayed to the user with the ring edge detection highlighted, so that the user can easily confirm correct image processing. This helps avoid artifacts and errors in processing that can sometimes be problematic in very irregular corneas, such as those following corneal transplantation. Figure 5-118 shows a typical Placido image capture verification screen with the edge detection clearly shown, confirming correct analysis to the user. Also, the user can obtain the K readings and refractive power readings from this immediate display following image capture.

The Corneal Topography Summary Displays can be customized to allow for any of the color maps available to be displayed with up to 4 maps at once.[143] The EyeSys Vista

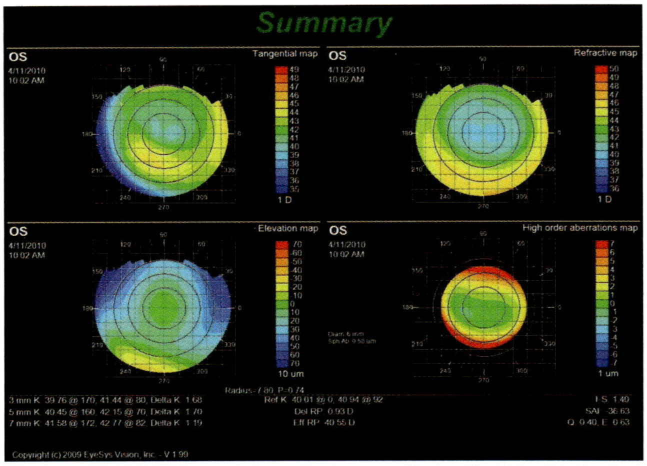


**Figure 5-116.** Comprehensive mapping display including tangential, refractive, elevation, and corneal wavefront aberrations maps.

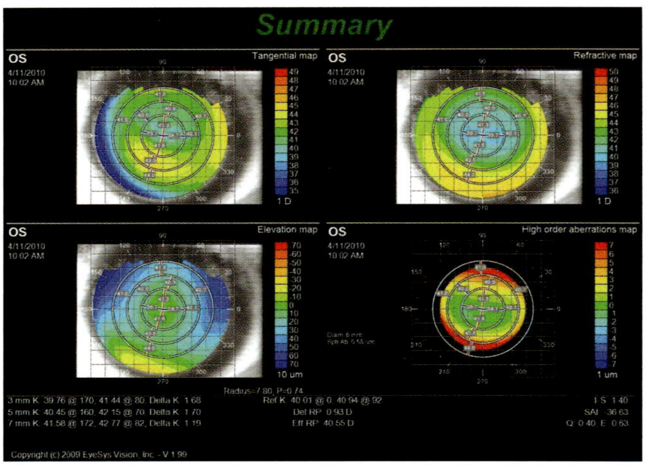


**Figure 5-117.** Comprehensive mapping display showing inferior steepening and coma on the wavefront map. The I-S value is 1.4, and this is suspicious for ectasia.

as well as the EyeSys 3000 is generally configured to show the Axial Map, Local Radius of Curvature Map, Refractive Map, and Z Elevation Map.[144] The Corneal Wavefront Map can be added as desired and positioned in any order, so there is full flexibility. The example of the corneal topography summary display in Figure 5-119 shows almost 4 D of with-the-rule astigmatism, where the steep corneal curvature is oriented vertically. As with all color maps, it is important to pay attention to scaling. With the EyeSys Vista as well as the EyeSys 3000, there is a choice to allow for auto-scaling features or user-defined fixed scaling units. Typically, 0.5-D step sizes are used to fulfill most of the needs to provide good corneal detail while also providing adequate range to most corneas. User choice is available to generate practically all scaling requirements.

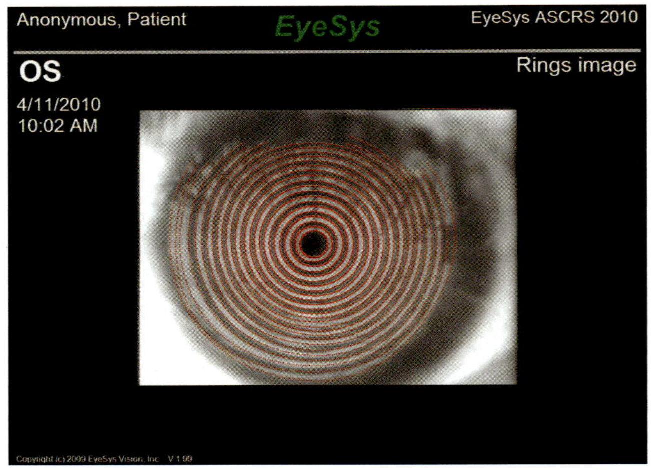


**Figure 5-118.** Verification display. The clinician is able to check the rings to ensure the capture if well done.

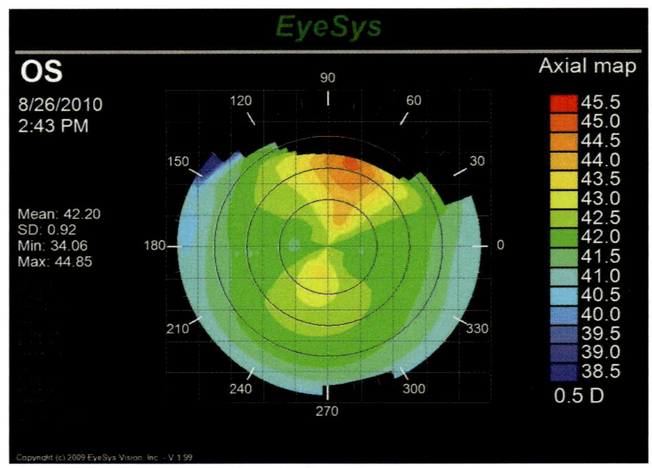


**Figure 5-119.** 1.5 D of with-the-rule astigmatism.

A Comparison Display Map is also available on each of the different color map displays available with both EyeSys systems. These maps are informative in revealing the differences that occur over time (ie, pre- and postsurgery), as well as over periods of healing or treatment. Figure 5-120 shows corneal stabilization after contact lens removal in a patient planning for excimer laser surgery. The refractive power difference between these 2 exams is much less than 0.25 D over most of the corneal surface, therefore indicating that the cornea has changed insignificantly between the 2 days examined. The difference map is overall green, indicating little or no change in corneal topography.

The Holladay Diagnostic Summary shown in Figure 5-121 demonstrates the power of corneal topography in diagnosing an early keratoconus case. This unique display generated by EyeSys software has been widely used for more than a decade in providing a single-page overview of the cornea with a number of valuable corneal indices. The

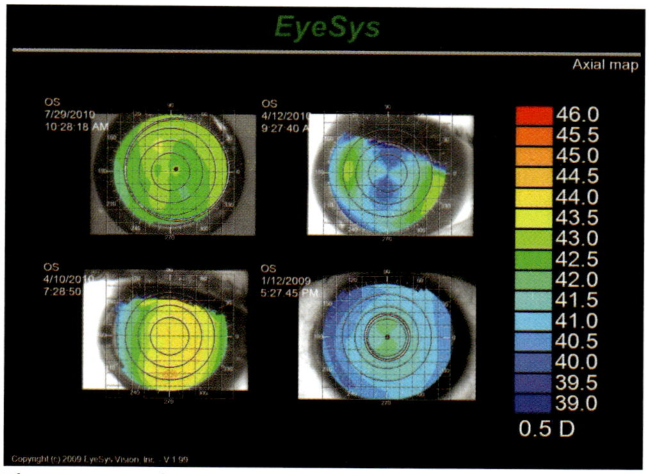


**Figure 5-120.** The comparison map compares topography over time, such as in this case of corneal stabilization after contact lens removal in a patient planning for excimer laser surgery.

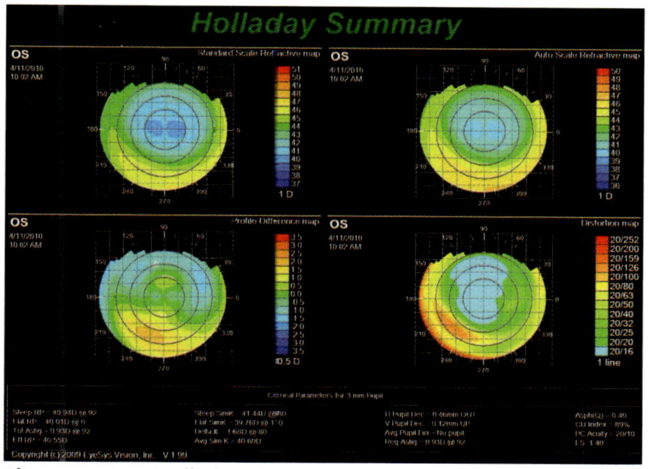


**Figure 5-121.** Holladay diagnostic summary in a patient with early keratoconus.

cornea displayed shows the classic pattern of inferior steepening in the Local Radius of Curvature Map in the upper right map and also a correlating change in the Asphericity Difference Map in the lower left demonstrating that the area of the keratoconus significantly alters the normal rate of flattening of the cornea from center to periphery. The Potential Corneal Acuity Map in the lower right reveals a pattern of inferior mire distortion expected in classic keratoconus as tear film break-up and irregularity over the ectasia is typical. The corneal indices at the bottom of the Holladay Diagnostic Summary are consistent with keratoconus having an I-S index greater than 1.0 (in this case 4.79) and a CUI of less than 60% (in this case 20%) with a degraded PCA of 20/100. With the data presented, a clinician only needs to complete the patient history to rule-out contact lens warpage in making the keratoconus diagnosis with a high degree of certainty.

# References


1. McKay T. *A Clinical Guide to the Humphrey Corneal Topography System*. Dublin, CA: Humphrey; 1998; Section 2:4-6.
2. *ATLAS Corneal Topography System: Model 9000 Instrument and ATLAS Review Software* [computer program]. Version 3.0. Jena, Germany: Carl Zeiss Meditec; 2007: Section 3:9.
3. Anderson D, Kojima R. Topography: a clinical pearl. *Optom Management*. 2007;42(2):35.
4. Roberts C. A practical guide to the interpretation of corneal topography. *CL Spectrum*. 1998;13(3):25-33.
5. Navarro R, Gonzalez L, Hernandez JL. Optics of the average normal cornea from general and canonical representations of its surface topography. *J Opt Soc Am A Opt Image Sci Vis*. 2006;23(2):219-232.
6. *ATLAS Corneal Topography System: Model 9000 Instrument and ATLAS Review Software* [computer program]. Version 3.0. Jena, Germany: Carl Zeiss Meditec; 2007: Section A:1-18.
7. Bagherinia H, Chen X, Flachenecker C, et al. Support vector machine (SVM)-based classification of corneal topography. Poster presented at: Association for Research in Vision and Ophthalmology (ARVO) Annual Meeting; April 27-May 1, 2008; Ft. Lauderdale, FL: 1023/D879.
8. Noble WS. What is a support vector machine? *Nature Biotech*. 2006;24(12):1565-1567.
9. *ATLAS Corneal Topography System: Model 9000 Instrument and ATLAS Review Software* [computer program]. Version 3.0. Jena, Germany: Carl Zeiss Meditec; 2007: Section B:1-30.
10. Gormley DJ, Gersten M, Koplin RS, Lubkin V. Corneal modeling. *Cornea*. 1988;7:30-35.
11. Mammone RJ, Gersten M, Gormley DJ, Koplin RS, Lubkin VL. 3-D corneal modeling system. *IEEE Trans Biomed Eng*. 1990;37:66-72.
12. Klyce SD. Computer-assisted corneal topography: high resolution graphical presentation and analysis of keratoscopy. *Invest Ophthalmol Vis Sci*. 1984;25:1426-1435.
13. Maguire LJ, Singer DE, Klyce SD. Graphic presentation of computer-analyzed keratoscope photographs. *Arch Ophthalmol*. 1987;105:223-230.
14. Swartz T, Marten L, Wang M. Measuring the cornea: the latest developments in corneal topography. *Curr Opin Ophthalmol*. 2007;18:325-333.
15. Konstantopoulos A, Hossain P, Anderson DF. Recent advances in ophthalmic anterior segment imaging: a new era for ophthalmic diagnosis? *Br J Ophthalmol*. 2007;91:551-557.
16. Wilson SE, Klyce SD, Husseini ZM. Standardized color-coded maps for corneal topography. *Ophthalmology*. 1993;100:1723-1727.
17. Dingeldein SA, Klyce SD, Wilson SE. Quantitative descriptors of corneal shape derived from computer-assisted analysis of photokeratographs. *Refractive & Corneal Surgery*. 1989;5:372-378.
18. Wilson SE, Klyce SD. Quantitative descriptors of corneal topography: a clinical study. *Arch Ophthalmol*. 1991;109:349-353.
19. Alimisi S, Miltsakakis D, Klyce S. Corneal topography for intraocular lens power calculations. *J Refract Surg*. 1996;12:S309-S311.

20. Maeda N, Klyce SD, Smolek MK, McDonald MB. Disparity of keratometry readings and corneal power within the pupil after refractive surgery for myopia. *Cornea.* 1997;16:517-524.
21. Mafra CH, Dave A, Wilson SE, Klyce SD. Extracapsular cataract surgery: corneal topographic alterations. *Invest Ophthalmol Vis Sci.* 1993;34:1248.
22. Maeda N, Klyce SD, Smolek MK, Thompson HW. Automated keratoconus screening with corneal topography analysis. *Invest Ophthalmol Vis Sci.* 1994;35:2749-2757.
23. Randleman JB, Russell B, Ward MA, Thompson KP, Stulting RD. Risk factors and prognosis for corneal ectasia after LASIK. *Ophthalmology.* 2003;110:267-275.
24. Holladay JT. Keratoconus detection using corneal topography. *J Refract Surg.* 2009;25:S958-S962.
25. Klyce SD. Chasing the suspect: keratoconus. *Br J Ophthalmol.* 2009;93:845-847.
26. Smolek MK, Klyce SD. Current keratoconus detection methods compared with a neural network approach. *Invest Ophthalmol Vis Sci.* 1997;38:2290-2299.
27. Hjortdal JO, Erdmann L, Bek T. Fourier analysis of video-keratographic data. A tool for separation of spherical, regular astigmatic and irregular astigmatic corneal power components. *Ophthalmic Physiol Opt.* 1995;15:171-185.
28. Olsen T, Dam-Johansen M, Bek T, Hjortdal JO. Evaluating surgically induced astigmatism by Fourier analysis of corneal topography data. *J Cataract Refract Surg.* 1996;22:318-323.
29. Tomidokoro A, Soya K, Miyata K, et al. Corneal irregular astigmatism and contrast sensitivity after photorefractive keratectomy. *Ophthalmology.* 2001;108:2209-2212.
30. Oshika T, Tanabe T, Tomidokoro A, Amano S. Progression of keratoconus assessed by Fourier analysis of videokeratography data. *Ophthalmology.* 2002;109:339-342.
31. Tanabe T, Tomidokoro A, Samejima T, et al. Corneal regular and irregular astigmatism assessed by Fourier analysis of videokeratography data in normal and pathologic eyes. *Ophthalmology.* 2004;111:752-757.
32. Hiraoka T, Furuya A, Matsumoto Y, et al. Quantitative evaluation of regular and irregular corneal astigmatism in patients having overnight orthokeratology. *J Cataract Refract Surg.* 2004;30:1425-1429.
33. Miyai T, Miyata K, Nejima R, et al. Visual acuity measurements using Fourier series harmonic analysis of videokeratography data in eyes after penetrating keratoplasty. *Ophthalmology.* 2005;112:420-424.
34. Szczotka LB, Reinhart W. Computerized videokeratoscopy contact lens software for RGP fitting in a bilateral postkeratoplasty patient: a clinical case report. *CLAO J.* 1995;21:52-56.
35. Bufidis T, Konstas AG, Mamtziou E. The role of computerized corneal topography in rigid gas permeable contact lens fitting. *CLAO J.* 1998;24:206-209.
36. Randleman JB, Woodward M, Lynn MJ, Stulting RD. Risk assessment for ectasia after corneal refractive surgery. *Ophthalmology.* 2008;115(1):37-50.
37. Bellucci R, Morselli S. Optimizing higher-order aberrations with intraocular lens technology. *Curr Opin Ophthalmol.* 2007;18(1):67-73.
38. Endl MJ. Contrast sensitivity & patient satisfaction: Softport AO Aberration-Free IOL vs. a wavefront-designed IOL. Paper presented at: American Society of Cataract and Refractive Surgery Annual Meeting; March 17-22, 2006; San Francisco, CA.
39. Fichte CM. A one year follow-up comparing two higher order aberration IOLs. In: *Current Concepts in Ophthalmology.* Paper presented at: Johns Hopkins Ophthalmology Meeting; March 10-12, 2007; Vail, CO.
40. American Academy of Ophthalmology. *Basic and Clinical Science Course, Section 8: External Disease and Cornea.* San Francisco, CA: Author; 2001-2002:305.
41. Rajan MS, Jaycock P, O'Brart D, et al. A long term study of photorefractive keratectomy; 12 year followup. *Ophthalmology.* 2004;111:1813-1824.
42. *Orbscan Keratoconus Screening Indices: Operators Manual and Procedural Recommendations.* Rochester, NY: Bausch & Lomb; July 2004.
43. Wilson SE, Lin DTC, Klyce SD, et al. Topographic changes in contact lens-induced corneal warpage. *Ophthalmology.* 1990;97:734.
44. McLellan JS, Marco S, Prieto PM, Burns SA. Imperfect optics may be the eye's defense against chromatic blur. *Nature.* 2002;417:174-176.
45. Marcos S, Barbero S, Jimenez-Alfaro I. Optical quality and depth of field of eyes implanted with spherical and aspheric intraocular lenses. *J Refract Surg.* 2005;21:223-235.
46. Wang L, Dai E, Koch DD, Nathoo A. Optical aberrations of the human anterior cornea. *J Cataract and Refract Surg.* 2003;29:1514-1521.
47. Price FW Jr. How important is it to reduce or eliminate spherical aberration and is there an advantage to having some present? In: Chang DF, ed. *Curbside Consultation in Cataract Surgery: 49 Clinical Questions.* Thorofare, NJ: SLACK Incorporated; 2007:37-42.
48. Levy Y, Segal O, Avni I, Zadok D. Ocular higher order aberrations in eyes with supranormal vision. *Am J Ophthalmol.* 2005;139:225-228.
49. Grimson JM, Schallhorn SC. Contrast sensitivity: establishing normative data for use in screening prospective naval pilots. *Aviat Space Environ Med.* 2002;73:28-35.
50. Wilson SE, Wang JY, Klyce SD. Quantification and mathematical analysis of photokeratoscopic images. In: Shanzlin DJ, Robin JB, eds. *Corneal Topography: Measuring and Modifying the Cornea.* New York, NY: Springer-Verlag; 1991:1-9.
51. Klyce SD, Wang JY. Considerations in corneal surface reconstruction from keratoscope images. In: Masters BR, ed. *Noninvasive Diagnostic Techniques in Ophthalmology.* New York, NY: Springer-Verlag; 1990:76.
52. Merlin U. I cheratoscopi: caratteristiche e attendibilita. In: Buratto L, Cantera E, Dal Fiume E, Genisi C, Merlin U, eds. *Topografia Corneale.* Milano, Italy: CAMO; 1995:43-56.
53. Klein SA, Mandell RB. Axial and instantaneous power conversion in corneal topography. *Invest Ophthalmol Vis Sci.* 1995;36:2155-2159.
54. Cohen KL, Tripoli NK, Holmgren DE, Coggins JM. Assessment of the power and height of radial aspheres reported by a computer-assisted keratoscope. *Am J Ophthalmol.* 1995;119:723-732.
55. Roberts C. Characterization of the inherent error in a spherically-biased corneal topography system in mapping a radially aspheric surface. *J Refract Corneal Surg.* 1994;10:103-116.
56. Koch DD, Foulks GN, Moran CT, Wakil JS. The corneal EyeSys system: accuracy analysis and reproducibility of first-generation prototype. *J Refract Corneal Surg.* 1989;6:423-429.
57. Gullstrand A. Photographic-ophthalmometric and clinical Investigations of corneal refraction. *Am J Optom Arch Am Acad Optom.* 1966;43:143-214.
58. Doss JD, Hutson RL, Rowsey JJ, Brown R. Method for calculation of corneal profile and power distribution. *Arch Ophthalmol.* 1981;99:1261-1265.
59. Wang J, Rice DA, Klyce SD. A new reconstruction algorithm for improvement of corneal topographical analysis. *J Corneal Refract Surg.* 1989;5:379-387.
60. van Saarloos PP, Constable IJ. Improved method for calculation of corneal topography for any photokeratoscopic geometry. *Optom and Vis Sci.* 1991;68:957-965.
61. Klein SA. A corneal topography algorithm that produces continuous curvature. *Optom Vis Sci.* 1002;69:829-834.
62. Campbell C. Reconstruction of the corneal shape with the MasterVue corneal topography system. *Optom Vis Sci.* 1997;74:901.

63. Mattioli R, Carones F, Cantera E. New algorithms to improve the reconstruction of corneal geometry on the Keratron videokeratographer. *Invest Ophthalmol Vis Sci* (suppl). 1995;36:1400.
64. El Hage SG. The computerized corneal topographer EH-270. In: Shanzlin DJ, Robin JB, eds. *Corneal Topography: Measuring and Modifying the Cornea*. New York, NY: Springer-Verlag; 1991:11-24.
65. El-Hage SG. Suggested new methods for photokeratoscopy: a comparison of their validities. I. *Am J Optom Arch Am Acad Optom*. 1971;48:897-912.
66. Brancato R, Carones F. *Topografia Corneale Computerizzata*. Milan, Italy: Fogliazza; 1994:2.12-17.3.
67. Chan WK, Carones F, Maloney RK. Corneal topographic maps: a clinical comparison. In: *International Society of Refractive Keratoplasty—Abstract Book*. Paper presented at: Pre-Academy meeting of the International Society of Refractive Keratoplasty; October 28-November 3, 1994; San Francisco, CA.
68. Mattioli R, Tripoli N. Corneal geometry reconstruction with the Keratron videokeratographer. *Optom Vis Sci*. 1997;74:881-894.
69. Hannush SB, Crawford SL, Waring GO III, Gemmill MC, Lynn MJ, Nizam A. Accuracy and precision of keratometry, photokeratoscopy and corneal modeling on calibrated steel balls. *Arch Ophthalmol*. 1989;107:1235-1239.
70. Maguire LJ, Wilson SE, Camp JJ, Verity S. Evaluating the reproducibility of topography systems on spherical surfaces. *Arch Ophthalmol*. 1993;111:259-262.
71. Wilson SE, Verity SM, Conger DL. Accuracy and precision of the Corneal Analysis System and the Topographic Modeling System. *Cornea*. 1992;11:28-35.
72. Carones F, Gobbi PG, Brancato R, Venturi E. Comparison between two computer-assisted keratoscopes in measuring aspheric surfaces. *Invest Ophtalmol Vis Sci* (suppl). 1994:3748.
73. Tripoli NK, Cohen KL, Holmgren DE, Coggins JM. Assessment of radial aspheres by the Keratron keratoscope using an arc-step algorithm. *Am J Ophthalmol*. 1995;120:658-664.
74. Cohen KL, Tripoli NK, Holmgren DE, Coggins JM. Assessment of the height of radial aspheres reported by a computer-assisted keratoscope. *Invest Ophthalmol Vis Sci* (suppl). 1993;34:1217.
75. Tripoli NK, Cohen KL, Obla P, Coggins JM, Holmgren DE. Height measurement of astigmatic test surfaces by a keratoscope that uses plane geometry reconstruction. *Am J Ophthalmol*. 1996;121:668-676.
76. Wang JY, Rice DA, Klyce SD. Analysis of the effects of astigmatism and misalignment on corneal surface reconstruction from photokeratoscopic data. *Refract Corneal Surg*. 1991;7(2):129-140.
77. Mattioli R, Carones F. How accurately can corneal profile heights be measured by Placido-based videokeratography? *Invest Ophthalmol Vis Sci* (suppl). 1996;37:4273.
78. Camellin M, Federici R, Federici S. Clinical applications of the aberrometric functions of the Keratron Scout. In: Caimi F, Brancato R, eds. *The Aberrometers*. Canelli, Italy: Fabiano; 2003:259-268.
79. Dekking HM. Zur photographie der hornhautoberfl-eche. *Graefes Arch Ophtalmol*. 1930;124:708-730.
80. Cantera E, Carones F, Brancato R, Cantera I, Neuschuler R. Evaluation of a new autofocus device for computer-assisted corneal topography. *Invest Ophtalmol Vis Sci*. 1994;35(suppl):2063.
81. Walsh G. The effect of mydriasis on the pupillary centration of the human eye. *Ophthalmic Physiol Opt*. 1988;8:178-182.
82. Wyatt HJ. The form of the human pupil. *Vision Res*. 1995;35:2021-2036.
83. Mattioli R, Carones F. An algorithm to recalculate topographic maps from any axis for computer assisted videokeratography. In: *International Society of Refractive Surgery—Abstract Book*. Paper presented at: International Society of Refractive Surgery Meeting; October 29-November 3, 1995; Atlanta, GA.
84. Mattioli R, Federici R. Intra-operatory corneal topography—Tools and applications. Acts from the congress "Refractive on Line," ICH-Milano, Sept. 2001. http://www.refractiveonline.com/eng/pages/edition.aspx?anno=2001. Accessed August 8, 2011.
85. Vinciguerra P, Camesasca FI. Smoothing in Excimer refractive surgery. In: Vinciguerra P, Camasasca FI, eds. *Refractive Surface Ablation*. Thorofare, NJ; SLACK Incorporated; 2007:3-16.
86. Mahmoud AM, Roberts C, Herderick EE, Lembach RG, Markakis G. The cone location and magnitude index (CLMI). *Invest Ophthalmol Vis Sci*. 2001;42:S898.
87. Twa MD, Parthasarathy S, Roberts C, Mahmoud AM, Raasch TW, Bullimore MA. Automated decision tree classification of corneal shape. *Optom Vis Sci*. 2005;82(12):1038-1046.
88. Mahmoud AM, Roberts CJ, Lembach RG, Twa MD, Herderick EE, McMahon TT; the CLEK Study Group. CLMI: The cone location and magnitude index. *Cornea*. 2008;27(4):480-487.
89. Mattioli R. CLMI (Cone Location + Magnitude) Indices in the *Keratron* Scout. Milano, Italy: AIM Congress srl - AIM Group. September 2005. http://www.refractiveonline.com/2005/eng/38mattioli/player.html. Accessed August 8, 2011.
90. Mattioli R. The Gaussian curvature map. Presented at Refractiveonline, Milano, Italy: September 2007. www.refractiveonline.com/2007/eng/04mattioli/player.html. Accessed August 8, 2011.
91. Barsky BA, Klein S, Garcia DD. Gaussian power, mean sphere and cylinder representations for corneal maps with applications to the diagnosis of keratoconus. *Invest Ophthalmol Vis Sci*. 1996;37(suppl):558.
92. Tang M, Shekhar R, Miranda D, Huang D. Characteristics of keratoconus and pellucid marginal degeneration in mean curvature maps. *Am J Ophthalmol*. 2005;140:993-1000.
93. Mattioli R. Representation of corneal wavefront from corneal topography. Milano, Italy: AIM Congress srl - AIM Group. September 2001. http://www.refractiveonline.com/eng/pages/edition.aspx?anno=2001. Accessed date August 8, 2011.
94. Mattioli R. Corneal topography and wavefront analysis. In: Caimi R, Brancato R, eds. *The Aberrometers*. Milan, Italy: Fabiano; 2003:113-132.
95. Mattioli R, Frondizi S, Rubeo A, Saldutti M. The *Keratron* Scout and wavefront analysis. In: Caimi F, Brancato R, eds. *The Aberrometers*. Milan, Italy: Fabiano; 2003:243-257.
96. Marcos S. Aberrations and optical quality of the eye: what the clinician needs to know In: Caimi F, Brancato R, eds. *The Aberrometers*. Milan, Italy: Fabiano; 2003:15-26.
97. Tripoli NK. The Zernike polynomials. In: Caimi F, Brancato R, eds. *The Aberrometers*. Milan, Italy: Fabiano; 2003:51-64.
98. Howland H, Buettner J, Applegate R. Computation of the shapes of normal corneas and their monochromatic aberrations from videokeratometric measurements. Vision science and its applications. *Technical Digest Series*. 1994;2:54-57.
99. Hemenger RP, Tomlinson A, Oliver K. Corneal optics from videokeratographs. *Ophthalmic Physiol*. 1995;15:63-68.
100. Schwiegerling J, Greivenkamp JE. Using corneal height maps and polynomial decomposition to determine corneal aberrations. *Optom Vis Sci*. 1997;74:906-916.
101. Marcos S. Aberrations and visual performance following standard laser vision correction. *J Refract Surg*. 2001;17:596-601.
102. Marcos S, Barbero B, Llorente L, Merayo-Lloves J. Optical response to LASIK for myopia from total and corneal aberrations. *Invest Ophthalmol Vis Sci*. 2001;42:3349-3356.
103. Artal P, Guirao A, Berrio E. Compensation of corneal aberrations by the internal optics in the human eye. *J Vision*. 2001;1:1-8.
104. Artal P, Berrio E, Guirao A, Piers P. Contribution of the cornea and internal surfaces to the change of ocular aberrations with age. *J Opt Soc Am A*. 2002;19:137-143.
105. Artal P, Guirao A, Contributions of the cornea and the lens to the aberrations of the human eye. *Optics Letters*. 1998;23:1713-1715.
106. Guirao A, Gonzalez C, Redondo M, Geraghty E, Norrby S, Artal P. Average optical performance of the human eye as a function of age in a normal population. *Inv Ophth Vis Sci*. 1999;40:203-213.

107. Guirao A, Artal P. Corneal wave aberration from videokeratography: accuracy and limitations of the procedure. *J Opt Soc Am A.* 2000;17:955-965.
108. Malacara D. *Optical Shop Testing.* 2nd ed. New York, NY: John Wiley & Sons; 1992:472-488.
109. Thibos LN, Applegate RA, Schwiegerling JT, Webb RH, VSIA Standards Taskforce Members. Standards for reporting the optical aberrations of eyes, vision science and its applications. *OSA Trends in Optics & Photonics.* 2000;35:110-130.
110. Thibos LN. Wavefront data reporting and terminology. *J Refract Surg.* 2001;17:S578-S583.
111. Thibos LN, Hong X, Bradley A, Cheng X. Statistical variation of aberration structure and image quality in a normal population of healthy eyes. *J Opt Soc Am A.* 2002;19:2329-2348.
112. Smith S. *Digital Signal Processing,* 2nd ed. San Diego, CA: California Technical Publishing; 1999.
113. Bonci P. Decentramenti in chirurgia rifrattiva. In: Buratto L, Picardo V, eds. *Focal Points su Chirurgia Refrattiva.* Canelli, Italy: Fabiano; 2003:11-25.
114. Arbelaez MC. Early work shows safety and efficacy. *Ophthalmology Management.* 2003:56-58.
115. Rummelt V. Selective corneal wavefront diagnosis and excimer laser treatment for vision improvement. *Highlights of Ophthalmology.* 2003;31(5):27-30.
116. Siganos D. Quality of vision improved with ORK-W system. *Euro Times.* May 16, 2003. http://www.escrs.org/eurotimes/May2003/quality.asp. Accessed August 8, 2011.
117. Munnerlyn CR, Koons J. Photorefractive keratectomy: a technique for laser refractive surgery. *J Cataract Refract Surg.* 1988;14:46-52.
118. Gatinel D, Hoang-Xuan T, Azar DT. Determination of corneal asphericity after myopia surgery with the excimer laser: a mathematical model. *Invest Ophthalmol & Vis Sci.* 2001;42:1736.
119. Mattioli R, Camellin M. La aberrometria corneale ed il link topo aberrometrico. In: Camellin M, ed. *LASEK and ASA.* Canelli, Italy: Fabiano; 2004:231-253.
120. Risoldi U, Venturini S, De Nicolò N. RGP contat lenses Horus e topografo corneale, una soluzione integrata, moderna ed efficace. *Professional Optometry.* 1996;8:32-41.
121. No7 Contact Lenses. *No7 Contact Lenses: Why Topography? Video.* http://www.no7contactlenses.com/index.php?option=com_hdflvplayer&Itemid=241&title=No7-Contact-Lenses:-Why-Topography?&compid=1&id=2&page=1. Accessed August 15, 2011.
122. Garcia D, Barsky B, Bolles B. *The OPTICAL Project at UC Berkeley: Computer Aided Cornea Modeling and Visualization.* 1996. http://www.eecs.berkeley.edu/~ddgarcia/optical/SIGGRAPH96_ET.html.
123. Manganotti A, Pedrotti E, Sbabo A. RGP contact lenses custom made links with topographical apex saving in keratoconus. Our experience and comparison with traditional lenses. *EuVision.* 2004:6-13.
124. Manfredini M. L'evoluzione applicativa delle lenti a contatto RGP: dalle lenti a contatto su misura tradizionali, alle LAC Custom Made realizzate mediante link informatico con topografo corneale *EuVision.* 2003:8-14. http://www.manganottioculista.it/Area_Professionisti/1%20APPLICAZIONE%20LAC%20e%20LENTI%20SPECIALI/3%20LAC%20CUSTOM-MADE%20da%20topografia%20corneale.pdf. Accessed August 8, 2011.
125. Manfredini M. Corneal topography in contact lens practice. In: Soper JW, ed. *A Comprehensive Study and Reference Guide.* Vol I. Herndon, VA; Contact Lens Society of America (CLSA); 2003:397-408.
126. Maller K. Using CAD/CAM lenses for orthokeratology. *Review of Contact Lenses.* 2004:16-20.
127. Linton G. Software increased one OD's RGP fit. *Contact Lens Spectrum.* 2000:60.
128. Brown K. Focal points: the power of computing in GP lens design and manufacturing. *Boston Update North American Edition.* 2005;16:4-9.
129. Stojanovic A. LaserSight alternatives in topography-based custom ablation. In: Wang M, ed. *Corneal Topography in the Wavefront Era: A Guide for Clinical Application.* Thorofare, NJ: SLACK Incorporated; 2006:146-154.
130. D'souza HM, Sarver EJ, Wakil YS, inventors; Eyesys Technologies Inc, assignee. Method of corneal analysis using a checkered Placido apparatus, US patent 5841511; November 24, 1998.
131. Liu DD, Santiago D, Wu L, et al. Irregular astigmatism: LaserSight ellipsoid model and topography-driven aspheric treatment. In: Wang M, ed. *Irregular Astigmatism Diagnosis and Treatment.* Thorofare, NJ: SLACK Incorporated; 2007:195-209.
132. Bueeler M, Mrochen M, Seiler T. Maximum permissible lateral decentration in aberration sensing and wavefront guided corneal ablation. *J Cataract Refract Surg.* 2003;29:257-263.
133. Stojanovic A, Suput D. Strategic planning in topography-guided ablation of irregular astigmatism after laser refractive surgery. *J Refract Surg.* 2005;21(4):369-376.
134. Bueeler M, Mrochen M, Seiler T. Maximum permissible torsional misalignment in aberration sensing and wavefront guided corneal ablation. *J Cataract Refract Surg.* 2004;30:17-25.
135. Falavarjani KG, Hashemi M, Modarres M, Sanjari MS, Darvish N, Gordiz A. Topography-guided vs wavefront-optimized surface ablation for myopia using the WaveLight platform: a contralateral eye study. *J Refract Surg.* 2011;27(1):13-17.
136. Cummings AB, Mascharka N. Outcomes after topography-based LASIK and LASEK with the WaveLight Oculyzer and Topolyzer Platforms. *J Refract Surg.* 2009:1-8.
137. Jankov MR, Panagopoulou SI, Aslanides IM, Hajitanasis GI, Pallikaris GI. Topography-guided treatments with WaveLight ALLEGRETTO WAVE for irregular astigmatism. *J Refract Surg.* 2006;22(4):335-344.
138. Cummings AB, Mascharka N. Outcomes after topography-based LASIK and LASEK with the WaveLight Oculyzer and Topolyzer Platforms. *J Refract Surg.* 2009;Sep 2:1-8.
139. Kanellopoulos AJ, Pe LH. Wavefront-guided enhancements using the WaveLight excimer laser in symptomatic eyes previously treated with LASIK. *J Refract Surg.* 2006;22(4):345-349.
140. González Pérez J, Cerviño A, Giraldez MJ, Parafita M, Yebra-Pimentel E. Accuracy and precision of EyeSys and Orbscan systems on calibrated spherical test surfaces. *Eye Contact Lens.* 2004;30(2):74-78.
141. McMahon TT, Anderson RJ, Joslin CE, Rosas GA; Collaborative Longitudinal Evaluation of Keratoconus (CLEK) Study Topography Analysis Group. Precision of three topography instruments in keratoconus subjects. *Optom Vis Sci.* 2001;78(8):599-604.
142. McCarey BE, Zurawski CA, O'Shea DS. Practical aspects of a corneal topography system. *CLAO J.* 1992;18(4):248-254.
143 Wang L, Koch DD. Corneal topography and its integration into refractive surgery: application in refractive surgery. *Medscape Reference Web site.* http://www.medscape.com/viewarticle/504198_2. Accessed February 25, 2011.
144. Fung MW, Raja D, Fedor P, Kaufman SC. Corneal topography and imaging. *Medscape Reference Web site.* http://emedicine.medscape.com/article/1196836-overview. Accessed February 25, 2011.

# Chapter 6

# Tomographers

## The Bausch & Lomb Orbscan II/IIz Anterior Segment Analysis System

Paul M. Karpecki, OD, FAAO

The Bausch & Lomb Orbscan II/IIz Anterior Segment Analysis system (Rochester, NY; Figure 6-1) performs a complete anatomical analysis of the anterior segment of the eye. The system combines 2 technologies: a calibrated video and scanning slit-beam system that measures anterior segment geometry and an advanced Placido disk system that measures the curvature of the anterior surface of the cornea.

During an examination, the patient fixates on a blinking light source, which is coaxial with a calibrated video imaging system. The video imaging system performs 40 scans through light slits projected at a 45-degree angle. In two 0.75-second periods, 20 slits are projected sequentially on the eye from the left and right sides of the video axis. The 5-mm central zone of the cornea is sampled twice, once in each direction, through these overlapping slits, as illustrated in Figure 6-2. Before the slit scans, an additional image is captured using the Placido rings.

The Orbscan performs noninvasive measurements of thousands of points on 4 surfaces of the anterior segment of the eye: the anterior cornea, posterior cornea, anterior iris, and anterior lens. An example of a raw image is shown in Figure 6-3. The system measures 9600 points (240 from each of the 40 slits). These point measurements are used to construct mathematical representations of the true topographic surfaces of the anterior segment, including maps of elevation (z) versus horizontal and vertical (x and y) coordinates. The mathematical surface representations, which typically have continuous second-order derivatives, are used to calculate slope and curvature at any point and in every direction. A tracking system measures involuntary eye movement and is used to accurately assemble the mathematical surface representation from the 40 slit images. The resulting calculations are used to describe 4 elements of the anterior segment: anterior and posterior corneal elevations, corneal power, and corneal thickness. Keratometric power is calculated using a standard keratometric index.

The Orbscan system acquires, analyzes, and presents the calculated data. Displays use a color scale to show relative elevations, providing a 3-dimensional view of surface topography. In all elevation maps, green is the reference surface, or zero level. Red is high, positive, and anterior to the reference surface, while blue is low, negative, and posterior to the reference surface. A commonly used view of surface topography is the quad map, which presents anterior elevation, posterior elevation, corneal power, and pachymetry maps in one view. Figure 6-4 is a quad map showing typical with-the-rule astigmatism. In this figure,



Wang M. *Corneal Topography: A Guide for Clinical Application in the Wavefront Era, Second Edition* (pp. 103-160)

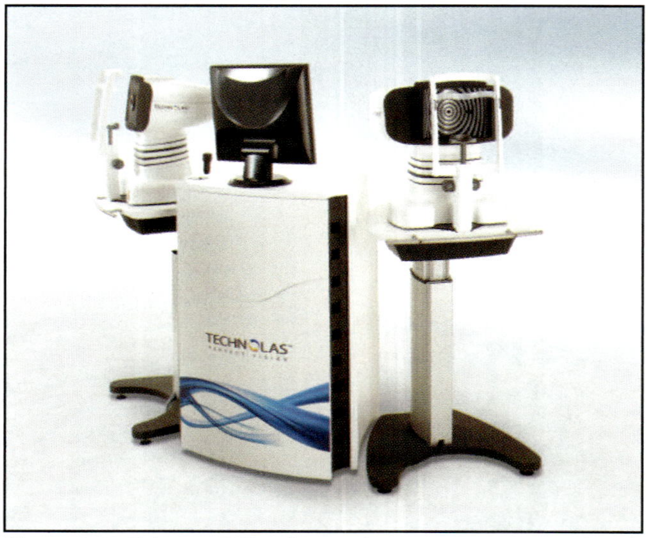

**Figure 6-1.** Orbscan II/IIz diagnostic systems. (Reprinted with permission of Bausch & Lomb.)

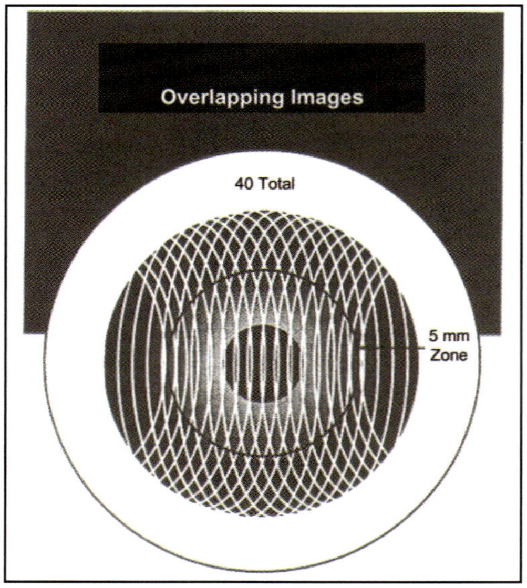


**Figure 6-2.** Slit scans used for data acquisition.

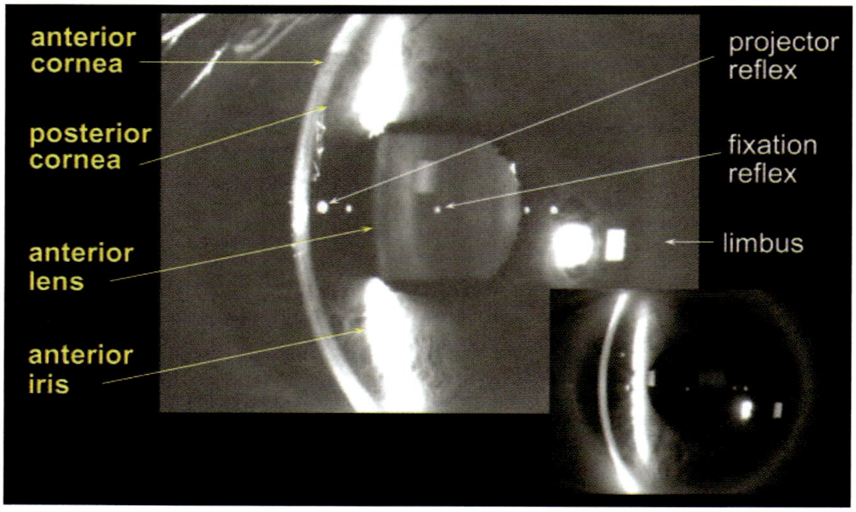


**Figure 6-3.** Structures of the anterior segment analyzed by Orbscan include the anterior cornea, posterior cornea, anterior lens, and anterior iris. (Reprinted with permission of Bausch & Lomb.)

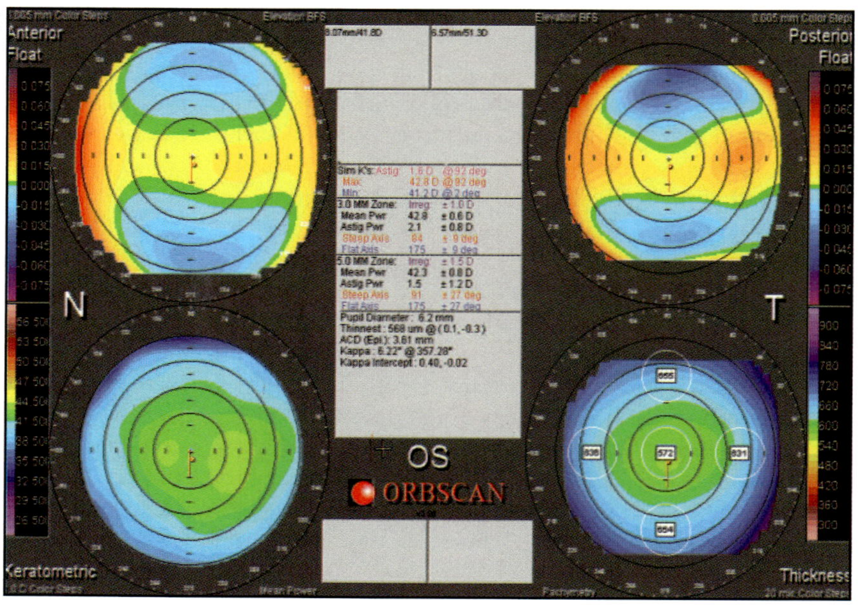


**Figure 6-4.** Orbscan quad map showing typical with-the-rule astigmatism. (Reprinted with permission of John Vukich, MD.)

the anterior corneal float (elevation) appears in the upper left corner, and the posterior float appears in the upper right corner. Keratometric topography is shown in the lower left, and corneal thickness is shown in the lower right.

# Theory of Measurement

The Orbscan system uses hybrid measurement technology. Specular reflection from a Placido disk is used to calculate the surface curvature of the cornea by measuring the specularly reflected image of a set of concentric mires. Slit scanning is used to measure the anterior segment geometry; its basic measurement is the absolute elevation of optical surfaces. These curvature and elevation measurements are combined to develop accurate maps of absolute anterior and posterior surface elevation and pachymetry. Curvature is displayed as a keratometric power.

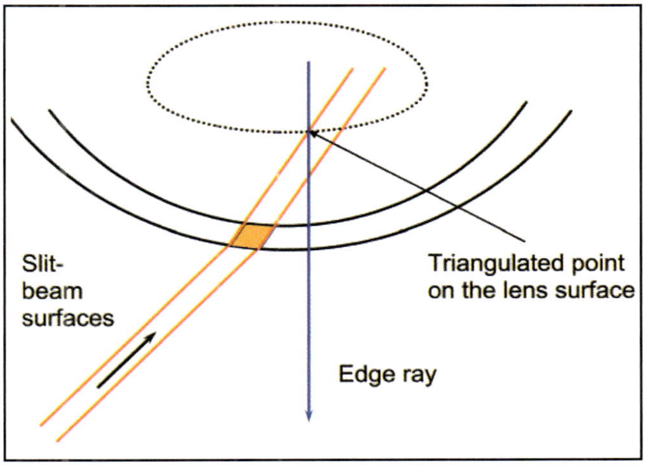


**Figure 6-5.** Orbscan raytrace triangulation. (Reprinted with permission of Bausch & Lomb.)

## Diffuse Reflections

When a slit beam intercepts an optically smooth surface, it is split into a specular reflection and a refracted beam that penetrates the surface and is volume scattered by internal scattering centers. Like surface diffuse reflection, volume scattering is omnidirectional. This important property allows surface points to be independently observed and triangulated and gives Orbscan the capability to measure arbitrary surface shapes—convex or concave, aspheric or irregular. Volume (or diffuse) scattering is typically negligible from liquids such as the tear film and aqueous humor because the constituent molecules are very small compared to the illuminating wavelength. In contrast, volume scattering is significant from the lens, the iris, and the cornea. For that reason, Orbscan sees through the tear film and captures the image of the diffusely scattered light from the corneal volume that is directly illuminated by the slit beam.

Because typical internal scatters are generally smaller than the wavelength of visible light, the magnitude of scattering is inversely proportional to the third or fourth power of the optical wavelength (Rayleigh scattering: $\lambda^4$ for spherical particles, $\lambda^3$ for cylindrical fibers). As a consequence, the diffusely scattered return consists of the shortest wavelengths found in the interrogating beam (the reasons that Tyndall reflections from the cornea appear blue). Calculations of the beam and ray refraction depend on the physiologic refractive indices of the various ocular tissues and humors. Orbscan assumes that the standard physiologic refractive index of air is 1.000; aqueous is 1.336; and cornea is 1.376.

## Triangulation of Complex Surfaces

Triangulation is required to map complex surfaces, such as those of the anterior eye. Raytrace triangulation is required to accurately locate internal surface points when they lie behind an optical interface that refracts the slit beams and the conjugate image rays. The planar slit beam, diffusely reflected from the convex corneal shell, appears as an annular arc in the video image. The outer and inner edges of this arc correspond to the anterior and posterior surfaces of the diffusely reflected volume, shown in Figure 6-5.

To locate a point on the anterior surface, an outer edge point is first detected to sub-pixel accuracy. From the video calibration, the detected edge point is then translated into its conjugate 3-space ray. An example is shown in Figure 6-6. This ray is represented mathematically as:

$$y = U + Vr$$

where the (x, y, z) vector U defines the ray origin at the principle/nodal point of the camera optics; the vector V defines its direction; and the scalar r specifies the distance of a ray point from the origin.

Direct triangulation is used to locate points on the external surface of the cornea. In direct triangulation, a ray is intersected with the calibrated outer surface of the illuminating slit beam. This surface can be mathematically represented as:

$$S(\mathbf{x}) = 0$$

where the vector **x** represents the (x, y, z) coordinates of any valid point on the outer beam surface. Direct triangulation finds r such that S(U + Vr) = 0.

Surfaces are triangulated one at a time, from front to back. Thus, all of the refracting surfaces in front of a desired surface point are known *a priori* and can be used to calculate all the necessary refractions.

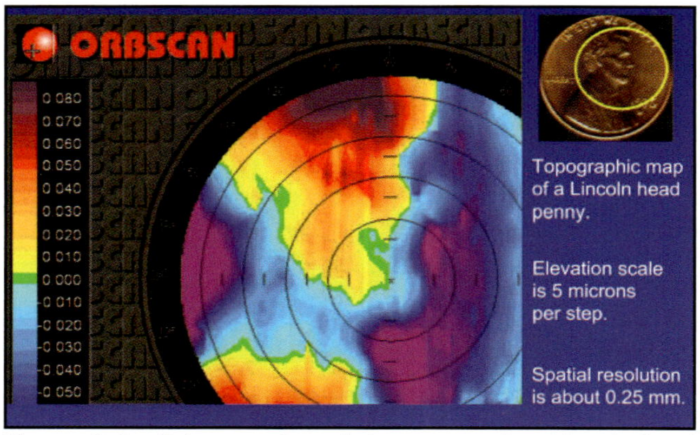


**Figure 6-6.** Orbscan triangulation map of a Lincoln-head penny (area in yellow circle is mapped). (Reprinted with permission of Bausch & Lomb.)

# Foundation for Analysis

## The Measurement of Topography

The Orbscan system's analysis produces a set of data describing the true topographic surfaces of the anterior and posterior cornea, the anterior iris, and the anterior lens. All other measures and displayed maps are derived from these true 3-space surfaces. This approach was taken because it avoids the pitfalls of high- and low-frequency noise generated by numerical transformation.

All numerical transformations generate noise. Mathematic extraction of curvature from elevation (differentiation) generates high-frequency noise, while the transformation required to deduce elevation from curvature or slope (integration) generates low-frequency noise. Although high-frequency noise is more apparent, low-frequency noise is more difficult to deal with; in addition, the most important optical aberrations are low-frequency. Consequently, direct measurement of elevation and computation of curvature were the methods selected to extract the geometric information of optical surfaces in Orbscan.

Another advantage of directly measured topography is that it facilitates surface analysis and display from other points of view. Like other corneal measurement systems, Orbscan aligns with the fixation-reflex axis of the eye, which is appropriate when examining optical properties in the visual zone. However, in contact lens fitting and other procedures in which the apical shape of the cornea is important, the viewpoint should be aligned with the axis of best symmetry of the anterior surface. This alignment can be easily and accurately achieved by rotating the directly measured topographic surfaces in physical space.

## Fixation-Reflex Alignment

During data acquisition with Orbscan, the eye is aligned by having the patient fixate on a blinking light source that is coaxial with the video system while the operator aligns the fixation light reflex with the instrument axis. As slit-scan technology is relatively insensitive to misalignment of the eye, some misalignment is expected. Following data acquisition, the system determines the properly aligned fixation-reflex axis and places it at the center of the map. This fixation-reflex alignment ensures that the map center is always a point of stationary elevation with zero surface slope; for convex surfaces, this point is always a local maximum. Thus, the local surface normal at the map center is aligned with the map axis. This form of alignment is crucial for determining many relative properties that are axis-based, such as axial and tangential curvature. Because the fixation-reflex axis is very sensitive to surface inclination, refractive surgery will almost always alter this axis; for this reason, standard alignment of a postoperative eye is unlikely to coincide exactly with the preoperative alignment.

## Surface Rotation

Surfaces measured by Orbscan can be rotated to any other point of view by selecting a view center, which becomes the surface point that is rotated to the map center. The view axis is automatically chosen to be coincident with the local surface normal. Because 3-dimensional rotations are not commutative, the meridional orientation of a rotated view generally depends on all the rotations that preceded it. To eliminate the ambiguity that order dependency might create and to ensure that the rotated meridians are as close as possible to the standard alignment meridians, all surface rotations are computed as simple single-axis rotations from the standard alignment position, which is always centered on the fixation-reflex axis.

## Relative Versus Absolute Properties

Relative properties depend on the alignment, size, and shape of a reference object; when the reference object changes, so does a relative measure. In contrast, absolute properties are intrinsic properties of the surface and are not alignment dependent; they are measured directly from the surface. Only absolute measurements can identify true ocular landmarks, such as optical axes. Although absolute properties are superior, most properties are relative by their nature. In Orbscan, both relative and absolute properties are mapped, as described in Table 6-1.

# Geometric Analysis

## Elevation

Looking at an irregular corneal surface is like looking at the mountains and valleys of the earth. When drawn to scale, the mean curvature of the earth overwhelms even the most significant topographic features. Hills and valleys are only apparent if elevation is shown with respect to the mean sea level. Similarly, corneal irregularities can only be

TABLE 6-1.

## Preview of Relative and Absolute Properties

| GEOMETRIC OR OPTICAL PROPERTY | TYPE | REFERENCE OBJECT (PARAMETERS) |
|---|---|---|
| Surface topography | Complete | |
| Normal elevation (floating alignment) | Relative | Surface (size and shape) |
| Normal elevation (axis alignment) | Relative | Axis + surface (size and shape) |
| Axial elevation | Relative | Axis + surface (size and shape) |
| Slope | Relative | Axis |
| Mean and astigmatic curvatures | Absolute | |
| Irregular curvature | Absolute | (Aperture size) |
| Axial pseudo-curvature | Relative | Axis |
| Tangential and sagittal curvatures | Relative | Axis |
| Axial thickness and depth | Relative | Axis |
| Normal thickness and depth | Absolute | |
| Optical power | Relative | Axis |
| Normal power | Absolute | |

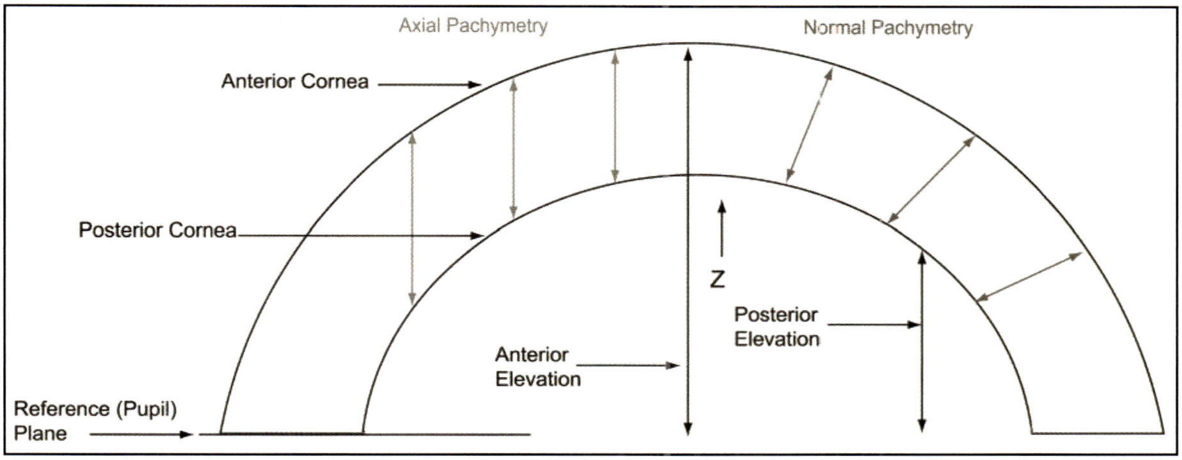


**Figure 6-7.** True elevation, also known as topographic elevation, is the perpendicular distance Z of a point on the cornea from the system reference plane. (Reprinted with permission of Bausch & Lomb.)

seen after a reference surface is mathematically removed. Changes in the reference surface, like changes in sea level, can dramatically affect the perceived topography of the corneal landscape, while its true topography (z as a function of x and y) remains unchanged. Figure 6-7 illustrates true elevation, also known as topographic elevation. It is the perpendicular distance Z of a point on the cornea from the system reference plane. True elevation data are used to determine pachymetry.

A reference sphere may be oriented with a surface in 3 different ways: floating, axial, or pinned, demonstrated in Figure 6-8. Floating alignment minimizes the surface fit error with no additional constraints. Axial and pinned alignments each add one additional constraint (indicated below by the X in Figure 6-8). Axial alignment forces the sphere center to lie on the view axis, while pinned alignment forces the sphere surface to include the view center. Axial pinned alignment employs both constraints.

The advantage of displaying elevation with respect to a best-fitting sphere is that a sphere is rotationally symmetric, and thus it is completely described by its radius and center. Unfortunately, corneal surfaces are not spherical. To view elevation asymmetries with respect to the axisymmetric surface that fits the cornea no matter what its shape, it is

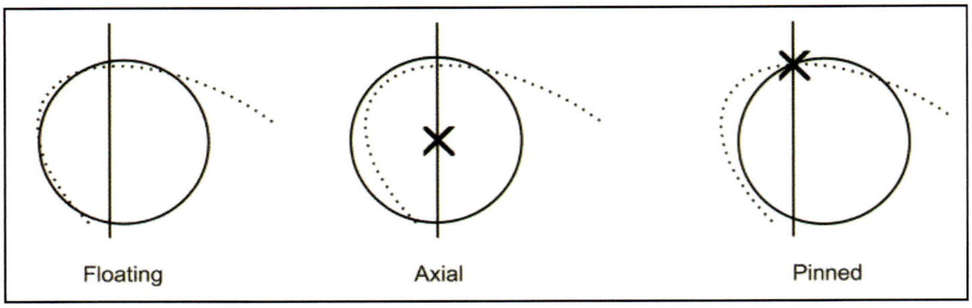


**Figure 6-8.** Reference sphere orientation. (Reprinted with permission of Bausch & Lomb.)

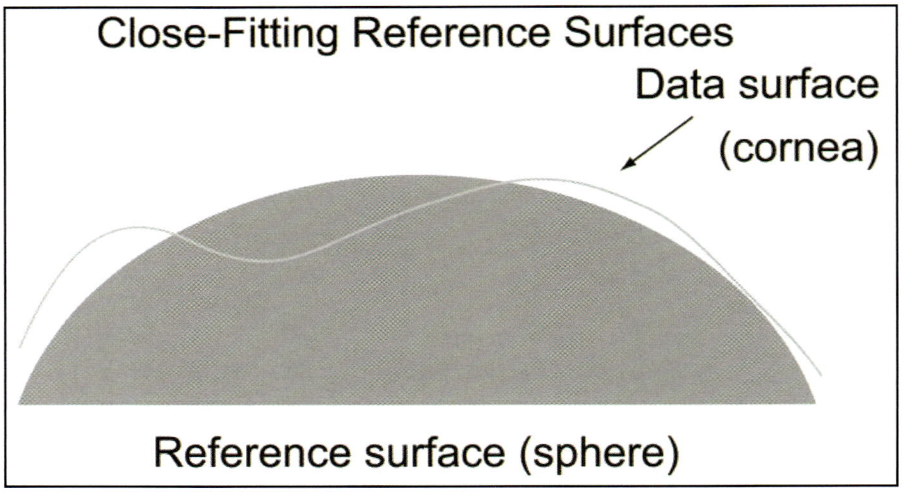


**Figure 6-9.** Close-fitting reference surfaces. (Reprinted with permission of Bausch & Lomb.)

necessary to select a rotor reference surface (Figure 6-9). The name *rotor* is derived from its method of construction, which is to find a surface of revolution by spinning the data surface around the view axis. A rotor (without modifiers) is the mean surface of revolution. The high rotor (or low rotor) is the surface of revolution lying just above (or below) the data surface. Orbscan setup options and parameters that affect the relative elevation of a single topographic surface include surface rotation from the instrument axis; reference surface type (plane, sphere, cone, or rotor); reference surface size, shape, and alignment (floating, axial, or pinned); and elevation direction (normal to the reference surface or axially directed).

## Pachymetry

Corneal thickness is calculated as the distance from the anterior to the posterior surface, in the direction perpendicular to the anterior surface. Orbscan pachymetry calculations have been correlated with manual ultrasound pachymetry; in general, Orbscan determinations of corneal thickness are several percent thicker than ultrasound measurements of the same corneas. Orbscan pachymetry measurements can be automatically converted to their acoustic equivalent values; the correlation factor can be set individually for each Orbscan system. The refractive surgeon can overlay the intended radial and astigmatic keratotomy (RK and AK) cuts on any Orbscan anterior corneal map. The values of minimum corneal thickness are shown on each incision.

## Anterior Segment and Chamber Depths

The anterior chamber depth (ACD) from the posterior cornea to the anterior lens or iris is calculated differently as the straight-line axial distance between anterior chamber surfaces. Anterior chamber volume is easily determined by integrating this distance across the cornea. In addition, the rate of change of this distance in radial directions can be used to estimate the anterior angle.

## Surface Slope and Surface Curvature

Surface slope measures the rate of change of surface elevation in a particular direction. Determination of the radially directed slope of the corneal surfaces is important in contact lens fitting and in the implantation of intracorneal rings for refractive correction. Surface curvature measures the bending (or rate of change of slope, or second derivative) intrinsic to a curve or a surface. Because curvature is inversely related to radius of curvature, a small radius sphere has a large curvature.

Surface curvature can be described as cutting the surface of an object with a plane and then fitting a circle to the plane intersection. The inverse radius of the circle gives the surface curvature in the direction of the plane. Obviously, the value measured is highly dependent on the orientation of the cutting plane. Every surface point has an infinite number of surface normal planes, each containing the local surface normal, but each cutting the surface in a

TABLE 6-2.

**Assumed Refractive Indices and Typical Spherical Curvatures**

| OCULAR SURFACE | INDEX TYPE | POSTERIOR INDEX | CURVATURE (GEOMETRIC) | CURVATURE (DIOPTERS) |
|---|---|---|---|---|
| Keratometric cornea | Standard keratometric | 1.3375 | 128 1/m | 43.2 D |
| Anterior cornea | Physiologic | 1.376 | 128 1/m | 48.1 D |
| Posterior cornea | Physiologic | 1.336 | 149 1/m | – 6.0 D |
| Anterior lens | Physiologic | 1.425 | 98 1/m | 8.7 D |

different direction. Thus, every point on a smooth surface has a direction-dependent curvature, whose complete description is captured by a mathematical object known as a tensor. Orbscan calculates the complete curvature tensor field from the derivatives of the fitted topographic surfaces. From this tensor field, the curvature at any surface point and in any direction can be directly calculated.

A theorem of differential geometry states that every point on a smooth surface has a minimum and a maximum curvature (called principle curvatures), which lie in perpendicular surface normal planes. Thus, the curvature at any smooth surface point can be completely specified by 3 independent quantities: the minimum and maximum (principle) curvatures and their direction. Two curvatures at a point in nonprinciple directions do not contain sufficient information to construct the complete curvature tensor.

Curvature of an optical surface is directly related to the focusing power of a normally incident bundle of light rays. Because of this property, curvature is often expressed in diopters (D; the unit of optical power) and is often referred to as power, which is a potential cause of confusion. Orbscan emphasizes the distinction between curvature and power by exclusively reserving the name *power* for optical properties. Curvature, whether expressed in standard geometric units (inverse meters, 1/m) or radius of curvature units (millimeters, mm), or scaled by D, is always called *curvature* by Orbscan.

Three concepts are important in understanding Orbscan's mapping of surface curvature. First, curvature applies only to a single surface. In contrast, optical power is generally calculated for a sequence of surfaces (always beginning with the anterior cornea). Second, surface curvature is not single-valued, but direction-dependent. A complete specification of curvature requires 3 values: the 2 principle curvatures and their orientation. As a color contour map (without overlays) can only show the variation of one value, many different curvature maps are used to display combinations of the 3 principle values in useful ways. These maps are grouped into 2 families: absolute local curvatures (mean, astigmatic, and irregular) and relative axis-based curvatures (axial, tangential, and sagittal). The third concept important to understanding Orbscan maps is that curvature expressed in D is proportional to an assumed refractive index difference. The assumed index difference may be physiologic (the real value averaged over the population), or it may be invented (eg, the standard keratometric index). Table 6-2 lists the assumed posterior indices (air = 1) for each optical surface in the anterior segment, together with their typical curvatures, expressed in both geometric and D units. Note that the curvature (in D) of the posterior cornea is negative, not because the geometric curvature is negative, but because the interfacial index difference is negative ($\Delta n$ = -0.040 = 1.336 – 1.376). The standard keratometric index is applicable only to the anterior cornea. When so applied, the anterior cornea is referred to as the keratometric cornea.

## Mean and Astigmatic Curvature

Mean curvature is a measure of absolute local sphericity. A local sphere is the one that best fits a point and its surface derivatives. The inverse radius of this sphere is an absolute measure of the local spherical component of curvature. Because it is absolute, mean curvature is intrinsic to the surface and is independent of surface alignment. Absoluteness is important in the diagnosis of certain corneal diseases like keratoconus, as it ensures that any geometric abnormality will appear as it exists. Hence, keratoconus appears as a symmetric local maximum because the mean curvature of a cone increases toward its apex.

Maps of mean curvature display the variation of local sphericity. Thus, the mean curvature of a normal cornea is typically very uniform, even when its astigmatism is significant. Mean curvature typically filters out global astigmatism in favor of the local spherical component. As a rule, any residual astigmatism seen in a mean curvature map is greatly reduced and rotated 90 degrees from the real astigmatism. To see the local axes of astigmatism, the principle directions overlay is used.

Astigmatic curvature is a measure of absolute local cylinder. Astigmatic curvature typically filters out the global spherical component in favor of astigmatism or local cylinder. As maps of astigmatic curvature display the variation of local cylinder, an eye with regular astigmatism will have a fairly uniform astigmatic map. The bow-tie pattern typically associated with astigmatism and seen in axis-based maps (eg, axial, tangential, and sagittal curvatures) is not physical, but is really an artifact of the measurement.

## Irregular Curvature

A normal but ametropic eye with regular astigmatism is correctable with spherocylindrical spectacles. Surface irregularity includes the curvature variation of an optical surface that cannot be corrected with a spherocylindrical lens, thereby producing an uncorrectable loss in visual acuity.

As the mean and astigmatic curvature maps of a normal eye are fairly uniform, the variation of these curvatures is a measure of surface irregularity. Irregular curvature is the statistical combination of the standard deviations of the mean and astigmatic curvatures, measured over a local aperture (typically, 1 mm in diameter). Surface irregularity caused by incisional keratotomy (such as the RK artifact) is recognizable in maps of irregular curvature.

## Axial, Tangential, and Sagittal Curvatures

Axial, tangential, and sagittal curvatures are relative properties measured with respect to the arbitrary view axis. Because the measurement directions radiate from or encircle this axis, these axis-based maps always contain a conspicuous axial artifact, the familiar bow-tie pattern seen in Figure 6-10. The direction of this artifact effectively locates the meridians of astigmatism, but only with respect to the view axis.

Unlike absolute curvature, which is a property of the surface and requires no reference object, axis-based curvature maps change dramatically when their axis is repositioned. Axis-based maps also distort corneal abnormalities, like keratoconus, making it impossible to locate the true conical apex.

The curvature of an aligned sphere is correctly determined by any of the axis-based curvatures and the mean curvature (which gives the correct value even when the sphere is off center). Axial curvature, however, is not a true measure of curvature but is a spherical equivalent not applicable to aspheres or to asymmetric surfaces. Tangential and sagittal maps, although true measures of curvature, do not contain sufficient information to construct the complete curvature tensor, except for the special case of aligned axisymmetric surfaces.

# Theory of Optical Analysis

## Optical Power

Optical power is defined as the posterior refractive index divided by the posterior focal length: $P = \frac{n_2}{f_2}$ (Figure 6-11, left panel). Light rays, originally parallel to an arbitrary power axis, are refracted by both surfaces of the cornea and are brought to focus on the power axis, which is also refracted. The refractive index is included in the definition so that power measured in either direction is the same. Optical performance can be calculated from topographic surface data when the material refractive indices are known (see Table 6-2).

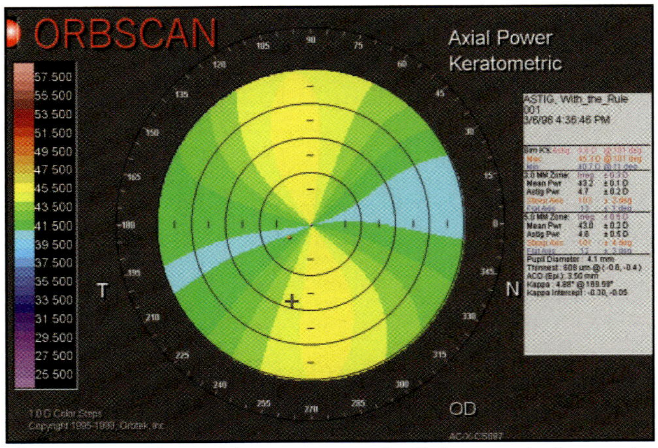


**Figure 6-10.** The axial power map in Orbscan, similar to the sagittal map from Placido systems, produces its image using only the Placido rings. (Reprinted with permission of Bausch & Lomb.)

Peripheral rays are brought to a shorter focus than central paraxial rays. This is illustrated in Figure 6-11. This spherical aberration is apparent in optical power maps of the cornea, which show increasing power peripherally. When astigmatism is present, the familiar bow-tie pattern will also be seen. This pattern arises from the interaction of light, collimated along the line of sight, with a smooth optical surface or sequence of surfaces. Optically, the bow-tie pattern is real, while geometrically it is an artifact.

## Normal Power

Normal power is a measure of the normally incident mean focusing power of a sequence of surfaces, beginning with the anterior cornea (see Figure 6-11, right panel). Unlike optical power, which is a relative property defined with respect to some arbitrary power axis, normal power is an attempt to define an optically relevant absolute measure.

Normal power can be calculated locally for any point on the anterior corneal surface by orienting a ray pencil (a tight bundle of paraxial rays) initially perpendicular to the point of interest. The ray pencil is mathematically propagated through the specified surface sequence and the mean paraxial focus calculated. The normal power is calculated from the mean focal length.

Because the normal power of an anterior surface point is independently calculated, neither a common focal point nor power axis exists. However, when the optical power axis is aligned to the local surface normal, normal power

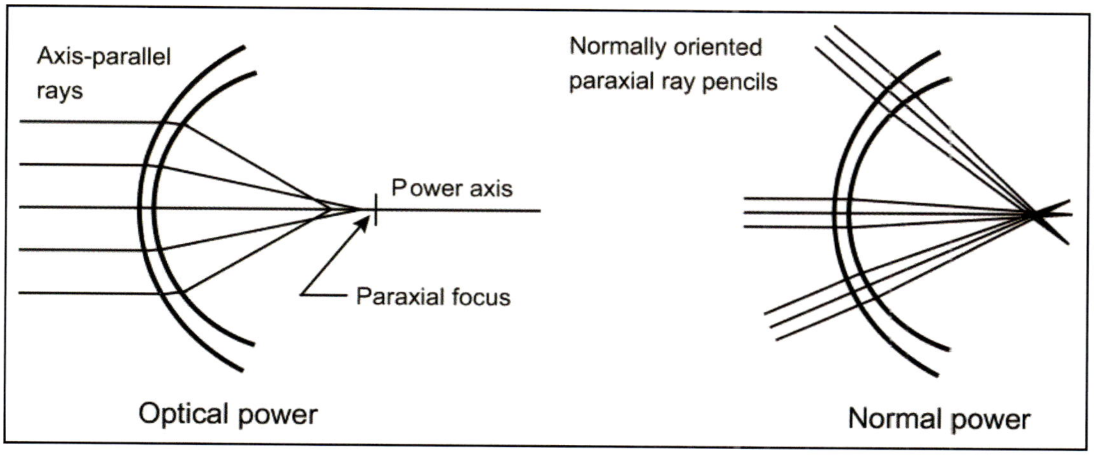


**Figure 6-11.** Optical power and normal power. (Reprinted with permission of Bausch & Lomb.)

and paraxial optical power are equivalent. Hence, normal power is the paraxial portion of optical power as seen from any point on the cornea.

## Optical Axes

An optical axis can be defined for any 2 surfaces by the alignment of a point source and its 2 catoptric images. Thus, an optical axis is the refracted light ray oriented perpendicular to both surfaces. In tilted optical systems, like the human eye, the optical axis is not a straight line, but is bent or curved by refraction occurring between the 2 defining surfaces.

Normal pachymetry and normal anterior segment depth are both distances measured along the refracted light ray that is initially perpendicular to the anterior corneal surface. Maps of these quantities each show a local extreme, which locates a 2-surface optical axis. The local minimum in corneal thickness is the origin of the corneal optical axis, as defined by its anterior and posterior surfaces. Similarly, the local maximum in anterior segment depth is the origin of the anterior optical axis, as defined by the anterior cornea and lens.

Both of these optical axes lie close to the traditional optical axis of the eye, which is defined by the confluence of the 4 Purkinje images. However, because 4 images cannot generally be brought into alignment, the traditional axis is undefined for many eyes. When the traditional axis exists, it is coincident with both the corneal and anterior segment optical axes, which always exist.

# Ocular Landmarks Used by Orbscan

In general, a surface center is any well-defined point on a surface—usually the anterior cornea. A landmark center is any uniquely defined physical or optical point of the eye, whereas a reference center is defined by the arbitrary reference object employed. Fixed centers are points on ocular surfaces that rotate with the eye and any reference objects, whereas movable centers are dependent on the rotational point of view (eg, entrance pupil center). Nine centers used by Orbscan are defined in Table 6-3. The tabulated accuracy reflects the theoretical precision with which these centers can be calculated from a set of topographic surfaces.

# Optical Surface Irregularity

*Irregularity* is a statistical term that describes the variation of values in a data set. Optical surface irregularity is proportional to the standard deviation of surface curvature. As applied to the Orbscan, it is a spatial variation in curvature, quantified as the statistical combination of the standard deviations of the mean and toric curvatures. Irregularity is calculated for a specific area using the following formula:

$$\text{Irregularity} = I = [(\sigma(\bar{\kappa}))^2 + (\sigma(\Delta\kappa))^2]^{1/2}$$

where

$\sigma$ = standard deviation

$\bar{\kappa}$ = mean curvature = $\frac{\kappa_1 + \kappa_2}{2}$

$\Delta\kappa$ = toric curvature = $|\kappa_1 - \kappa_2|$

$\kappa_1$ and $\kappa_2$ represent the principle curvatures

The Orbscan system calculates irregularity using the following method. First, initial parameters are set using default values that can be changed in an initialization file. The beginning default pupil diameter is 3 mm, and the increment for increasing the diameter is 2 mm. With these settings, there are 4 possible irregularity zones on the pupil (3, 5, 7, and 9 mm). Next, the algorithm defines the sampling rules for each zone. Nine concentric rings are defined in the 3-mm zone; each ring is divided into segments using a formula to ensure uniform sampling density (eg, the center ring has 3 segments, the second ring has 9 segments, the third has 15 segments, etc.) The center point of each segment is defined. In the third step, the algorithm calculates all of the map zone statistics at each center point, including the principle and mean, toric curvatures, etc. Then, the

Table 6-3.

### Ocular Landmarks (Surface Centers) Used by Orbscan

| Surface Center | Definition | Type | Accuracy | Map mark (typically white) |
|---|---|---|---|---|
| Fixation reflex | Corneal reflex point of a fixating patient, measured by a coaxial optical system and corrected for acquisition misalignment | Fixed landmark | High | Oblique cross, x |
| Pachymetry minimum | Anterior corneal point with minimum normal thickness; defines the 2-surface optical axis of the cornea | Fixed landmark | Low | C |
| Anterior segment maximum | Anterior corneal point with maximum normal anterior segment depth; defines the 2-surface optical axis of the anterior cornea and lens combination | Fixed landmark | Low | S |
| Anterior corneal apex | Geometric center of the cornea, or the location where the axis of best anterior symmetry intersects the anterior surface | Fixed landmark | Low | Triangle |
| Entrance pupil | Physical pupil of the eye imaged through the cornea. Its center is taken to be the geometric centroid of the pupil image | Movable landmark | Medium | Dot |
| Sphere center (of an axisymmetric reference object) | View-axis projection of its apical center of curvature | Movable reference | Exact | Circle |
| View center | Point at which the view axis pierces the surface; placed at the map center in standard alignment | Movable reference | Exact | Black cross (map center) |
| Summit | Highest surface point measured with respect to the current view axis; placed on the view center (and therefore at map center) in standard alignment of a convex surface | Movable reference | High | |
| Instrument or system center | Point at which the instrument axis (defined by the video camera) pierces the data surface; if located on the unrotated anterior cornea, is a measure of acquisition misalignment | Fixed reference | High | |

algorithm calculates the standard deviation of these values for the first zone and applies the formula for calculating irregularity. These calculations are repeated for each zone.

Optical surface irregularity is proportional to the standard deviation of surface curvature. Consequently, only axis-independent surface curvatures are used in the calculation, as only they are true surface properties. These include the mean curvature, which is a measure of local surface sphericity, and astigmatic curvature, which is a measure of local cylinder. As both curvature variations are important, the standard deviations of the mean and astigmatic curvature are statistically combined (their variances are added) to yield the irregularity in standard curvature units (reciprocal meters). Curvature in reciprocal meters can be converted to D by multiplying it by the surface refractive index difference, which is 0.3375 for the keratometric surface. Thus, the D equivalent of irregularity is about one-third the curvature measure in reciprocal meters.

## Clinical Implications of Irregularity Calculations

Optical surface irregularity is important to the refractive surgeon because it often represents a loss in best-corrected visual acuity (BCVA). Regular astigmatism has a low irregularity, while irregular astigmatism has a high degree of irregularity. Higher-order aberrations (HOAs) may also have a high degree of irregularity. Measures of irregularity may also be useful as a supporting indicator (but not the sole indicator) in evaluating keratoconus. A 3-mm

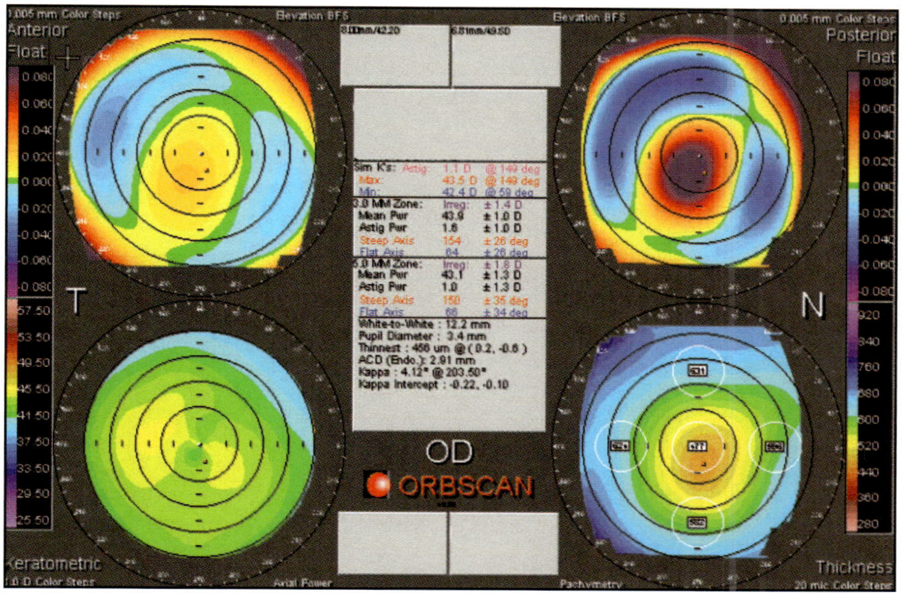


**Figure 6-12.** This Orbscan quad map shows a posterior float of approximately 0.063 D, a strong red flag for forme fruste keratoconus or pellucid marginal degeneration (PMD). (Reprinted with permission of John Vukich, MD.)

irregularity greater than 1.5 or a 5-mm irregularity greater than 2.0 may be an early sign of keratoconus, while a 3-mm irregularity greater than 2.0 or a 5-mm irregularity greater than 2.5 may indicate full keratoconus. Irregularity cannot be corrected with spherocylindrical lenses or with current surgical techniques.

# Clinical Examples

## Risk of Ectasia

One of the most frequent uses of Orbscan is in the screening of patients for LASIK surgery. The risk of ectasia can be accurately assessed using 5 indices: the number of abnormal maps using the normal band scale, a variance of more than 1.00 D in astigmatism between the eyes, keratometric or corneal steepness on the mean power map, a posterior surface float greater than 0.05 D (the difference between the highest and lowest spots; Figure 6-12), 3-mm and 5-mm irregularity (Figure 6-13), and a minimum peripheral corneal thickness that is not at least 20 μm greater than the thickness of the central cornea (Figure 6-14).

Figure 6-12 shows a posterior float of approximately 0.063 D, indicated by the dark reddish color near the center of the posterior elevation map (upper right). A posterior float greater than 0.050 raises a strong red flag for forme fruste keratoconus or pellucid marginal degeneration (PMD) and confirms the diagnosis if supported by other maps and measurements. Note that when the posterior float is greater than 0.050, posterior elevation is rarely the only abnormal map. In this example, the pachymetry map shows a significant irregularity in corneal thickness, with a central area whose thickness is only approximately 0.050 mm—2 indices suggesting that LASIK may not be appropriate for this patient.

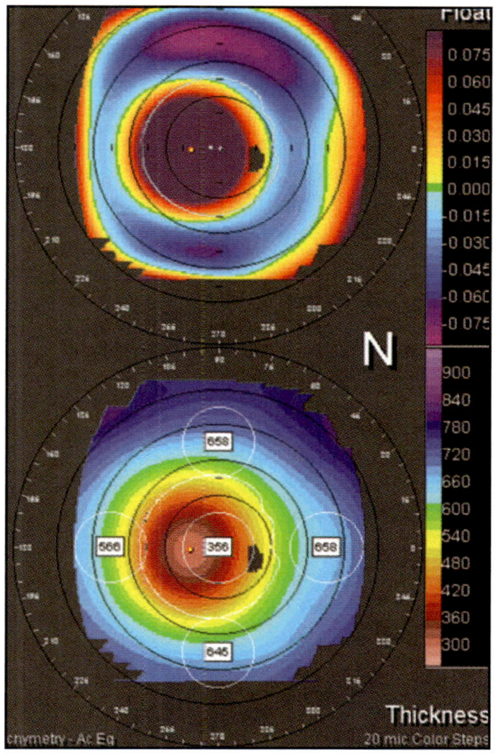


**Figure 6-13.** This Orbscan quad map shows surface irregularity of 2.1 D in the 3-mm zone and of 2.2 D in the 5-mm zone, suggesting the clinician look for other signs, such as the number of abnormal maps or a posterior float greater than 0.050 mm (50 μm).

Figure 6-13 shows surface irregularity of 2.1 D in the 3-mm zone and of 2.2 D in the 5-mm zone, indicated by the circled scores in the gray area in the center of the screen. It does not indicate forme fruste keratoconus in and of itself

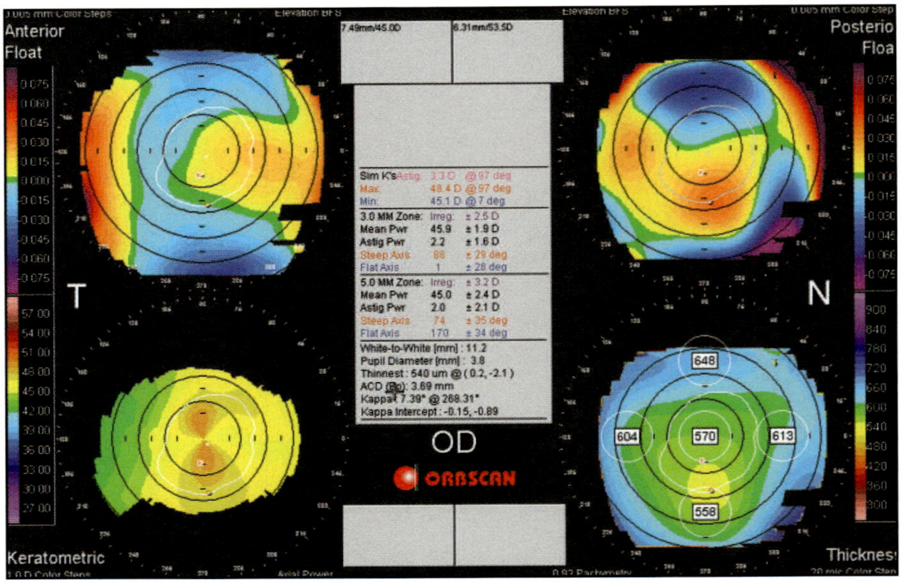


**Figure 6-14.** In the pachymetry map at the lower right corner of this quad map, the thinnest area is 30 µm thinner than the central cornea.

but raises suspicion to look for other signs, such as the number of abnormal maps or a posterior float greater than 0.050 mm (50 µm). Irregularity at 3.00 and 5.00 mm may simply indicate the presence of HOAs without pathology, so this index should only be used in conjunction with other findings to diagnose keratoconus.

In the pachymetry map, shown in Figure 6-14, the lower left corner of this quad map, the thinnest area is more than 30 µm thinner than the central cornea (marked in red). Peripheral pachymetry measurements in which the peripheral cornea is not at least 20 µm thicker than the central cornea may be a sign of keratoconus, which should be corroborated with other observations. Another potential source of concern is a cornea in which the thinnest point is outside the central 5 mm of the cornea.[1]

One abnormal map on the Orbscan normal band scale does not usually indicate forme fruste keratoconus, but requires patient education or having the patient return for monitoring of changes in 6 to 12 months. Two abnormal maps may indicate early keratoconus; or, if the posterior float is abnormal with a slightly thinner cornea (less than 500 µm), 2 abnormal maps may still indicate keratoconus depending on other variables described in this chapter. If a patient has 2 abnormal maps but no indication of forme fruste keratoconus, surface ablation would likely be a better procedure than LASIK for this patient. Three or more abnormal maps is a contraindication to corneal surgery and often indicates a high risk of post-LASIK ectasia.[2]

A difference of more than 1.00-D cylinder between the eyes or increasing cylinder over time is also a risk factor for keratoconus that can be detected with the Orbscan.[3] Because keratoconus is known to be an asymmetric condition, one eye usually progresses faster than the other.[4] A higher risk of keratoectasia is also suggested by a K reading of more than 46.00 D at the steepest point on the Orbscan keratometric mean power map.

## Anterior Chamber Map

The anterior chamber map, which shows the depth of the anterior chamber, can be useful in surgical planning for phakic intraocular lenses (IOLs). The endothelial anterior map (Figure 6-15) shows the true available space. This map is likely to grow in its usefulness in the future as the use of phakic IOLs increases.

## Post-LASIK Follow-Up

Approximately 1 month following LASIK, the Orbscan system may be used to assess problems such as dry eye and corneal edema and to map the change in corneal shape as a reference for an enhancement procedure. Earlier than 1 month, reflections from the recovering tear film or corneal edema may produce an Orbscan reading that incorrectly suggests ectasia.

## Dry Eye and Corneal Edema

Dry eye that continues for more than 1 month after LASIK can be evaluated in a distinctive Orbscan map, shown in Figure 6-16. Note the irregularity on the keratometric mean power map as well as the significant missing data points. These anomalies confirm that the maps are not reliable. After artificial tears were instilled, the images were normal. An Orbscan map with irregularity on the anterior elevation map and thinning on pachymetry are indicators of dry eye.[5]

Corneal edema also produces a distinctive Orbscan map (Figure 6-17). The specular reflection from corneal edema might be interpreted as Descemet's layer, and, therefore, the edema will often look similar to a case of ectasia.

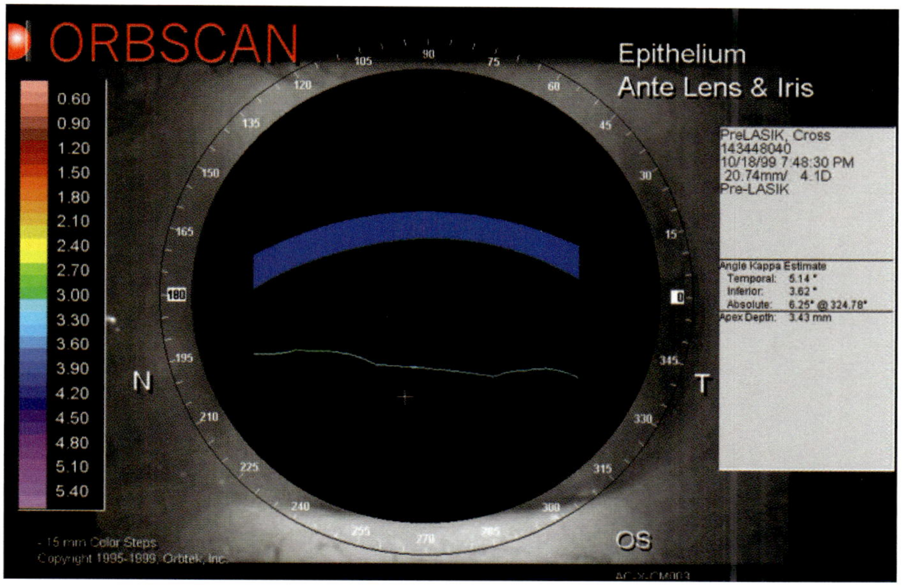


**Figure 6-15.** The endothelial anterior chamber map shows the depth of the anterior chamber.

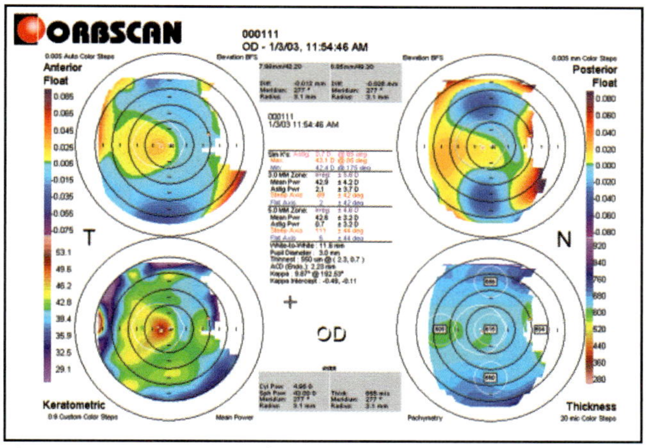


**Figure 6-16.** Post-LASIK dry eye.

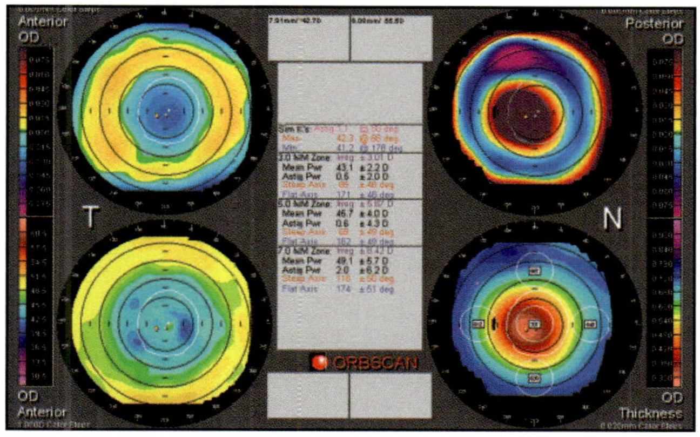


**Figure 6-17.** Post-LASIK corneal edema. (Reprinted with permission of Dan Durrie, MD.)

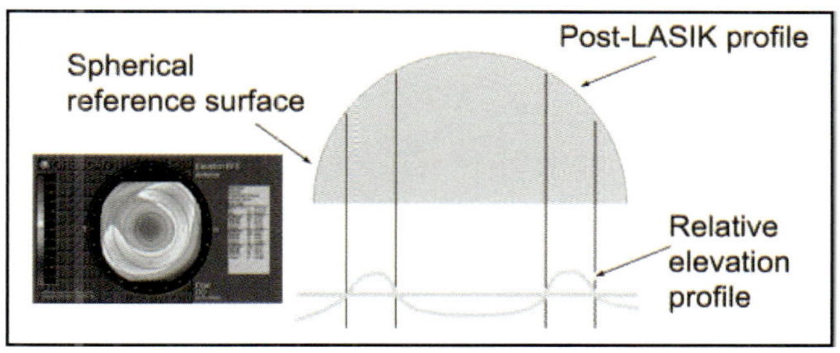


**Figure 6-18.** Corneal topography S/P myopic LASIK. (Reprinted with permission of John Vukich, MD.)

## Post-LASIK Enhancement Planning

LASIK surgery results in significant changes to the corneal surface geometry (Figure 6-18). The blue areas in the center and at the edges of the Orbscan map show the changes in the cornea that result from LASIK, including a flattening of the center and sides of the cornea with respect to the reference sphere. Although the map appears to show that the cornea is concave, this is not the case; the depression in the center of the cornea is lower than the reference sphere, but not lower than the outer corneal edges. A 3-dimensional Orbscan map of the post-LASIK cornea provides the surgeon with a means to visualize the cornea and determine an enhancement strategy when an enhancement procedure is desired.

## Pellucid Marginal Degeneration

PMD is a rare form of corneal ectasia, with an arcuate band of corneal thinning in the inferior cornea. The Orbscan system can be used in the diagnosis of patients with this disorder. PMD typically presents with topography similar to Figure 6-19. Note the classic kissing birds appearance in the bottom left keratometric axial map, as well as the extreme peripheral elevation on the anterior and posterior floats (upper right and left maps). Note also that the steepest part of the cornea is located more inferiorly in PMD, and the axial topography shows a bending of the bow-tie pattern. The keratometric mean map shows a localized inferior corneal steepening, especially in the peripheral areas.

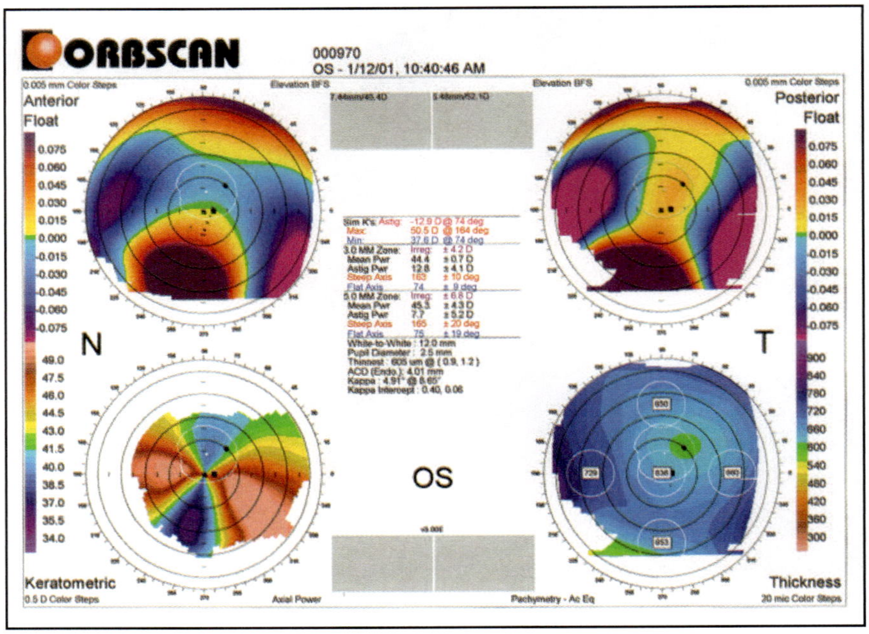


**Figure 6-19.** PMD. (Reprinted with permission of Tim Cavanaugh, MD.)

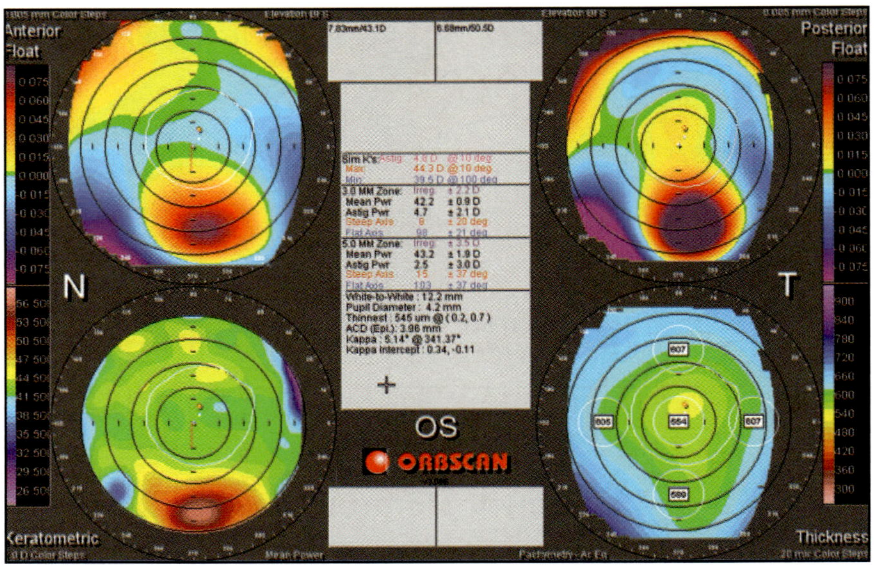


**Figure 6-20.** Keratoconus.

## Keratoconus

Diagnosis of keratoconus is facilitated by the use of Orbscan maps, which show the magnitude and location of corneal thinning and protrusion (Figure 6-20). Orbscan maps can also be used to detect early keratoconus (which always appears initially on the posterior surface) and document the progression of the disorder. Note the normal pachymetry map and the irregularity in the 3- and 5-mm zones and the deeper cone on the posterior surface. The mean power map shows Ks in the inferior cornea greater than 54 D. Indices for the detection of keratoconus are described above, in the discussion of the risk of post-LASIK ectasia.

## Raytrace Analysis as a Diagnostic Tool

Raytrace analysis can calculate optical properties even more informative than power. The retinal point spread function (PSF) is the retinal image of a point of light. It contains all the information needed to reconstruct what the patient sees. The PSF describes how an object point is aberrated (spread out) in the retinal image. PSF size and shape indicate the ocular aberration. In an emmetropic, unaberrated eye, the image is concentrated at one point. In an astigmatic eye, the image takes on an elongated shape, while in monocular diplopia, the image is double peaked. Figure 6-21 shows an original picture and a simulated retinal image, produced with the retinal PSF, in a patient with monocular diplopia.

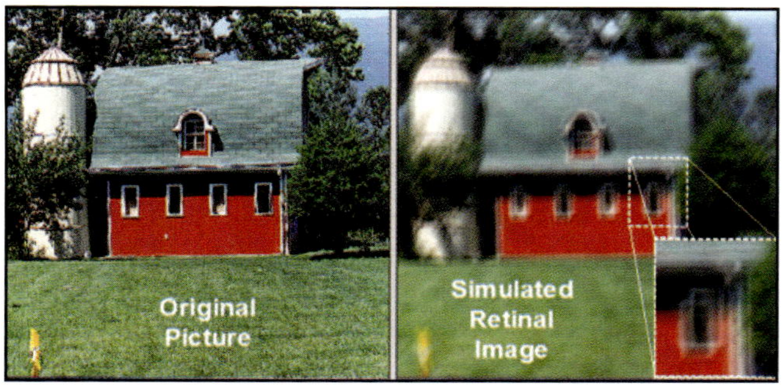


**Figure 6-21.** Reconstruction of patient's view of an object using retinal PSF in raytrace analysis. (Reprinted with permission of Bausch & Lomb.)

The patient complained of double vision, halo, and night driving difficulties, but only for the left eye. Raytrace analysis through the anterior corneal surface did not reveal any visual impairment. When both corneal surfaces were raytraced, the left eye showed several ghost images, which are associated with the posterior corneal surface. An analysis of posterior elevation maps showed that each eye had a posterior cone, but the off-axis eccentricity of the OS cone resulted in the optical aberrations reported by the patient. Retreatment was not undertaken because of concern that it would increase the posterior ectasia and the associated visual impairment.

### Orbscan Diagnostics and Wavefront Technology

A unique aspect of the Bausch & Lomb Zyoptix Diagnostic Workstation is that it combines wavefront aberrometry information with data from the Orbscan system. This allows for potential greater data capture and potential optimal results based on those data. Taking into consideration variables such as pachymetry and the new placement of 2- to 1-mm laser flying spot placement are factors that allow the Zyoptix system to be one of the few systems that is tissue paring when moving from conventional to wavefront. Furthermore, it is becoming apparent that wavefront data can also enhance topography diagnostic capabilities. In a study reported by Pepose,[6] posterior float signs of ectasia noted on the Orbscan Diagnostic System were differentiated from PMD and keratoconus based on wavefront data. Patients with PMD tended to have higher degrees of peripheral aberrations on the Zywave system including trefoil, whereas patients with keratoconus tended to have higher degrees of coma. Combining the Wavefront data with the Orbscan data will enhance diagnostic capabilities and wavefront data, potentially improving outcomes.

## Conclusion

This section has described the Bausch & Lomb Orbscan Anterior Segment Analysis System, focusing on the principles underlying its measurement and analysis technology. The Orbscan system provides unique tools for the refractive surgeon to use in the evaluation and diagnosis of visual disorders of the anterior segment.

## Acknowledgment

The author thanks Barry Eagan, Director, Optical Systems Design & Numerical Analysis, Bausch & Lomb, Rochester, NY for his assistance in the development of this section.

# *OCULUS PENTACAM*

Stephen S. Khachikian, MD and Michael W. Belin, MD, FACS

With the increased popularity of refractive surgery and the high success rates for corneal transplantation, there has been an increasing need to understand corneal contour. Computerized corneal topography has advanced our knowledge of the complex corneal surface beyond what was previously possible with earlier examination equipment. Traditional computerized corneal analysis relied on the processing of a Placido-type reflected image. This precludes obtaining data from the posterior corneal surface. True topography implies shape and requires the generation of an x, y, and z coordinate system. Placido-based systems create such a coordinate system from curvature data by making geometric assumptions about the cornea and its position relative to the Placido disk.[7]

There are significant limitations in trying to describe the cornea with a Placido-based curvature map (Figure 6-22). The area of corneal coverage is limited to about 60% of the corneal surface, eliminating important data for many peripheral or paracentral pathologies. Placido maps provide no information about the posterior corneal surface. Without measurement of the anterior and posterior surfaces, pachymetric maps depicting the distribution of corneal thickness cannot be made. Additionally, there are limitations in attempting to

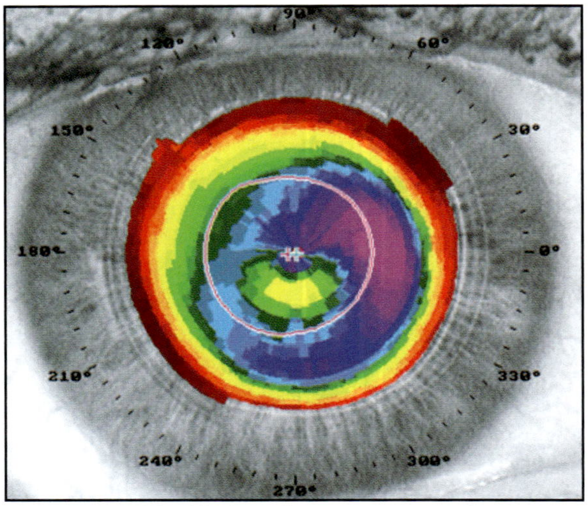


**Figure 6-22.** Placido-based curvature map demonstrating limited corneal coverage.

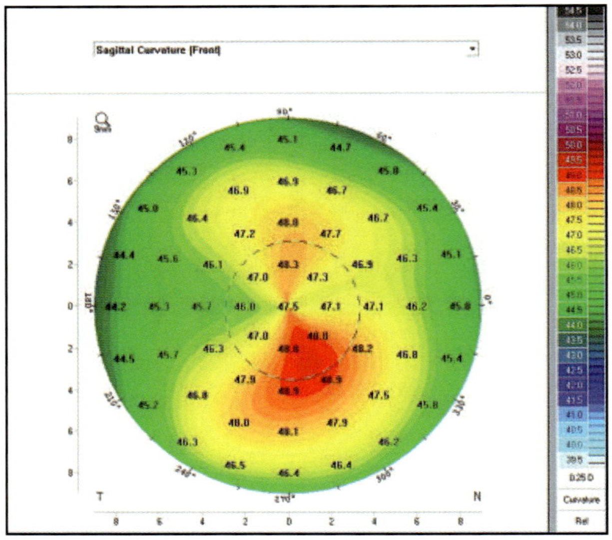


**Figure 6-24.** Pentacam-generated elevation-based curvature map on the same eye as shown in Figure 6-23.

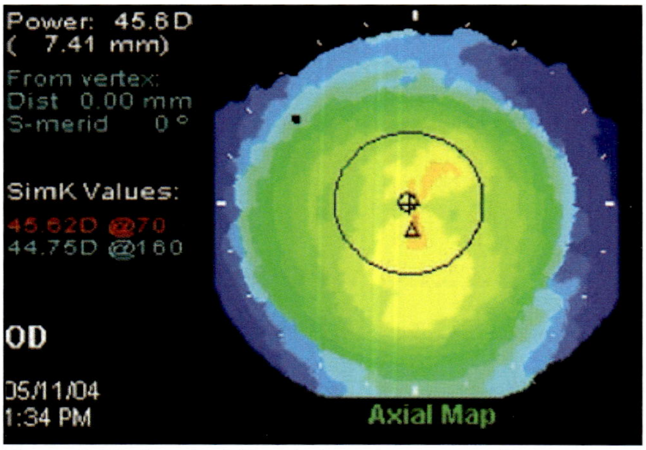


**Figure 6-23.** Standard Placido-based curvature display.

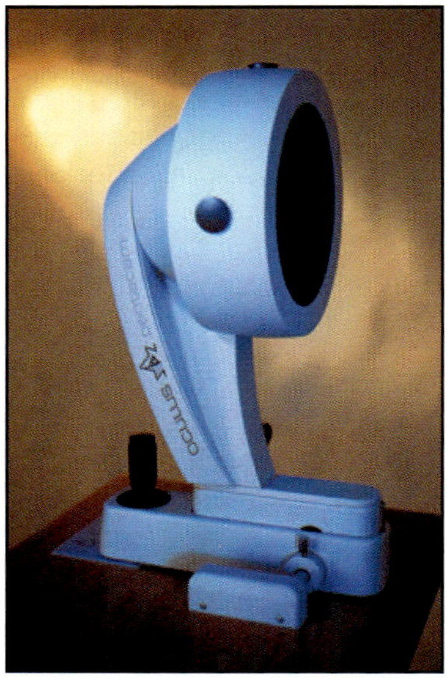

**Figure 6-25.** Pentacam Anterior Segment Analysis System.

reconstruct the corneal surface based on curvature measurements.[8]

The standard topographic curvature (axial or sagittal) is a reference-based measurement (Figure 6-23). It is not a unique property of the cornea. The same shape can have many different "curvatures" depending on which axis is used to make the measurement. Most of us visualize the eye as a Gullstrand-reduced eye, assuming that the eye is symmetric, with the line of sight, visual axis, center of pupil, and corneal apex all crossing at a common point. This, however, is not the case.[9,10] Furthermore, we assume that the measurement axis of the Placido system also coincides. Most people do not look through the center of the cornea. The line of sight and the measurement axis of the videokeratoscope are not the same.[11,12] In contrast to the reflection-based Placido measurement, each elevation system uses a direct triangulation technique to measure the anterior corneal surface. Curvature data are directly calculated from the elevation data using second-order derivatives (Figure 6-24).[13]

The Pentacam Anterior Segment Analysis System (OCULUS, Wetzlar, Germany) is an elevation-based topographer that represents a significant advancement in corneal and anterior segment imaging (Figure 6-25). The Pentacam uses 2 cameras to obtain imaging of the anterior segment. The central camera is used for fixation monitoring and pupil measurement, and the second Scheimpflug camera captures optical cross-sections of the anterior segment.[14]

The Scheimpflug principle, the photographic technique on which the camera is based, was first described in 1875 by Theodore Scheimpflug as a way to minimize distortion in aerial photographs. Scheimpflug photography is an alternative method of capturing images by adding an angle between the lens and the film (Figure 6-26). Scheimpflug cameras capture images with a better spatial accuracy than a traditional camera containing a coaxial lens and film

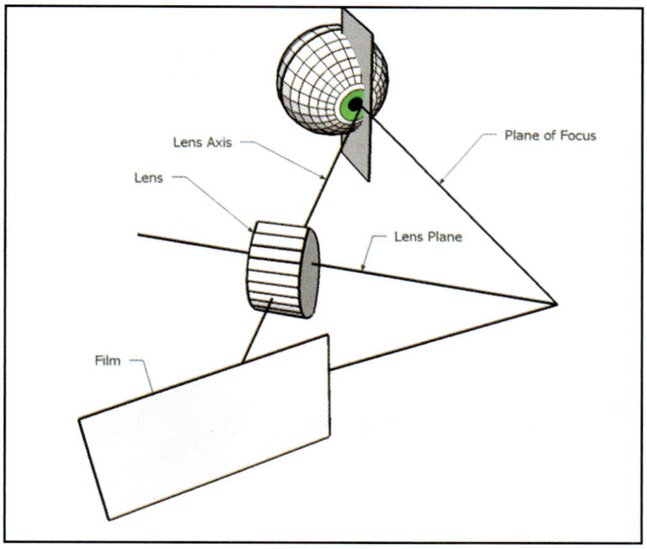


**Figure 6-26.** Diagram of Scheimpflug-generated corneal cross-section, showing plane of focus and lens position.

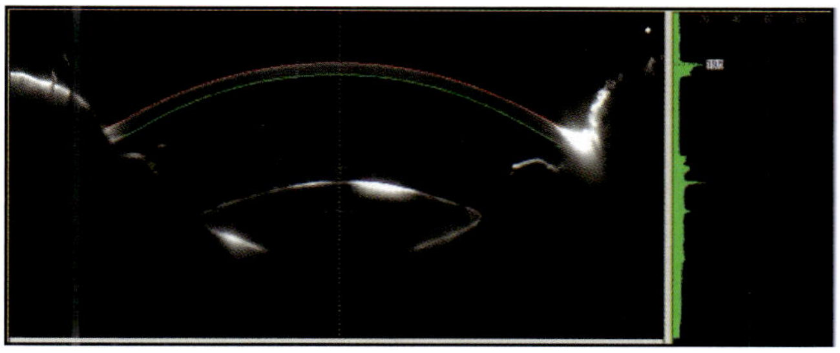

**Figure 6-27.** Pentacam-generated corneal cross-section with edge detection lines.

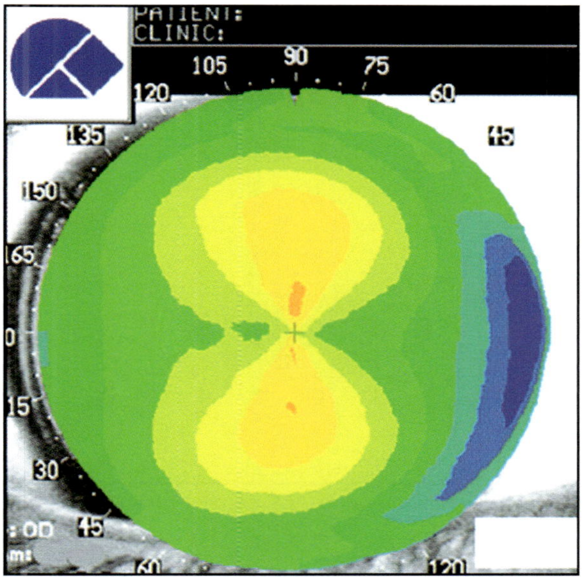


**Figure 6-28.** PAR CTS grid projected onto fluorescein-stained tear film.

optical system. By rotating around the point of fixation, the Scheimpflug system reduces the artifact created by small movements during image acquisition.[15,16] The Scheimpflug camera rotates 360 degrees around a single point of fixation as the patient focuses on a central light source. The camera completes several rotations before coming to a steady speed. It then obtains images over a 2-second period without vibrations and image artifact that might occur during acceleration or deceleration. The slit images are photographed on an angle from 0 to 180 degrees to avoid shadows from the nose. Every picture is a complete image through the cornea in the specific angle, so a real 360-degree image of the anterior segment of the eye is acquired. The camera provides 25 or 50 images during a scan of less than 2 seconds duration. Each image typically contains approximately 500 elevation points, which are then analyzed to yield 12,500 to 25,000 total data points. The images generated by the rotating Scheimpflug camera are used to locate the anterior and posterior corneal surfaces as well as the iris and anterior lens surface. By taking a series of cross-sectional images around a common central point, a 3-dimensional reconstruction of the anterior segment can be created. While the Pentacam is primarily a topography instrument, the cross-sectional Scheimpflug photographs obtained also have clinical importance (Figure 6-27).

The OCULUS Pentacam was neither the first elevation-based corneal analysis system nor the first to use optical cross-sectioning. Elevation-based systems were first reported to have benefits over Placido-based systems in 1991.[13] The PAR CTS used a projection grid system to measure anterior corneal elevation (Figure 6-28). It had advantages over Placido-based systems in that accurate measurements were possible on distorted corneas that could not be fully analyzed by reflective systems and offered complete corneal coverage. The PAR CTS required the instillation of fluorescein onto the tear film for the grid to be viewed and relied on the distortion of the grid pattern to determine elevation by a technique similar to triangulation called *raster-photogrammetry*. Because it was a projection-based system, measurement of the posterior corneal surface or anterior segment was not possible. Optical cross-sectioning was first introduced commercially in the mid 1990s. The Orbscan used parallel segmental cross-sectioning (no shared points) and relied on a Placido image to augment the anterior surface measurements and reportedly to assist in image registration. The rotating system used by the Pentacam offers certain advantages. Because each image shares a common point (center of rotation), image registration should be more accurate (Figure 6-29).

Precise image registration is a prerequisite for accurate topographic data. Because the distance travelled during rotation is less in the center, the point density is greatest in the central cornea and decreases in the periphery. Additionally, the edge detection software on the Pentacam appears less susceptible to corneal haze than the Orbscan, and the system does not suffer from the inaccuracy in locating the posterior corneal surface common to the Orbscan in the acute postoperative cornea.[17]

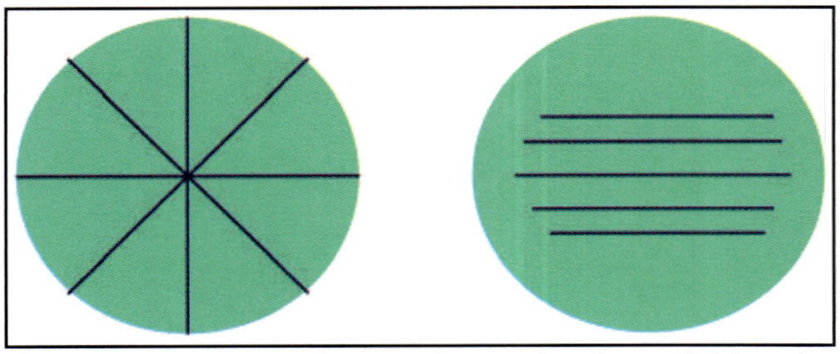

**Figure 6-29.** Diagram showing the overlapping radial imaging of the Pentacam (left) and parallel imaging of the Orbscan (right).

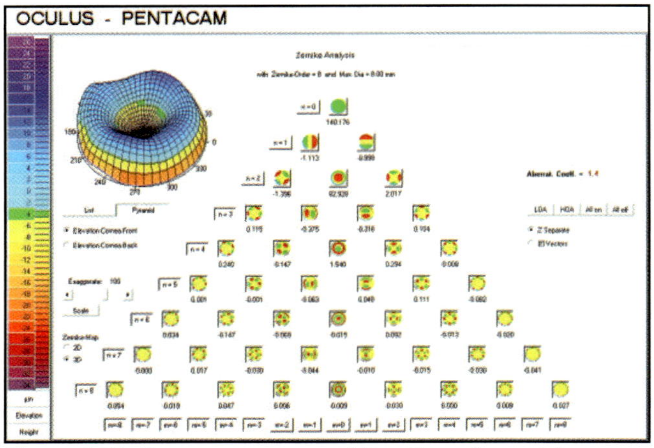


**Figure 6-30.** Pentacam-generated Zernike polynomials.

While primarily designed as a topographic unit, the Pentacam also provides cross-sectional visualization of the cornea and the anterior chamber, as well as an objective lens densitometry assessment. It calculates the pachymetry of the cornea from limbus to limbus with an accuracy of ±5 µm. True elevation measurements allow for computations of anterior and posterior sagittal (axial) and tangential curvature, anterior and posterior elevation maps, ACD measurement, angle approximation, corneal and anterior chamber volumes, and anterior surface-derived Zernike polynomials (Figure 6-30).

## Clinical Applications

Refractive surgical screening is the most common clinical application of the Pentacam. Screening should be rapid, technician friendly, and accurate. The vast majority of patients can be quickly and safely screened with the 4-map refractive display (Figure 6-31). The recommended maps in the composite display include anterior and posterior corneal elevation using a best-fit sphere (BFS), pachymetric distribution, and anterior sagittal curvature. Screening requires consistent scales, colors, and settings to allow the practitioner to rapidly evaluate the preoperative map.

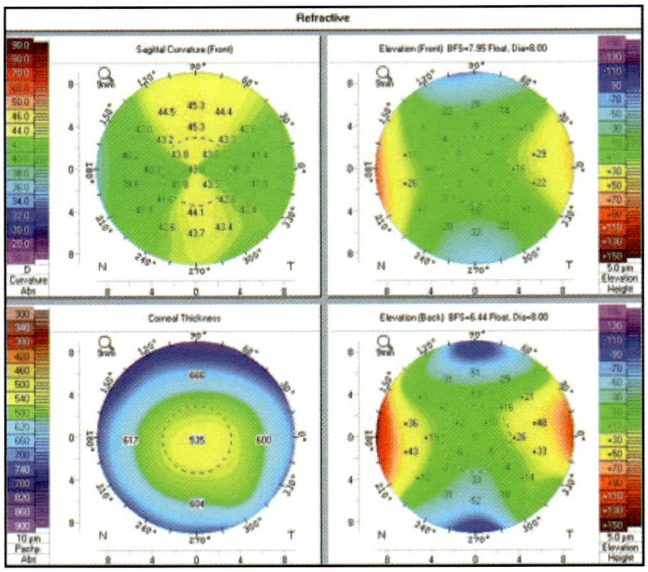


**Figure 6-31.** Four-view refractive display on the Pentacam.

For routine use, it is recommended to use the manual setting with the BFS set to sphere, float, and the diameter set to 8.5 mm. We also suggest that, for routine screening, the overall area of the map displayed on the screen be limited to the central 9.0-mm zone. This does not eliminate the peripheral coverage; it just masks it from the screening view and makes the inspection of the maps easier. When viewing the maps limited to the central 9.0-mm area, a valid map would have no or very minimal extrapolated data. In the authors' experience, in all but markedly abnormal corneas, it is possible to obtain maps free of extrapolated data. For refractive screening, we are dealing with presumed normal corneas, and quality images should almost always be obtained. These settings are chosen to maximize sensitivity and allow for a quick visual screening based on color and pattern recognition. It should be understood that when screening for refractive surgery, the goal is to identify patients who are not "normal." The recommended settings are designed for that purpose.

It is important to realize that what we call an "elevation" map does not really display the actual raw elevation data, but shows the elevation data against some reference surface. The most commonly used reference surface is a BFS. The shape, scales, and colors should be chosen to simplify screening. Different scales, shapes, and color bars may be appropriate for other uses. Others have proposed using a toric-ellipsoid as the base reference surface for screening patients under the premise that a toric-ellipsoid more closely follows the normal prolate shape of the cornea. While this is true (ie, toric-ellipsoid more closely mimics the shape of the cornea), this is exactly opposite of what a functional reference surface should do when screening normal patients. The purpose of the reference surface is to highlight or magnify surface features to allow the clinician to identify things

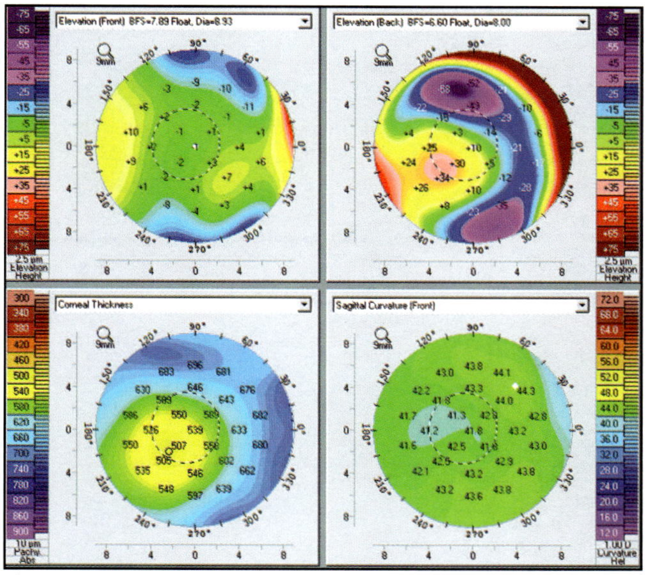

**Figure 6-32.** Four-view refractive display of a cornea with isolated posterior elevation.

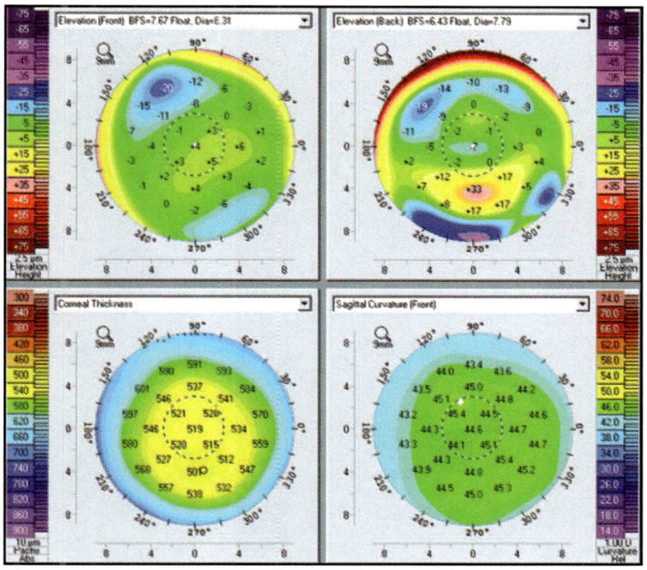

**Figure 6-33.** Four-view refractive display of a cornea showing an abnormal displacement of the thinnest point.

such as astigmatism or conical protrusion (ectasia or keratoconus). A reference surface, such as a toric-ellipsoid, will more closely fit the astigmatic cornea or the conical cornea and will effectively mask the pathology. Keratoconus, for example, is a progressive disorder, the hallmarks of which are stromal thinning, conical protrusion, corneal scarring, decreased spectacle-corrected visual acuity, Fleischer ring, and, in advanced cases, Vogt's striae.[18] The composite screening display outlined previously (see Figure 6-31) has significant advantages for identifying ectatic change.

Figure 6-32 is a 4-view composite map of an asymptomatic patient presenting for refractive surgical evaluation. The map demonstrates the importance of both the posterior corneal surface and the pachymetric distribution map. The patient had 20/20 best spectacle-corrected vision, normal Placido topography, and central ultrasound pachymetry of 540 µm. The Pentacam composite display reveals the limitations of relying on anterior curvature and central corneal thickness measurements alone. The anterior elevation (upper left) and anterior sagittal curvature (lower right) are all normal, both maps displaying a small amount of astigmatism. The pachymetric map (lower left) shows a normal central reading of 539 µm. The pachymetric distribution is significantly displaced, however, where the thinnest region (501 µm) is inferotemporal to the central cornea. The difference between the thinnest reading and the apical reading is 38 µm. The posterior elevation (upper right) is distinctly abnormal. The posterior map shows a well-demarcated, paracentral island of positive elevation (>34 µm) off the BFS representing an ectatic change. The pachymetric distribution also corresponds to the area of posterior elevation, further increasing its significance.

Similarly, the patient depicted in Figure 6-33 would have a completely normal exam if one relied solely on ultrasound pachymetry and Placido-based topography. The sagittal curvature (lower right), the map most commonly displayed on a Placido system, is completely normal. The curvature map is symmetric and shows minimal astigmatism. The simulated keratometry readings are in the mid 40s. Central ultrasound pachymetry readings were 520 µm. All of these values would be considered well within the normal range. This is, however, an incomplete picture. The pachymetric distribution is distinctly abnormal with a marked inferior displacement of the thinnest region. The thinnest area of the cornea is 499 µm, significantly thinner than the central reading. The posterior elevation map shows a well-circumscribed, clearly demarcated, island of positive elevation representing the area of ectatic change. The area of posterior ectasia and the thinnest corneal region coincide. This patient has subclinical keratoconus in spite of normal Placido topography and normal ultrasound pachymetry. The Pentacam clearly reveals the shortcomings of the original incomplete corneal analysis.

## Refractive Screening

While the basis for the development of ectasia may ultimately be a structural, genetic, or biochemical abnormality of the cornea, measurable structural components, such as elevation and pachymetry, should be thoroughly evaluated. With subclinical disease, curvature alone may not provide enough information to detect early corneal abnormality.

The goal of the Belin/Ambrósio Enhanced Ectasia display (Figure 6-34) is to combine elevation-based and pachymetric corneal evaluation in an all-inclusive display. This gives the clinician a global view of the structure of the cornea and allows the physician to quickly and effectively

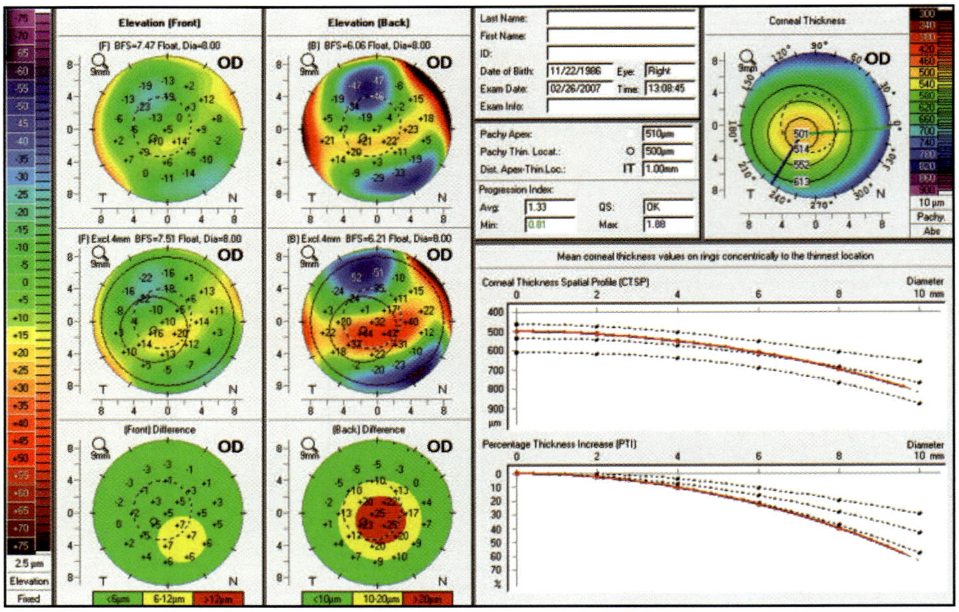


**Figure 6-34.** The Belin/Ambrósio Enhanced Ectasia screening display.

screen patients for ectatic disease. The elevation maps and pachymetric data are placed side-by-side in a comprehensive display. By evaluating these measurements from different perspectives, the ability to identify abnormalities is increased. The elevation and pachymetric components of the display are designed to be complimentary.

The creation of a pachymetric map allows for the identification of the true thinnest point and can contrast the thinnest point with the geometric center of the cornea. In 12% of normal patients, the pachymetry difference between the thinnest point and the geometric center of the cornea is more than 10 μm.[19] The distance between the thinnest point and the geometric central point is significantly higher in keratoconus patients. A reliable pachymetric map is therefore essential for determining the localization and value of the cornea's thinnest point. Along with the thinnest point evaluation, the data from a full pachymetric map enable characterization of the thickness profile of the cornea. Because the absolute central (or thinnest) pachymetry value varies significantly among a normal population, the relationship between the central and peripheral cornea can be an indicator of pathologic thinning. The normal cornea is thinner at the center, with a gradual increase in thickness toward the periphery.[20-22] These concepts and the ability to accurately measure the corneal thickness limbus-to-limbus add significantly to our diagnostic capability. These data can only be obtained with an elevation-based topographer and accurate measurement of the posterior corneal surface.

The Belin/Ambrósio display allows the clinician to view the pachymetric profile and view the corneal elevation as it appears with an optimized reference surface. The literature is replete with numerous articles of iatrogenic post-LASIK ectasia in patients reportedly with normal preoperative exams.[23] How many of these so-called "normal" exams are truly normal and how many had undiagnosed changes on their posterior corneal surface is unknown. Additionally, reported residual bed computations based on central ultrasound readings may significantly overestimate the actual residual bed. Like flap thickness unpredictability, pachymetric distribution inconsistency may represent a previously unrecognized confounding variable.

# Corneal Morphology

The Pentacam's complete corneal analysis is also advantageous in characterizing keratoconus morphology. Traditionally, the morphology of the cone was categorized by descriptions based solely on anterior curvature analysis. Sagittal curvature, however, is a very poor indicator of cone location and morphology. Figure 6-35 reveals the limitations of curvature analysis in the assessment of cone location. Sagittal curvature maps, whether generated by Placido systems or by elevation systems, do not depict shape nor do they accurately locate the cone. One can see that the sagittal curvature map (lower right) would incorrectly place the apex of the cone below the limits of the 9.0-mm display. The true apex of the cone, however, is slightly below the pupillary margin as shown in both the pachymetry map and the anterior and posterior elevation maps. Accurately identifying cone location and size are crucial in planning Intacs surgery and corneal transplantation. Elevation maps are inherently more accurate than sagittal curvature displays in depicting the morphology of the cone and should be used to classify keratoconus.

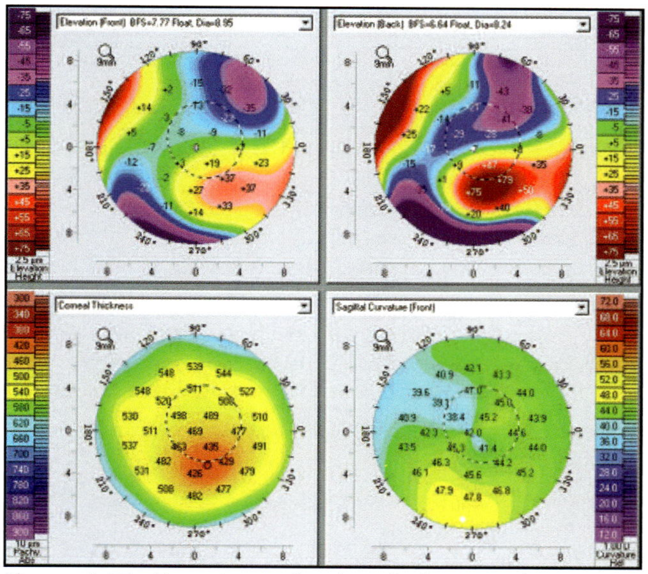

Figure 6-35. Four-view refractive display revealing proper cone localization on the elevation and pachymetric maps.

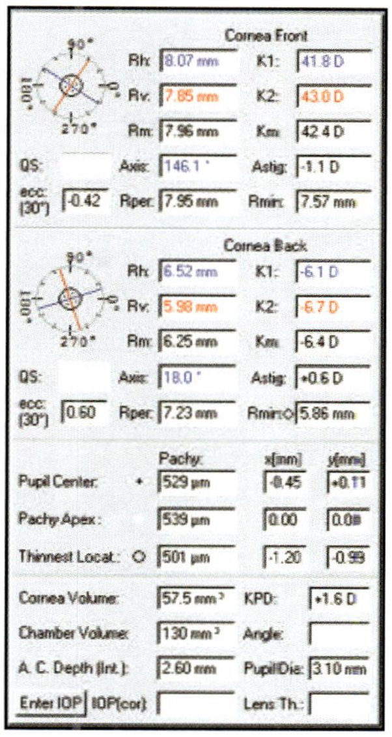


Figure 6-36. Corneal indices calculated by the Pentacam.

## Individual Displays

Single map displays are available for corneal thickness, anterior and posterior elevations, and anterior and posterior sagittal and tangential curvatures. They are selected by choosing the "1 Large Color Map" option and then selecting the map from the drop-down list. All of the single maps share a common presentation of corneal indices, which is shown on the left side of the display (Figure 6-36).

## Corneal Indices

The steep (K2/Rs) and the flat (K1/Rf) simulated keratometry values are shown for both the anterior and posterior surfaces. These are computed at the central 3-mm zone and are always orthogonal (ie, 90 degrees apart). The orientation of the major and minor meridians is shown in the small diagram on the left side of the field. It should be noted that, even in highly irregular corneas, the simulated K values will be reported as orthogonal and that this does not suggest that the cornea is regular. Other values depicted are listed in Table 6-4.

## Compare Exams

These displays allow the user to show different exams from the same patient to compare and to observe the differences between exams such as pre- and post-LASIK (Figure 6-37). Any of the available single maps may be selected, and their differences will be computed. Additionally, the user may left-click on any of the maps, and the corresponding individual point value will be displayed on all the maps. This display is particularly useful for showing surgical effect or following a progressive disease.

TABLE 6-4.

### Pentacam Corneal Indices

| |
|---|
| **Steep (K2/Rs):** Simulated keratometry value for the steepest meridian on both the anterior and posterior surfaces computed at the central 3-mm zone. |
| **Flat (K1/Rf):** Simulated keratometry value for the flatest meridian on both the anterior and posterior surfaces computed at the central 3-mm zone. |
| **Rf/K1:** Flat central radii in the 3-mm zone. |
| **Rs/K2:** Steep central radius in the 3-mm zone. |
| **Rm/Km:** Mean central radius, arithmetic average of Rf and Rs. |
| **QS:** Stands for "quality statement" and is a check on the image acquisition quality. Here "OK" means the acquired image was of sufficient quality. |
| **Axis:** Axis of corneal astigmatism (red for steep, blue for flat and user selectable). |
| **Astig.:** Corneal astigmatism in the central 3 mm. |
| **Q-val.:** Corneal shape factor of the cornea in 30 degrees. |
| **Rper:** The mean radii of the zone between the 7- and 9-mm ring. |
| **Rmin:** Minimum radii of the cornea. |

For the conversion of the curvature readings into refractive power on the anterior surface, a refractive index of n = 1.3375 is used and for the posterior surface the refractive index n = 1.376 for cornea and 1.336 for aqueous is used.

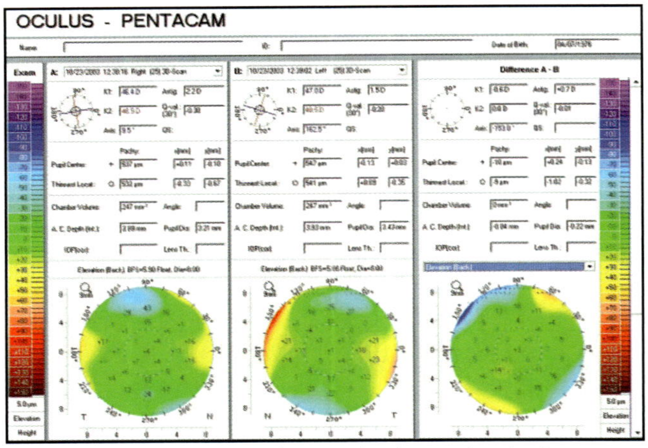


**Figure 6-37.** Comparison of 2 examinations using the Pentacam.

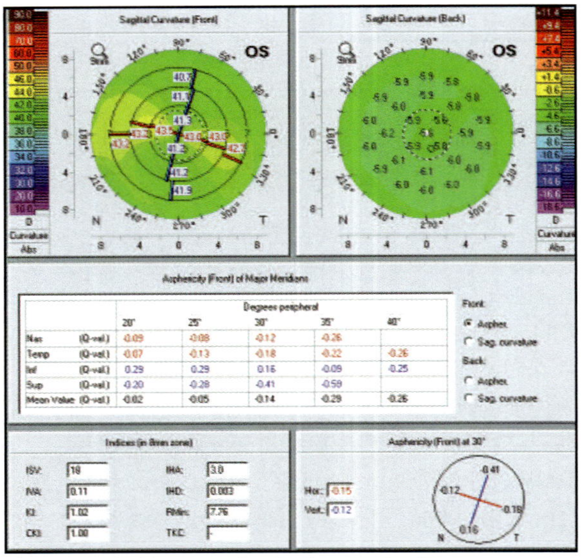


**Figure 6-38.** Topometric display on the Pentacam.

TABLE 6-5.

## Curvature Indices

**Index of Surface Variance (ISV):** Gives the deviation of individual corneal radii from the mean value. This index is elevated in all types of irregularity of the corneal surface (scars, astigmatism, deformities caused by contact lenses, keratoconus, etc).

**Index of Vertical Asymmetry (IVA):** Gives the degree of symmetry of the corneal radii with respect to the horizontal meridian as axis of reflection. Elevated in cases of oblique axes of astigmatism, in keratoconus, or in limbal ecstasies.

**Keratoconus Index (KI):** Elevated especially in keratoconus.

**Center Keratoconus Index (CKI):** Elevated especially in central keratoconus.

**Index of Height Asymmetry (IHA):** Gives the degree of symmetry of height data with respect to the horizontal meridian as axis of reflection. Analogous to IVA, although sometimes more sensitive.

**Index of Height Decentration (IHD):** This index is calculated from Fourier analysis of height and gives the degree of vertical decentration. Steeper in keratoconus.

**Radii minimum (RMin):** Gives the smallest radius of curvature in the entire field of measurement. Elevated in keratoconus.

**Topographical Keratoconus Classification (TKC):** Based on anterior corneal data the keratoconus is classified based on the Amsler/Muckenhirn staging.

Note: This classification ignores the degree of thinning and ectatic changes on the posterior surface. This classification would classify as normal eyes with significant posterior changes associated with thinning if the anterior surface was uninvolved and is also prone to false positives in corneas with a displaced apex.

## Topometric Display

The Topometric display (Figure 6-38) is designed to analyze the cornea based on anterior and posterior curvature data. This display presents a number of anterior curvature values commonly found on Placido-based systems. The display shows anterior and posterior sagittal curvature with their associated simulated K values, pachymetry, true net power, and asphericity values. Additionally, it displays the 8 curvature indices listed in Table 6-5. Note that these indices, which were derived from Placido-based data only, consider the anterior corneal surface. Their predictive and descriptive abilities are limited by not evaluating either the posterior surface or the pachymetric distribution.

## Pachymetric Display

The individual pachymetric display (Figure 6-39) provides the color map of the distribution of corneal thickness, the thickness of the cornea at the apex, the pupillary center, and the thinnest corneal point. It provides the corneal volume calculated at the 10-mm optical zone centered on the apex, the chamber volume at the 12-mm zone centered at the apex, and the ACD. The 2 large graphs (Corneal Thickness Spatial Profile [CTSP] and Percentage Thickness Increase [PTI]) and the progression index show how the corneal thickness changes relative to data from a normal population. The graphs show the "average" normal values and ±2 SD (95% confidence interval). Pachymetric progression data are very useful in screening for ectatic disease.

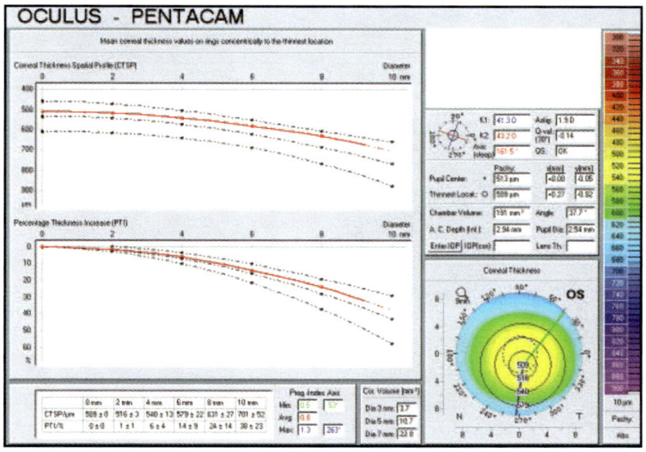


Figure 6-39. Pentacam Individual Pachymetric display.

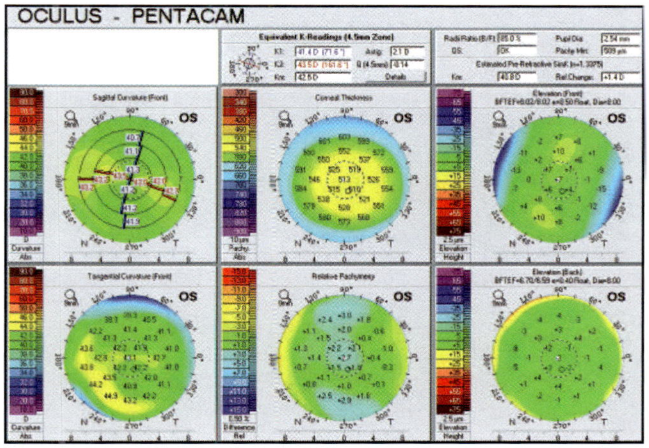


Figure 6-40. The Holladay Equivalent Keratometry Readings detailed report.

## Holladay "Equivalent K" Detail Report

As more and more of the early refractive surgery patients develop cataracts, the need for accurate postrefractive IOL calculations increases. Unfortunately, many of these patients do not have their prerefractive corneal measurements available, making the historical method of IOL calculation impossible. Standard keratometry assumes normal spherocylindrical optics and assumes a constant relationship between the anterior and posterior corneal surfaces. Standard keratometry predicts overall corneal power based solely on anterior curvature measurements. These assumptions are usually accurate in "normal" eyes, and this explains the excellent refractive results typically seen with modern cataract surgery. After refractive surgery, however, these assumptions no longer hold true, and using standard "K" values in IOL formulas may lead to a significant deviation from the desired refractive result.

Because the relationship between the anterior and posterior corneal surfaces deviates from typical after refractive surgery, the optical approximation of the corneal power requires data from both anterior and posterior surfaces as well as the index of refraction of the cornea and aqueous. Additionally, the power change from the corneal center to the periphery may change dramatically after refractive surgery, and the overall power may be more dependent (postoperatively) on the pupillary size. The Equivalent Keratometer Reading (EKR) uses all of the above information to produce a graphic and tabular representation of the "adjusted" postsurgical "K" readings at varying pupil sizes (Figure 6-40). In the absence of historical data, the use of the EKR (at an appropriate pupillary size) in standard IOL formulas may allow for more precise postrefractive IOL calculation.

## Phakic Intraocular Lens Simulation Program

The 3-dimensional simulation program for phakic IOLs was designed to assist surgeons in the preoperative planning for the implantation of phakic IOLs into the anterior chamber and to determine whether adequate clearances are present for safe implantation (Figure 6-41).

The specific phakic IOL type and power can be chosen from the database. The selected lens is located on the iris automatically. The minimum distances between phakic IOL and endothelium and natural crystalline lens are calculated in all dimensions and automatically displayed. The phakic IOL alignment can be modified by the user. The phakic IOL simulation software offers an automatic calculation of the refractive power of the phakic IOL with reference to the subjective refraction of the patient.

Additionally, due to the normal growth of the lens with age and subsequent shallowing of the anterior chamber, an aging prediction module was incorporated. The age of the patient can be changed while clicking on the arrow keys or typing in a specific age. The software assumes a growing of 18 μm per year for the crystalline lens. The outcome of this is an anterior movement of the iris toward the cornea. Depending on the predicted age, the clearances in the Scheimpflug image change. The minimum clearances in the anterior chamber are shown on the lower right-hand side of the display.

## Contact Lens Fitting Display

The complex interaction between a rigid contact lens and the corneal surface can only be simulated if you know the true corneal shape (elevation) and if the system is capable

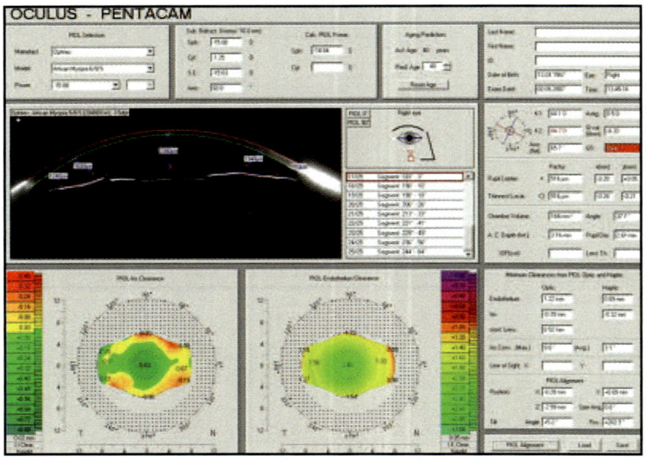


**Figure 6-41.** Pentacam phakic IOL simulation program.

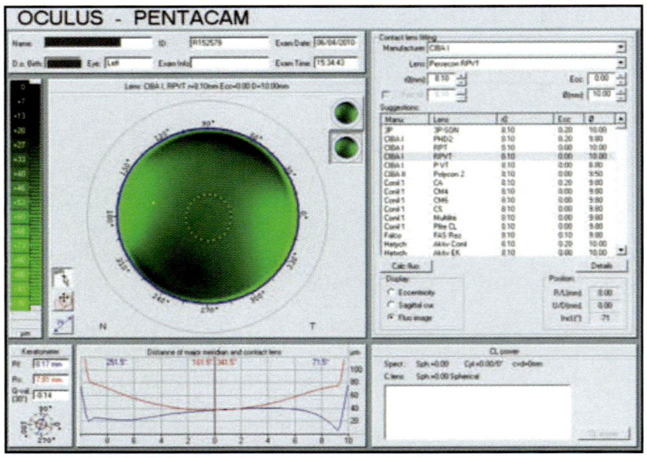


**Figure 6-42.** Contact Lens Fitting display on the Pentacam.

of imaging more of the corneal surface that is typical of a reflective Placido-based system. If the total corneal shape is known, rigid gas-permeable lenses can be "fit" to the corneal surface and the lens/corneal relationship can be predicted. The lenses can be adjusted both in overall diameter, base curve, and peripheral curves, and a simulated fluorescein pattern can be produced.

The Contact Lens Fitting Display (Figure 6-42) allows the practitioner to either design a custom lens or to select from a large number of commercially available rigid lens designs. The lens selection can then be modified based on the simulated lens/cornea alignment and predicted fluorescein pattern.

The development of elevation-based imaging systems that allow assessment of both the anterior and posterior corneal surfaces marks an evolutionary change in computerized corneal analysis. Accurate assessment of both corneal surfaces and complete pachymetric distribution significantly enhances our knowledge and should allow for better and more complete corneal and refractive evaluations.

# Precisio Surgical Tomographer

Aleksandar Stojanovic, MD and Xiangjun Chen, MD, MS

Precisio (Figure 6-43) is a modern corneal topographer/tomographer that measures limbus-to-limbus elevation of the anterior and posterior corneal surfaces, corneal pachymetry, as well as the ACD, using the Scheimpflug principle. It is designed as a custom surgical data acquisition device to be used as a part of the iVIS-Suite laser system. Its resolution, sensitivity, and specificity are fine-tuned for detecting the details of corneal morphology with accuracy and repeatability suited for use in custom ablation treatments.

During the examination, Precisio projects a rotating slit onto the anterior segment of the eye at an angle of 20 degrees from its rotational axis, which coincides with the visual axis of the examined eye. The slit image is captured by 2 integrated CCD cameras—the main camera and the focus camera—and is further converted to a digital format for analysis. The main camera is mounted on a rotational wheel, perpendicular to the projection of the slit, to capture the images of the anterior and posterior surfaces of the cornea, the anterior surface of the iris, and the crystalline lens, while the focus camera, mounted on the rotational axis, detects the positional data of the examined eye and monitors the fixation (Figure 6-44). For each examination lasting 1 second, the main camera acquires 50 images during its 360-degree rotation, generating 39,000 data points on both the anterior and posterior surfaces. The elevation data captured by the main camera are paired with the positional data from the focus camera. The focus camera also captures the iris and limbal vessel architecture with the help of a secondary illumination system consisting of 4 infrared

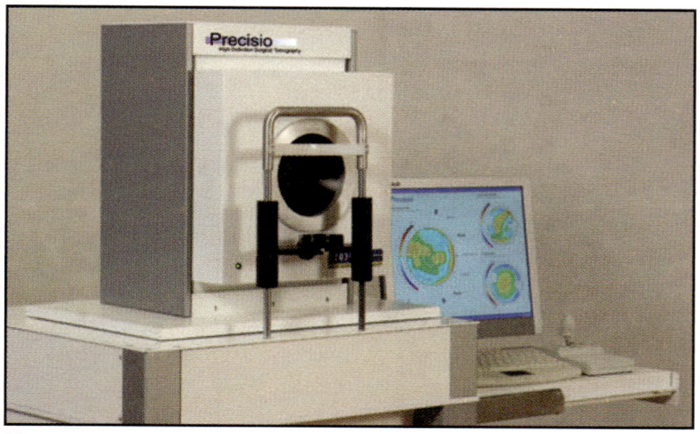


Figure 6-43. Precisio topo/tomographer.

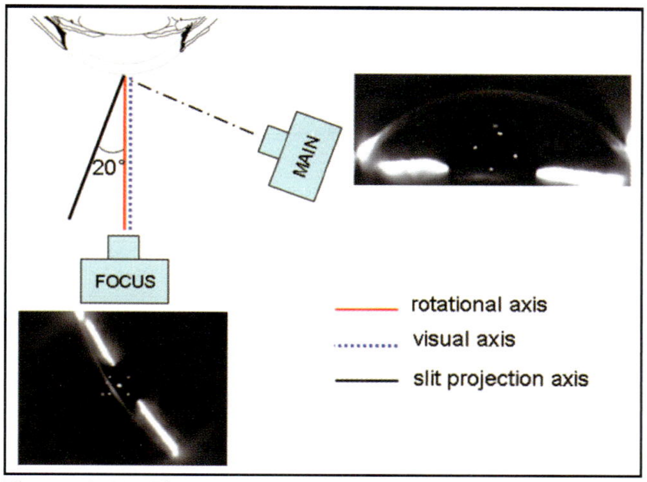


Figure 6-44. The main camera captures a perpendicularly projected slit during a 360-degree rotation, while the focus camera, located on the rotational axis, detects the positional data.

LEDs and 4 white LEDs for illumination of a concentric area from 8 to 14 mm from the pupil center (Figure 6-45). The image of the iris and limbal vessel architecture is used for eye registration and for cyclotorsional tracking during the surgery with the iVIS-Suite laser system.

As a surgical data acquisition device, Precisio shows some clear differences compared to the other Scheimpflug topo/tomographers, designed primarily for diagnostic purposes (eg, Pentacam). To maximize the accuracy of the data from the cornea, the main camera of Precisio uses a higher optical magnification compared to the Pentacam (Figure 6-46), thus covering only the space between the cornea and the anterior surface of the lens. Consequently, a higher resolution image is obtained, sacrificing, however, information on the structure behind the surface of the crystalline lens. In order to maximize the repeatability of the data, the following unique features are implemented:

- A heavy and rigid mechanical construction to minimize vibration induced by the rotating structure during the acquisition

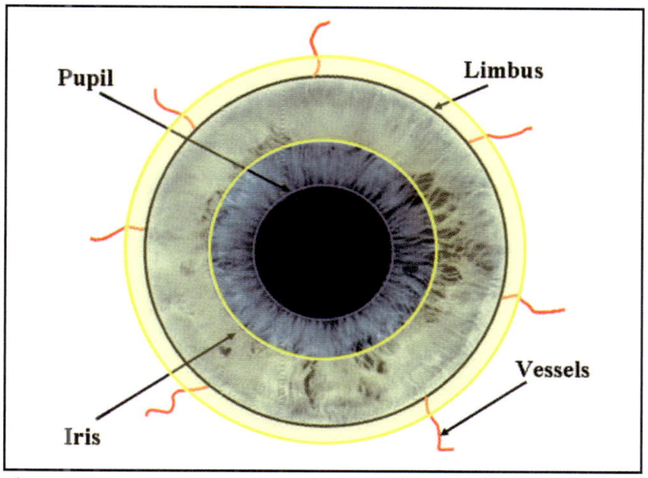


Figure 6-45. Yellow shaded concentric area from 8 to 14 mm from the pupil center showing iris and limbal vessel architecture used for eye registration and cyclotorsional tracking.

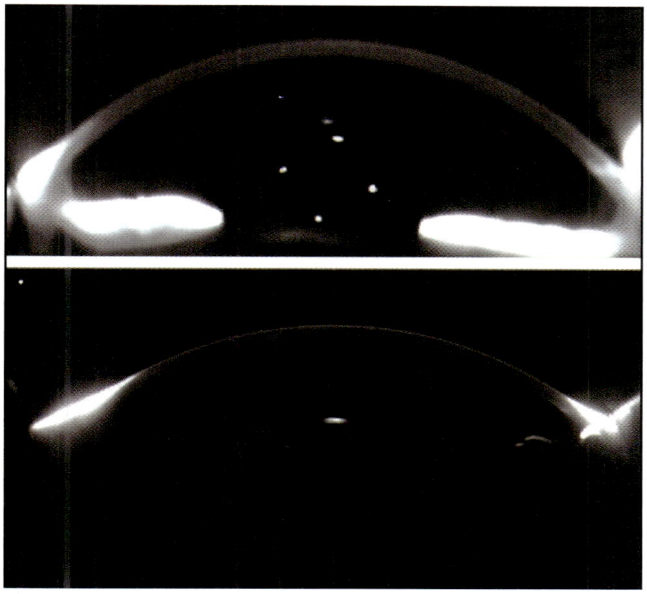

Figure 6-46. Precisio (top) uses a higher optical magnification compared to Pentacam (bottom) and consequently covers a smaller space.

- A fully automated acquisition process based on 4 software-aided motors, which allows an examination without introduction of any operator's vibration to the system
- An eye tracker, which compensates for x, y micro movements and cyclotorsion of the eye during the examination

Finally, Precisio provides quality control of the surgical data by not allowing export to the custom ablation planning software until the requirement for repeatability of ±3 µm for the anterior elevation examinations within the central 6 mm is reached.

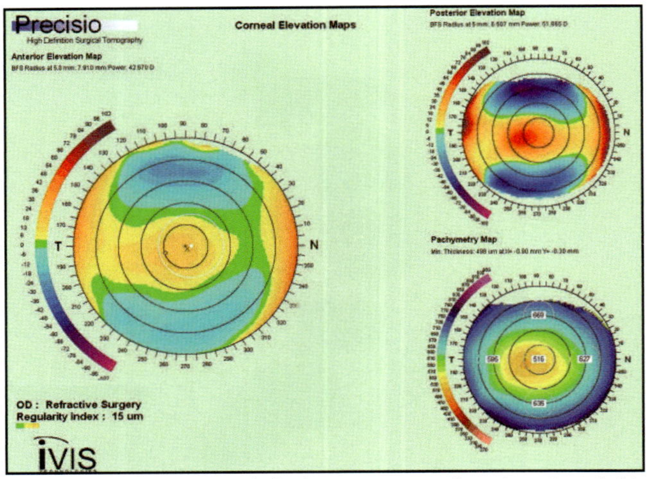


**Figure 6-47.** Precisio's default maps—anterior elevation (left), posterior elevation (right superior), and pachymetry (right inferior) in a case of preclinical keratoconus.

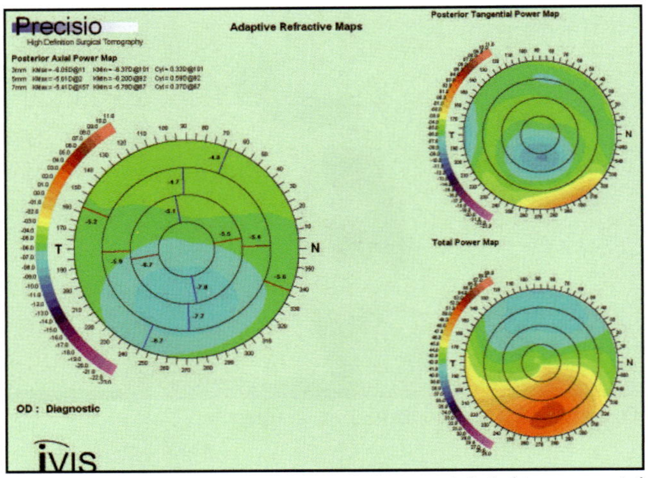


**Figure 6-49.** Posterior curvature maps—axial (left), tangential (right superior), and total power (right inferior).

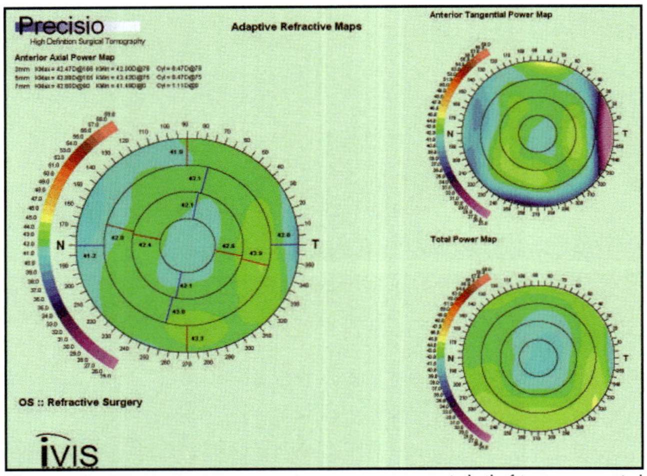


**Figure 6-48.** Anterior curvature maps—axial (left), tangential (right superior), and total power (right inferior).

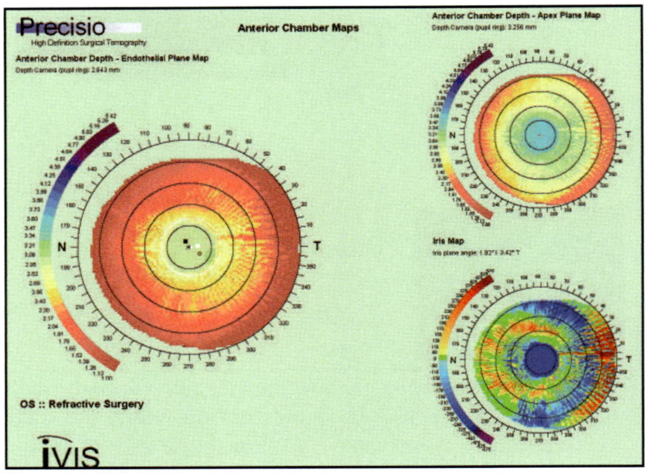


**Figure 6-50.** ACD maps.

Precisio's default display presents anterior elevation, posterior elevation, and pachymetry maps in one view (Figure 6-47). The curvature maps (axial, tangential, and mean power) of the anterior and posterior corneal surfaces are also available (Figures 6-48 and 6-49), as well as ACD map (Figure 6-50) and a 3-dimensional view of the cornea.

Clinically, Precisio can be used as an instrument for diagnostic purposes, for topography-guided refractive and therapeutic treatments, as well as for analysis of the effectiveness of the refractive treatments.

## Diagnostics

Probably the most important task of preoperative evaluation in refractive surgery is the early detection of keratoconus. Before the development of scanning slit systems, the diagnosis of keratoconus was mainly dependent on the Placido-based systems' detection of localized increases in curvature.[24,25] Although such measurements are reproducible in normal corneas, this is not the case in extremely irregular corneas, such as in keratoconus, where a deviation in the tear film thickness will significantly affect the measurements. A thin tear film will cause nonexisting surface irregularities to show as artifacts, whereas a thick tear film may prevent some real irregularities from showing. Even more importantly, the Placido-based systems do not measure the posterior surface of the cornea, which as a rule shows keratoconus changes before the anterior surface. The early keratoconus changes do not show on the anterior surface due to epithelial remodeling, which causes a masking effect by initially smoothing the keratoconic changes of the anterior corneal surface.[26,27] The Precisio's high-resolution Scheimpflug images provide precise anterior and posterior elevation and pachymetry maps of the cornea and represent a solid base for identification of preclinical keratoconus (see Figure 6-47).

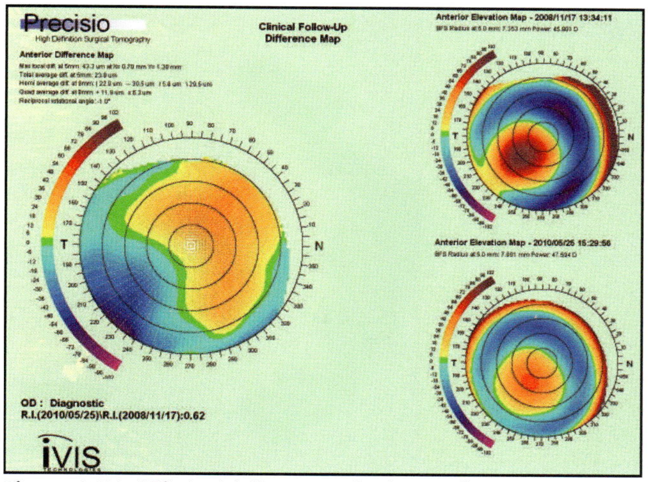


**Figure 6-51.** "Clinical follow-up" display: Difference map (left) between anterior elevation maps before (right superior) and after (right inferior) CXL treatment in a keratoconus eye.

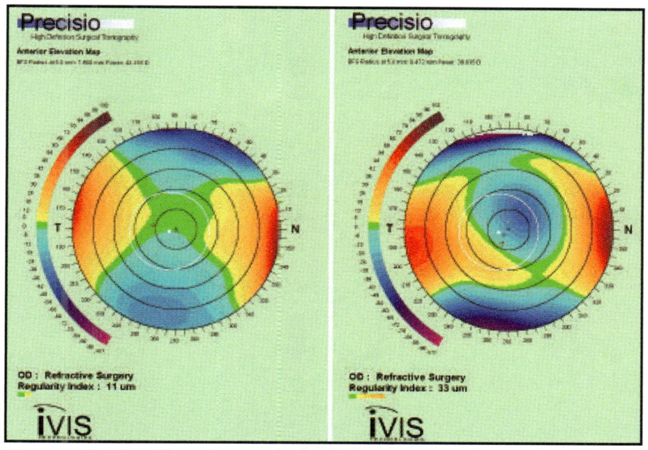


**Figure 6-52.** "Regularity index" represents an indication of irregularity of the corneal surface. Normal virgin cornea (left) and a cornea after a decentered LASIK (right).

To monitor progression of corneal shape changes, Precisio's "clinical follow-up" mode provides comparison of 2 examinations of the same eye performed at different times (Figure 6-51).

Precisio also provides so-called "Regularity index," which represents an indication of irregularity of the corneal surface compared to its best aconic surface within the central 6-mm area (Figure 6-52).

## Surgical Design

Any excimer laser treatment is based on an ablation plan expressed in µm of corneal tissue to be removed at any particular coordinate of its surface. This implies that, independent of the type of the information used for the custom ablation planning (wavefront aberrometry, corneal curvature, corneal elevation topography, or corneal wavefront), a final calculation must be performed to find the depth of ablation expressed in µm on the corneal level. Placido-based topography measures corneal curvature in D. To obtain the necessary corneal elevation data, a mathematical conversion from D to µm is needed, resulting in "secondary data" prone to cumulative error. Precisio, however (along with other Scheimpflug-based topographers), measures the corneal shape directly in µm of corneal elevation, providing high-quality "primary data" for topography-guided custom ablation planning.

Precisio is designed to provide data for the iVIS-Suite custom ablation system. In order to accomplish this, corneal anterior elevation and pachymetry data are fed to Corneal Interactive Program Topographic Ablation (CIPTA) planning software, while the iris and limbal vessel architecture data are transferred to the laser and are used for eye registration and cyclotorsional eye tracking during the surgery. The details of the working principle of CIPTA have been described by Alessio.[28] Basically, to program a refractive surgery, pupillometry and the patient's refraction are also fed to the CIPTA software, which then compiles a custom ablation plan with the aim of transforming the actual corneal shape into a regular aspheric shape of desired curvature, within the treatment zone suggested by pupillometry. The volume of the ablation is defined by the intersection between the corneal anterior surface as detected by Precisio and the targeted aspheric surface determined by CIPTA. The curvature of the targeted surface is determined by subtracting the amount of desired dioptric change from the preoperative curvature. Excimer laser-based lamellar corneal transplantation programmed by Corneal Lamellar Ablation for Transplantation (CLAT) software is also built around the corneal topography/tomography information imported from Precisio. CLAT first defines an "Ideal Corneal Bed" with uniform thickness of residual healthy corneal tissue, based on the thinnest point of the pachymetry map provided by Precisio. CLAT ablation of the host cornea is performed to achieve this uniform bed, which then takes on membrane properties and assumes a regular shape. Finally, a trephine is used to cut the donor's cornea to the diameter of the receiving bed, while the laser adjusts the thickness of donor cornea to suit the residual thickness of the receiving bed by performing an even thickness ablation from the endothelial surface of the donor cornea. Figure 6-53 shows the principle of the CLAT, while Figure 6-54 shows an example of topographic outcome after CLAT transplantation.

Precisio's "Surgical follow-up mode—iVerify" evaluates the effect of the laser ablation by comparing the delivered (real) ablation map with the planned (expected) ablation map. The real ablation map is calculated by subtracting the postoperative elevation map from the preoperative elevation map, while the expected ablation map is imported from CIPTA. Thanks to the Precisio's registration information, any cyclotorsional or x, y misalignment between the preoperative and the postoperative maps is accounted for.

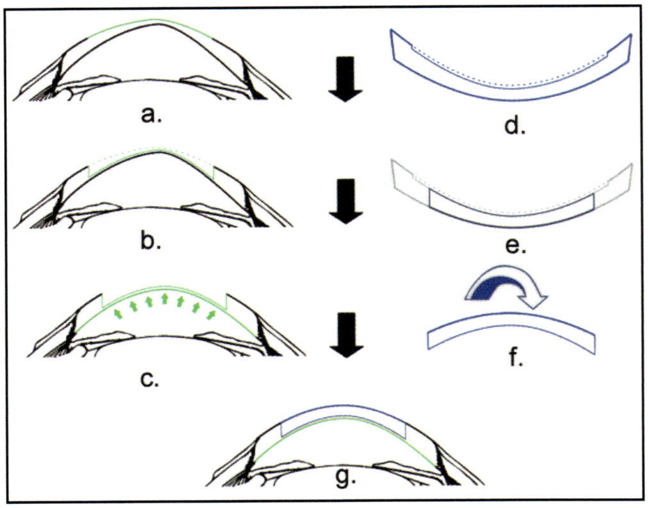


**Figure 6-53.** (A) CLAT performed in a keratoconus eye. (B) An "Ideal Corneal Bed" with uniform thickness of healthy corneal tissue is obtained by pachymetry-guided laser ablation. (C) A uniform bed assumes a regular shape after the ablation. (D) The thickness of donor cornea is then reduced to suit the residual thickness of the receiving bed by a laser ablation from the endothelial surface. (E) A trephine is used to cut the donor's cornea to the diameter of the receiving bed. (F) The button is turned around with the endothelial side facing the host bed and (G) sutured in place.

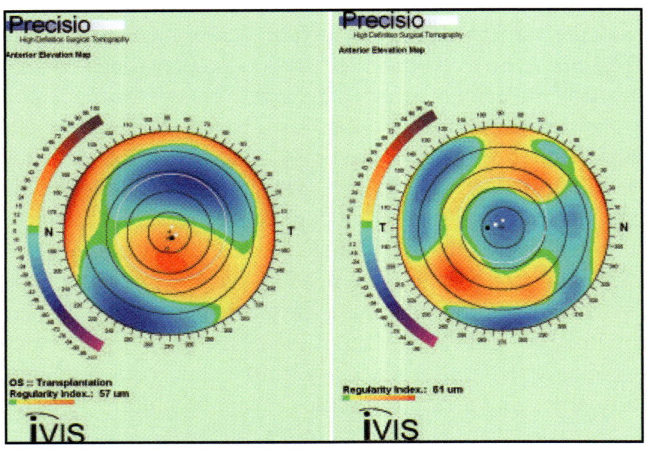


**Figure 6-54.** Anterior elevation map in an eye with keratoconus, before (left) and after (right) the CLAT treatment.

The ablation difference map shows the differences in the maximum ablation depth, the volume, and the achieved change in spherical equivalent and cylinder between the real and the expected ablation (Figures 6-55 and 6-56). These differences are the result of the efficiency of the laser and the corneal biological and biomechanical factors. Thus, iVerify is meant to be used as a tool for sophisticated nomogram building.

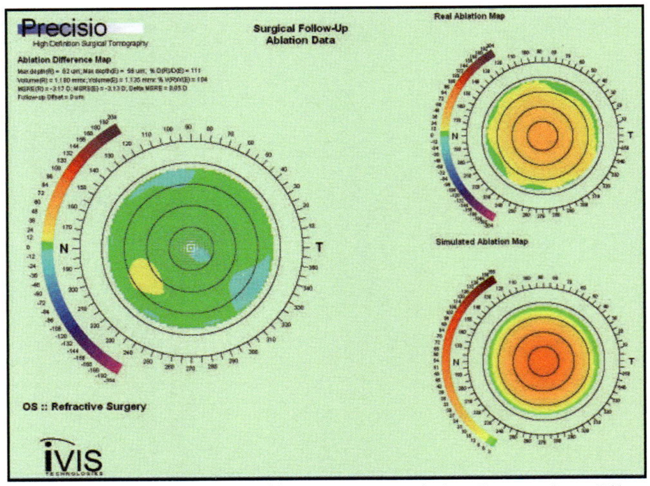


**Figure 6-55.** Ablation difference map (left) shows the difference between the real (right superior) and the expected (simulated) ablation (right inferior), in an eye with excellent results after treatment for low myopia.

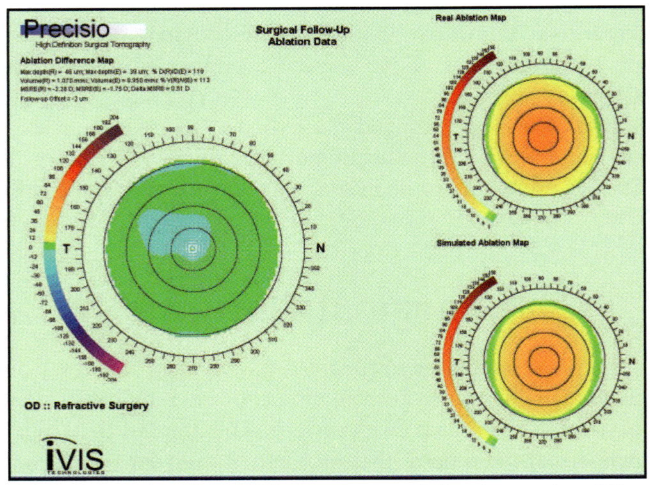


**Figure 6-56.** Ablation difference map (left) shows the difference between the real (right superior) and the expected (simulated) ablation (right inferior), in an overcorrected eye after treatment for low myopic astigmatism.

# Conclusion

Precisio is a unique topographer/tomographer, especially designed to provide precise surgical data for topography-guided custom ablation and laser-assisted corneal lamellar transplantation, to analyze the results of refractive surgery and to provide reliable diagnostic information for corneal evaluation and presurgical screening.

# VISANTE OMNI

Amin Ashrafzadeh, MD

A new era was ushered in with the advent of optical coherence tomography (OCT). Initially, the OCT was recognized for the diagnostic capabilities in the treatment of retinal disorders. The Stratus OCT has an 820-nm diode that was optimized to reach the retina and reduce light scatter. The 820-nm light, however, is not optimal for anterior segment. The 1310-nm light has increased water absorption, allowing the Visante OCT to have a 20-fold increase in light intensity with decreased retinal exposure. This allows for faster scanning at the same signal-to-noise ratio, reducing motion artifacts. Additionally, the 1310-nm light has reduced scattering of the light, allowing for better penetration into turbid and more opacified tissue. This increased signal-to-noise ratio allows for a faster processing with increased detail of structures, such as the cornea, sclera, and the anterior chamber angle.[29]

## Technical Information

### Visante Anterior Segment OCT

The Visante Anterior Segment OCT (Carl Zeiss Meditec, Dublin, CA) is a real-time, low-energy infrared laser, time domain OCT employing a 1310-nm light. Images may be acquired using 3 modes. The Anterior Segment Mode, referred to as "Ant Seg," is a 16-mm by 6-mm image with 256 optical "A Scans" in a span of 0.125 seconds. The High Resolution Mode, referred to as the "Hi Res" mode, is a 10-mm by 3-mm image with 512 optical "A Scans," in a span of 0.25 seconds. The Pachymetry Mode is a modified Hi Res Mode, 10-mm by 3-mm image, however, with only 128 optical "A Scans" in a span of 0.0625 seconds. The axial (depth) resolution of the Visante OCT is 18 μm, and the lateral (transverse) resolution is 60 μm. This information is presented in Table 6-6.

The Visante is capable of rotating the OCT drum 360 degrees. The images can then be acquired using 2 modes: Ant Seg or Hi Res Scans may also be performed in the "Enhanced" mode where 4 sequential images are acquired and then compressed into a single image. Additionally, the Ant Seg or the Hi Res modes can also be performed in a dual- or quad-scan mode. The dual-scan mode is performed at the 20- to 200-degree axis and at the 160- to 340-degree axis. This dual-scan mode is also capable of being rotated, but the degree separation remains constant. In the quad scan mode, the 4 scans are in equal 45-degree separations. The Visante 3.0 software also allows for customization of the scan in terms of the number of scans and also the degrees and the type of scans.

TABLE 6-6.

**Maps Included in the Predefined Themes**

| STANDARD | ALTERNATE | HOLLADAY |
|---|---|---|
| Anterior axial curvature (ATLAS) | Anterior mean curvature (ATLAS) | Anterior axial curvature (ATLAS) |
| Pachymetry (Visante OCT) | Pachymetry (Visante OCT) | Pachymetry (Visante OCT) |
| Anterior elevation sphere (ATLAS) | Anterior elevation toric ellipsoid (ATLAS) | Anterior elevation toric ellipsoid (ATLAS) |
| Anterior mean curvature (ATLAS) | Posterior mean curvature (Both) | Anterior mean curvature (ATLAS) |
| Relative pachymetry (Visante OCT) | Relative pachymetry (Visante OCT) | Relative pachymetry (Visante OCT) |
| Posterior elevation sphere (Both) | Posterior elevation toric ellipsoid (Both) | Posterior elevation toric ellipsoid (Both) |

The pachymetry scans are performed in either the standard pachymetry mode, which performs 8 sequential images in rotating fashion spaced every 22.5 degrees apart, or a Global Pachymetric Map, where 16 sequential pachymetric images are acquired spaced every 11.25 degrees apart. The Pachymetric Map is acquired in 0.5 seconds, and the Global Pachymetric Map is acquired in 1.0 seconds. The repeatability of the pachymetric map in the standard mode was noted to be 7 μm standard deviation in the center and 14 μm standard deviation in the periphery.[30] The central corneal 10-mm circular pachymetric map provides 2048 data points.

The relative pachymetric map compares the patient's corneal pachymetric map against a standard normal cornea with a central pachymetry of 550. This relative pachymetric map produces a percent deviation compared to the norm. This map provides a rapid visual analysis of abnormality. This information is directly calculated by the Visante and is presented in the middle, lower position.

The Visante is also equipped with an optometer that ranges from +20 to -35 D. The optometer is used to bring the focusing reticle into view for patients with refractive error.

Table 6-7.

**Scan Modes**

| | Ant Seg | Hi Res | Pachy |
|---|---|---|---|
| **Scan Size** | 16 mm by 6 mm | 10 mm by 3 mm | 10 mm by 3 mm |
| **# of A-Scans** | 256 | 512 | 128 |
| **Acquisition time** | 0.125 seconds | 0.25 seconds | 0.0625 seconds per B-scan; 0.5 seconds for regular pachymetry, 1.0 second for global pachymetry |
| **Modes** | Single, double, quad, single enhanced | Single, double, quad, single enhanced | 8 scan regular pachymetry or 16 scan global pachymetry |

Additionally, it can also be used to induce accommodation. The ability to induce accommodation allows for studying the movement of the anterior surface of the crystalline lens or the accommodating IOLs. The capacity to evaluate the anterior surface lens information in the setting of phakic IOLs is important as the vault distance may dramatically change with accommodation.

The Visante is also equipped with several software modules. The refractive module allows for placement of "Residual Stromal Bed" line in the Hi Res modes using standard, enhanced, or combined scans that can be adjusted to the desired amount as a set distance from the endothelial surface. This module may be either used for surgical planning, patient education, or postoperative evaluation of outcomes.

In the Anterior Segment (Ant Seg) modes, the "Anterior Chamber Rainbow" provides standardized lines of 0.5, 1.0, and 1.5 mm distances into the anterior chamber from the endothelial surface. This tool is very useful for the evaluation of the anterior chamber when considering phakic IOLs.

The "Phakic IOL" tool has a list of Artisan lenses (Ophthec, Groningen, Netherlands) and models including the 202 (5-mm Verisyse) and 204 (6-mm Verisyse) that are approved by the US FDA. The "Safety Distance" tools measure the distance from the endothelial surface to the edge of either the model or the real postoperative anterior chamber implant. Additionally, the "Vault Distance" tools are used to measure the distance from the posterior surface of the implant to the anterior surface of the crystalline lens.

The "Irido-Corneal" tools allow for measurement of the angles with more precise tools. The tool is manually placed at the scleral spur. Once placed, the Visante will automatically calculate the distance along the internal corneal surface at 500 and 750 μm. Then, the tool will continue to calculate the appropriate angle-opening distance (AOD) at 500- and 750-μm marks along with the trabeculo-iris surface area (TISA) at the 500- and 750-μm areas.

## ATLAS Corneal Topographer

The ATLAS corneal topographer is a Placido disk-based system. Models 993, 995, and 9000 are capable of linking with the Visante 3.0. The ATLAS topographers have a 22-ring Placido disk, 18 superior, and 22 inferior to the point of fixation. The latest model, the 9000, uses a 950-nm light source, which is not visible to the patient, is well-tolerated by dilated or light-sensitive patients, and does not induce any alteration in pupil size.

Because the information obtained by the ATLAS topographer is from the reflection of light from the Placido disk, all data pertain to the anterior surface. The Visante 3.0 version is upgraded with a tracking device to ensure corneal pachymetric mapping occurs with sequential scans centered to the same location. Additionally, the vertex of the cornea is recognized as the point with greatest signal in a vertical scan. The vertex of the ATLAS scans and the Visante pachymetric scans are matched to represent the same location. By using the corneal thickness map (pachymetric data), with known anterior surface curvature data from the ATLAS, the posterior corneal curvature data are calculated.

# Displays

To ease clinical use, various displays may be chosen. The ATLAS supplies the axial, tangential, mean curvature, anterior elevation, corneal refractive, and corneal wavefront maps. The Visante supplies pachymetry data and enables calculation of posterior surface topography and power. Table 6-7 presents preset formats of presentation; however, they can also be personalized.

## The Holladay Report

In cooperation with Jack T. Holladay, MD, MSEE, Houston, TX, the *Holladay Report* has been created to produce a single page of information that provides all pertinent information in evaluating candidacy for refractive

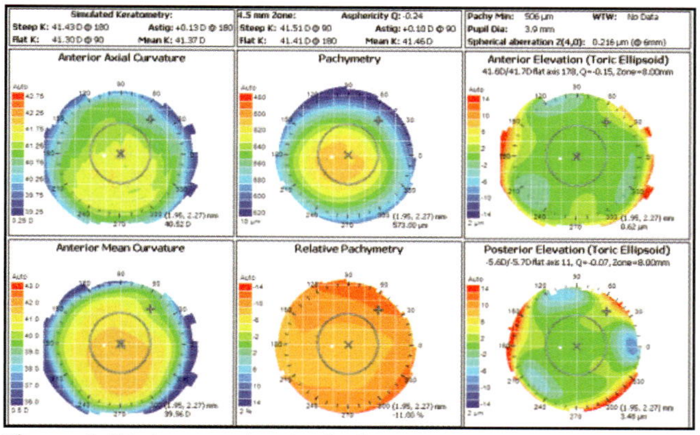


**Figure 6-57.** A normal, spherical cornea.

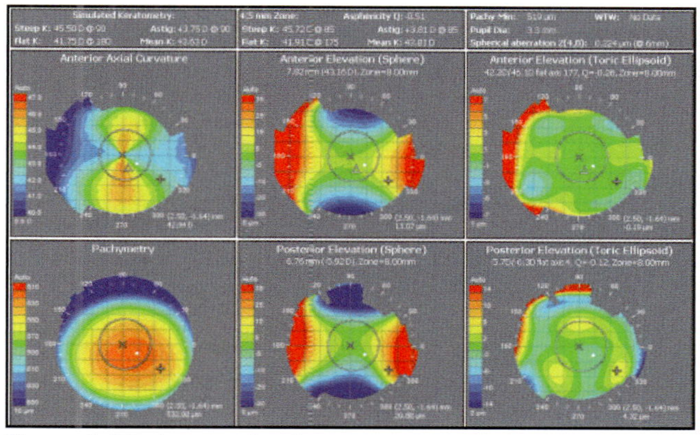


**Figure 6-58.** A normal toric cornea.

procedure. The axial curvature map, placed in the top left corner, is imported directly from the ATLAS. The mean curvature map, placed in the bottom left corner, is also imported directly from the ATLAS. The anterior elevation map is directly imported from the ATLAS and is presented in the top right corner. The elevation data, combined with the pachymetric data, allow for calculation of the posterior surface, and the posterior elevation map is presented in the right lower corner. The pachymetry map is in the middle.

## Refractive Evaluation

The evaluation of the LASIK patient both preoperatively and postoperatively is enhanced with the Visante Omni. Accurate posterior surface information may detect early ectasia in candidates as well as those who are postkeratorefractive surgery.

A normal, spherical cornea is presented in Figure 6-57. The *Holladay Report* of a 25-year-old White woman with plano refraction and 20/15 visual acuity in both eyes is shown. It is to be noted that because her corneal pachymetry is 506 µm by the Visante, her relative corneal pachymetric map uniformly shows an 11% deviation from the normal 550-µm cornea. Clearly, her corneas are normal, but the percent deviation data are used to spot not only eyes with uniform deviation, but more importantly the eyes with abnormal pattern deviation.

A normal toric cornea is presented in Figure 6-58. A 33-year-old White woman presented with a history of stable refraction. Her manifest refraction resulted in 20/15 in each eye with -0.50 -4.00 x 003 OD and -0.50 -4.00 x 180 OS. Corneal ultrasound pachymetry was 550 µm OD and 549 µm OS. The Visante Omni presented a regular bow-tie astigmatism with a regular pachymetry map. Mean curvature and the anterior elevation maps were unremarkable. The calculated posterior elevation presented the highest elevation point at 4.32 µm in the best-fit toric ellipsoid map.

The purpose of the elevation map is to compare a patient's cornea to some theoretically perfect geometric surface that should nearly match. Deviation from such surface is then represented as points of elevation above (red) or below (blue) such theoretical best-fit surface. Sphere and toric ellipsoid are 2 such surfaces, and they provide variable data. Figure 6-58 illustrates the variations between the BFS and the best-fit toric ellipsoid for both the anterior and the posterior surfaces. The BFS model over such astigmatic cornea has areas that fall below (blue) such sphere surface on the vertical meridian and areas that are above (red) such sphere surface on the horizontal meridian. By taking such reference surface and altering it to a best-fit toric ellipsoid, the curvatures of the astigmatic cornea are now compared to a more similar geometric surface shape. This example for this patient points out the lack of ease in "user friendliness" of BFS data. The best-fit toric ellipsoid represents a modified model that takes into account a regular astigmatic cornea.

Figure 6-59 demonstrates forme fruste keratoconus. A 36-year-old Hispanic woman presented for consideration of refractive surgery. Her manifest refraction was -0.50 -3.25 x 018 in her right eye (20/20) and -1.25 -2.75 x 175 in her left eye (20/25) Her ultrasound corneal pachymetry values were 531 µm OD and 521 µm OS. Despite a relatively normal axial map, the Visante Omni demonstrated an elevation of greater than 10 µm above the reference best fit toric ellipsoid on posterior elevation maps. The threshold for concern on the posterior elevation map is 10 µm. Note the correlation between the slightly heavier inferior bow tie on the axial map, highlighted inferior temporal area on the mean curvature map, the inferotemporal displacement of the thinnest point, and the elevation inferotemporally on the anterior and posterior elevation maps. The plus sign on all 6 maps indicates the same anatomical location. Typically, 3 indicators of ectasia contraindicate LASIK, and this patient has 6. The patient was diagnosed with forme fruste keratoconus.

Figure 6-60 demonstrates keratoconus. A 37-year-old White man presented for consideration of refractive surgery. His manifest refractions were -1.00 -1.50 x 025 OD (20/25) and -1.50 -1.25 x 152 OS (20/30). Ultrasound corneal pachymetry found 430 µm OD and 427 µm OS.

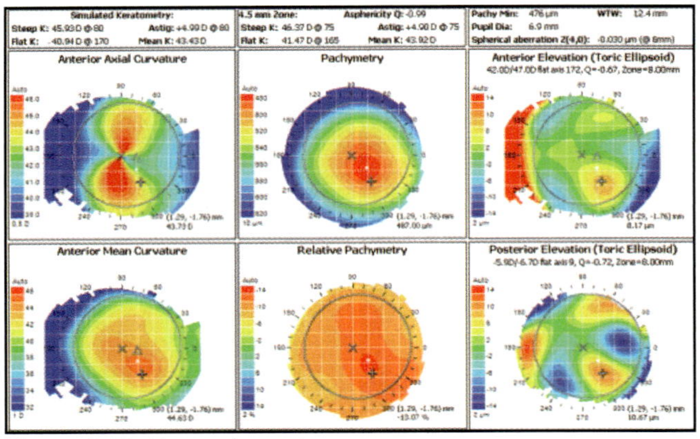


**Figure 6-59.** Forme fruste keratoconus.

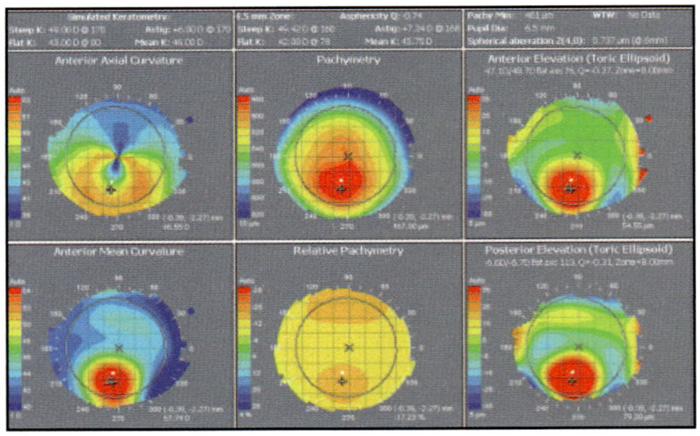


**Figure 6-61.** PMD.

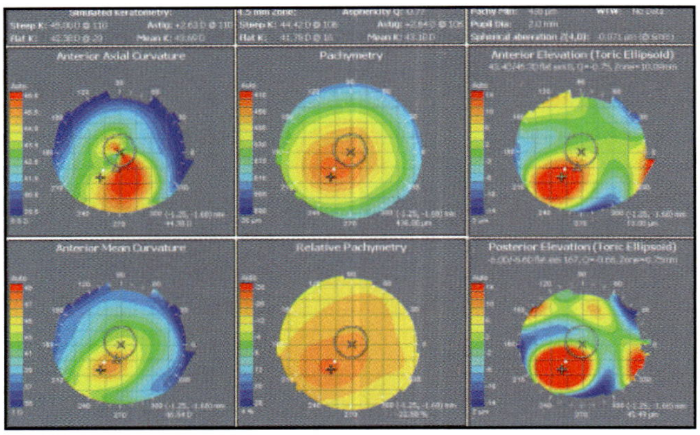


**Figure 6-60.** Keratoconus.

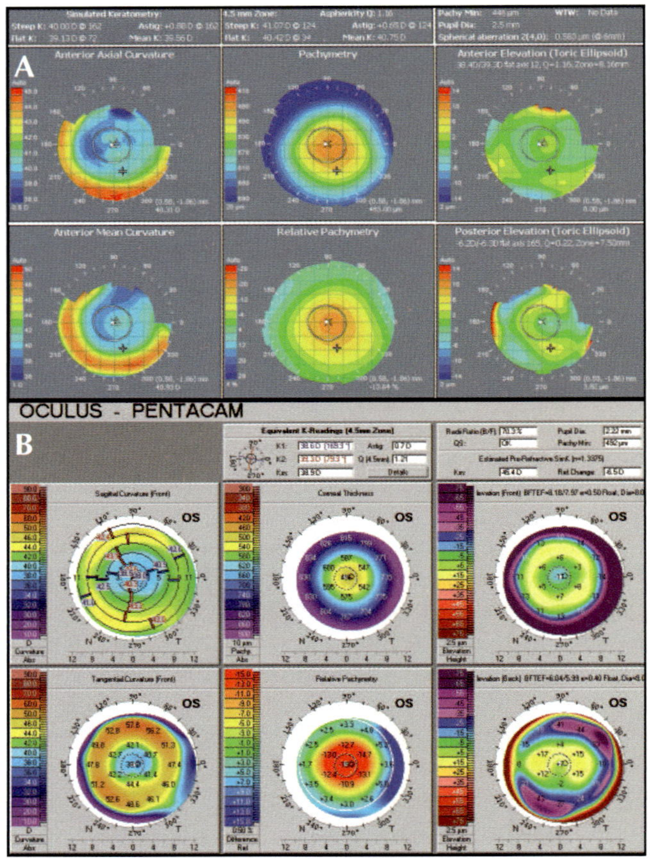


**Figure 6-62.** (A) A patient with a history of myopic LASIK. Original prescription was -6.00 -1.25 x 178. The posterior surface appears normal using the Visante Omni. (B) In the same patient, the Pentacam suggested several areas were elevated.

Note the 19 µm of anterior elevation on the anterior best fit toric ellipsoid surface and 45.49 µm of protrusion above the posterior surface. This disparity is noted as a consequence of the corneal epithelial thinning noted at the tip of the cone, which masks the stromal protrusion, yet there are no compensatory mechanisms on the endothelial surface.

Figure 6-61 demonstrates PMD. A 54-year-old Black woman had a refraction of +2.50 -3.75 x 093 (20/30) and +1.50 -4.00 x 093 (20/40) with central ultrasound corneal pachymetry of 515 µm OD and 503 µm OS. Note the Holladay Report OD shows a 54.55-µm anterior corneal surface elevation above the best fit toric ellipsoid and a 79.20-µm anterior elevation above the posterior surface elevation.

Figure 6-62 demonstrates a patient with a history of myopic LASIK. A 23-year-old White woman presented following treatment for -6.00 -1.25 x 178 due to residual refractive error. The Visante revealed a cornea with normal posterior surface. In comparison, the Pentacam found several elevated areas (more than 10 µm) on the posterior corneal surface best-fit toric ellipsoid. Over a period of 2 years with repeated exams, the refraction as well as the Visante Omni exams were stable.

Figure 6-63 demonstrates a patient 9 years post-LASIK, now suffering from post-LASIK ectasia. Her left eye was evaluated using the Visante Omni and the Pentacam. Over the course of 1 year, the Visante presented a consistent, slowly progressive ectasia OS. The Pentacam results were less suggestive.

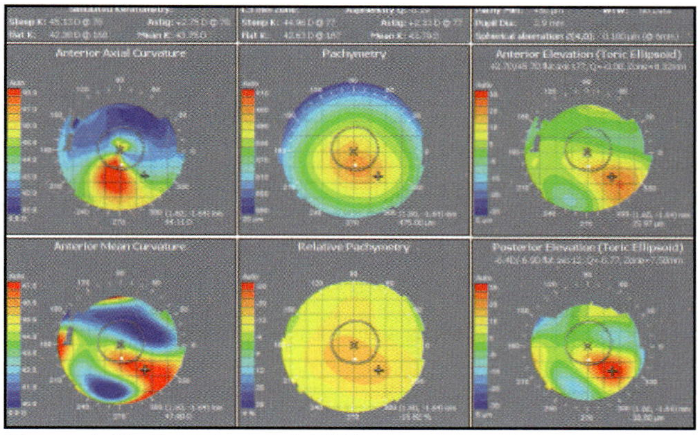


**Figure 6-63.** Ectasia post-LASIK.

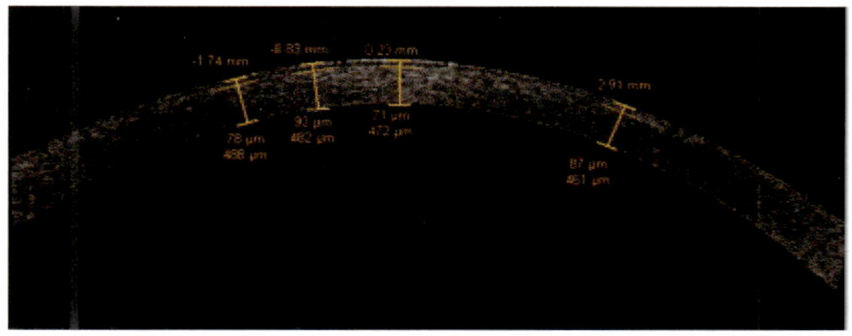

**Figure 6-64.** LASIK flap in patient who presented for enhancement. The flap was measured to be thin, and the patient chose to undergo PRK rather than relift the flap.

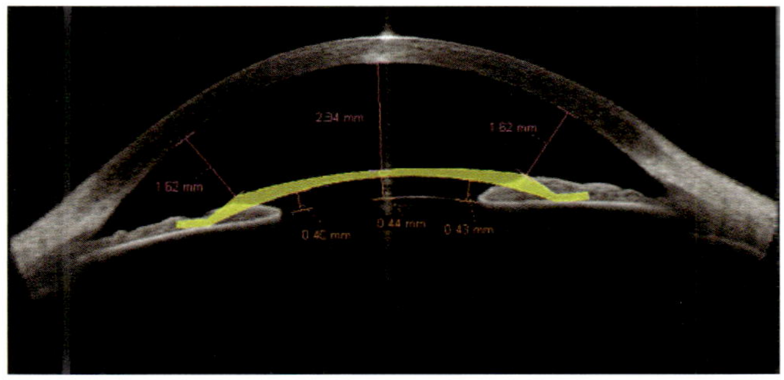


**Figure 6-65.** A model for Verisyse lens placement. The -10.00-D implant decreased the endothelial clearance to 1.5 mm, so a -7.00-D implant was used.

Figure 6-64 demonstrates the Visante Omni's ability to evaluate LASIK flap morphology. Microkeratome blades create variable thickness flaps. Thin flaps are difficult to lift and may tear. In rare cases, the flap is too thick, with insufficient residual stromal bed for further enhancement. In these cases, PRK may be more appropriate. This patient was evaluated using the Visante, was found to have a thin LASIK flap, and underwent PRK enhancement.

## Phakic Intraocular Lenses

At the time of this writing, there are only 2 types of phakic intraocular implants that are approved by the US FDA: the Verisyse/Artisan and the Visian lens. The Verisyse/Artisan-type implants are anterior chamber, iris fixed lenses. The Visian lens is implanted into the posterior chamber. One of the key issues with the Verisyse/Artisan-type implants is the endothelial clearance of the implant. The current standard is to maintain a minimum of 1.5 mm from the edge of the implant to the endothelium.

The rise of the crystalline lens above a straight line from the deepest portion of the angle is a concept that Dr. George Baikoff described as "crystalline lens rise" (CLR).[31] He noted that a high CLR is a contraindication for the phakic IOLs due to increased risk of complications, such as pigmentary dispersion. With an increasing lens rise of 18 µm per year, the age of the patient must be considered. Thus, implantation of Verisyse/Artisan implants for patients with more than 300 µm of CLR is contraindicated (personal communication, G. Baikoff, September 21, 2010).

The Visante has a set of models of the Verisyse/Artisan implants. After the Ant Seg view is acquired, the endothelial clearance Rainbow Tool allows for a quick visualization and a guide to center the Verisyse/Artisan implant. The implant models 202 or 204 with 5- and 6-mm optics, respectively, need to be placed with the flat portion of the implant slightly anterior to the posterior pigmented iris line. Once the model is in place, safety tools can be placed to measure the endothelial clearance, and vault tools allow measurement of the distance from the phakic IOL to the anterior crystalline lens surface.

Figure 6-65 illustrates the Visante Omni's ability to model the implantation and check for safety issues prior to surgery. A 42-year-old woman with the prescription of -11.00 -2.75 x 021 (20/30) and central corneal ultrasound pachymetry of 556 was evaluated for the Verisyse implant in conjunction with an IntraLase LASIK for residual refraction. VeriCalc suggested the endothelial clearance of a -12 D, 6-mm implant would be 2.00 mm. The Visante, however, showed less than 1.5 mm of clearance. This required a change in planning.

Although the -10.0 D, 6-mm implant had just 1.5 mm of clearance, one has to allow for a slightly decentered implant surgically, as the pupil is a dynamic structure. I opted for a -7.0 D, 6-mm implant that had a 1.60-mm endothelial clearance on the model. Postoperatively, the Visante Omni measured a 1.60-mm endothelial clearance. The residual refractive error was corrected using iLASIK (Abbott Medical Optics, Mellpitas, CA).

Figure 6-66 demonstrates postoperative analysis for Intacs for keratoconus. Intrastromal corneal ring segments, such as Intacs, were originally devised as a reversible alternative to LASIK surgery. Currently, Intacs are used for the treatment of ectasia. Visante measures peripheral pachymetry, guiding the IntraLase channel placement. Once the implant is inserted intrastromally, the Visante can confirm postoperative results. Using the pachymetric maps or the Holladay Report in such patients requires special attention to the "surface fit lines." The Visante follows the normal contour of the cornea to set the surface fit lines (in blue) to

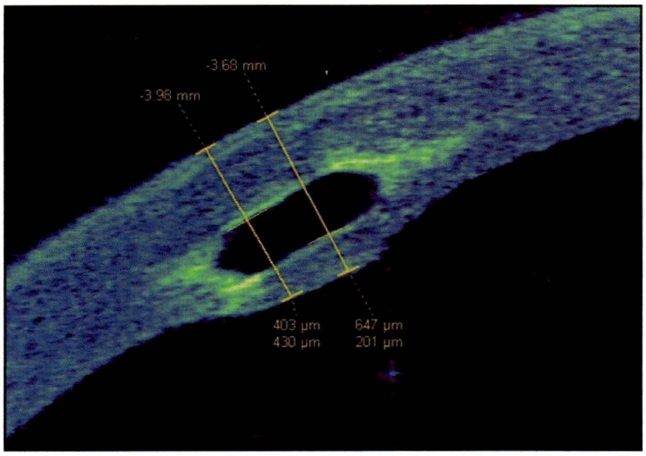


**Figure 6-66.** Evaluation of INTACS placed for keratoconus.

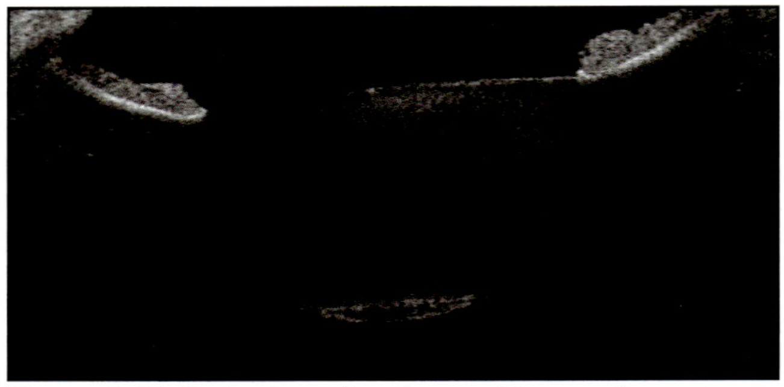

**Figure 6-67.** Evaluation of patients with complex cataracts such as a posterior polar cataract with adhesion to the posterior capsule can reduce surgical complications.

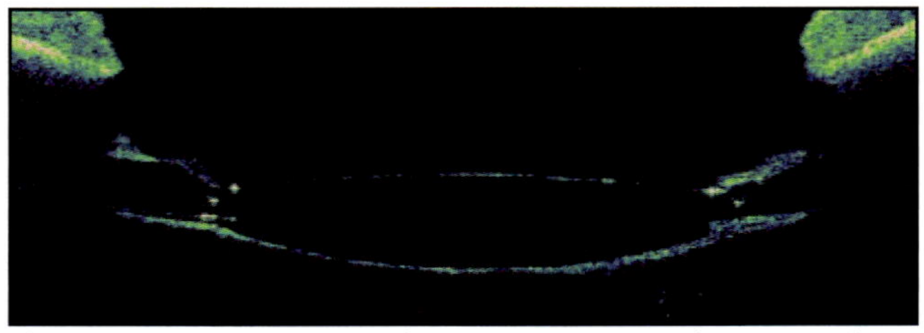

**Figure 6-68.** A patient with a CrystaLens implant, seen here where there is no movement of the optics when provoked with the optometer to induce "accommodation."

calculate the pachymetric data. A sudden change as seen with Intacs may not be recognized automatically and may need manual adjustment of such surfaces.

## Cataract Evaluation and Surgical Planning

Cataract is the clouding of the crystalline lens. It is the most commonly performed refractive procedure with more than 2 million surgeries per year in the United States. Although cataract is not the main central focus of this section, it is important to note a few cases.

In postcorneal refractive surgery patients, the ATLAS corneal topography can provide data for the 0-, 1-, 2-, and 3-mm zones, which can be used on the postrefractive surgery calculators such as the one on the American Society of Cataract and Refractive Surgery Web site (www.ascrs.org).[32]

The Visante can also be used to evaluate the postkeratorefractive surgery patients, as well as those with complex cataracts, such as a posterior polar cataract with adhesion to the posterior capsule (Figure 6-67). Additionally, new technologies can be evaluated. A patient with a CrystaLens (Bausch & Lomb) implant is noted here, and there is no movement of the optics that can be noted even when provoked with the optometer to induce "accommodation" (Figure 6-68).

## Future Developments

Visante anterior segment OCT gained FDA approval in 2005. Its limitations are accentuated by the rapidly growing field of technological advances in the OCT field. The Visante is a time domain technology capable of 2048 A-scans in 1 second. Competing technologies such as the spectral domain instruments provide 10 times or more scans, resulting in an exquisitely more-detailed image. The current commercially available spectral domain OCTs, however, are all 820- to 840-nm light technology with some limitations in what structures they can observe. With the 820- to 840-nm technology, the ability to view intraocular implants, the healed LASIK flaps, and healed endothelial keratoplasty interfaces are significantly reduced compared to the 1310-nm light technology.

The other limitation of the 820- to 840-nm technologies is the size of the acquired image. For example, the Cirrus OCT is, at the time of the writing, limited to 2- by 4-mm images. That image size is far too limiting to fully evaluate the cornea. The Spectralis (Heidelberg Engineering, Vista, CA), although not FDA approved for anterior segment OCT at the time of this writing, is providing claims of ability to provide 16- by 3-mm images. Such images become invariably difficult in acquiring as the narrow window requires exquisite patient cooperation. With the capacity to provide the 16- by 6-mm images, the Visante still remains the most comprehensive imaging device.

The side viewing screen and the small footprint of the instrument also make it a practical device. The ability to scan the patient as the family watches and to analyze the images along with the patient creates a very sophisticated, elegant real-time patient evaluation and education tool. Visante's capacity to link with the ATLAS topographer along with refractive and iridocorneal software capabilities makes this instrument truly unique and the most comprehensive anterior segment imaging device.

# The Oculyzer

Renato Ambrósio Jr, MD, PhD; Diogo L. Caldas, MD; Ana Laura C. Canedo, MD; Leonardo N. Pimentel, MD; Bruno F. Valbon, MD; and Mirko R. Jankov II, MD, PhD

The Oculyzer (Alcon-WaveLight, Fort Worth, TX; Figure 6-69) is a comprehensive cornea and anterior segment analyzer based on the same hardware platform as the Pentacam, with customized software capability for planning customized corneal photoablations based on corneal front elevation data. The system uses a rotating Scheimpflug camera for a 3-dimensional scanning of the cornea and anterior segment, which is aligned to a second frontal pupil camera.

The Scheimpflug image is based on the principle named after the Austrian Captain Theodor Scheimpflug (1865-1911). In 1904, Cap. Scheimpflug described and patented a geometric rule that describes an innovative orientation of the plane of focus of a camera, in which the lens plane is not parallel to the image plane. The technique uses the 3 imaginary planes: the film plane, the lens plane, and the plane of sharp focus in nonparallel manner, so that they intersect in a line (Scheimpflug intersection), with a virtual point of intersection (Figure 6-70A). Thereby, in a Scheimpflug camera, the lens is tilted in a way that the resulting lens plane intersects the film plane and the plane of focus in a form of a line. This setup extends the depth of focus, providing more sharpness to points of the image located at different planes, with the cost of having minor distortion of the image (Figure 6-70B), which is, in the case of the Pentacam and Oculyzer exams, compensated by the software calculations.

In a normal or ordinary camera, the film plane, the lens plane, and the plane of sharp focus are all parallel to each other, and, therefore, all 3 planes are perpendicular to the lens axis (Figure 6-71). This generates a limited depth of focus when compared to the Scheimpflug image (Figure 6-72).

The Oculyzer is a corneal tomography system, from the Greek words "to cut or section" (tomos) and "to write" (graphein), because it provides a 3-dimensional reconstruction of the corneal picture. It is capable of capturing 25 (in 1 second) or 50 (in 2 seconds) Scheimpflug images during 1 scan for a 3-dimensional tomographic reconstruction. It is also capable of acquiring single Scheimpflug images for documentation (Figure 6-73). Up to 500 points are measured per single image during a scan, which generates up to 25,000 true elevation points that are measured and analyzed by the Oculyzer software. The system integrates a second frontal pupil camera, which serves the purposes of controlling fixation and alignment compensation, as well as the correction of eye movements. The frontal pupil camera is also important for the acquisition mode and enables the detection of the size and orientation of the pupil image.

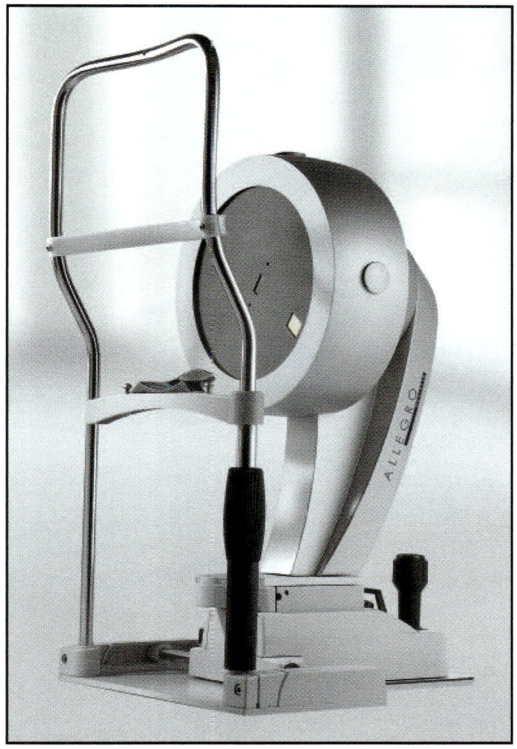


**Figure 6-69.** The Oculyzer Instrument (Alcon-WaveLight).

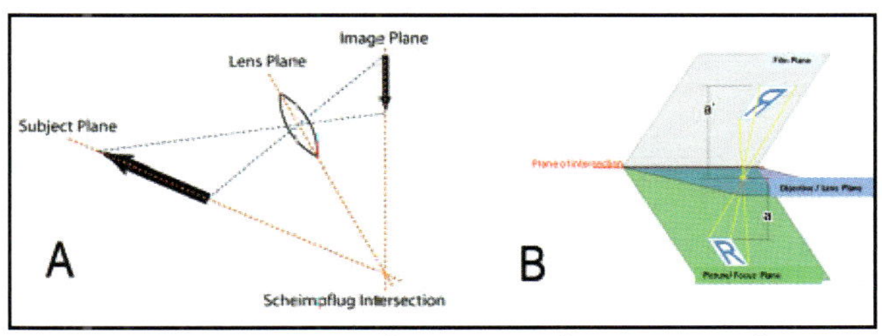


**Figure 6-70A.** (A) Scheimpflug's principle. (B) Image distortion by the Scheimpflug system.

The images are obtained in slit thickness of 80 μm and the range of 14 mm, allowing a complete image through the cornea (Figure 6-74). To avoid the shadows of the nose, the slit images are photographed from the temporal side at angles from 0 to 180 degrees (Figure 6-75), in order to reconstruct a 3-dimensional model of the anterior segment of the eye (Figure 6-76). More measurements are performed around the corneal center because this is the point of intersection of the images. The range for corneal radius

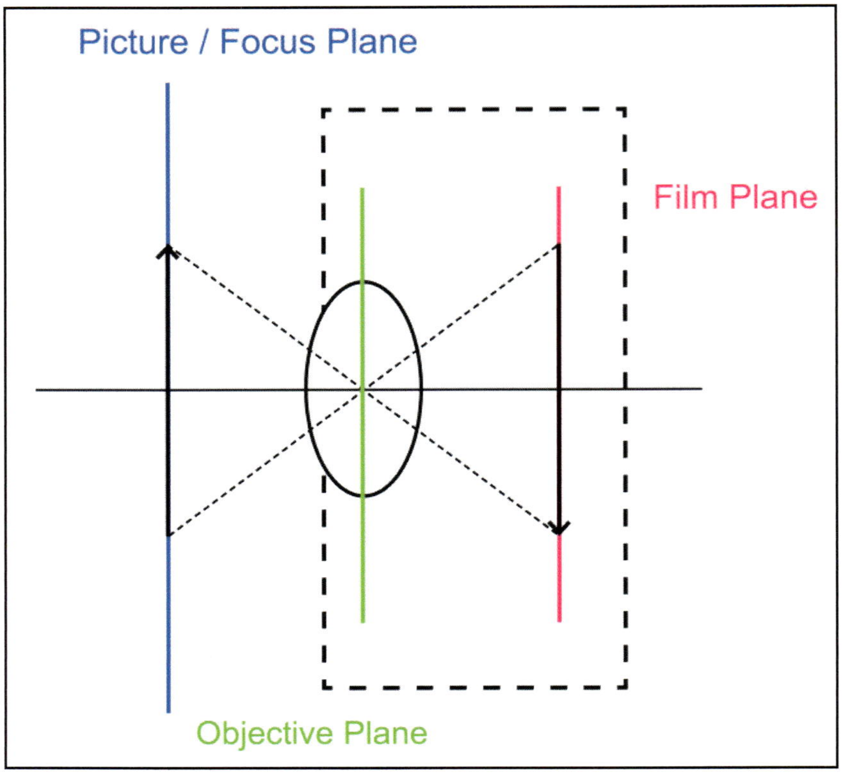


**Figure 6-71.** Ordinary camera schematics. (Reprinted with permission of Thomas Auer.)

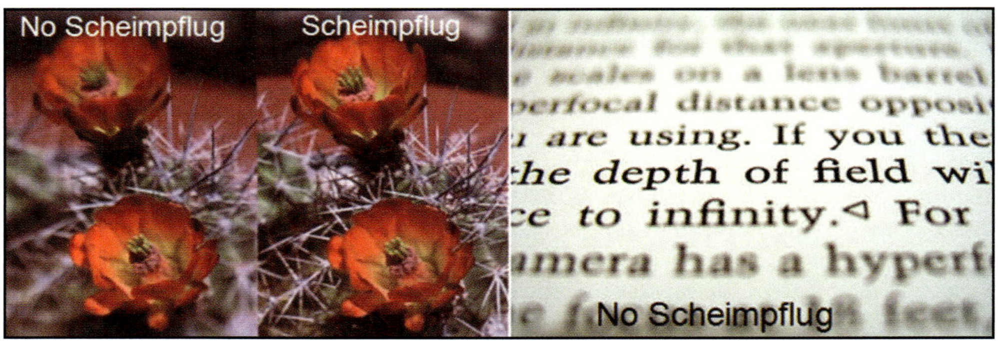


**Figure 6-72.** Comparison of Scheimpflug and ordinary images. Note the expanded depth of field.

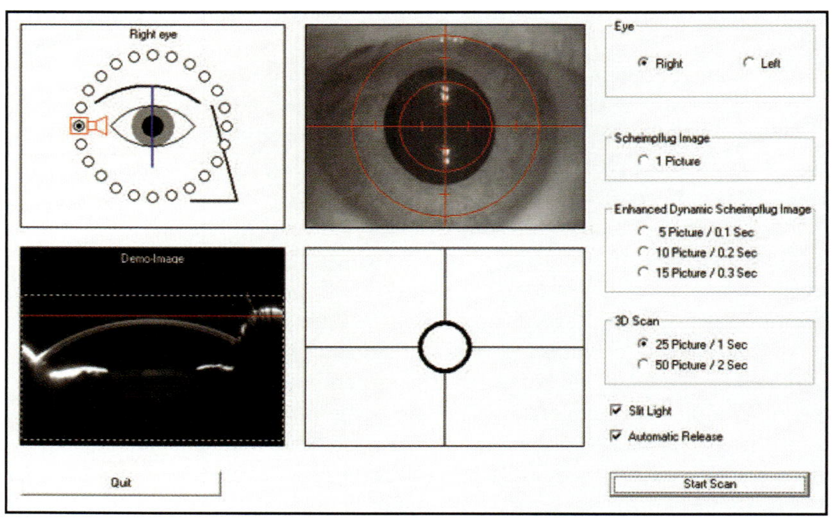


**Figure 6-73.** Acquiring scan display with options for exams on the Oculyzer software.

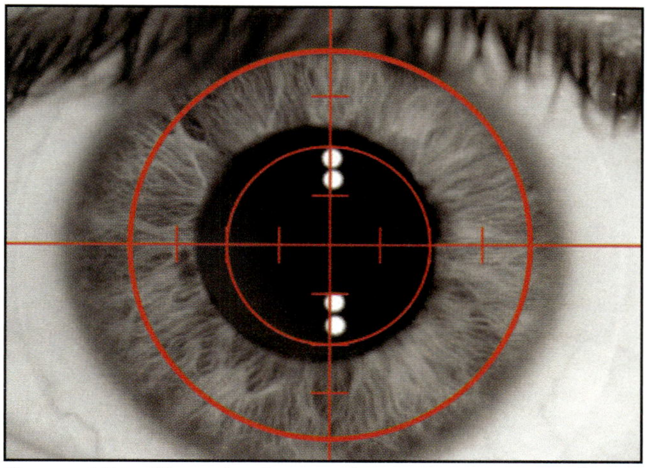

**Figure 6-74.** Slit projection on the cornea. (Reprinted with permission of Thomas Auer.)

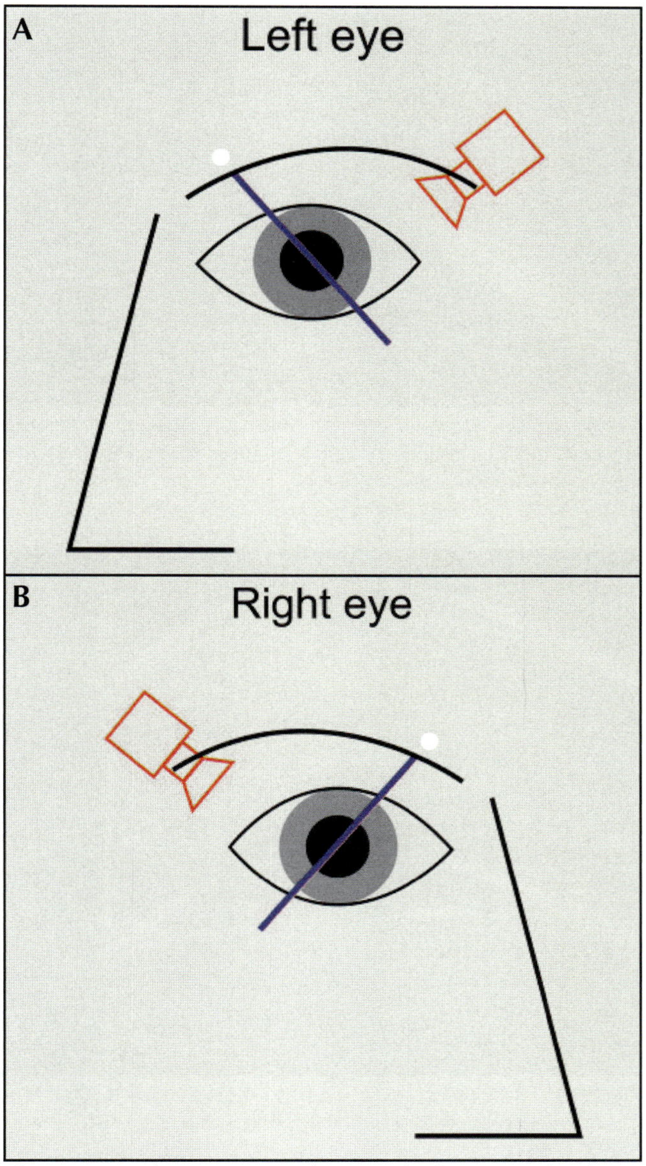


**Figure 6-75.** Slit images are photographed at an angle of 0 to 180 degrees. (Reprinted with permission of Thomas Auer.)

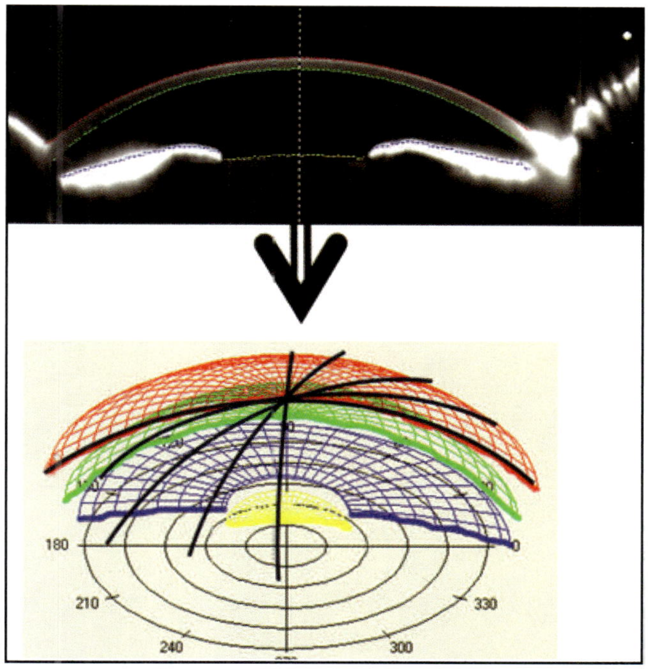


**Figure 6-76.** Three-dimensional tomographic reconstruction of the cornea and anterior segment picture from Scheimpflug images.

measurement is from 3 to 38 mm, and its refractive power measurement range is from 9 to 99 D. The repeatability of the thickness measurements is 3 µm, while for the curvature measurements, it is 0.2 D.

During the examination, the patient should be comfortably positioned at the instrument with adjustment of height and proper placement on the chin rest and forehead strap. The patient is asked to blink normally and to open both eyes and stare at the fixation target. After alignment is close to perfect, the patient is asked to blink a couple of times, and the final alignment is done for the automatic release mode in order to start the scan. We advise using the 25 single Scheimpflug images 3-dimensional scan as a routine.

Image quality should be checked right after the exam is taken, and only images with an acceptable quality should be considered. The quality specification shows several parameters separately for the front and back surfaces of the cornea: the area of coverage of the measurements (analyzed area), blinking (lost segments), alignment (x, y, and z axis), and fixation of the eye (Figure 6-77). If the case is considered for customized topography-guided ablation treatment (T-CAT), at least 4 (and up to 8) scans should be taken sequentially. The exam can be taken in the manual release mode, but such scans are not accepted by T-CAT software for treatment planning.

The exams are sensitive to any drops previously applied to the cornea, mainly ocular surface dyes such as fluorescein. These would lead to artifacts of the slit images and result in false calculations. Pupil dilation is also not advised because it may also affect the centration of T-CAT

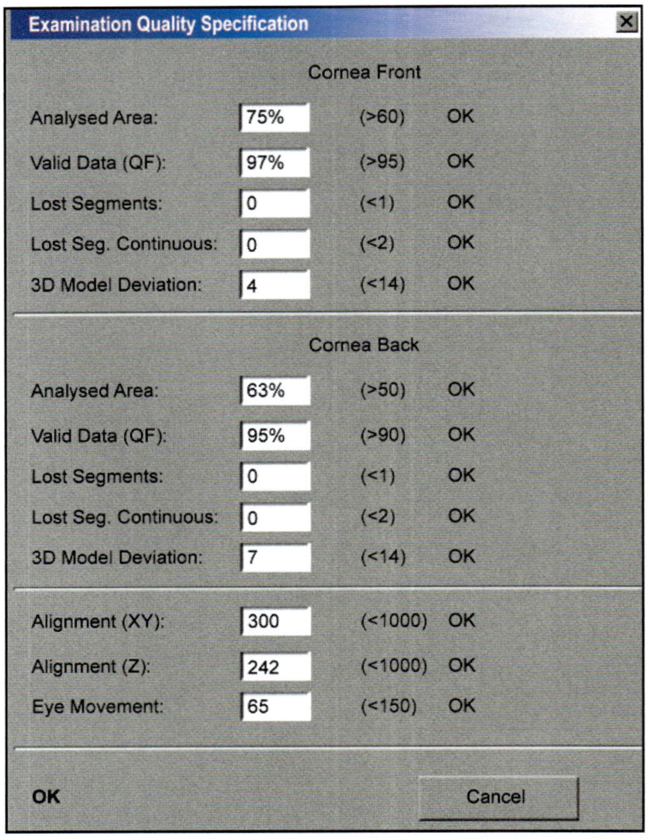


**Figure 6-77.** Quality assessment of the scan box. (Reprinted with permission of Thomas Auer.)

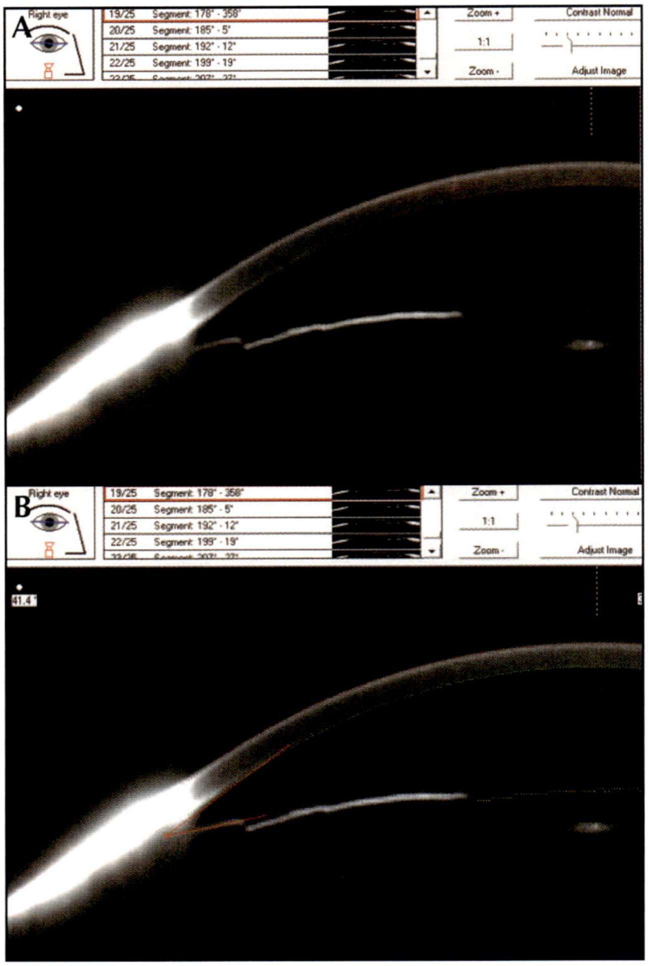


**Figure 6-78.** (A) Total internal reflection of light at the iris-corneal angle. (B) Extrapolation of edge detection from the software for angle measurements.

treatments, unless the T-CAT treatment is planned immediately afterward, presumably with the same pupil size. Dilation of the pupil is necessary only for diagnostic purposes in the case with interest in examining IOLs or the crystalline lens.

The 3-dimensional Scheimpflug image scanning provides data from the anterior and posterior surfaces of the cornea, the anterior iris, and the lens (see Figure 6-73). Because the system uses the visible blue light (custom-designed 475-nm, UV-free), it is sensitive to any corneal opacity rendering hyper-reflective images and inaccurate contour analyses by the Oculyzer software. This also makes the images optically sensitive to total internal reflection at the peripheral cornea, thus not enabling visualization of the anterior chamber angle, as well as anything posterior to the iris (Figure 6-78A). Although the exam does not provide a direct visualization of the iris-corneal angle, the sophisticated extrapolation software is capable of providing a value for angle estimation with high accuracy. Very importantly, the clinician should re-evaluate the extrapolation calculation on the Scheimpflug image for ensuring proper clinical evaluation of the anterior chamber angle (Figure 6-78B). However, this approach has been successfully used in clinical practice to screen narrow angle cases and to document the improvement after cataract surgery (Figure 6-79).

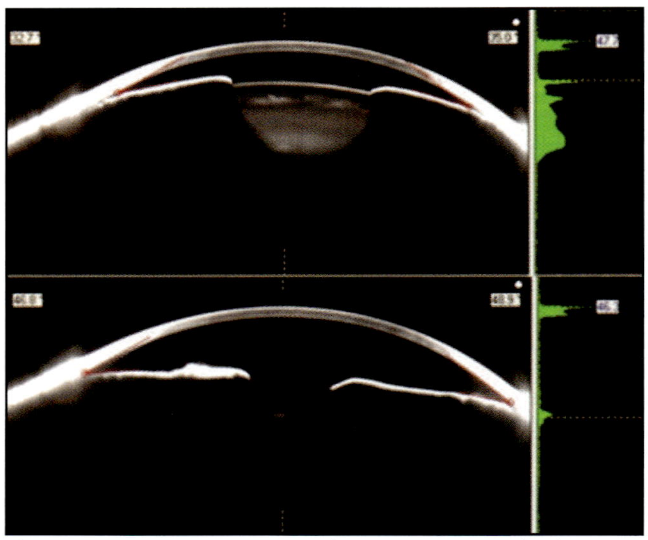

**Figure 6-79.** (Top) Narrow angle in a patient with glaucoma prior to cataract surgery. (Bottom) The same eye post-cataract surgery. Note the widening of the angle in the absence of the crystalline lens.

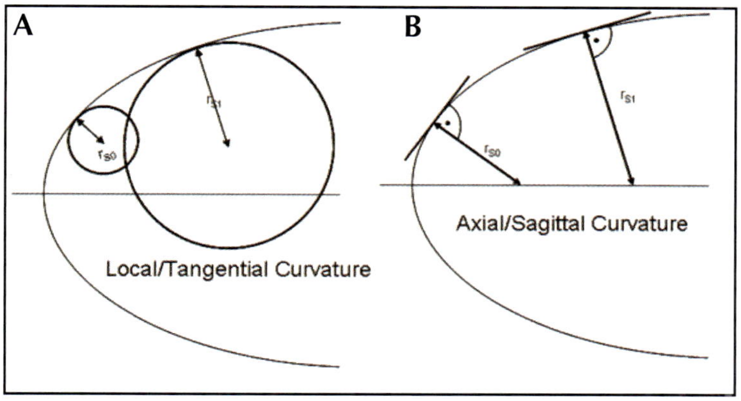


**Figure 6-80.** Diagram scheme for (A) local/tangential (or instantaneous) curvature and (B) axial/sagittal curvature calculations.

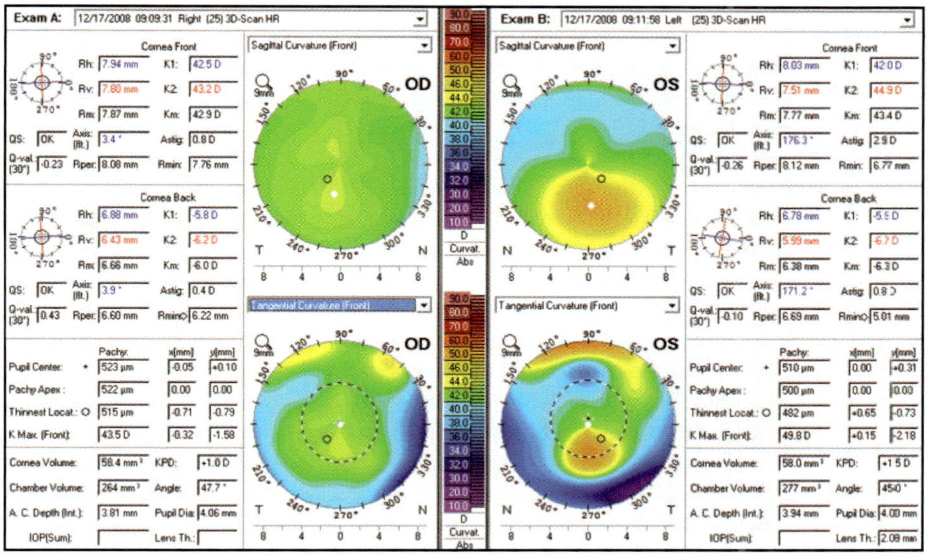


**Figure 6-81.** Sagittal (superior) and tangential (inferior) maps from both eyes of a refractive candidate with very asymmetric keratoconus (not unilateral). Scale used was American Scale with 61 colors, absolute (normal). Note the tangential maps highlighting the cone are surrounded by a flatter zone. Both corneas were prolate with average asphericity (Q) for 30 degrees of -0.23 in OD and -0.26 in OS. Interestingly, the topometric indices for the 8-mm front curvature zone did not detect a keratoconic pattern in OD and detected KC stage 2 in OS.

The Oculyzer is a powerful diagnostic tool that also serves therapeutic purposes. The exam provides detailed corneal tomographic information, along with anterior chamber maps and Scheimpflug images for optical scattering densitometry of the cornea and crystalline lens.

The Oculyzer is a corneal tomography system, and the Scheimpflug scanning provides considerably larger area measurement of the cornea compared with Placido's topography systems. It is also not sensitive to irregularities on the corneal reflex and interference from the tear film. Having measured the true elevation raw data of the front and back corneal surfaces, this exam generates curvature maps using a sagittal (axial) and tangential (instantaneous) algorithm. In the sagittal map, the curvature of the cornea is determined at each measured point at a normal (90-degree) angle to its surface referenced to the mid-line (axis), while tangential maps evaluate the local radius at each measured point of data (Figure 6-80). This highlights differences among the measured points and results in a more "noisy" color pattern for the tangential maps, which facilitates diagnosis of keratoconus (Figure 6-81). Sagittal curvature maps have been more popular for screening refractive candidates and served as the basis for classic screening parameters such as the Rabinowitz-McDonnell,[33,34] which are based on the steepness of the cornea, superior-inferior asymmetry, and between-eyes asymmetries.

The clinical value for the curvature maps from the posterior corneal surface relies on the more accurate corneal power measurements, mainly for assessing IOL calculations. There are, however, different approaches for calculating the relationship between the radii of curvature of the anterior and posterior cornea. The BESST formula,[35] the true net power, the keratometric power deviations, and other methods[36,37] have been described. However, it still remains controversial if K values from Scheimpflug photography do improve accuracy for routine IOL power calculations.[38]

The Oculyzer provides a corneal thickness map with accuracy and repeatability within less than 3 µm.[39] Central thickness and thinnest pachymetry data are provided. In addition, the CTSP and the PTI graphs are calculated from the pachymetry map (Figure 6-82). Starting from the thinnest point outward, the CTSP describes the rate of increase of corneal thickness by noting the averages of pachymetric values within imaginary annular rings concentric to the

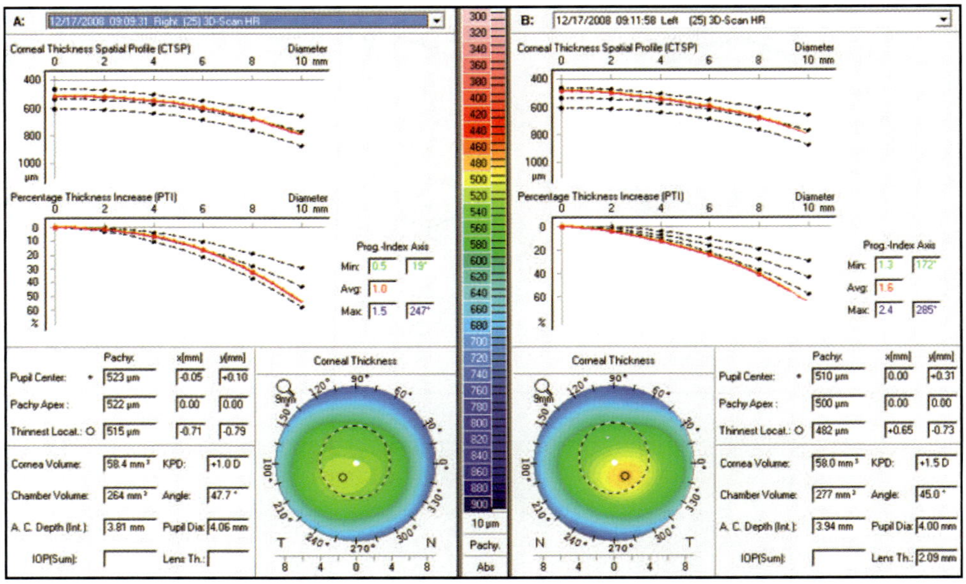


**Figure 6-82.** Pachymetric maps and CTSP and PTI graphs from the same case as in Figure 6-81.

thinnest point with increasing diameters in 0.1-mm steps. The PTI takes the percentage of increase from the thinnest point for the average at each ring.[22,40,41]

A pachymetric progression index (PPI) is also calculated for every 1-degree meridian along the complete 360 degrees, starting at the thinnest point. The average of all meridians and the one with lower and higher values are presented. In a normal population, the averages and SD of PPI of the minimal, maximal, and average of all meridians (PPI-Ave, PPI-Max, PPI-Min) are 0.58 ± 0.3, 0.85 ± 0.18, and 0.13 ± 0.33.[22,40] The pachymetric index will be higher if the cornea gets thicker more abruptly from the thinnest point out to the periphery (PTI and CTSP graphs falling down). The graphs enable the diameter zone where the increase in thickness is higher than the mean of a normal population.

The best parameters developed for diagnosing keratoconus are the "relational" thinnest, which is the thinnest pachymetric value divided by the pachymetric progression. The "Ambrósio Relational Thinnest" (ART) is thereby calculated for the minimal (ART-Min), average (ART-Mid), and maximal (ART-Max). The "ART" concept combines thinnest with the pachymetric distribution, which facilitates the identification of an abnormal cornea despite its thinnest value. The ART-Mid and ART-Max have AUROC of 0.98 and 0.99, with cut-offs of 426 and 339 µm, respectively.[42,43] For practical reasons, we have opted not to perform LASIK if ART-Max is lower than 400 µm. This tomographic approach for pachymetric characterization has been useful for increasing the sensitivity to detect very subtle abnormalities in refractive candidates who may be at higher risk for ectasia.[44,45]

The anterior and posterior elevation maps are a generalized form of comparing the true corneal shape with a reference shape, usually a (best fit) sphere or toric ellipsoid. The diameter of the cornea used for calculating the best fit impacts the calculation. We advise setting a fixed zone of 9 mm or preferably 8 mm. Guidelines for interpretation of elevation maps have been well-described by Belin.[46,47]

The Oculyzer exam also provides an analysis of corneal wavefront. Zernike polynomial decomposition of the anterior and posterior surfaces of the cornea provides lower-order aberrations and HOAs. The understanding of corneal spherical aberrations may be used for customizing aspheric IOLs in cataract surgery.[48] The impact of the posterior corneal wavefront is still not well understood. Also, coma and other HOA terms may be useful for diagnosing keratoconus and related conditions.

From the 3-dimensional model created, the Oculyzer allows a detailed assessment of anterior chamber angle, height, volume, and depth,[49] becoming a useful tool to complement the study of glaucoma and for planning the implantation of anterior chamber lenses.[50-52]

The Scheimpflug images also enable the documentation and quantification of corneal and lens opacity and other abnormalities. For example, the increased reflectivity in the posterior surface of the cornea may be an indication of cornea guttata ("sign of the camel" in the densitogram).[53] Scheimpflug documentation of cataract has also been very useful for supporting and also planning refractive lens surgery indications.[54]

The Oculyzer is a very powerful diagnostic tool, but one of the most important applications of the Oculyzer is planning customized ablations for laser vision corrections with the Alcon WaveLight laser system. Although the exam provides a 3-dimensional model of the cornea, the link for customization currently only considers front elevation and corneal apex-pupil centroid relation data. We have used this approach for all therapeutic cases as well as for most hyperopic procedures with very successful outcomes.[55]

# Optovue—Fourier Domain Anterior Segment Optical Coherence Tomography

Karolinne Maia Rocha, MD, PhD and J. Bradley Randleman, MD

Optical coherence tomography (OCT) is a real-time, high-resolution, high-speed, noninvasive, and noncontact optical device that provides 2- and 3-dimensional visualization of anterior segment morphology. This technique generates unique imaging capabilities for the cornea and anterior segment and provides valuable information for both keratorefractive and lenticular surgery, including flap architecture analysis, residual stromal bed thickness determination, keratoconus screening, and IOL power calculations.

## Principles of Optical Coherence Tomography

OCT images are acquired by measuring the intensity and time delay of wave lights diffracted from anatomical structures passing through an established reference path. Low-coherence light from a super-luminescent diode source is reflected off ocular structures at different axial depths and is processed to create an axial scan.[56] OCT systems provide cross-sectional scans of anterior segment structures such as the cornea, iris, anterior chamber angle, and lens as well as the retina and optic nerve. However, the pigmentation on the posterior side of the iris blocks the high-resolution visualization of the ciliary body.[57-60]

Initial time-domain OCT technologies used detection of backscattered light from the tissues by mechanically sweeping a mirror in a known reference position. A commercially available time domain OCT (Visante OCT, Carl Zeiss Meditec, Jena, Germany) operates at a scan rate of 2048 axial scans per seconds, axial resolution of 18 μm, and transverse resolution of 60 μm. Anterior segment OCT system operates at 1310 nm to attenuate the signal from highly scattering structures (eg, sclera),[61] contrary to the retinal imaging system that operates at 830 nm.[62]

With the advent of a spectral-domain OCT (Fourier domain) in 2002, the image acquisition speed has consistently increased. The spectral-domain OCT systems use a charge-coupled device camera to register the diffraction grating of wave lights returning from the eye structures. The intensity and time delay of the wave lights are calculated using a mathematical formula, a Fourier transformation. The images in Fourier domain OCT systems (Optovue RTVue-100, Optovue Inc, Fremont, CA) are acquired up to 100 times more quickly when compared to the standard time-domain OCT devices.[63] A Cornea/Anterior Segment Module (CAM) for the Optovue RTVue-100 OCT was approved in 2007, and it provides full-range, artifact-free high-pixel density cross-sectional imaging of the anterior segment.[64,65]

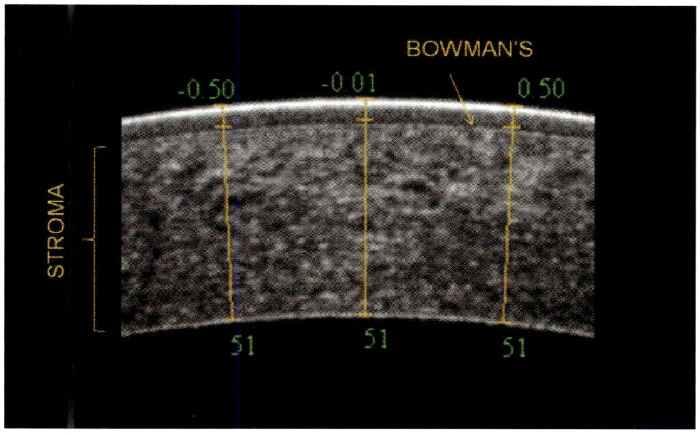

**Figure 6-83.** Fourier domain OCT CAM-L raster module scan of a normal cornea. All anatomical layers are visible.

The higher-resolution anterior segment images obtained with Fourier domain OCT systems result from a scan rate of 26,000 axial scans per second, axial resolution of 5 μm, and transverse resolution of 15 μm compared with a scan rate up to 2048 axial scans per seconds, axial resolution of 18 μm, and transverse resolution of 60 μm of the time-domain OCT systems. Furthermore, the increased axial resolution of spectral-domain OCT allows visualization of anatomical details that are not observed with time-domain OCT, including discreet epithelial thickness profiles and Bowman's layer, among others (Figure 6-83).[64,66]

## Imaging and Examination Techniques

The add-on Cornea/Anterior Segment Module lens (CAM mode) should be adjusted prior to anterior segment high-resolution scan acquisition. Two anterior segment models are available: a wide-angle lens (long lens or CAM-L) and a high-magnification lens (short lens or CAM-S) for anterior segment imaging. Select either CAM-L or CAM-S mode to assess the tab contents. The wide-angle lens (CAM-L, 6.0 to 2.0 mm) is the most commonly used because it balances depth of field with transverse image capture. The currently available anterior segment maps for the Optovue

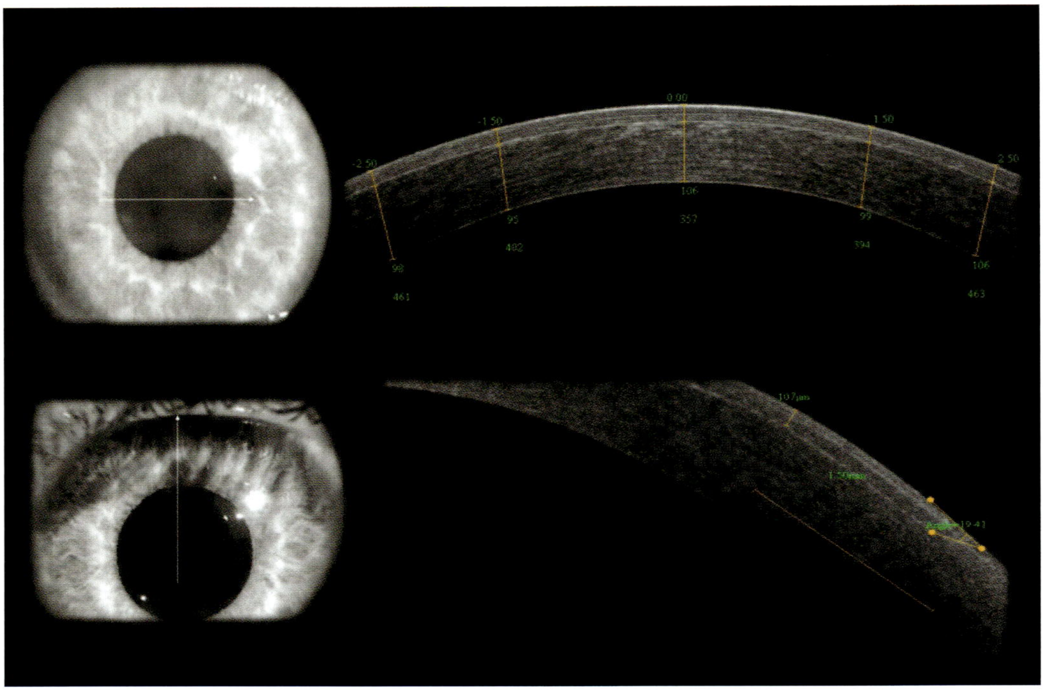

**Figure 6-84.** Fourier domain OCT of thin LASIK flap for myopia, revealing a uniform flap thickness.

are pachymetry map, cornea power validation, cross-sectional scan line (CL-line), cross line (CL-cross line), anterior chamber angle (CL-angle), raster scan (CL-raster), and 3-dimensional view of all corneal layers (CL-3D Cornea). Users can program a series of scan types for imaging strategies such as clinical trials, specific corneal diseases, and postoperative follow-up.

Image acquisition is obtained while the patient sits in front of the scanning device with the forehead and chin stabilized by a head rest. External illumination and scan optimization can be adjusted by clicking "Auto P," which automatically adjusts for differences in polarization. Patients are asked to fixate on the target light source, and consecutive scans are performed of the operated eye using the high-resolution scanning mode.

The "Analyze" menu activates the view and tools for manual measurements of the captured images. Editing tools include removal of tracing lines, area of interest selection, zoom, and "Undo/Redo." Measurement tools include distance tool, area tool, point line, text annotation, zoom, OCT noise level, snapshot, and video. Diagnostic tools include progression, symmetry, and comparison analysis.

# Clinical Applications

## Refractive Surgery

Fourier domain OCT is a useful tool when evaluating LASIK flaps, stromal bed thickness prior to enhancement, and preoperative evaluation for keratoectasia. The posterior edge of the LASIK flap is determined by direct visualization of the area of increased reflectivity corresponding with the flap-stroma interface.[67-69] The flap tool of the high-resolution cross-line scan may be used with the add-on lens to measure flap thickness. The anterior surface of the cornea and the flap-stroma interface are used as anatomical landmarks for this purpose. In addition to the central flap thickness, the overall flap architecture can be evaluated (Figure 6-84). Using the OCT, a recent study demonstrated that some modern mechanical microkeratomes make essentially planar flaps, similar in architecture to flaps created with the femtosecond laser.[69]

Previous studies have suggested actual residual stromal bed (RSB) thickness may vary significantly from predicted values due to variation in flap thicknesses.[70-73] Further, a nonuniform meniscus-shaped mechanical microkeratome flap can lead to deeper disruption of collagen lamellae in the corneal periphery, resulting in peripheral corneal steepening and central corneal flattening.[74] The OCT can provide important information, such as the overall RSB, and may prove especially useful when determining if there is sufficient RSB for LASIK retreatments. Some cases of ectasia after LASIK may be due to excessive, irregular flap thickness (Figure 6-85).

Although many topographic indices have been described for the diagnosis and progression of keratoconus,[24,75-78] one of the most important findings in keratoconus detection is focal corneal thinning.[34,79,80] The OCT pachymetry maps have shown high reproducibility in detecting eccentric and asymmetric corneal thinning.[81] Li and coworkers have demonstrated higher repeatability in the 0- to 5-mm central area of the OCT pachymetry map and have suggested keratoconus

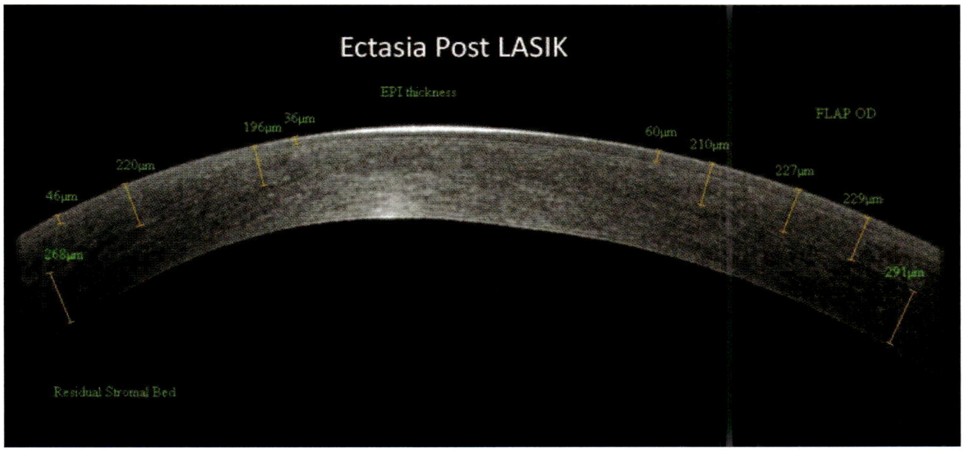


**Figure 6-85.** Fourier domain OCT of an ectatic cornea post-LASIK. Note the highly variable residual stromal bed thickness, flap thickness, and the meniscus shape of the flap.

analysis of the central 5-mm diameter zone.[81,82] The Optovue RTVue-CAM pachymetry map is divided into 8 zones and 2-, 5-, and 6-mm annular rings. The map is obtained in 0.32 seconds and comprises 8 meridional scans. The average of 6-mm paracentral pachymetry measurements of superior (S), inferior (I), temporal (T), nasal (N), superotemporal (ST), superonasal (SN), inferotemporal (IT), and inferonasal (IN) zones are displayed. The central measurement corresponds to the average pachymetry of the central 2 mm. The pachymetry map also includes minimum corneal thickness and location; anterior and posterior corneal power and curvature radius; and total corneal power (Figure 6-86).

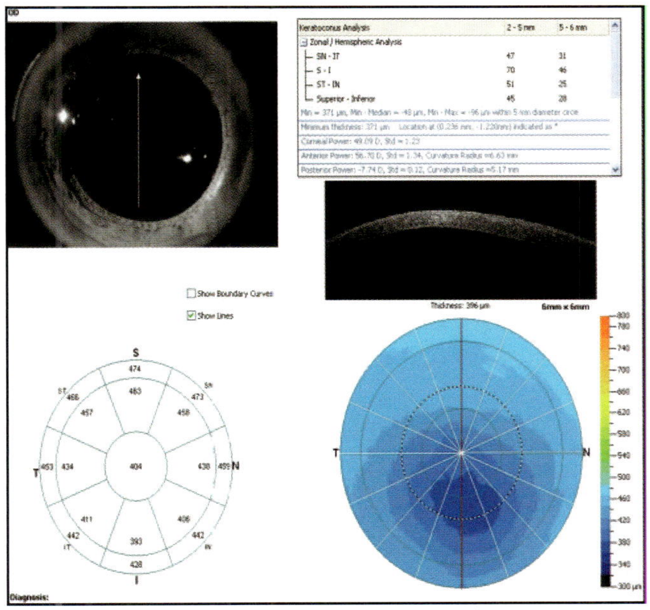

**Figure 6-86.** Optovue RTVue-CAM OCT pachymetry map.

RTvue CAM-L mode (CL-line) scans provide high-resolution imaging of the corneal architecture and the epithelial thickness profile of keratoconic eyes. Specific areas of reactive epithelial hyperplasia and residual stromal bed can be precisely assessed. Reinstein and coauthors have demonstrated that the epithelium is thinner in the apex of the cone and thicker surrounding the apex of the stromal cone (creating a "doughnut" shape) using the Artemis very high-frequency (VHF) digital ultrasound.[27,83] The authors also suggested that the epithelial compensation of areas surrounding the cone can interfere with the interpretation of anterior corneal surface topography. An advantage of the Fourier domain OCT is cross-sectional high-resolution scans that demonstrate specific areas of epithelial changes overlying the corneal stroma. The epithelium can be significantly thinner in the apex of the cone with reactive thickening compensation immediately inferior to the conical apex in severe keratoconus as demonstrated in Figure 6-87.

### Lens Surgery

With the OCT, true corneal power can also be assessed for IOL calculation. Contrary to other devices that only analyze the anterior corneal surface or curvature, this program compares both the anterior and posterior corneal surfaces. Errors in measuring true corneal power affect IOL calculation outcomes, especially in cataract patients who had previous refractive surgery. Standard keratometry and topography measurements of the cornea power (K) after refractive surgery tend to overestimate the K readings following laser corrections for myopia and underestimate for hyperopia, frequently resulting in significant hyperopia in eyes with previous myopic surgery and myopic error in eyes with previous hyperopic surgery.[84-92]

Very high-speed OCT can directly measure both anterior and posterior corneal power and should increase the accuracy of the corneal power calculation. OCT-based formulas for calculating IOL powers are in active clinical trials.

## Advanced Diagnostic Imaging

The high resolution of the Fourier domain OCT and the ability to visualize all cornea layers is extremely useful for diagnosis, management, and follow-up of complex corneal cases. Figure 6-88 shows a patient who presented with significant visual symptoms and irregular astigmatism

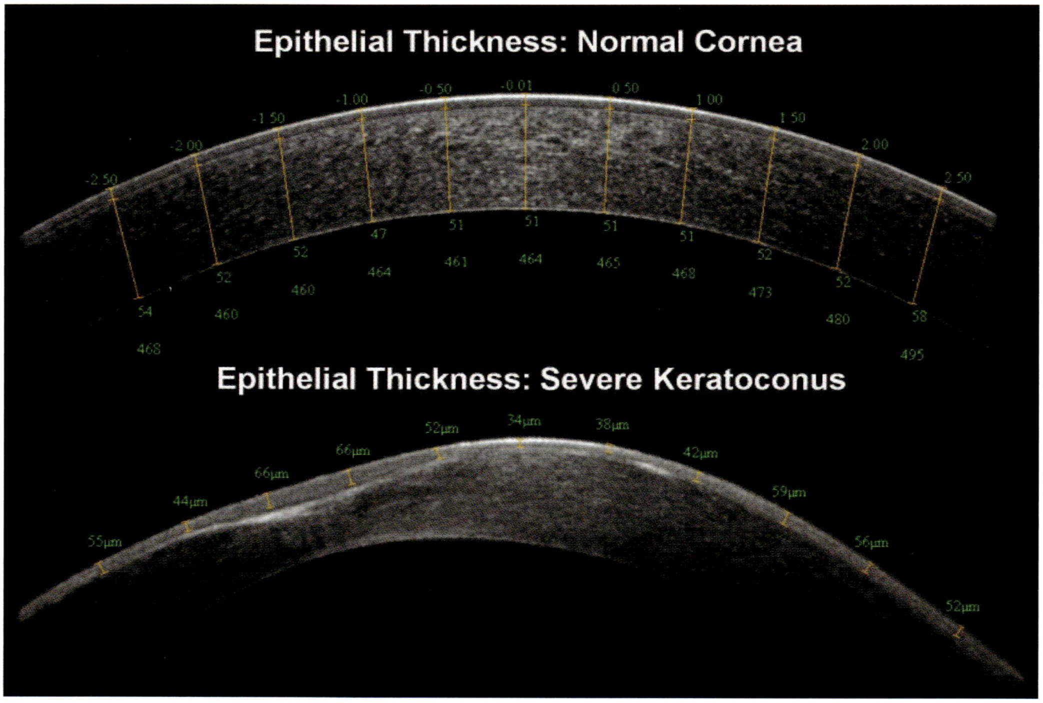


**Figure 6-87.** Fourier domain OCT of a normal cornea (top) and severe keratoconus (bottom).

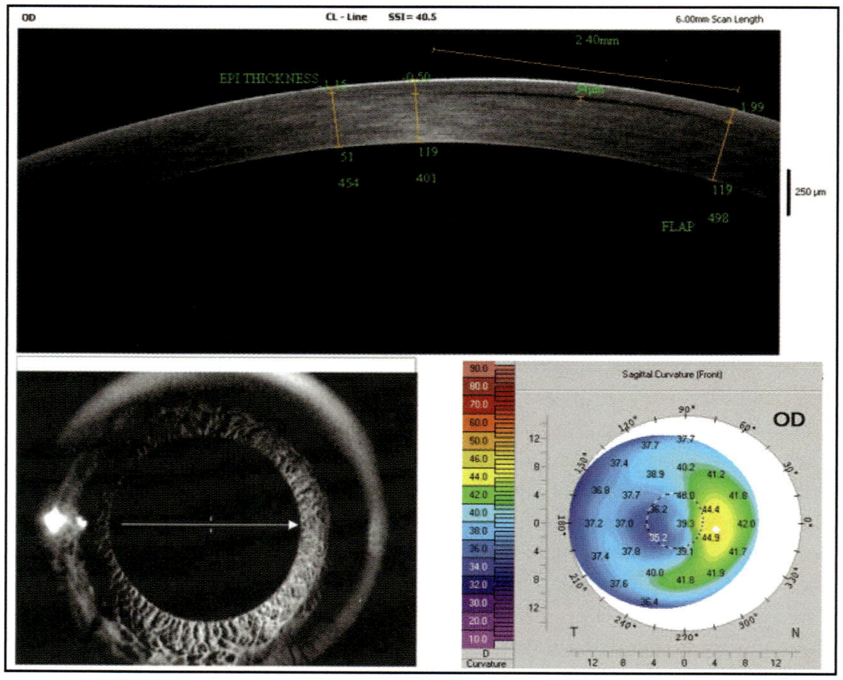


**Figure 6-88.** Fourier domain OCT of LASIK interface fluid causing topographic irregular astigmatism as demonstrated by the Pentacam (bottom right).

7 months post-LASIK despite a normal clinical appearance. The diagnosis of interface fluid was made with OCT. Figure 6-89A illustrates a case of a patient who developed progressive irregular astigmatism after phakic IOL implantation. Fourier domain high-resolution CL-line scan demonstrated irregular wound healing. After wound revision, the patient's symptoms resolved. The apposition of the surgical wound 1-week postwound revision is demonstrated in Figure 6-89B.

Optovue RTVue-CAM can also produce high-resolution images of intrastromal corneal rings, allowing for accurate depth and position of the intrastromal ring. Superficial implant of corneal ring segments may cause epithelial-stromal breaks, fibrosis, and extrusion, while very deep implants can result in anterior chamber perforation. Figure 6-90 illustrates a case where the corneal ring segment was placed too deep (bottom) and one example of stromal and epithelial irregularities surround the implant (top).

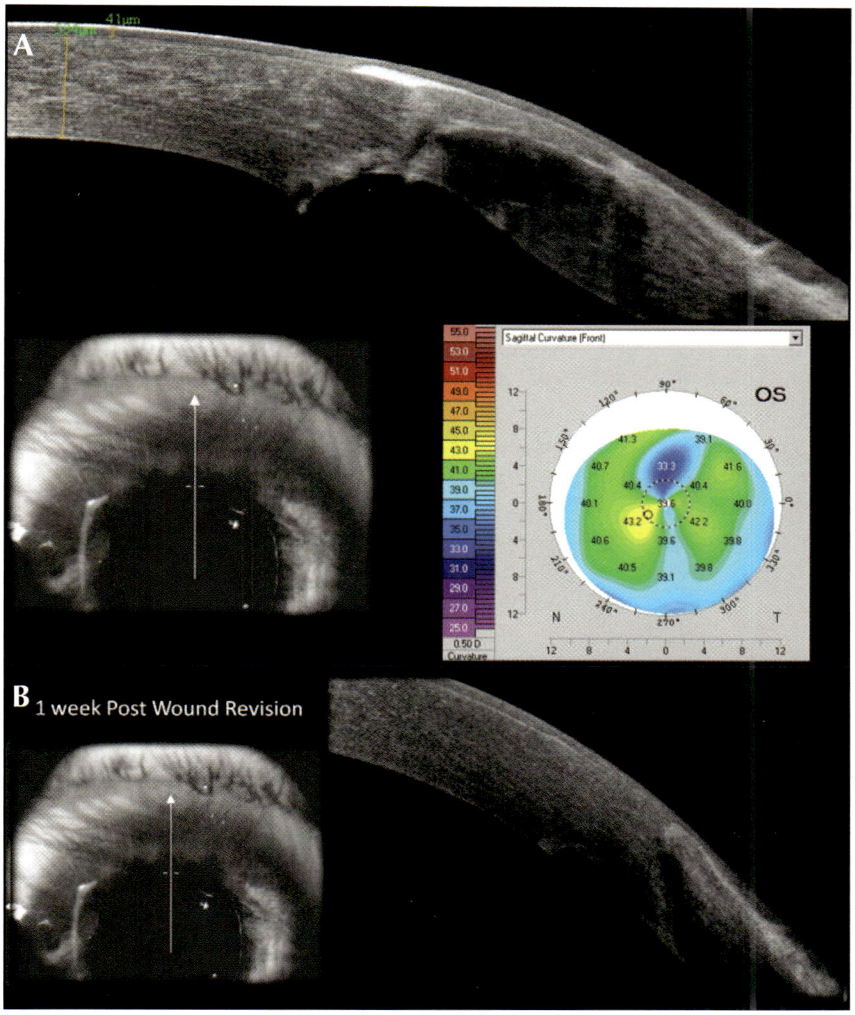


**Figure 6-89.** (A) Fourier domain OCT of apposition of the surgical wound after phakic IOL implant; Pentacam (bottom right) shows irregular astigmatism. (B) One week after wound revision.

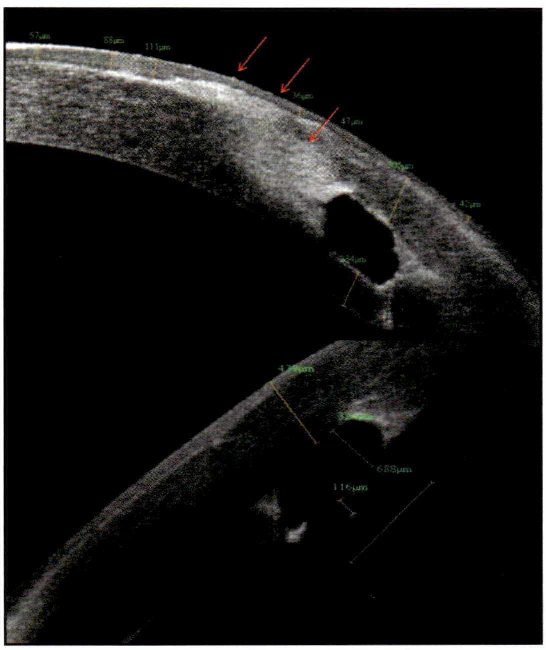

**Figure 6-90.** Fourier domain OCT demonstrating depth and position of the corneal intrastromal rings.

# Conclusion

Fourier domain OCT provides accurate assessment of the anterior segment with applications including corneal diagnostic procedures, treatment planning, and monitoring outcomes. Certainly, high-resolution anterior segment OCT can help anterior segment surgeons to improve their clinical evaluation and surgical techniques.

# Artemis Epithelial Thickness Profile: A Surrogate for Stromal Surface Topography

Dan Z. Reinstein, MD, MA(Cantab), FRCSC, FRCOphth; Timothy J. Archer, MA(Oxon), DipCompSci(Cantab); and Marine Gobbe, MST(Optom), PhD

The corneal epithelium is a highly active, self-renewing layer; a complete turnover occurs in approximately 5 to 7 days.[93] Despite this high turnover rate, the epithelium must maintain the same thickness profile over time to maintain corneal power and, hence, ocular refraction. The epithelium accounts for an average of 1.03 D of corneal power at the central 2-mm diameter zone.[94] The corneal epithelium is known to have the ability to alter its thickness profile to try and re-establish a smooth, symmetrical optical surface to compensate for changes to the stromal surface.[95,96] For example, central epithelial thickening after myopic excimer laser ablation has been widely reported,[97-101] while epithelial breakdown over an advanced cone in keratoconus demonstrates that the epithelium must have thinned over the cone.[26,102-104] Epithelial changes such as these will have an impact on the ocular refraction; however, the biggest clinical impact of epithelial changes is to corneal front surface topography. Because the epithelium compensates for stromal irregularities, the presence of an irregular stromal surface is either partially or totally masked from corneal front surface topography. Therefore, corneal front surface topography does not always tell the whole story and in some cases does not provide the necessary information to establish a correct diagnosis.

Ideally, we would like a method of directly measuring stromal surface topography. Some have suggested measuring topography after epithelial removal and have shown an increase in irregularity.[105] However, this is not a clinically feasible test. Alternatively, the anterior stromal surface shape can be appreciated by an examination of its proxy—the epithelial thickness profile. Based on an understanding of the pattern of the normal epithelial thickness profile, any localized abnormal epithelial changes can be relied upon as a mirror of a relative localized stromal surface irregularity. Therefore, the epithelial thickness profile can be thought of as a form of stromal surface topography.

Different methods have been used to measure corneal epithelial thickness: OCT,[106,107] slit-lamp-adapted OCT,[108] confocal microscopy,[109,110] optical pachymetry,[111] and focusing confocal microscopy.[112] However, these techniques only allow single-point measurement of epithelial thickness, so they cannot be used to investigate the epithelial thickness profile. Most studies have reported central epithelial thickness measurements, and a few studies also provided epithelial thickness in the peripheral cornea, but the number of points measured in the periphery is limited.[111,113,114]

Currently, the only validated method capable of measuring epithelial thickness continuously over a 10-mm area is VHF digital ultrasound.[115,116] The first confirmed measurement of the epithelium of the cornea in vivo was reported by our group in 1993 using VHF digital ultrasound, demonstrating that acoustic interfaces that were being detected were indeed located spatially at the epithelial surface and at the interface between epithelial cells and the surface of Bowman's layer.[117] In 1994, we reported the first high-precision 3-dimensional thickness mapping of the corneal epithelium for the central 3-mm diameter.[118] The area of acquisition was increased to 10 mm using the Artemis VHF digital ultrasound (ArcScan Inc, Morrison, CO) in 2000.[115]

The Artemis has since been used to measure the epithelial thickness in a wide variety of situations, the majority of which are summarized in this section, and the effect these changes have on ocular refraction and the implications for misdiagnosis by corneal front surface topography are discussed. This section will focus on the diagnosis of early keratoconus, epithelial thickness changes after refractive surgery and Intacs, and establishing a true diagnosis after complicated LASIK.

## Artemis Technology

All the epithelial thickness data set out in this section were obtained using the Artemis 1 VHF digital ultrasound arc-scanner. Artemis VHF digital ultrasound is carried out using an ultrasonic standoff medium, and so provides the advantages of immersion scanning (eg, the tear film is not incorporated into the corneal or epithelial thickness measurement, and there is no physical contact of the transducer with the cornea). The patient sits and positions the chin and forehead into a headrest while placing the eye in a soft-rimmed eye-cup. Warm sterile normal saline (33°C) is filled into the darkened scanning chamber. The patient fixates on a narrowly focused aiming beam, which is coaxial with the infrared camera, the corneal vertex, and the center of rotation of the scanning system. The technician adjusts the center of rotation of the system until it is coaxial with the corneal vertex. In this manner, the position of each scan plane is maintained about a single point on the cornea, and corneal mapping is therefore centered on the corneal vertex. A speculum is not required as patients find it comfortable to open the eye without blinking in the warm saline bath and voluntary elevation of the upper lid produces exposure of the central 10 mm of cornea in virtually all patients. Performing a 3-dimensional scan set with the Artemis 1 takes approximately 2 to 3 minutes per eye.

A broadband 50-MHz VHF ultrasound transducer (bandwidth approximately 10 to 60 MHz) is swept by a reverse arc high-precision mechanism to acquire B-scans as arcs that follow the surface contour of anterior or posterior segment structures of interest. The Artemis possesses a unique scan-arc adjustment mechanism to enable maximum perpendicularity (and signal-to-noise ratio) to be obtained for scanning any of the different curvatures within the globe (ie, cornea, iris plane, and retina). The resolution of the system is 21 μm, meaning that distinct echo-peaks can be seen on the I-scan for a corneal layer thicker than 21 μm.

For 3-dimensional scan sets, the scan sequence consists of 4 meridional B-scans at 45-degree intervals. Each scan sweep takes about 0.25 seconds and consists of 128 scan lines or pulse echo vectors. During the acquisition of each scan, data are converted (in near real-time) to a B-scan displayed on the computer screen.

Ultrasound data are digitized and stored. The digitized ultrasound data are then transformed using patented Cornell University (Ithaca, NY) digital signal processing technology I-scan. A linear polar/radial interpolation function is used to interpolate between scan meridians to produce a Cartesian matrix over a 10-mm diameter in 0.1-mm steps. The interpolation function also includes auto-correlation of back surface curvatures to center and align the meridional scans. This is our standard scanning protocol as it provides sufficiently high-density information in the central cornea with lower density of information in the periphery where it is less needed.

Interfaces between tissues are detected at the location of the maximum change in acoustic impedance (the product of the density and the speed of sound). It was first demonstrated in 1993 that acoustic interfaces being detected in the cornea were located spatially at the epithelial surface and at the interface between epithelial cells and the anterior surface of Bowman's layer.[117] The posterior boundary of the stroma with VHF digital ultrasound is located at the interface between the endothelium and the aqueous as this is the location of the maximum change in acoustic impedance. Therefore, stromal thickness with VHF digital ultrasound is measured from the front surface of Bowman's layer to the back surface of the endothelium.

Figure 6-91 shows an example B-scan of a patient 6 months after LASIK, including the following:

- A geometrically corrected B-scan after readjusting the data to account for the arc-scan motion of the transducer
- A redline image that represents the result after digital signal processing by a computer algorithm on the I-scan
- A nongeometrically corrected B-scan, which magnifies the image to make the interfaces easier to identify. The nongeometrically corrected B-scan is the initial output and appears relatively flat because the arc-scan motion of the transducer keeps it perpendicular to the cornea.

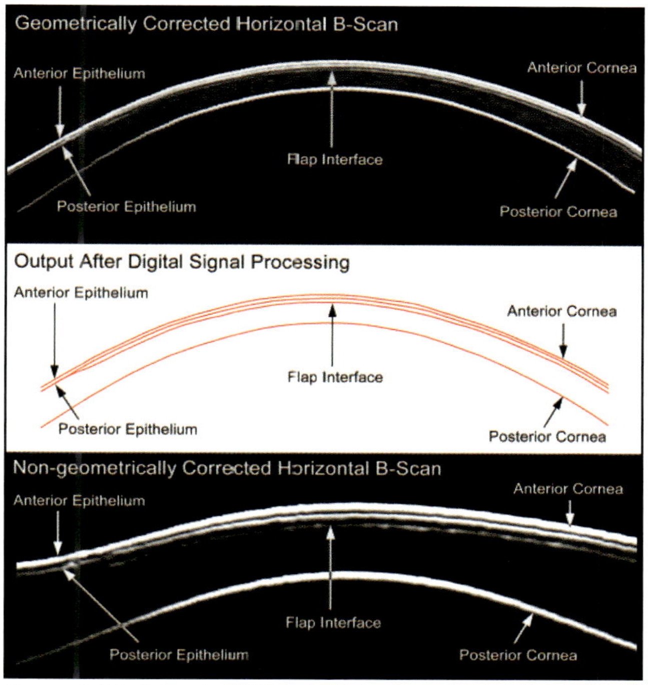


**Figure 6-91.** Artemis VHF digital ultrasound horizontal B-scan of a cornea 6 months after LASIK with a flap created using the VisuMax femtosecond laser. (Top) A geometrically corrected B-scan after readjusting the data to account for the arc-scan motion of the transducer. (Middle) Digital signal processing is performed on the B-scan signal, and layer thickness measurements are obtained by a computer algorithm on the I-scan, resulting in the red line image of the interfaces. (Bottom) Nongeometrically corrected B-scan, which magnifies the image to make the interfaces easier to identify. The nongeometrically corrected B-scan is the initial output and appears relatively flat because the arc-scan motion of the transducer keeps it perpendicular to the cornea.

We have previously published the 3-dimensional repeatability of thickness measurements using the Artemis VHF digital arc-scanner and demonstrated very high repeatability of 3-dimensional wide-area pachymetry for the epithelium, stroma, cornea, flap, and residual stromal bed.[116] The repeatability at the corneal vertex was 0.58 μm for epithelium, 1.78 μm for stroma, 1.68 μm for cornea, 1.68 μm for flap, and 2.27 μm for residual stromal bed. The region-repeatability within the central 1-mm radius was 1.01 μm for epithelium, 3.44 μm for stroma, 3.35 μm for cornea, 2.81 μm for flap, and 3.97 μm for residual stromal bed.

Therefore, the Artemis is capable of reliably detecting changes in epithelial thickness of less than 1 µm. This compares favorably with the other methods of single-point epithelial thickness measurement; the repeatability has been reported to be 3.24 µm using SL-OCT,[108] 3.33 µm using Humphrey Zeiss OCT,[112] and 3.41 µm using the OptoVue OCT (unpublished data, DZ Reinstein). Therefore, these other instruments are only capable of reliably measuring a change of more than 6 µm.

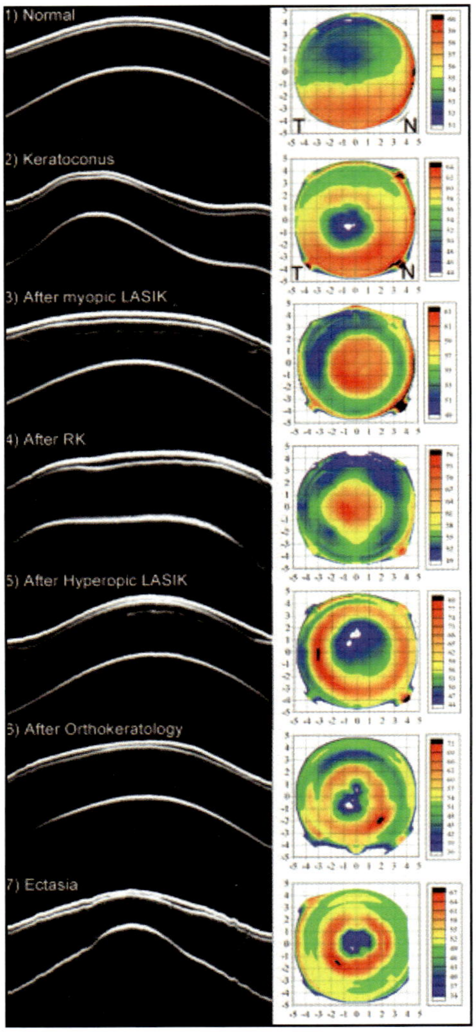


**Figure 6-92.** Artemis nongeometrically corrected B-scan and epithelial thickness profile for 1) a population of 110 normal untreated eyes, 2) a population of 54 keratoconic eyes, 3) a population of 24 eyes after myopic LASIK, 4) a population of 14 eyes after radial keratotomy, 5) a population of 65 eyes after hyperopic LASIK, 6) a case example of an eye after 2 weeks of wear of an orthokeratology lens, and 7) a case of post-LASIK ectasia.

## Epithelial Thickness Profile in Normal Eyes

Before we look at changes to the epithelium, it is important to obtain a baseline measurement in a normal population so that epithelial changes can be confirmed and quantified. We have previously published a study that characterized the in vivo epithelial thickness profile in a population of normal eyes with no ocular pathology other than refractive error.[119] In this study, the epithelial thickness profile was measured across the central 10-mm diameter of the cornea for 110 normal eyes of 56 patients, and these data were averaged. Epithelial thickness values for left eyes were reflected in the vertical axis and were superimposed onto the right eye values so that nasal/temporal characteristics could be combined.

The average epithelial thickness map (Figure 6-92) revealed that the epithelium was not a layer of homogeneous thickness as had previously been thought, but followed a very distinct pattern; on average, the epithelium was 5.7-µm thicker inferiorly than superiorly and 1.2-µm thicker temporally than nasally. The pattern of thicker epithelium inferiorly than superiorly and thicker epithelium nasally than temporally was consistent across a majority of eyes in the population sampled. The average central epithelial thickness was 53.4 µm, and the standard deviation was only 4.6 µm (range: 43.5 to 63.6 µm). This indicated that there was little variation in central epithelial thickness in the population. The thinnest epithelial point within the central 5 mm of the cornea was displaced 0.33 mm (±1.08) temporally and 0.90 mm (±0.96) superiorly with reference to the corneal vertex.

Figure 6-92 also shows an example of a B-scan of a normal cornea. The epithelium appears regular in thickness. The finding that the epithelium was thinner superiorly, rather than being a uniform thickness throughout, was a surprising result; however, we have recently suggested that eyelid mechanics and blinking might be responsible for the nonuniform epithelial thickness profile seen in normal corneas. In 1994, we originally suggested that eyelid blinking and friction onto the corneal surface may regulate the epithelial thickness profile.[117] We postulated that the eyelid might effectively be chafing the surface epithelium during blinking and that the posterior surface of the semi-rigid tarsus provides a template for the outer shape of the epithelial surface. During blinking, which occurs on average between 300 to 1500 times per hour,[120] the vertical traverse of the upper lid is much greater than that of the lower lid. Doane[121] studied the dynamics of eyelid anatomy during blinking and found that during a blink, the descent of the upper eyelid reaches its maximum speed at about the time it crosses the visual axis. As a consequence, the eyelid might effectively be chafing the surface epithelium during blinking, with greater forces applied on the superior cornea than on the inferior cornea. This could explain why the epithelium was found to be thinner superiorly.

# Epithelial Thickness Profile in Keratoconic Eyes

In keratoconus, the epithelium is known to thin in the area overlying the cone, and in advanced keratoconus, there may be excessive epithelial thinning leading to a breakdown in the epithelium. Epithelial thinning over the cone has been demonstrated using histopathologic analysis of keratoconic corneas,[102] while Haque and colleagues[103] found that central epithelial thickness was thinner in keratoconus than in normal corneas using OCT. Transmission electron microscopy (TEM) has demonstrated that the epithelium was irregular in thickness in keratoconus.[104]

In 2009, we published a study that characterized the in vivo epithelial thickness profile in a population of 54 keratoconic eyes.[26] The subjects included for study had previously been diagnosed with keratoconus, and the diagnosis was confirmed by clinical signs such as microscopic signs at the slit-lamp, corneal topographic changes, high refractive astigmatism, reduced best-corrected visual acuity and contrast sensitivity, and significant level of HOAs, in particular vertical coma. The epithelial thickness profile was measured across the central 10-mm diameter of the cornea for 54 keratoconic eyes of 30 patients, and the data were averaged. Epithelial thickness values for left eyes were reflected in the vertical axis and were superimposed onto the right eye values so that nasal/temporal characteristics could be combined.

The average epithelial thickness profile in keratoconus (see Figure 6-92) revealed that the epithelium was significantly more irregular in thickness compared to the normal population. The epithelium was thinnest at the apex of the cone, and this thin epithelial zone was surrounded by an annulus of thickened epithelium. The location of the thinnest epithelium within the central 5 mm of the cornea was displaced 0.48 mm (±0.66 mm) temporally and 0.32 mm (±0.67 mm) inferiorly with reference to the corneal vertex. The mean epithelial thickness for all eyes was 45.7 ± 5.9 µm (range: 33.1 to 56.3 µm) at the corneal vertex, 38.2 ± 5.8 µm at the thinnest point (range: 29.6 to 52.4 µm), and 66.8 ± 7.2 µm (range: 54.1 to 94.4 µm) at the thickest location. The epithelial thickness was outside the range observed in the normal population in both the thinnest and thickest regions, demonstrating the extent of the change in epithelial thickness in keratoconus.

While all eyes exhibited the same epithelial doughnut pattern, characterized by a localized central zone of thinning surrounded by an annulus of thick epithelium, the thickness values of the thinnest point and the thickest point as well as the difference in thickness between the thinnest and the thickest epithelium varied greatly between eyes. There was a significant correlation between the thinnest epithelium and the steepest keratometry (D), indicating that as the cornea became steeper, the epithelial thickness minimum became thinner. In addition, there was a significant correlation between the thickness of the thinnest epithelium and the difference in thickness between the thinnest and the thickest epithelium. This indicated that, as the epithelium thinned, there was an increase in the irregularity of the epithelial thickness profile. These factors demonstrate that the degree of potential epithelial compensation is dependent on the severity of the keratoconus and that the epithelium changes with the progression of the disease.

Figure 6-92 also shows a B-scan for a keratoconic cornea, which demonstrates the lack of homogeneity in epithelial thickness as well as central corneal thinning. There is epithelial thinning over the cone and relative epithelial thickening adjacent to the stromal surface cone.

As with the epithelial thickness profile seen in a normal population, the reason for the presence of an epithelial doughnut pattern in keratoconus could also be explained by eyelid mechanics and blinking. In keratoconus, because the cone is protruding, the apex would be the first point of contact with the eyelid, resulting in increased chafing and therefore thinning of the epithelium at the apex of the cone. As the cone becomes more severe and the protrusion becomes more pronounced, it makes sense that the epithelium at the apex of the cone becomes thinner. This theory is supported by the finding that the thinnest epithelium in the central zone of the epithelial doughnut pattern was thinner for eyes with steeper keratometry (more advanced keratoconus). As the cone becomes more severe, we also found that the surrounding annulus of epithelium in the epithelial doughnut pattern is thicker. The presence of annular epithelial thickening suggests that the eyelid is applying less force during blinking around the sides of the cone, allowing the epithelium to grow up to the inner surface template of the eyelid; in a sense, the eyelid inner surface is tented over the apex of a bulging cone, producing lateral valleys that are then filled with thickened epithelium. The epithelial reaction can be thought of in terms of draping a cloth over an irregular surface with the edges pulled taut. A taut cloth would not lie evenly across the surface; rather, it would be in contact with the peaks of the irregular surface and tent-shaped above the surface on either side of the peaks before gradually returning to the surface in areas without irregularities. The anterior surface of the cornea can be seen to be similar to such a tent shape in the B-scan in Figure 6-92.

## Diagnosing Early Keratoconus Using Epithelial Thickness Profiles

As we have just shown in the previous 2 sections, there is a distinct difference in the epithelial thickness profile in keratoconus compared to that of normal corneas. We have also shown that the epithelial thickness profile changes with the progression of the disease. Therefore, we can assume that the epithelial doughnut pattern would be observed in early keratoconus, where the degree of epithelial thickness changes would be expected to be relatively small, and epithelial thickness profiles can be used as a screening tool for keratoconus. We have recently proposed this method of using epithelial thickness profile maps as a new adjunctive diagnostic tool, with the aim to provide both higher specificity and higher sensitivity to diagnose early cases of keratoconus when topography is equivocal.[27]

In keratoconus, the cone is often represented by a high, eccentric apex on both anterior and posterior elevation BFS.[122,123] Our hypothesis is that front and back corneal surfaces are yoked, meaning that any back surface ectatic change will therefore be accompanied by a front stromal surface ectatic change. The epithelial doughnut pattern that we have observed in keratoconus will act to minimize the extent of the cone on anterior elevation BFS. Therefore, epithelial changes could potentially fully compensate the stromal surface irregularity for small amounts of stromal front surface ectasia and render a completely normal anterior elevation BFS, while the ectasia would still be apparent on the posterior surface elevation BFS.

Therefore, mild keratoconus might be picked up earlier on posterior surface elevation BFS than anterior surface elevation BFS; something that early adopters of Orbscan became convinced of in the mid- to late 1990s and was first presented by our group in 2003.[124] However, this does not necessarily mean that posterior elevation BFS changes are the first anatomical morphological changes in keratoconus, just that these are the first detectable changes. Interestingly, it was not until 2008 that a paper suggesting this concept actually came to press; Schlegel and colleagues[125] suggested that early posterior surface changes could be occurring in patients with no symptoms and with anterior surface modifications that are so small that they would not be detected. The authors concurred with our previously presented hypothesis that the corneal epithelium could remodel itself and mask or minimize some early anterior surface topographical changes. However, not all posterior elevation BFS changes will be due to keratoconus, which is why there is a need for a diagnostic tool to confirm or exclude a diagnosis of keratoconus in eyes with an eccentric posterior elevation BFS. The key to detecting keratoconus by geometric anatomical changes appears to be the ability to examine the anterior and posterior stromal surfaces.

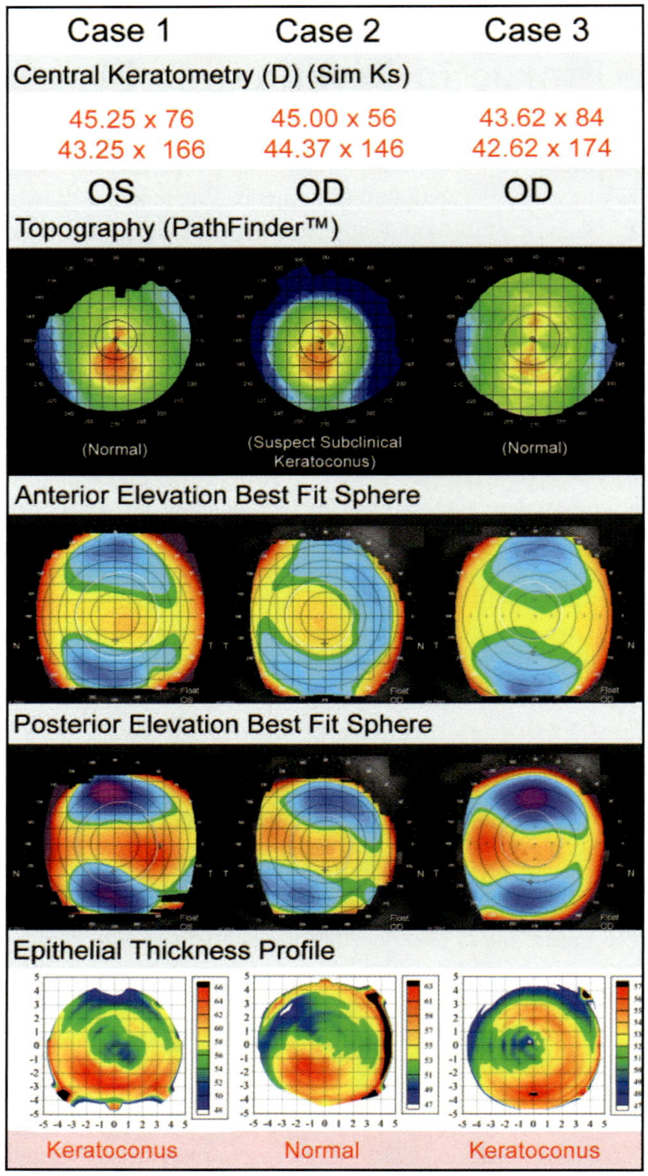


**Figure 6-93.** Central keratometry, ATLAS front corneal surface topography, and PathFinder corneal analysis (indicated below the topography map), Orbscan anterior and posterior elevation BFS, and Artemis epithelial thickness profile for 3 example eyes where the diagnosis of keratoconus might be misleading from topography. The final diagnosis based on the epithelial thickness profile is shown at the bottom of each example. OD = right eye, OS = left eye.

## Case Examples

Figure 6-93 shows 3 selected examples where epithelial thickness profiles helped to interpret and diagnose anterior and posterior elevation BFS abnormalities. In each case, the epithelial thickness profile appears to be able to differentiate cases where the diagnosis of keratoconus is uncertain from normal.[27]

Case 1 (OS) represents a 25-year-old man with a manifest refraction of -1.00 -0.50 x 150 and a best spectacle-corrected visual acuity of 20/16. ATLAS corneal topography demonstrated inferior steepening, which would traditionally indicate keratoconus. The keratometry was 45.25/43.25 D x 76, and PathFinder corneal analysis classified the topography as normal. Orbscan II posterior elevation BFS showed that the posterior elevation BFS apex was decentered inferotemporally. Corneal pachymetry minimum by handheld ultrasound was 479 µm. Contrast sensitivity was slightly below the normal range measured using the CSV-1000 (Vector Vision Inc, Greenville, OH). There was -0.30 µm (OSA notation) of vertical coma on WASCA aberrometry. Corneal hysteresis was 7.5 mm Hg, and corneal resistance factor was 7.1 mm Hg, which are low, but these could be affected by the low corneal thickness. The combination of inferior steepening, an eccentric posterior elevation BFS apex, and thin cornea raised the suspicion of keratoconus, although there was no suggestion of keratoconus by refraction, keratometry, or PathFinder corneal analysis. Artemis epithelial thickness profile showed a pattern typical of keratoconus with an epithelial doughnut shape characterized by a localized zone of epithelial thinning displaced inferotemporally over the eccentric posterior elevation BFS apex, surrounded by an annulus of thick epithelium. The coincidence of an area of epithelial thinning with the apex of the posterior elevation BFS, as well as the increased irregularity of the epithelium, confirmed the diagnosis of early keratoconus.

Case 2 (OD) represents a 31-year-old woman with a manifest refraction of -2.25 -0.50 x 88 and a best spectacle-corrected visual acuity of 20/16. Atlas corneal topography demonstrated a very similar pattern to case 1 of inferior steepening, therefore suggesting that the eye could also be keratoconic. The keratometry was 44.12/44.75 D x 148, and PathFinder corneal analysis classified the topography as suspect subclinical keratoconus. Orbscan II posterior elevation BFS showed that the apex was slightly decentered nasally. Corneal pachymetry minimum by handheld ultrasound was 538 μm. Contrast sensitivity was in the normal range. There was 0.32 μm (OSA notation) of vertical coma on WASCA aberrometry. Corneal hysteresis was 10.1 mm Hg, and corneal resistance factor was 9.8 mm Hg, which are well within normal range. The combination of inferior steepening, against-the-rule astigmatism, and high degree of vertical coma raised the suspicion of keratoconus, which was also noted by PathFinder corneal analysis. Artemis epithelial thickness profile showed a typical normal pattern with thicker epithelium inferiorly and thinner epithelium superiorly. Thicker epithelium inferiorly over the suspected cone (inferior steepening on topography) was inconsistent with an underlying stromal surface cone, and therefore the diagnosis of keratoconus was excluded. This patient would have been rejected for surgery given a documented PathFinder corneal analysis warning of suspect subclinical keratoconus, but given the epithelial thickness profile, this patient was deemed a suitable candidate for LASIK.

The anterior corneal topography in case 3 (OD) bears no features related to keratoconus. The patient is a 35-year-old woman with a manifest refraction of -4.25 -0.50 x 4 and a best spectacle-corrected visual acuity of 20/16. The refraction had been stable for at least 10 years, and the contrast sensitivity was within normal limits. The keratometry was 43.62/42.62 D x 74, and PathFinder analysis classified the topography as normal. Orbscan II posterior elevation BFS showed that the apex was slightly decentered inferotemporally, but the anterior elevation BFS apex was well-centered. Corneal pachymetry minimum by handheld ultrasound was 484 μm. Pentacam keratoconus screening indices were normal. WASCA ocular HOAs were low (RMS = 0.19 μm) as well as the level of vertical coma (coma = 0.066 μm). Corneal hysteresis was 8.9 mm Hg, and corneal resistance factor was 8.8 mm Hg, both within normal limits. In this case, only the slightly eccentric posterior elevation BFS apex and the low-normal corneal thickness were suspicious for keratoconus, while all other screening methods gave no indication of keratoconus. However, the epithelial thickness profile showed an epithelial doughnut pattern characterized by localized epithelial thinning surrounded by an annulus of thick epithelium, coincident with the eccentric posterior elevation BFS apex. Epithelial thinning with surrounding annular thickening over the eccentric posterior elevation BFS apex indicated the presence of probable subsurface keratoconus. In this case, it seems that the epithelium had fully compensated for the stromal surface irregularity so that the anterior surface topography of the cornea appeared perfectly regular. Given the regularity of the front surface topography and the normality of nearly all other screening parameters, it is feasible that this patient could have been deemed suitable for corneal refractive surgery and subsequently developed ectasia. As we were able to also consider the epithelial thickness profile, this patient was rejected for corneal refractive surgery. This kind of case may explain some reported cases of ectasia "without a cause."[27]

Knowledge of the differences in epithelial thickness profile between the normal population and the keratoconic population allowed us to identify several features of the epithelial thickness profile that might help to discriminate between normal eyes and keratoconus-suspect eyes. Mapping of the epithelial thickness profile may increase sensitivity and specificity of screening for keratoconus compared to current conventional corneal topographic screening alone and may be useful in clinical practice in 2 very important ways.

First, epithelial thickness mapping can exclude the appropriate patients by detecting keratoconus earlier or confirming keratoconus in cases where topographic changes may be clinically judged as being "within normal limits." Epithelial information allows an earlier diagnosis of keratoconus as epithelial changes will occur before changes on the front surface of the cornea become apparent. Epithelial thinning coincident with an eccentric posterior elevation BFS apex, and in particular if surrounded by an annulus of thicker epithelium, is consistent with keratoconus. Excluding early keratoconic patients from laser refractive surgery will reduce and potentially eliminate the risk of iatrogenic ectasia of this etiology and therefore increase the safety of laser refractive surgery. From our data, 136 eyes out of 1532 consecutive myopic eyes screened for refractive surgery demonstrated abnormal topography suspect of keratoconus. All 136 eyes were screened with Artemis VHF digital ultrasound arc-scanning, and individual epithelial thickness profiles were mapped. Out of 136 eyes with suspect keratoconus, only 22 eyes (16%) were confirmed as keratoconic.[126]

Second, epithelial thickness profiles may be useful in excluding a diagnosis of keratoconus despite suspect topography. Epithelial thickening over an area of topographic steepening implies that the steepening is not due to an underlying ectatic surface. In such cases, excluding keratoconus using epithelial thickness profiles appears to allow patients who otherwise would have been denied treatment due to suspect topography to be deemed suitable for surgery. From our data, out of the 136 eyes with suspect keratoconus screened with Artemis VHF digital ultrasound arc-scanning, 114 eyes (84%) showed normal epithelial thickness profile and were diagnosed as nonkeratoconic and were deemed suitable for corneal refractive surgery. One year post-LASIK, follow-up data[126] and preliminary 2-year follow-up data[127] on these demonstrated equal stability and refractive outcomes as matched control eyes.

Randleman et al, in their paper assessing risk factors for ectasia, reported that ectasia might still occur after uncomplicated surgery in appropriately screened candidates.[128] Mapping of epithelial thickness profiles might provide an explanation for these cases; it could be that a stromal surface cone was masked by epithelial compensation and the front surface topography appeared normal.

## Epithelial Changes After Refractive Surgery

The importance of epithelial changes in corneal refractive surgery has probably been underestimated. Significant changes in epithelial thickness profiles in both PRK[97,98] and LASIK[99-101] have been demonstrated and implicated in regression as well as the inaccuracy of topographically guided excimer laser ablation.[129] The curvature of Bowman's layer in the center of the normal cornea is on average greater than that of the epithelial surface.[130] As the refractive index of epithelium and stroma are sufficiently different (1.401 versus 1.377),[131] the epithelial-stromal interface constitutes an important refractive interface within the cornea, with a mean power contribution estimated at approximately -3.60 D.[130] Thus, unpredicted changes in the epithelial lenticule after surgery will result in unplanned refractive shifts. This is one of the reasons why current ablation depths and profiles ("nomograms") differ from theoretical ablation profiles—they incorporate the average change of epithelial power for a given level of stromal surface flattening (level of myopia treated). Thus, the understanding of epithelial dynamics and their patterns begins to unfold,[100,101] and these factors may potentially be used to improve the accuracy of corneal refractive outcomes.

## Epithelial Thickness Profile After Myopic LASIK

We have characterized the epithelial thickness profile in a population of 24 eyes 12 months after myopic LASIK. The mean preoperative spherical equivalent was -3.40±1.63 D (range: -0.75 to -6.00 D). The average post-LASIK epithelial pachymetric map in the population (see Figure 6-92) showed that the epithelium was thicker in a central, circular region approximately 6 mm in diameter. The central epithelial thickening can also be seen on the B-scan. The central zone of epithelial thickening was surrounded by an annulus of epithelial thinning between the 6- and 8-mm diameter. The mean thickest epithelial thickness for all eyes was 64.3±2.7 µm (range: 58.7 to 69.1 µm). The thickest epithelial point was displaced 0.45±0.68 mm temporally and 0.66±0.70 mm inferiorly on average with reference to the corneal vertex. Measurement of epithelial thickness profile provided evidence that the epithelium appears to behave as to reverse the change in stromal curvature and return the cornea to its preoperative curvature by remodeling itself to mirror the volume of stromal tissue removed.

In a separate study, we investigated changes in epithelial thickness profile as a function of myopia treated in a group of 37 eyes after myopic LASIK. The eyes were split into low myopia (-1.00 D to -4.00 D), moderate myopia (-4.25 to -6.00 D), and high myopia (-6.25 to -13.50 D).[132] We demonstrated that the amount of epithelial thickening was dependent on the level of myopia. There was more epithelial thickening for high myopia than for low myopia with maximum thickening centrally and progressively less thickening centrifugally in the low myopia group, whereas a more homogenous thickening in the moderate myopia and high myopia groups within the 5-mm diameter was noted. Knowledge of the epithelial thickness profile change between the pre- and postoperative epithelium is of interest as it will affect the refractive power of the epithelium. The increased epithelial thickening at the corneal vertex could partly explain the myopic shift described in the early period after myopic LASIK. Interestingly, we demonstrated that the myopic refractive shift due to epithelial profile changes was more significant for low than high myopic ablations because the gradient of epithelial thickening from center to periphery was steeper for low myopia than moderate and high myopia, although the epithelium thickened progressively with increasing central ablation depth.

These studies show that consideration of epithelial thickness changes might help improve the accuracy of myopic LASIK as epithelial healing and thickness changes play a role in the final refractive result.

## Longitudinal Epithelial Thickness Changes After Myopic LASIK

The epithelial thickness profile was measured in a population of 24 eyes at 1 day, 1 month, 3 months, 6 months, and 12 months after myopic LASIK. The mean preoperative spherical equivalent was -3.40±1.63 D (range: -0.75 to -6.00 D). The average epithelial thickness map at each time point (Figure 6-94) demonstrated a large change in epithelial thickness overnight, characterized by a central

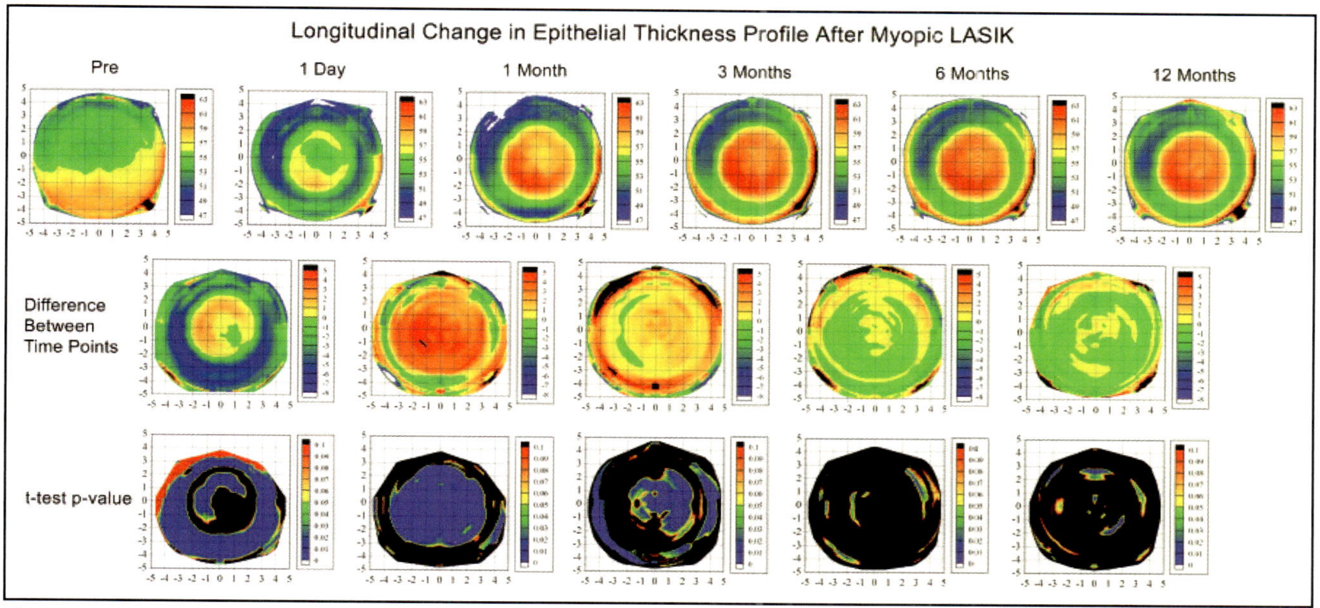


**Figure 6-94.** Top row: Maps of the average epithelial thickness before and 1 day, 1 month, 3 months, 6 months, and 12 months after myopic LASIK. Middle row: Maps of the change in epithelial thickness between each pair of time points. Bottom row: Maps of the t-test *p*-value comparing the change between each pair of time points; the areas in blue indicate a statistically significant change ($p<0.05$). The difference maps show that there was a change overnight with central epithelial thickening and peripheral epithelial thinning, followed by epithelial thickening until 3 months, after which the epithelial thickness stabilized.

zone of thickening of approximately 1 to 2 µm within the 5-mm diameter, surrounded by an annulus of epithelial thinning of approximately 4 to 6 µm between the 5- and 8-mm diameters. This demonstrates the speed at which the epithelium responds to stromal surface changes. Between 1 day and 1 month, the epithelium had thickened across the 7-mm diameter zone by up to 5 µm, with more pronounced thickening within the central 4 mm. Between 1 and 3 months, the epithelium had continued to thicken in the central 7-mm diameter zone by approximately an additional 1 µm. The t-test *p*-value maps shown in Figure 6-94 highlight the regions where the changes were statistically significant between each pair of time points. There were no further changes in epithelial thickness at the 6- and 12-month visits, supported by the t-test difference map that showed no regions of statistically significant difference between 3 and 6 months and between 6 and 12 months. This demonstrated that the epithelium had become stable 3 months after LASIK. These epithelial changes partially explain the regression seen after myopic LASIK in the first 3 months and agree with the common finding that refractive stability is attained after 3 months.[133]

## Epithelial Thickness Changes After Radial Keratotomy

The epithelial thickness profile was measured in a population of 14 eyes after radial keratotomy for myopia. The mean time of measurement after surgery was 17±6 years (range: 1.6 to 26 years). The mean preoperative spherical equivalent was -5.45±3.0 D (range: -2.00 to -9.50 D), although preoperative data were not available for 4 eyes. The average epithelial pachymetric map in the population (see Figure 6-92) showed that the epithelium became thicker in a central, circular region approximately 4 mm in diameter. The central zone of epithelial thickening was surrounded by an annulus of epithelial thinning. Interestingly, the epithelial thickness profile was very similar to that of eyes after myopic LASIK ablation, although the surgical techniques were completely different; the epithelium responded to changes in curvature alone after RK without tissue removal. The exaggerated change in curvature after RK can be visualized in the B-scan shown in Figure 6-92, where the cornea appears like a tabletop. The central zone of epithelial thickening was slightly smaller for eyes after RK than for eyes after LASIK, indicating that the size of the optical zone was smaller for eyes after RK than for eyes after LASIK.

## Epithelial Thickness Profile After Hyperopic LASIK

We have previously published a study that characterized the epithelial thickness profile in a population of 65 eyes at least 3 months after hyperopic LASIK using a 7-mm ablation zone with the MEL80 excimer laser (Carl Zeiss Meditec).[134] The average epithelial pachymetric map in the population (see Figure 6-92) showed that the epithelium was thinner in a central, circular region approximately 4 mm in diameter with the thinnest epithelium in the superior half of this region. The mean thinnest epithelial thickness for all eyes was 39.7±5.6 μm (range: 26.9 to 52.7 μm). The thinnest epithelial point was displaced -0.19±0.64 mm temporally and 0.93±0.82 mm superiorly on average with reference to the corneal vertex. The central, thin epithelium was surrounded by an annulus of thicker epithelium, with the thickest epithelium temporally. The mean thickest epithelial thickness for all eyes was 89.3±14.6 μm (range: 63.6 to 124.6 μm). The thickest epithelial point was displaced -2.49±1.04 mm temporally and -0.73±1.42 mm inferiorly on average with reference to the corneal vertex. The mean radial distance of the location of the thickest epithelium from the corneal vertex was 3.12±0.25 mm (range: 2.3 to 3.6 mm). The diameter of the annular zone of maximum epithelial thickening was 6.8 mm in the horizontal meridian and 6.7 mm in the vertical meridian, which matches the programmed laser ablation optical zone diameter of 7 mm where the maximum ablation depth was at the 7-mm diameter. This demonstrates that the epithelium was compensating for the paracentral stromal tissue removal due to the hyperopic ablation. Knowledge of the epithelial thickness profile after hyperopic LASIK may partly explain hyperopic regression and could be used to improve the accuracy of hyperopic ablation, particularly with respect to induced cylinder.

In this study, we also suggested that central epithelial thickness may be a more useful indicator than keratometry to determine whether further treatment may be attempted. There was a statistically significant and strong correlation between the attempted spherical equivalent refraction and both the thinnest ($R^2 = 0.350$, $p<0.001$) and thickest epithelium ($R^2 = 0.765$, $p<0.001$). This indicated that the minimum epithelial thickness was thinner and the maximum epithelial thickness was thicker in eyes after higher refractive ablations. It is currently assumed that hyperopic LASIK should be limited according to postoperative curvature as too much steepening can result in epitheliopathy or apical syndrome; it is generally accepted that the postoperative curvature should not exceed 49.00 to 50.00 D.[135] However, the results from the present study suggest that epithelial thickness might be a better indicator. Whereas the thinnest epithelium is correlated with the postoperative curvature ($R^2 = 0.210$, $p<0.001$), the postoperative curvature alone can be misleading. In an example case from the study,[134] the maximum simulated keratometry of 50.80 D would most likely prevent the surgeon from treating further hyperopia; however, the central epithelial thickness of 41.7 μm would suggest that the cornea could be steepened further without resulting in epithelial breakdown. On the other hand, another case from the present study demonstrates that the epithelial thickness can be thin (33.7 μm) although the cornea was still relatively flat postoperatively (46.40 D). The curvature limit would allow further hyperopic ablation, whereas the thin, central epithelium would indicate that further steepening might increase the risk of apical syndrome. Therefore, using epithelial thickness measurements, hyperopic retreatments might be performed without risk of apical syndrome while also allowing some patients to have retreatment who would otherwise have been rejected for further surgery due to high keratometry postoperatively.

## Orthokeratology

We previously described epithelial, stromal, and corneal thickness changes in a patient before and during orthokeratology treatment and were able to demonstrate that refractive changes were mainly due to epithelial thickness changes.[136] The epithelial thickness changes appeared to reveal the pattern of compression produced by orthokeratology lenses. In both eyes, there was a zone of central epithelial thinning within the central 1.5-mm radius, surrounded by a midperipheral annulus of epithelial thickening at the 2-mm radius. The Artemis epithelial thickness profile and B-scan of the right eye is shown in Figure 6-92. There also appeared to be a degree of central stromal thickening and midperipheral stromal thinning, although the magnitude of the stromal changes was less than one-third of the magnitude of the epithelial changes. Using epithelial thickness mapping, we were able to differentiate epithelial thickness changes from stromal thickness changes to understand the mechanism of refractive changes and demonstrate that the majority of the refractive correction in orthokeratology is caused by changes to the epithelial thickness profile, which explains the temporary nature of the effect.

The epithelial thickness changes observed add more weight to the theory that the epithelium remodels to fit the template in front of the cornea. In orthokeratology, the template normally provided by the posterior surface of the semi-rigid tarsus is replaced by a contact lens that is designed to fit tightly to the center of the cornea and loosely paracentrally. Therefore, the epithelium is chafed and squashed by the lens centrally while the epithelium is free to thicken paracentrally where the lens is not so tightly fitted.

## Ectasia Diagnosis

Ectasia is one of the most devastating potential consequences of LASIK, and it behooves us to prevent it from happening in every possible way. In the first section, we described the use of epithelial thickness mapping for the early diagnosis of keratoconus as an aid in the determination of candidacy for LASIK with the aim of avoiding ectasia given that the majority of post-LASIK ectasia has been caused by undetected keratoconus.[128,137-140] Epithelial thickness maps can also be used to confirm and monitor the diagnosis of post-LASIK ectasia. The example in Figure 6-92 shows the epithelial thickness profile of an eye with post-LASIK ectasia. The epithelial thickness profile demonstrates similar features to that of a keratoconic eye, characterized by localized central thinning coincident with the back surface cone on topography, surrounded by an annulus of thick epithelium.

We have also hypothesized that epithelial thickness profile maps could be a useful adjunct to topography in monitoring patients after collagen corneal cross-linking (CXL) treatment. We have used Artemis to measure epithelial thickness profile in vivo across the central 10-mm corneal diameter of a patient before CXL for post-LASIK corneal ectasia and at intervals up to 2 years after CXL. The epithelial thickness profile was altered, with a slight reduction of the area of epithelial thinning and decreased peripheral thickening. This resulted in minimizing the difference between the thinnest and thickest epithelium and might indicate an improvement of the condition. However, little change was seen on front corneal surface topography, which suggests that the epithelium remodeling masked the stromal surface changes. This suggests that epithelial thickness profiles might be a more sensitive tool to monitor changes in ectasia than front corneal surface topography and keratometry alone.

## Intracorneal Ring Segments

We have also previously published a case report showing the epithelial thickness changes that occur after the insertion of intracorneal ring segments.[141] The Artemis scan showed that the epithelium was thinner directly over the intracorneal ring segment and thicker to the side of the ridge caused by the intracorneal ring segment. The epithelial reaction is another example of the eyelid tenting effect of a ridge, which allows the epithelium to grow into the space created on either side of the ridge, while also thinning on top of the ridge due to the localized eyelid contact.

## Epithelial Thickness Mapping for True Diagnosis of Irregular Astigmatism

While LASIK and PRK are already relatively safe procedures today, we are constantly striving to make them even safer. We need to prevent complications, and when these do occur, we need methods for correcting them and restoring visual function. In keeping with basic principles of surgery, accurate imaging and biometry will be the cornerstone of these goals because accurate diagnosis enables optimal treatment planning.

Surface topography has been the mainstay of diagnostic testing in complicated LASIK. Recently, the introduction of aberrometry has greatly enhanced our diagnostic capabilities in being able to understand in a quantitative way how irregular astigmatism and other shape irregularities produce visual complaints. However, neither the understanding of the optical defect nor the surface shape of the cornea will necessarily provide a diagnosis for the cause of the problem.[129] This is due to the fact that internal corneal refractive interfaces (such as epithelial-stromal interface) are not being measured independently. The anatomical cause of a surface abnormality may only be understood at an internal corneal level (eg, irregularities in the flap versus the stromal bed). With burgeoning surgical rates of PRK and LASIK worldwide, it is becoming increasingly evident that there is a distinct need for a method of determining the layered anatomy of the changes induced. Without an accurate anatomical diagnosis, topography or wavefront-guided treatments may lead to a suboptimal treatment plan.

Here, we show some examples where the epithelium masked true topographic and/or wavefront error to be corrected, and the Artemis provided essential information for treatment planning.

### Case 1: Phototherapeutic Keratectomy Treatment for Irregular Epithelial Thickness Profile

We have previously published a case of a 60-year-old male NASA employee who was referred to our clinic with severe visual difficulties in his dominant left eye.[95] The patient complained that the vision in the left eye was not compatible with that of the right eye and that he felt as if "everything is coming in from the side." The patient also complained of reduced contrast sensitivity. These symptoms meant that the patient preferred to keep his left eye closed, sometimes wearing an eye patch. His original manifest refraction in his left eye was -6.25 -0.50 × 180. He underwent automated lamellar keratoplasty (ALK), which resulted in a residual astigmatism of -1.50 D. He was later retreated by arcuate keratotomy (AK) procedures. He then underwent LASIK with a newly created flap to treat residual compound hyperopic astigmatism of +2.50 -1.75 × 95 and a second LASIK procedure with a further flap cut to treat -1.00 -0.75 × 75. Finally, he underwent a LASIK enhancement by relifting a flap to treat a refraction of +1.00 -1.00 × 65.

His UCVA in the left eye was 20/32, improving to 20/25 with -0.50 -0.50 × 80. Topography was irregular with a central flattened optical treatment zone of approximately 4 mm in diameter, slightly displaced inferiorly (Figure 6-95A). Within this central zone, there was an outer ring of extreme flattening to a power of about 37.5 D surrounding a central area with a power of about 39 D at a diameter of approximately 1.5 mm. Higher-order aberrations were significantly raised. The Artemis epithelial profile (see Figure 6-95A) revealed a central area of thin epithelium (44 µm) covering a diameter of approximately 1 mm surrounded by concentric rings of thick (up to 75 µm) and thin (down to 32 µm) epithelium. The horizontal cross-sectional B-scan (Figure 6-95B) shows the undulations of the surface of Bowman's layer accompanied by partial epithelial compensation within the troughs. It was found that each ring of thickened epithelium coincided with the rings of flattening on topography. This is an example of the known phenomena of the epithelium remodeling itself to try to regularize the front surface of the cornea[142]; it had become thicker to fill in troughs in the stromal surface and thinner over peaks in the stromal surface. However, the irregular topography shows that the epithelium had not been able to completely compensate for the stromal irregularities.

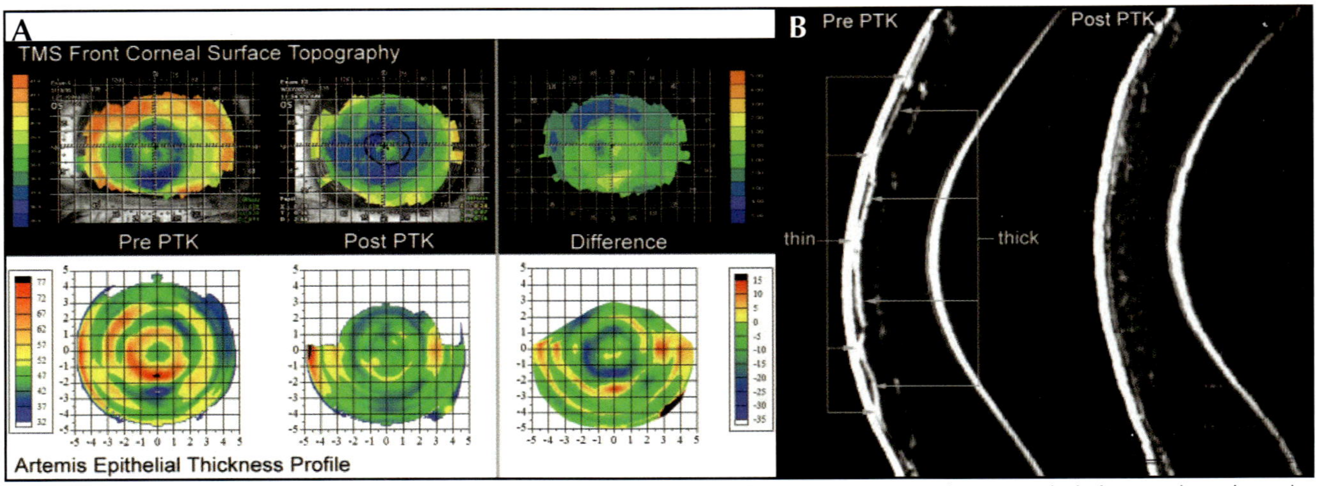


**Figure 6-95.** (A) TMS-3 front corneal surface topography before and after Artemis-assisted transepithelial PTK plotted on the same scale. The topography is significantly more regular postoperatively, with a relatively normal optical zone. The map on the right shows the change in the topography following the PTK treatment. Bottom row: Artemis epithelial thickness profile before and after Artemis assisted transepithelial PTK plotted on the same scale. The concentric rings of thin and thick epithelium have been significantly regularized. The map on the right shows the change in the epithelium following the PTK treatment. (B) Non-geometrically corrected horizontal B-scans through the visual axis of a cornea before and 3 months after Artemis assisted transepithelial PTK. There is a large z-axis zoom in scale (2.1 mm represented horizontally on the image) relative to lateral distance (10 mm represented vertically on the image). The concentric rings of epithelial thinning and epithelial thickening are marked on the pre-PTK B-scan. The epithelium has become significantly more regular as a consequence of the Artemis-assisted trans-epithelial PTK smoothing of the stromal surface irregularities.

In this case, topography and wavefront analysis did not provide information on the etiology of the surface irregularities. Mapping of the epithelial thickness map allowed the diagnosis of irregular stromal surface to be made. The visual symptoms were most probably due to micro-optical scattering within the cornea as well as HOAs. Therefore, the treatment plan was split into 2 parts: (1) perform a VHF digital ultrasound-assisted transepithelial phototherapeutic keratectomy (PTK) using the epithelium as a mask to focus the laser ablation on the areas of raised stroma in order to regularize the stromal surface and (2) remove any remaining epithelium and perform a wavefront-guided ablation to attempt to correct the higher-order aberrations also present. The treatment successfully regularized the stromal surface, confirmed by the regularization of the epithelial thickness profile (see Figure 6-95A), which can also be seen on the postoperative B-scan (see Figure 6-95B). The HOAs were dramatically reduced, the contrast sensitivity was improved from below normal to high normal, and the BSCVA was improved to 20/20.

### Case 2: Phototherapeutic Keratectomy Treatment for Irregular Epithelial Thickness Profile

A 50-year-old man was referred to our clinic complaining of poor vision in his left eye following several refractive procedures. His original manifest refraction was approximately -5.50 D. He underwent a radial keratotomy procedure in June 1982, followed by another surgery 2 months later consisting of trapezoid stromal incisions inferiorly and superiorly of the pupil margins with the aim of improving the near function, similar to a presbyopic correction. Six months after the second procedure, the surgeon recommended a lamellar graft, which the patient refused. Since then, the patient sought advice from several surgeons to improve his quality of vision in the left eye.

On presentation to the London Vision Clinic in February 2009, the patient's refraction was +6.50 -8.00 x 110 achieving CDVA of 20/50. ATLAS front corneal surface topography was irregular showing an asymmetric bow-tie pattern decentered superiorly (Figure 6-96A). Simulated central keratometry was 42.12 x 4/36.75 x 94. The bow-tie pattern was surrounded inferiorly by a crescent-shaped zone of corneal steepening, extending nasally and temporally. Higher-order aberrations were raised. The Artemis epithelial thickness profile (see Figure 6-96A) was very irregular in thickness with up to 35 μm variation within the central 4-mm corneal diameter. The epithelial thickness map demonstrated 2 small zones of thin epithelium (40 μm), approximately 1 mm in diameter each, at a 2-mm radius inferiorly and superiorly from the corneal vertex; these regions of thin epithelium were coincident with the trapezoidal incisions. The epithelium was thicker (up to 75 μm) along the horizontal meridian centrally, extending nasally, and at the 3-mm radius inferonasally. In this case, the epithelial thickness profile was masking a significant proportion of the stromal irregularity from front corneal surface topography, meaning that this proportion of the stromal irregularity would not be taken into account by a topography-guided ablation algorithm. Therefore, the optimal treatment plan was to

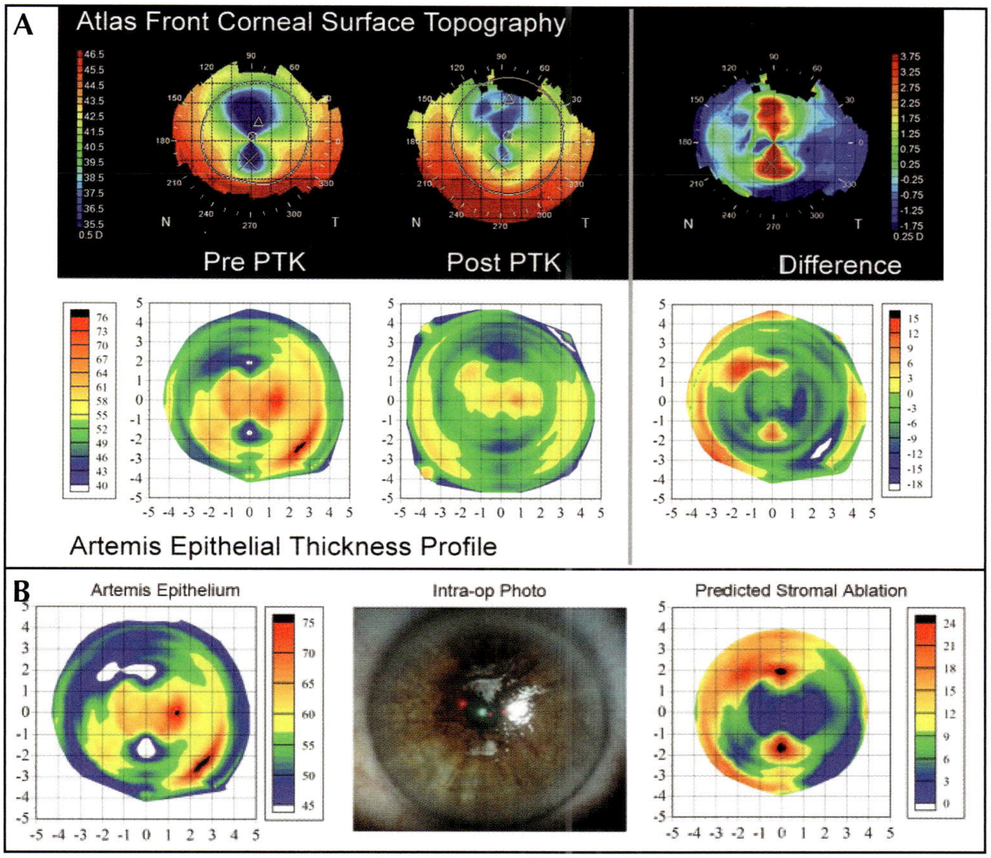


**Figure 6-96.** (A) Atlas front corneal surface topography before and after Artemis-assisted transepithelial PTK plotted on the same scale. The superior astigmatic flattening has been significantly reduced postoperatively, highlighted by the bow-tie pattern seen on the difference map showing up to 3.50 D of steepening. Bottom row: Artemis epithelial thickness profile before and after Artemis-assisted transepithelial PTK plotted on the same scale. The superior and inferior regions of thin epithelium have become thicker postoperatively, and the epithelium has also become thinner centrally, resulting in a significantly smoother epithelial thickness profile. The map on the right shows the change in the epithelium following the PTK treatment that highlights the 10 µm to 15 µm of thickening in the regions where the epithelium was thinnest before surgery. (B) Artemis digital subtraction pachymetry simulation of the pattern of remaining epithelium after 45 µm of epithelial tissue removal by PTK. The white areas indicate where the stromal surface would be exposed (ie, the areas where stroma would be ablated). The stromal surface would first be exposed in these areas because the epithelium was thinner to compensate for the raised areas on the irregular stromal surface. Middle: Intraoperative photograph showing the epithelial pattern after 45 µm of PTK ablation. On inspection, the pattern of exposed stroma closely resembles the Artemis-predicted pattern. Right: Predicted stromal ablation profile calculated based on the Artemis epithelial thickness data. The stromal ablation profile shows the greatest ablation of 25 µm was in the superior and inferior regions where the epithelium was thinnest, coincident with the location of the extra trapezoidal incisions performed during the second RK procedure.

perform an Artemis-assisted transepithelial PTK procedure to target the component of the stromal irregularity compensated for by the epithelium. Once the irregularity is reduced, the epithelium should become sufficiently smooth for a topography-guided ablation to be used to correct the remaining irregularity.

The epithelial thickness profile was used to generate a simulation of the pattern of epithelium after regular intervals of ablation, which were used to monitor the progress of the PTK ablation during the procedure. Figure 6-96B shows the simulated epithelial pattern next to the actual intraoperative photograph of the cornea after 45 µm of ablation. These images show that the pattern of remaining epithelium matched that predicted by the Artemis epithelial maps, with stroma exposed in the 2 regions where the epithelium was thinnest, 2 mm superiorly and inferiorly of the corneal vertex. The concentration of stromal ablation superiorly and inferiorly in the vertical meridian meant that the stromal ablation pattern (see Figure 6-96B) was similar to a hyperopic astigmatic ablation.

Nine months after the procedure, the astigmatism had been halved so that the manifest refraction was +4.50 -4.50 x 101 and the CDVA had improved to 20/20. The postoperative Artemis epithelial thickness profile (see Figure 6-96A) showed that the epithelium was much more regular in thickness. The epithelial thickness difference map (see Figure 6-96A) demonstrated that the epithelium had become thicker in the superior and inferior regions where the maximum ablation was performed and had become thinner centrally where the epithelium was thickest before the procedure. The change could also be seen on ATLAS front corneal surface topography (see Figure 6-96A) where the difference map showed a significant astigmatic change. The PTK procedure had succeeded in reducing the stromal irregularity, and the presence of a smoother epithelium meant that the impact of epithelial masking on front corneal surface topography was also reduced. Therefore, the patient was then suitable for treatment using a topography-guided ablation as the majority of the remaining irregularity was apparent on front corneal surface topography.

This case demonstrates the influence the epithelium can exert on the manifest refraction; in this case, a refraction change of +2.24 -3.97 x 120 was achieved with a transepithelial PTK ablation alone. This example shows that the pattern of irregular epithelium and the associated refractive effect must be taken into account when planning PTK and/or custom ablation (topography guided or wavefront guided).

### Case 3: Topographic Diagnosis of Decentration: Is It Really a Laser Decentration?

Decentration is a diagnosis made postoperatively by inspection of topography. Decentration denotes off-center ablation. We have found that what appears to be decentration by topography is not always due to off-center ablation.

In the following example, a patient presented to us complaining of monocular double vision after LASIK. The initial refraction was -6.50 D. Treatment was carried out with the Moria LSK-One microkeratome and the Nidek EC5000. Preoperative corneal thickness by Orbscan was measured as 516 µm. With an ablation depth of 90 µm, the predicted postoperative residual stromal thickness was 266 µm. On examination, UDVA was 20/70, and manifest refraction was +3.00 -3.75 x 96, yielding a CDVA of 20/40+2. Slit-lamp examination showed a clear cornea, with an unremarkable flap possessing a few very faint, faded shallow-appearing vertical microfolds. Orbscan anterior elevation BFS map (Figure 6-97A) provided a differential diagnosis of decentration of the ablation zone or ectasia. Aberrometry demonstrated coma-like HOAs.

Horizontal 3D Artemis VHF digital ultrasound B-scan cross-section of the cornea revealed anatomical features that provided further diagnostic information. Figure 6-97B shows the B-scan demonstrating a flatter (F) nasal side of the cornea, with a raised (R) surface temporally as found also on the Orbscan BFS surface shape map. Beneath the raised (R) area, the epithelial thickness is seen to be reduced, due to invagination by the underlying Bowman's layer (B). Bowman's (B) is highly irregular, showing 3 major ultrasonic discontinuities (*) representing either cracks or microfolds in the flap surface. Pachymetric maps of the epithelium, residual stroma, and stromal component of the flap are shown in Figure 6-97A. The epithelial thickness profile is seen to vary continuously, filling in and smoothing out the surface of Bowman's layer. The thinnest point within the residual stromal bed, determined by 3-dimensional thickness mapping, was 223 µm. The residual stromal layer thickness profile appears slightly asymmetric or decentered in the nasal direction. Inspection of the stromal component of the flap map showed the reason for this—the stromal component of the flap was thicker temporally than nasally.

A diagnosis was made of flap malposition and possible asymmetric biomechanical shift. In addition, the residual stromal thickness was noted to be too thin for further under-the-flap ablation, despite the fact that the preoperative parameters would have implied that there was room for further treatment.

This case clearly illustrates the importance of anatomical diagnosis, in contrast to a topographical description, in planning the management of LASIK complications. By topography alone, this case may well have been diagnosed as a decentration. The eye may well have then undergone a topographically guided treatment under the flap. Given the low residual stromal thickness, it is conceivable that further tissue removal would have led to further mechanical shifts and an unpredictable result, with a high possibility of inducing progressive ectasia.[143]

## Conclusion

In this section, we have demonstrated that knowledge of the epithelial thickness profile is a useful tool in understanding and planning corneal refractive procedures. We have shown that the epithelium always remodels itself to fit a template (normally provided by the eyelid) and that this mechanism results in compensation for stromal irregularity, which then impacts the validity of front corneal surface topography. Therefore, the epithelial thickness profile needs to be considered alongside front corneal surface topography to build a picture of true stromal irregularity.

We have described the major areas where the epithelium can make a significant difference. Mapping of the epithelial thickness profile may increase sensitivity and specificity of screening for keratoconus compared to conventional front corneal surface topography. This should help reduce cases of post-LASIK ectasia and therefore improve the safety of LASIK. Knowledge of epithelial thickness profile changes after myopic and hyperopic LASIK may partly explain refractive regression and could be used to improve the

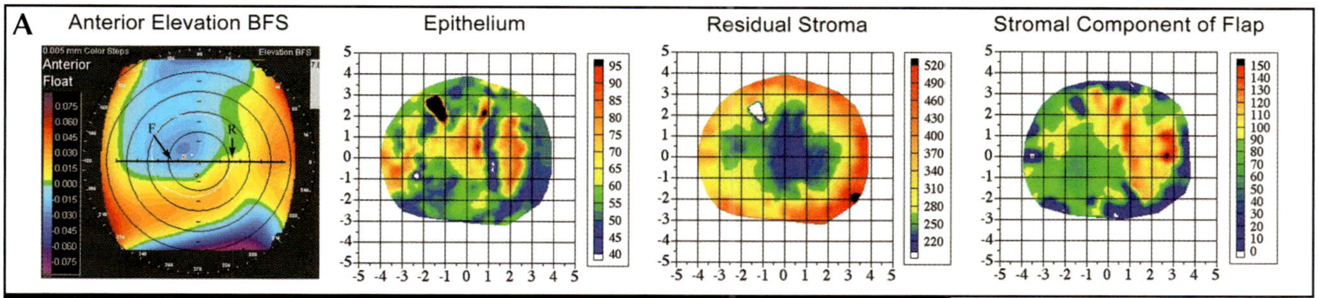


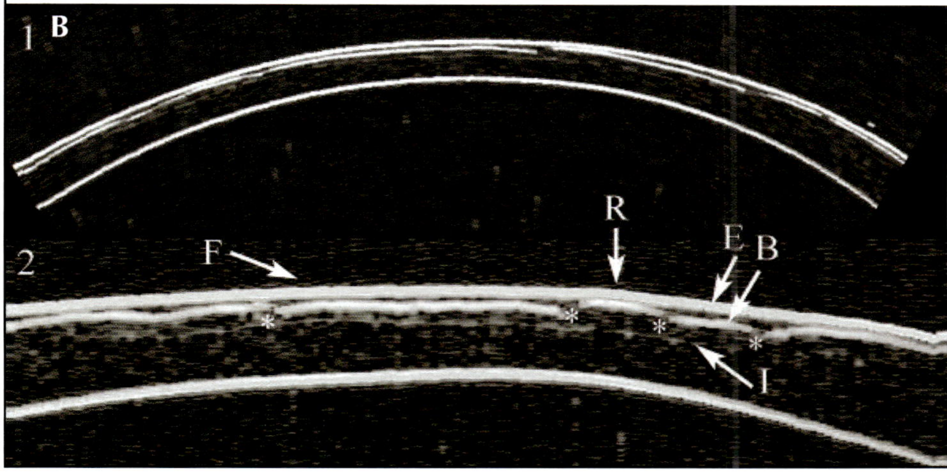


**Figure 6-97.** (A) Orbscan anterior BFS (default 10-mm zone fit) plot of the cornea in a patient presenting with monocular diplopia and a topographic diagnosis of "decentered ablation," proved incorrect by B-scan imaging in the plane represented by the horizontal black line. Flatter (F) and raised (R) areas are correlated to the ultrasound B-scan in Figure 6-97B. Right: Artemis pachymetric maps of the epithelium, residual stroma, and stromal component of the flap. Inspection of the epithelial thickness profile demonstrates the error introduced by epithelial compensation if one were to attempt topography-guided or wavefront-guided ablation to correct the optical defect. The residual stromal layer thickness profile appears slightly asymmetric or decentered in the nasal direction. Inspection of the stromal component of the flap map showed the reason for this—the stromal component of the flap was thicker temporally than nasally. B-scan imaging (Figure 6-97B) confirms that laser ablation would be a less optimal management strategy in this case, in which there is extreme flap bunching due to inadequate distension. (B) Horizontal VHF digital ultrasound corneal B-scan through the visual axis of the right cornea of the patient in Figure 6-97A. The upper image (1) shows the geometrically corrected image, while the lower image (2) shows the raw ultrasound data with axial zoom to better appreciate the interfaces. The surface of epithelium (E), Bowman's (B), and the keratectomy interface (I) are labeled. It is clearly noted that Bowman's surface is highly irregular, with numerous true microfolds (*), which were only very faintly visible on slit-lamp examination, due to the impressive epithelial compensation producing excellent smoothing of the corneal surface. The diagnosis of "decentered ablation" is clearly less likely than that of an inadequately distended flap, producing surface asymmetry. Appropriate management would most likely involve flap distension and repositioning, not further laser ablation.

accuracy of corneal ablations. In cases of complicated corneal refractive surgery, knowledge of epithelial thickness profile is crucial in establishing the correct diagnosis and planning further treatment.

There are numerous other situations where the epithelium should be taken into account that have not been covered in this chapter. We have also published numerous other reports demonstrating epithelial compensation for stromal irregularities in cases of asymmetric resection in automated lamellar keratoplasty,[129] asymmetric LASIK flaps,[129,144,145] microfolds,[144,145] flap malposition,[144-146] short flap,[144-146] and free cap malrotation.[147] This weight of evidence for epithelial compensation proves that it always occurs and that the epithelium must be considered in relation to any corneal interaction.

Consideration of epithelial changes also applies to corneal measurements. For example, an estimation of achieved ablation depth derived from the change in corneal pachymetry will be skewed by the epithelial changes that will have occurred after tissue removal (eg, achieved depth after a myopic ablation will be underestimated due to the epithelial thickening that will have occurred).[148] Epithelial changes should also be considered in flap thickness measurement after excimer laser ablation. A postoperative measurement of flap thickness will include epithelial changes; therefore, a more accurate method of measuring flap thickness at the time of flap creation is to combine the stromal component of the flap (measured postoperatively) with the preoperative epithelium.[149,150] This method effectively resets the epithelium to the thickness profile at the time of surgery.

Orthopedic surgery was practiced without pre- and postoperative anatomical imaging until the discovery of X-ray imaging in 1895, by Wilhelm Konrad Roentgen. Perhaps, epithelial imaging will have a similar impact on corneal refractive surgery.

# References


1. Pflugfelder SC, Liu Z, Feuer W, Verm A. Corneal thickness indices discriminate between keratoconus and contact lens-induced corneal thinning. *Ophthalmology*. 2002;109(12):2336-2341.
2. Tanabe T, Oshika T, Tomodokoro A, et al. Standardized color-coded scales for anterior and posterior elevation maps of scanning slit corneal topography. *Ophthalmology*. 2002;109(7):1298-1302.
3. Davis LJ, Schechtman KB, Begley CG, Shin JA, Zadnik K. Repeatability of refraction and corrected visual acuity in keratoconus. The CLEK Study Group. Collaborative Longitudinal Evaluation of Keratoconus. *Optom Vis Sci*. 1998;75(12):887-896.
4. Zadnik K, Steger-May MA, Fink BA, et al. Between-eye asymmetry in keratoconus. *Cornea*. 2002;21:671-679.
5. Liu Z, Pflugfelder SC. Corneal thickness is reduced in dry eye. *Cornea*. 1999;18(4):403-407.
6. Pepose JS, Applegate RA. Making sense out of wavefront sensing. *Am J Ophthalmol*. 2005;139(2):335-343.
7. Belin MW. Intraoperative raster photogrammetry—the PAR Corneal Topography System. *J Cataract Refract Surg*. 1993;19:188-192.
8. Belin MW, Zloty P. Accuracy of the PAR Corneal Topography System with spatial misalignment. *CLAO J*. 1993;19:64-68.
9. Arffa RC, Klyce SD, Busin M. Keratometry in refractive surgery. *J Refract Surg*. 1986;2:6.
10. Rubin ML. *Optics for Clinicians*. Gainesville, FL: Triad Publishing Company; 1993.
11. Mandell RB. The enigma of the corneal contour. *CLAO J*. 1992;18:267-273.
12. Arffa RC, Warnicki JW, Rehkopf PG. Corneal topography using rasterstereography. *Refract Corneal Surg*. 1989;5:414-417.
13. Litoff D, Belin MW, Winn SS, et al. PAR Technology Corneal Topography System. *Inv Ophthalmol Vis Sci*. 1991;32:922.
14. Swartz T, Marten L, Wang M. Measuring the cornea: the latest developments in corneal topography. *Curr Opin Ophthalmol*. 2007;18:325-333.
15. Wegener A, Laser H. Image analysis and Scheimpflug photography of anterior segment of the eye--a review. *Klin Monatsbl Augenheilkd*. 2001;218:67-77.
16. Müller-Breitenkamp U, Hockwin O. Scheimpflug photography in clinical ophthalmology. A review. *Ophthalmic Res*. 1992;24:47-54.
17. Ciolino J, Belin MW. Changes to the posterior cornea after LASIK and PRK. *J Cataract & Refract Surg*. 2006;32:1426-1431.
18. Miller D, Greiner JV. Corneal measurements and tests. In: Albert DM, Jakobiec FA, eds. *Principles and Practice of Ophthalmology*. Philadelphia, PA: WB Saunders; 1994:7.
19. Ambrósio R Jr, Klyce SD, Wilson SE. Corneal topographic and pachymetric screening of keratorefractive patients. *J Refract Surg*. 2003;19:24-29.
20. Jonsson M, Behndig A. Pachymetric evaluation prior to laser in situ keratomileusis. *J Cataract Refract Surg*. 2005;31:701-706.
21. Ciolino JB, Khachikian SS, Belin MW. Comparison of corneal thickness measurements by ultrasound and Scheimpflug photography in eyes that have undergone laser in situ keratomileusis. *Am J Ophthalmol*. 2008;145:75-80.
22. Ambrósio R, Alonso RS, Luz A, Coca Velarde LG. Corneal-thickness spatial profile and corneal-volume distribution: tomographic indices to detect keratoconus. *J Cataract Refract Surg*. 2006;32(11):1851-1859.
23. Klein SR, Epstein RJ, Randleman JB, Stulting RD. Corneal ectasia after laser in situ keratomileusis in patients without apparent preoperative risk factors. *Cornea*. 2006;25:388-403.
24. Rabinowitz YS. Videokeratographic indices to aid in screening for keratoconus. *J Refract Surg*. 1995;11:371-379.
25. Binder PS, Lindstrom RL, Stulting RD, et al. Keratoconus and corneal ectasia after LASIK. *J Refract Surg*. 2005;21:749-752.
26. Reinstein DZ, Gobbe M, Archer TJ, Silverman RH, Coleman DJ. Epithelial, stromal, and total corneal thickness in keratoconus: three-dimensional display with Artemis very-high frequency digital ultrasound. *J Refract Surg*. 2010;26:259-271.
27. Reinstein DZ, Archer TJ, Gobbe M. Corneal epithelial thickness profile in the diagnosis of keratoconus. *J Refract Surg*. 2009;25(7):604-610.
28. Alessio G, Boscia F, La Tegola MG, Sborgia C. Topography-driven photorefractive keratectomy: results of corneal interactive programmed topographic ablation software. *Ophthalmology*. 2000;107(8):1578-1587.
29. Huang D, Izatt JA. Physics and fundamentals of anterior segment optical coherence tomography. In: Steinert RF, Huang D, eds, *Anterior Segment Optical Coherence Tomography*. Thorofare, NJ: SLACK Incorporated; 2008:3-10.
30. *Visante OCT User Manual System Software* [computer program]. Version 3.0. Jena, Germany: Carl Zeiss Meditec; 2009.
31. Baïkoff G. Anterior segment OCT and phakic intraocular lenses: a perspective. *J Cataract Refract Surg*. 2006;32:1827-1835.
32. Hill W, Wang L, Koch DD. IOL power calculation in eyes that have undergone LASIK/PRK/RK. http://iol.ascrs.org. Accessed July 18, 2011.
33. Rabinowitz YS, McDonnell PJ. Computer-assisted corneal topography in keratoconus. *Refract Corneal Surg*. 1989;5(6):400-408.
34. Rabinowitz YS. Keratoconus. *Surv Ophthalmol*. 1998;42(4):297-319.
35. Borasio E, Stevens J, Smith GT. Estimation of true corneal power after keratorefractive surgery in eyes requiring cataract surgery: BESSt formula. *J Cataract Refract Surg*. 2006;32(12):2004-2014.
36. Holladay JT, Hill WE, Steinmueller A. Corneal power measurements using scheimpflug imaging in eyes with prior corneal refractive surgery. *J Refract Surg*. 2009;25(10):862-868.
37. Jin H, Rabsilber T, Ehmer A, et al. Comparison of ray-tracing method and thin-lens formula in intraocular lens power calculations. *J Cataract Refract Surg*. 2009;35(4):650-662.
38. Shammas HJ, Hoffer KJ, Shammas MC. Scheimpflug photography keratometry readings for routine intraocular lens power calculation. *J Cataract Refract Surg*. 2009;35(2):330-334.
39. Amano S, Honda N, Amano Y, et al. Comparison of central corneal thickness measurements by rotating Scheimpflug camera, ultrasonic pachymetry, and scanning-slit corneal topography. *Ophthalmology*. 2006;113(6):937-941.
40. Ambrosio R Jr. Percentage thickness increase and absolute difference from thinnest to describe thickness profile. *J Refract Surg*. 2010;26(2):84-86; author reply 86-87.
41. Luz A, Ursulio M, Castaneda D, Ambrosio R Jr. [Corneal thickness progression from the thinnest point to the limbus: study based on a normal and a keratoconus population to create reference values]. *Arq Bras Oftalmol*. 2006;69(4):579-583.
42. Ambrósio R Jr, Nogueira LP, Caldas DL, et al. Evaluation of corneal shape and biomechanics before LASIK. *Int Ophthalmol Clin*. 2011;51(2):11-38.
43. Ambrósio Jr R, Caiado ALC, Guerra FP, et al. Novel pachymetric parameters based on corneal tomography for diagnosing keratoconus. *J Refract Surg*. 2011; in press
44. Ambrosio R Jr, Dawson DG, Salomao M, Guerra FP, Caiado AL, Belin MW. Corneal ectasia after LASIK despite low preoperative risk: tomographic and biomechanical findings in the unoperated, stable, fellow eye. *J Refract Surg*. 2010:1-6.
45. Belin MW, Ambrosio R Jr. Corneal ectasia risk score: statistical validity and clinical relevance. *J Refract Surg*. 2010;26(4):238-240.
46. Belin MW, Khachikian SS. An introduction to understanding elevation-based topography: how elevation data are displayed—a review. *Clin Experiment Ophthalmol*. 2009;37(1):14-29.

47. Ciolino JB, Belin MW. Changes in the posterior cornea after laser in situ keratomileusis and photorefractive keratectomy. *J Cataract Refract Surg.* 2006;32(9):1426-1431.
48. Packer M, Fine IH, Hoffman RS. Aspheric intraocular lens selection based on corneal wavefront. *J Refract Surg.* 2009;25(1):12-20.
49. Rabsilber TM, Khoramnia R, Auffarth GU. Anterior chamber measurements using Pentacam rotating Scheimpflug camera. *J Cataract Refract Surg.* 2006;32(3):456-459.
50. Tehrani M, Dick HB. Scheimpflug biometry of the anterior segment after implantation of foldable iris-fixated lenses. *J Refract Surg.* 2006;22(3):243-246.
51. Lovisolo CF, Reinstein DZ. Phakic intraocular lenses. *Surv Ophthalmol.* 2005;50(6):549-587.
52. de Souza RF, Allemann N, Forseto A, Barros PS, Chamon W, Nose W. Ultrasound biomicroscopy and Scheimpflug photography of angle-supported phakic intraocular lens for high myopia. *J Cataract Refract Surg.* 2003;29(6):1159-1166.
53. Kwon RO, Price MO, Price FW Jr, Ambrosio R Jr, Belin MW. Pentacam characterization of corneas with Fuchs dystrophy treated with descemet membrane endothelial keratoplasty. *J Refract Surg.* 2010:1-8.
54. Nixon DR. Preoperative cataract grading by Scheimpflug imaging and effect on operative fluidics and phacoemulsification energy. *J Cataract Refract Surg.* 2010;36(2):242-246.
55. Cummings AB, Mascharka N. Outcomes after topography-based LASIK and LASEK with the WaveLight Oculyzer and Topolyzer Platforms. *J Refract Surg.* 2009:1-8.
56. Huang D, Swanson EA, Lin CP, et al. Optical coherence tomography. *Science.* 1991;254(5035):1178-1181.
57. Radhakrishnan S, Goldsmith J, Huang D, et al. Comparison of optical coherence tomography and ultrasound biomicroscopy for detection of narrow anterior chamber angles. *Arch Ophthalmol.* 2005;123(8):1053-1059.
58. Müller M, Dahmen G, Pörksen E, et al. Anterior chamber angle measurement with optical coherence tomography: intraobserver and interobserver variability. *J Cataract Refract Surg.* 2006;32(11):1803-1808.
59. Dada T, Sihota R, Gadia R, Aggarwal A, Mandal S, Gupta V. Comparison of anterior segment optical coherence tomography and ultrasound biomicroscopy for assessment of the anterior segment. *J Cataract Refract Surg.* 2007;33(5):837-840.
60. Wong HT, Lim MC, Sakata LM, et al. High-definition optical coherence tomography imaging of the iridocorneal angle of the eye. *Arch Ophthalmol.* 2009;127:256-260.
61. Radhakrishnan S, Rollins AM, Roth JE, et al. Real-time optical coherence tomography of the anterior segment at 1310 nm. *Arch Ophthalmol.* 2001;119(8):1179-1185.
62. Hee MR, Izatt JA, Swanson EA, et al. Optical coherence tomography of the human retina. *Arch Ophthalmol.* 1995;113(3):325-332.
63. Keane PA, Bhatti RA, Brubaker JW, Liakopoulos S, Sadda SR, Walsh AC. Comparison of clinically relevant findings from high-speed Fourier-domain and conventional time-domain optical coherence tomography. *Am J Ophthalmol.* 2009;148(2):242-248.e1.
64. Sarunic MV, Asrani S, Izatt JA. Imaging the ocular anterior segment with real-time, full-range Fourier-domain optical coherence tomography. *Arch Ophthalmol.* 2008;126:537-542.
65. Wojtkowski M, Bajraszewski T, Targowski P. A realtime in vivo imaging by high-speed spectral optical coherence tomography. *Opt Lett.* 2003;28:1745-1747.
66. Wylegała E, Teper S, Nowińska AK, Milka M, Dobrowolski D. Anterior segment imaging: Fourier-domain optical coherence tomography versus time-domain optical coherence tomography. *J Cataract Refract Surg.* 2009;35(8):1410-1414.
67. Kim JH, Lee D, Rhee KI. Flap thickness reproducibility in laser in situ keratomileusis with a femtosecond laser: optical coherence tomography measurement. *J Cataract Refract Surg.* 2008;34:132-136.
68. Stahl JE, Durrie DS, Schwendeman FJ, Boghossian AJ. Anterior segment OCT analysis of thin IntraLase femtosecond flaps. *J Refract Surg.* 2007;23:555-558.
69. Rocha KM, Randleman JB, Stulting RD. Analysis of thin microkeratome flap architecture using Fourier-domain optical coherence tomography. Paper presented at: American Society of Cataract and Refractive Surgery (ASCRS) meeting; April 9-14, 2010; Boston, MA.
70. Das S, Sullivan LJ. Comparison of residual stromal bed and flap thickness in primary and repeat laser in situ keratomileusis in myopic patients. *J Cataract Refract Surg.* 2006;32(12):2080-2084.
71. Reinstein DZ, Srivannaboon S, Archer TJ, Silverman RH, Sutton H, Coleman DJ. Probability model of the inaccuracy of residual stromal thickness prediction to reduce the risk of ectasia after LASIK part I: quantifying individual risk. *J Refract Surg.* 2006;22(9):851-860.
72. Randleman JB, Hewitt SM, Lynn MJ, Stulting RD. A comparison of 2 methods for estimating residual stromal bed thickness before repeat LASIK. *Ophthalmology.* 2005;112(1):98-103.
73. Prandi B, Baviera J, Morcillo M. Influence of flap thickness on results of laser in situ keratomileusis for myopia. *J Refract Surg.* 2004;20(6):790-796.
74. Dupps WJ Jr, Roberts C. Effect of acute biomechanical changes on corneal curvature after photokeratectomy. *J Refract Surg.* 2001;17(6):658-669.
75. Maeda N, Klyce SD, Smolek MK, Thompson HW. Automated keratoconus screening with corneal topography analysis. *Invest Ophthalmol Vis Sci.* 1994;35:2749-2757.
76. Schwiegerling J, Greivenkamp JE. Keratoconus detection based on videokeratoscopic height data. *Optom Vis Sci.* 1996;73:721-728.
77. Rabinowitz YS, Rasheed K. KISA% index: a quantitative videokeratography algorithm embodying minimal topographic criteria for diagnosing keratoconus. *J Cataract Refract Surg.* 1999;25:1327-1335.
78. Tang M, Shekhar R, Miranda D, Huang D. Characteristics of keratoconus and pellucid marginal degeneration in mean curvature maps. *Am J Ophthalmol.* 2005;140:993-1001.
79. Krachmer JH, Feder RS, Belin MW. Keratoconus and related noninflammatory corneal thinning disorders. *Surv Ophthalmol.* 1984;28:293-322.
80. Vinciguerra P, Camesasca FI. Prevention of corneal ectasia in laser in situ keratomileusis. *J Refract Surg.* 2001;17:S187-S189.
81. Li Y, Meisler DM, Tang M, et al.Keratoconus diagnosis with optical coherence tomography pachymetry mapping. *Ophthalmology.* 2008;115(12):2159-2166.
82. Li Y, Shekhar R, Huang D. Corneal pachymetry mapping with high-speed optical coherence tomography. *Ophthalmology.* 2006;113:792-799.
83. Reinstein DZ, Archer TJ, Gobbe M. Stability of LASIK in topographically suspect keratoconus confirmed non-keratoconic by Artemis VHF digital ultrasound epithelial thickness mapping: 1-year follow-up. *J Refract Surg.* 2009;25(7):569-577.
84. Randleman JB, Loupe DN, Song CD, Waring GO III, Stulting RD. Intraocular lens power calculations after laser in situ keratomileusis. *Cornea.* 2002;21:751-755.
85. Koch DD. New options for IOL calculations after refractive surgery. *J Cataract Refract Surg.* 2006;32:371-372.
86. Chokshi AR, Latkany RA, Speaker MG. IOL calculations after refractive surgery. *J Cataract Refract Surg.* 2006;32:1984.
87. Seitz B, Langenbucher A. Intraocular lens calculations status after corneal refractive surgery. *Curr Opin Ophthalmol.* 2000;11:35-46.
88. Gimbel HV, Sun R. Accuracy and predictability of intraocular lens power calculation after laser in situ keratomileusis. *J Cataract Refract Surg.* 2001;27:571-576.
89. Aramberri J. Intraocular lens power calculation after corneal refractive surgery: double-K method. *J Cataract Refract Surg.* 2003;29:2063-2068.

90. Speicher L. Intra-ocular lens calculation status after corneal refractive surgery. *Curr Opin Ophthalmol.* 2001;12:17-29.
91. Odenthal MT, Eggink CA, Melles G, Pameyer JH, Geerards AJ, Beekhuis WH. Clinical and theoretical results of intraocular lens power calculation for cataract surgery after photorefractive keratectomy for myopia. *Arch Ophthalmol.* 2002;120:431-438.
92. Arce CG, Soriano ES, Weisenthal RW, et al. Calculation of intraocular lens power using Orbscan II quantitative area topography after corneal refractive surgery. *J Refract Surg.* 2009;25(12):1061-1074.
93. Hanna C, O'Brien JE. Cell production and migration in the epithelial layer of the cornea. *Arch Ophthalmol.* 1960;64:536-539.
94. Simon G, Ren Q, Kervick GN, Parel JM. Optics of the corneal epithelium. *Refract Corneal Surg.* 1993;9:42-50.
95. Reinstein DZ, Archer T. Combined Artemis very high-frequency digital ultrasound-assisted transepithelial phototherapeutic keratectomy and wavefront-guided treatment following multiple corneal refractive procedures. *J Cataract Refract Surg.* 2006;32:1870-1876.
96. Vogt A. *Textbook and Atlas of Slit Lamp Microscopy of the Living Eye.* Bonn: Wayenborgh Editions; 1981.
97. Gauthier CA, Holden BA, Epstein D, Tengroth B, Fagerholm P, Hamberg-Nystrom H. Factors affecting epithelial hyperplasia after photorefractive keratectomy. *J Cataract Refract Surg.* 1997;23:1042-1050.
98. Lohmann CP, Reischl U, Marshall J. Regression and epithelial hyperplasia after myopic photorefractive keratectomy in a human cornea. *J Cataract Refract Surg.* 1999;25:712-715.
99. Srivannaboon S, Reinstein DZ, Sutton HFS, Silverman RH. Effect of epithelial changes on refractive outcome in LASIK. *Invest Ophthalmol Vis Sci.* 1999;40:S896.
100. Reinstein DZ, Srivannaboon S, Silverman RH, Coleman DJ. Limits of wavefront customized ablation: biomechanical and epithelial factors. *Invest Ophthalmol Vis Sci.* 2002;43:E-Abstract 3942.
101. Reinstein DZ, Srivannaboon S, Silverman RH, Coleman DJ. The accuracy of routine LASIK; isolation of biomechanical and epithelial factors. *Invest Ophthalmol Vis Sci.* 2000;41(Suppl):S318.
102. Scroggs MW, Proia AD. Histopathological variation in keratoconus. *Cornea.* 1992;11:553-559.
103. Haque S, Simpson T, Jones L. Corneal and epithelial thickness in keratoconus: a comparison of ultrasonic pachymetry, Orbscan II, and optical coherence tomography. *J Refract Surg.* 2006;22:486-493.
104. Aktekin M, Sargon MF, Cakar P, Celik HH, Firat E. Ultrastructure of the cornea epithelium in keratoconus. *Okajimas Folia Anat Jpn.* 1998;75:45-53.
105. Gatinel D, Racine L, Hoang-Xuan T. Contribution of the corneal epithelium to anterior corneal topography in patients having myopic photorefractive keratectomy. *J Cataract Refract Surg.* 2007;33:1860-1865.
106. Wang J, Fonn D, Simpson TL, Sorbara L, Kort R, Jones L. Topographical thickness of the epithelium and total cornea after overnight wear of reverse-geometry rigid contact lenses for myopia reduction. *Invest Ophthalmol Vis Sci.* 2003;44:4742-4746.
107. Feng Y, Simpson TL. Comparison of human central cornea and limbus in vivo using optical coherence tomography. *Optom Vis Sci.* 2005;82:416-419.
108. Wirbelauer C, Pham DT. Monitoring corneal structures with slitlamp-adapted optical coherence tomography in laser in situ keratomileusis. *J Cataract Refract Surg.* 2004;30:1851-1860.
109. Ladage PM, Yamamoto K, Ren DH, et al. Effects of rigid and soft contact lens daily wear on corneal epithelium, tear lactate dehydrogenase, and bacterial binding to exfoliated epithelial cells. *Ophthalmology.* 2001;108:1279-1288.
110. Moller-Pedersen T, Vogel M, Li HF, Petroll WM, Cavanagh HD, Jester JV. Quantification of stromal thinning, epithelial thickness, and corneal haze after photorefractive keratectomy using in vivo confocal microscopy. *Ophthalmology.* 1997;104:360-368.
111. Perez JG, Meijome JM, Jalbert I, Sweeney DF, Erickson P. Corneal epithelial thinning profile induced by long-term wear of hydrogel lenses. *Cornea.* 2003;22:304-307.
112. Sin S, Simpson TL. The repeatability of corneal and corneal epithelial thickness measurements using optical coherence tomography. *Optom Vis Sci.* 2006;83:360-365.
113. Li HF, Petroll WM, Moller-Pedersen T, Maurer JK, Cavanagh HD, Jester JV. Epithelial and corneal thickness measurements by in vivo confocal microscopy through focusing (CMTF). *Curr Eye Res.* 1997;16:214-221.
114. Patel SV, McLaren JW, Hodge DO, Bourne WM. Confocal microscopy in vivo in corneas of long-term contact lens wearers. *Invest Ophthalmol Vis Sci.* 2002;43:995-1003.
115. Reinstein DZ, Silverman RH, Raevsky T, et al. Arc-scanning very high-frequency digital ultrasound for 3D pachymetric mapping of the corneal epithelium and stroma in laser in situ keratomileusis. *J Refract Surg.* 2000;16:414-430.
116. Reinstein DZ, Archer TJ, Gobbe M, Silverman RH, Coleman DJ. Repeatability of layered corneal pachymetry with the Artemis very high-frequency digital ultrasound arc-scanner. *J Refract Surg.* 2010;26(9):646-659.
117. Reinstein DZ, Silverman RH, Coleman DJ. High-frequency ultrasound measurement of the thickness of the corneal epithelium. *Refract Corneal Surg.* 1993;9:385-387.
118. Reinstein DZ, Silverman RH, Trokel SL, Coleman DJ. Corneal pachymetric topography. *Ophthalmology.* 1994;101:432-438.
119. Reinstein DZ, Archer TJ, Gobbe M, Silverman RH, Coleman DJ. Epithelial thickness in the normal cornea: three-dimensional display with Artemis very high-frequency digital ultrasound. *J Refract Surg.* 2008;24:571-581.
120. Bentivoglio AR, Bressman SB, Cassetta E, Carretta D, Tonali P, Albanese A. Analysis of blink rate patterns in normal subjects. *Mov Disord.* 1997;12:1028-1034.
121. Doane MG. Interactions of eyelids and tears in corneal wetting and the dynamics of the normal human eyeblink. *Am J Ophthalmol.* 1980;89:507-516.
122. Rao SN, Raviv T, Majmudar PA, Epstein RJ. Role of Orbscan II in screening keratoconus suspects before refractive corneal surgery. *Ophthalmology.* 2002;109:1642-1646.
123. Lim L, Wei RH, Chan WK, Tan DT. Evaluation of keratoconus in Asians: role of Orbscan II and Tomey TMS-2 corneal topography. *Am J Ophthalmol.* 2007;143:390-400.
124. Reinstein DZ. High-frequency ultrasound versus optical coherence tomography. Paper presented at: American Academy of Ophthalmology 2003 Annual Meeting; November 15-18, 2003; Anaheim, CA.
125. Schlegel Z, Hoang-Xuan T, Gatinel D. Comparison of and correlation between anterior and posterior corneal elevation maps in normal eyes and keratoconus-suspect eyes. *J Cataract Refract Surg.* 2008;34:789-795.
126. Reinstein DZ, Archer TJ, Gobbe M. Stability of LASIK in corneas with topographic suspect keratoconus, with keratoconus excluded by epithelial thickness mapping. *J Refract Surg.* 2009;25:569-577.
127. Reinstein DZ, Archer TJ, Gobbe M. Stability of LASIK in corneas with topographic suspect keratoconus confirmed non-keratoconic by epithelial thickness mapping: 2-years follow-up. Paper presented at: American Academy of Ophthalmology 2009 Annual Meeting; October 24-27, 2009; San Francisco, CA.
128. Randleman JB, Woodward M, Lynn MJ, Stulting RD. Risk assessment for ectasia after corneal refractive surgery. *Ophthalmology.* 2008;115:37-50.
129. Reinstein DZ, Silverman RH, Sutton HF, Coleman DJ. Very high-frequency ultrasound corneal analysis identifies anatomic correlates of optical complications of lamellar refractive surgery: anatomic diagnosis in lamellar surgery. *Ophthalmology.* 1999;106:474-482.

130. Patel S, Reinstein DZ, Silverman RH, Coleman DJ. The shape of Bowman's layer in the human cornea. *J Refract Surg.* 1998;14:636-640.
131. Patel S, Marshall J, Fitzke FW. Refractive index of the human corneal epithelium and stroma. *J Refract Surg.* 1995;11:100-105.
132. Reinstein DZ, Srivannaboon S, Gobbe M, et al. Epithelial thickness profile changes induced by myopic LASIK as measured by Artemis very high-frequency digital ultrasound. *J Refract Surg.* 2009;25:444-450.
133. Reinstein DZ, Archer TJ, Gobbe M. LASIK for myopic astigmatism and presbyopia using non-linear aspheric micro-monovision with the Carl Zeiss Meditec MEL80 platform. *J Refract Surg.* 2011;27(1):23-37.
134. Reinstein DZ, Archer TJ, Gobbe M, Silverman RH, Coleman DJ. Epithelial thickness after hyperopic LASIK: three-dimensional display with Artemis very high-frequency digital ultrasound. *J Refract Surg.* 2010;26(8):555-564.
135. Varley GA, Huang D, Rapuano CJ, Schallhorn S, Boxer Wachler BS, Sugar A. LASIK for hyperopia, hyperopic astigmatism, and mixed astigmatism: a report by the American Academy of Ophthalmology. *Ophthalmology.* 2004;111:1604-1617.
136. Reinstein DZ, Gobbe M, Archer TJ, Couch D, Bloom B. Epithelial, stromal, and corneal pachymetry changes during orthokeratology. *Optom Vis Sci.* 2009;86:E1006-1014.
137. Barraquer JI. *Queratomileusis y queratofakia.* Bogotá, Colombia: Instituto Barraquer de America; 1980:342.
138. Wellish KL, Glasgow BJ, Beltran F, Maloney RK. Corneal ectasia as a complication of repeated keratotomy surgery. *J Refract Corneal Surg.* 1994;10:360-364.
139. Seiler T, Koufala K, Richter G. Iatrogenic keratectasia after laser in situ keratomileusis. *J Refract Surg.* 1998;14:312-317.
140. Randleman JB, Trattler WB, Stulting RD. Validation of the Ectasia Risk Score System for preoperative laser in situ keratomileusis screening. *Am J Ophthalmol.* 2008;145:813-818.
141. Reinstein DZ, Srivannaboon S, Holland SP. Epithelial and stromal changes induced by Intacs examined by three-dimensional very high-frequency digital ultrasound. *J Refract Surg.* 2001;17:310-318.
142. Lazzaro DR, Aslanides IM, Belmont SC, et al. High frequency ultrasound evaluation of radial keratotomy incisions. *J Cataract Refract Surg.* 1995;21:398-401.
143. Reinstein DZ, Srivannaboon S, Sutton HFS, Silverman RH, Shaikh A, Coleman DJ. Risk of ectasia in LASIK: revised safety criteria. *Invest Ophthalmol Vis Sci.* 1999;40(Suppl):S403.
144. Reinstein DZ, Silverman RH. Artemis VHF digital ultrasound technology. In: Wang M, ed. *Corneal Topography in the Wavefront Era.* Thorofare, NJ: SLACK Incorporated; 2006:207-226.
145. Reinstein DZ, Silverman RH, Archer TJ. VHF digital ultrasound: Artemis 2 scanning in corneal refractive surgery. In: Vinciguerra P, Camesasca FI, eds, *Refractive Surface Ablation: PRK, LASEK, Epi-LASIK, Custom, PTK and Retreatment.* Thorofare, NJ: SLACK Incorporated; 2006 315-330.
146. Reinstein DZ, Archer TJ. Evaluation of irregular astigmatism with Artemis very high-frequency digital ultrasound scanning. In: Wang M, ed. *Irregular Astigmatism: Diagnosis and Treatment.* Thorofare, NJ: SLACK Incorporated; 2007:29-42.
147. Reinstein DZ, Rothman RC, Couch DG, Archer TJ. Artemis very high-frequency digital ultrasound-guided repositioning of a free cap after laser in situ keratomileusis. *J Cataract Refract Surg.* 2006;32:1877-1882.
148. Reinstein DZ, Archer TJ, Gobbe M. Corneal ablation depth readout of the MEL80 excimer laser compared to Artemis three-dimensional very high-frequency digital ultrasound stromal measurements. *J Refract Surg.* 2010;26(12):949-959.
149. Reinstein DZ, Sutton HF, Srivannaboon S, Silverman RH, Archer TJ, Coleman DJ. Evaluating microkeratome efficacy by 3D corneal lamellar flap thickness accuracy and reproducibility using Artemis VHF digital ultrasound arc-scanning. *J Refract Surg.* 2006;22:431-440.
150. Reinstein DZ, Archer TJ, Gobbe M, Johnson NF. Accuracy and reproducibility of Artemis central flap thickness and visual outcomes of LASIK with the Carl Zeiss Meditec VisuMax femtosecond laser and MEL 80 excimer laser platforms. *J Refract Surg.* 2010;26(2):107-119.

# Chapter 7

# Topography and Wavefront Combined Systems

## The iTrace Combination Corneal Topography and Wavefront System

Tracy Schroeder Swartz, OD, MS, FAAO and Joe S. Wakil, MD

The iTrace system manufactured by Tracey Technologies Corp (Houston, TX) is uniquely designed to combine full-surface Placido corneal topography with the advantages of ray-tracing aberrometry, a robust wavefront technology to measure quality of vision. The iTrace incorporates the Placido components manufactured by EyeSys Vision, Inc, (Houston, TX) with integrated software application produced by Tracey Technologies to deliver corneal topography and total eye aberrometry data acquisition and analysis (Figure 7-1).

At the core of this instrument is the unique technology providing optical ray tracing of the eye, as is evidenced by the product name, the iTrace. A sequential series of thin, infrared beams or rays of light on the order of 100 μm each is projected into the entire entrance pupil of the eye using a software-programmable, scanning pattern measuring hundreds of points within milliseconds. Each of these points represents the entrance of parallel, sampling light rays into the eye, which become refracted by the eye's optical power eventually focusing on the retina. By locating the spot on the retina where each thin beam of light is focused, a direct aberration measurement is made leading to calculations for a complete aberration profile and optical performance examination of the eye. This technology stems from former Soviet military applications and was developed by scientist Vasyl Molebny, PhD,[1] and his team of engineers in Kiev, Ukraine in collaboration with ophthalmic surgeon Ioannis Pallikaris, MD, and his colleagues in Crete, Greece. The combination of this aberrometry information with corneal topography in a compact, cost-efficient package provides valuable clinical information in elucidating the ocular sources of aberrations, primarily as to whether they are corneal or lenticular for added diagnostic power.

### iTrace Engineering Advantages

Important in any system design is the philosophy behind it and the utility goals for its practice and use. The iTrace features a dual-purpose system with full corneal topography and wavefront capabilities along with integrated software analysis on a single computer platform. This device demonstrates the far greater power of the combination of these 2 technologies.

In addition, the slim engineering allows the eye under measurement to fixate directly through the instrument's transparent optics at a distance target. For example, the



Wang M. *Corneal Topography: A Guide for Clinical Application in the Wavefront Era, Second Edition* (pp. 167-198)

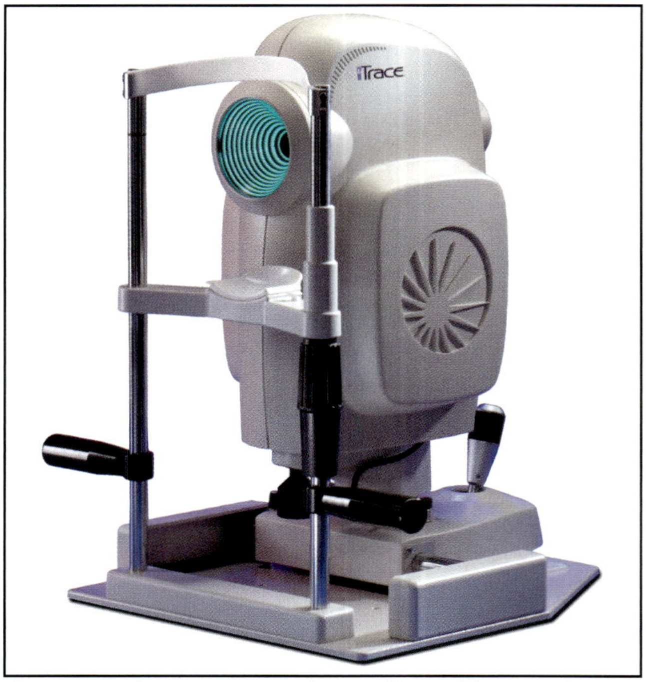


**Figure 7-1.** The iTrace unit's slim profile enables true distance target measurement binocularly for strong control of accommodation. (Reprinted with permission of Joe S. Wakil, MD.)

instrument may be placed such that the patient looks through an office window at a tree across the street while the fellow eye also has an unobstructed view of the same target. This helps provide an important and proprietary feature in allowing for binocular open field fixation of a real object at a truly far distance much greater than 20 feet during wavefront measurement. Natural binocular vision overcomes instrument myopia, a phenomenon where monocular fixation on an optically simulated "far" target results in excessive myopia. This phenomenon plagues all conventional autorefraction systems in measuring, particularly in younger patients.

## Corneal Topography Features of the iTrace System

The corneal topography displays are generated from Placido images of the cornea and are fully customizable within the iTrace software. Using advanced edge detection software, the Placido image of the cornea is analyzed across all the ring edges from center to periphery (Figure 7-2). The binocular display is shown in Figure 7-3. This display is often preferred by cataract surgeons due to its content. Simulated keratometry values, spherical aberrations, and corneal astigmatism (delta value) are easily located on the printout and facilitate intraocular lens (IOL) selection.

Additionally, a refractive power reading of the cornea is calculated for the 3-mm zone in similar fashion to the

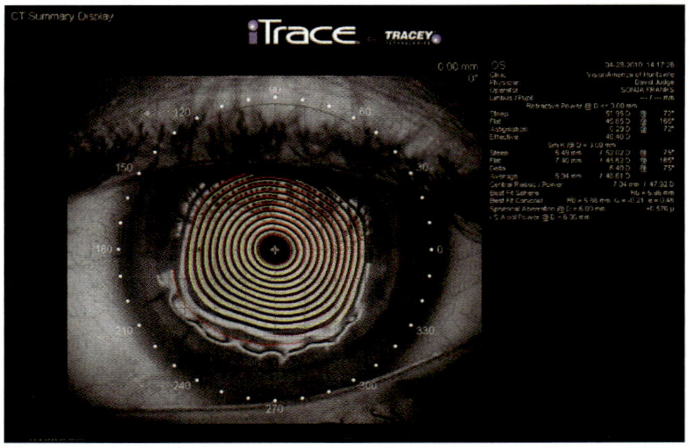


**Figure 7-2.** Default topographic display upon data capture. Note the distortion of the mires secondary to a corneal graft.

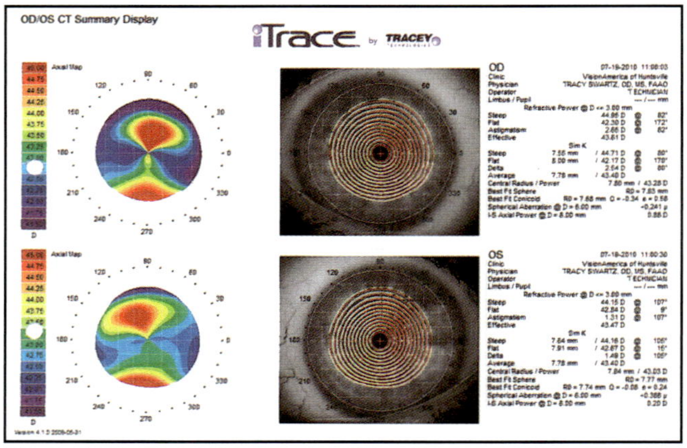


**Figure 7-3.** Binocular topographic display includes 2 maps (customized) and various indices valuable to refractive and cataract surgeons.

K readings, but based on Snell's Law of Refraction to more accurately describe the refractive power of the central cornea. A single effective refractive power reading is given for the entire central 3-mm zone of the cornea to be used primarily for IOL calculations. This number has been popularized by Jack Holladay, MD, as an improvement in understanding central corneal refractive power contribution in more accurately calculating the necessary IOL power for eyes postrefractive surgery.[2]

Beyond the numeric data of K readings, refractive power readings, and other corneal indices, color maps are provided to depict the unique features of each cornea. For both 2- and 3-dimensional color maps, a number of algorithms are available providing complete corneal analysis. These include the Axial Map, Local Radius of Curvature Map, Refractive Map, Z Elevation Map, and Wavefront Map.

The standard Axial map (Figure 7-4) is based on the keratometric formula wherein the curvature of the cornea is presented with respect to the optical axis of the instrument. This color map has been commonly used over the years as an extension of the keratometer to the entire corneal surface.

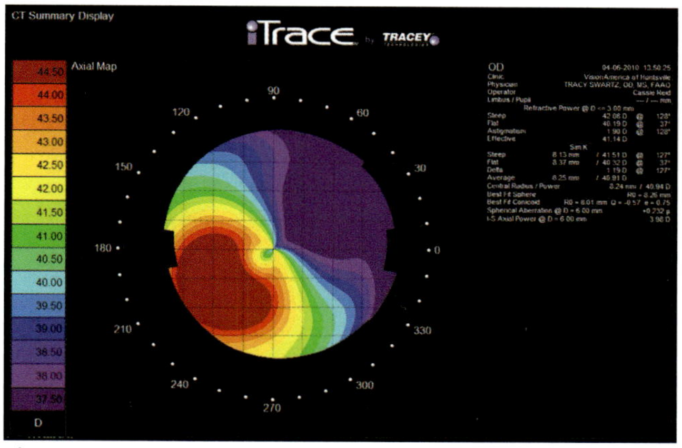


**Figure 7-4.** Axial map in a patient with keratoconus.

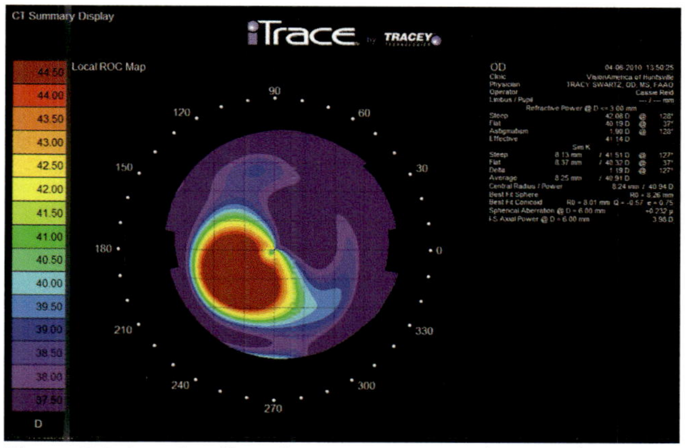


**Figure 7-5.** Local radius of curvature map, otherwise known as the tangential or instantaneous radius of curvature map, in a patient with keratoconus.

However, in applying the simple keratometric formula, this map only provides accurate curvature data and corneal refractive power data in the central corneal region. The data outside of the 3-mm zone is simply not accurate in terms of either the true curvature of the cornea or the refractive power generated in the peripheral cornea.

The Local Radius of Curvature Map, otherwise known as the Tangential Map or Instantaneous Radius of Curvature Map (Figure 7-5), is used to accurately depict the true corneal shape in terms of millimeter radius of curvature from center to periphery. This map is a mathematical derivative of the axial color map and can be most useful in appreciating the detail of corneal surface features both centrally and peripherally. Contact lens fitters will derive more accurate curvature measurements in the periphery to better fit contact lenses, while refractive surgeons will better appreciate the sharpness of transition zone edges from excimer laser ablations that commonly generate halos and glare to postsurgical eyes with small effective optical zones using this map. Also, for the critical diagnosis of keratoconus, the Local Radius of Curvature Map will emphasize the true size and nature of an ectasia as observed in the slit-lamp microscope. This is very important to note as it is necessary to know the actual apex location and severity of curvature generated by the keratoconus to treat appropriately. The Local Radius of Curvature Map is typically the best source of information for such corneal shape information.

The Refractive Map (Figure 7-6) accurately calculates the refractive power across the entire corneal surface as it applies Snell's Law of Refraction instead of the basic keratometric formula, which once again is only correct for the limited central corneal region. The Refractive Map is always presented in diopter units. The Refractive Map provides the clinician with appreciation for the greater refractive power of the normal cornea in the periphery than in the center despite the fact that the normal cornea does flatten in the periphery. This map is an accurate source of data to truly understand corneal optics and their contribution to the total ocular power.

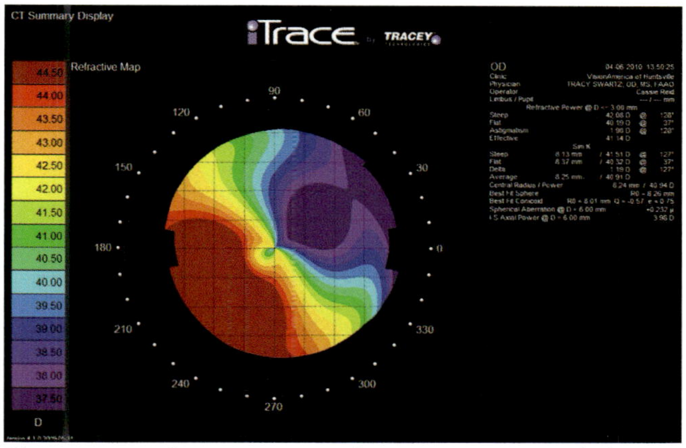


**Figure 7-6.** Refractive map in the same patient with keratoconus.

The Z Elevation Map (Figure 7-7) illustrates the physical nature of the cornea in terms of its height difference in microns from a reference sphere. The algorithms used to choose a reference sphere are important, as one can generate a number of different elevation measurements based solely upon the particular reference sphere. iTrace uses an algorithm that uses a reference sphere based on the best fit to the central cornea. The Z Elevation Map illustrates depressions and elevations from a best-fit sphere. The user can modify the reference sphere to obtain more detail in some cases. Without providing a reference sphere, the ability to discern the very subtle height differences across the cornea would be difficult. Because the cornea is generally aspheric, there will always be some differences in the height from a sphere. Elevation mapping is critical for planning excimer laser enhancement surgeries, including surgical correction of decentered ablations, and in studying corneal disease progression.

The corneal wavefront (CW) map (Figure 7-8) is an extension of wavefront analysis of the eye applied strictly

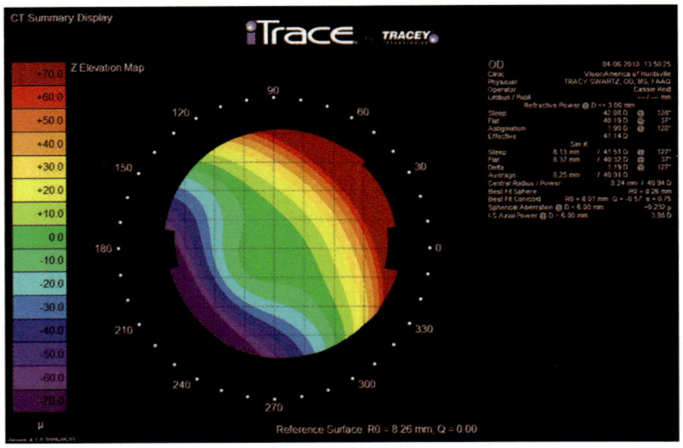


**Figure 7-7.** Z elevation map in the same patient with keratoconus.

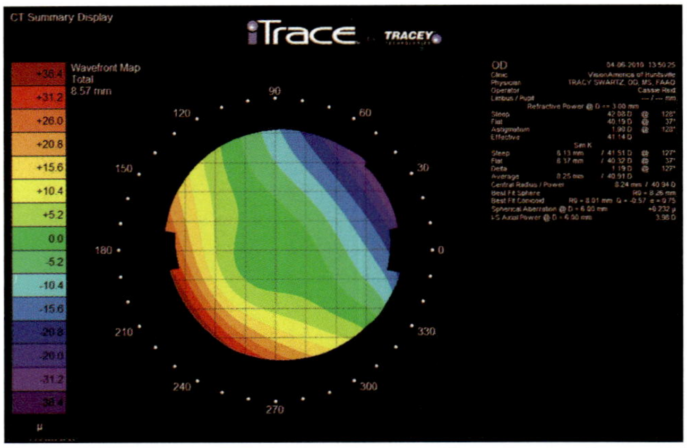


**Figure 7-8.** CW map showing coma in the same patient with keratoconus.

to the cornea. It is a Zernike calculation of the wavefront errors generated by the corneal surface. This is useful in understanding the cornea's contribution to the overall aberrations in the eye. Subtracting the CW contributions from the entire ocular wavefront (OW) measurement to elucidate aberrations generated in the internal eye structures is a powerful diagnostic tool. This Wavefront Map is described in micron units of wavefront error and must not be confused with corneal height determination. There is a direct correlation of the CW Map, which only applies to the area of the cornea within the entrance pupil, to that of the Refractive Map in the same corneal area.

## Corneal Topography Verification and Analysis Displays

The iTrace system captures the Placido image automatically upon centering and focusing of the video image as the patient fixates upon a coaxial fixation point. This automatic

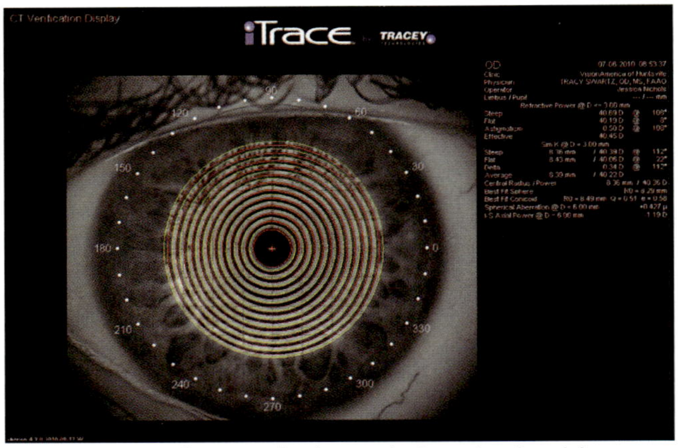


**Figure 7-9.** Verification display including simulated keratometry, spherical aberration values, and corneal astigmatism (delta) value to aid IOL selection.

capture occurs through triangulation of a low-power laser beam reflected off of the corneal apex at a calibrated distance from the Placido. Once captured, the Placido image is displayed with the ring edge detection highlighted to confirm correct image processing. This helps avoid artifacts and errors in processing that can sometimes be problematic in very irregular corneas, such as those following corneal transplantation. Figure 7-9 shows a typical Placido image capture verification screen with the edge detection clearly shown confirming correct analysis. Keratometry and refractive power readings are also displayed following image capture.

The Corneal Topography Summary Display can be customized to allow for up to 4 of any of the available color maps to be displayed. The iTrace is generally configured to show the Axial, Local Radius of Curvature, Refractive, and Z Elevation. The example in Figure 7-10 shows significant keratoconus.

Within the displays, scaling is also customizable. Autoscaling features or user-defined fixed scaling units may be used. Typically, 0.5-D step sizes are used to provide good corneal detail while also providing adequate range. User choice is available to generate practically all scaling requirements.

An example of the Z Elevation Map in 3 dimensions is shown in Figure 7-11. This effect can be applied to all maps and is included in the summary display.

A Comparison Display reveals differences that occur over time. This may be useful in patients with contact lens distortion preoperatively (Figure 7-12) or to monitor treatment (Figure 7-13). The difference map is overall green, indicating little or no change in corneal topography.

The caliper tool can be used to determine the axis of toric IOL when marked prior to surgery and scanned. The landmarks of the eye can be used to indicate the proper placement (Figure 7-14).

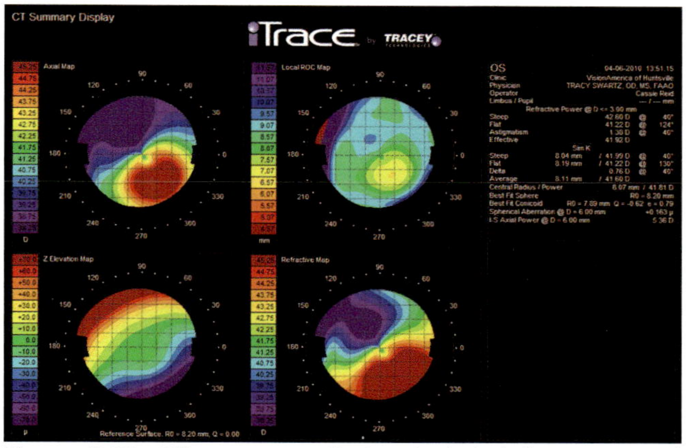


**Figure 7-10.** CT summary display included for maps and commonly used indices. This is an example of a patient with keratoconus.

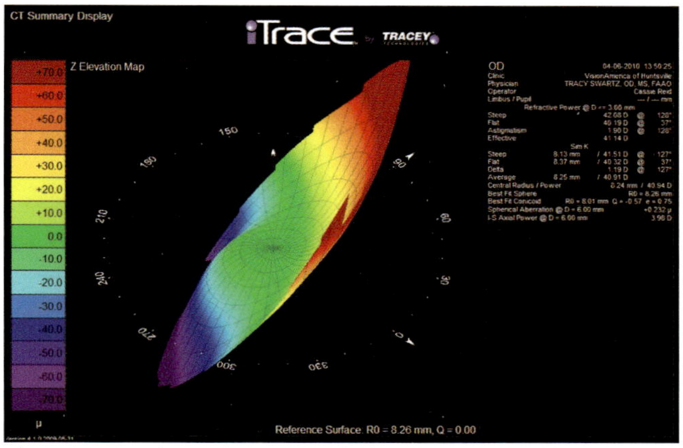


**Figure 7-11.** Three-dimensional elevation map. All maps may be viewed in 2 or 3 dimensions.

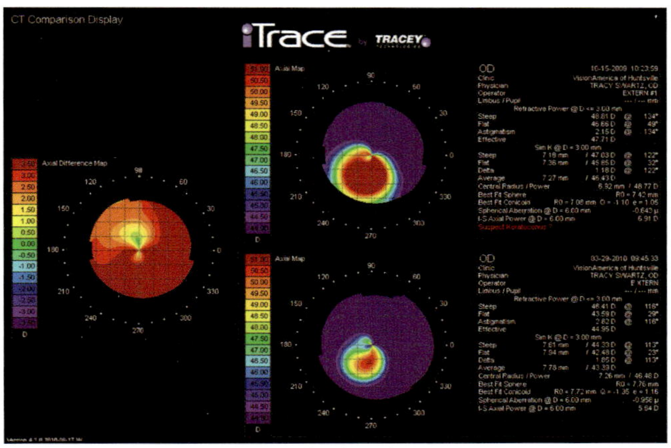


**Figure 7-12.** Comparison display for a keratoconic patient who had underworn his gas permeable lenses. Immediately after removal, the cone was larger. After cessation of lenses, the vision improved to 20/20 best corrected with improved topography.

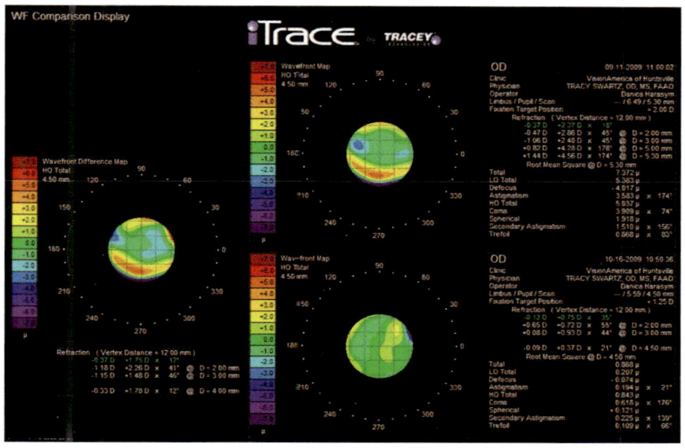


**Figure 7-13.** Corneal topography comparison display of higher order aberrations in a LASIK patient prior to (top) and following (bottom) dry eye treatment. The improvement in the inferior portion of the cornea was significant enough to bring the uncorrected acuity from 20/30 to 20/20.

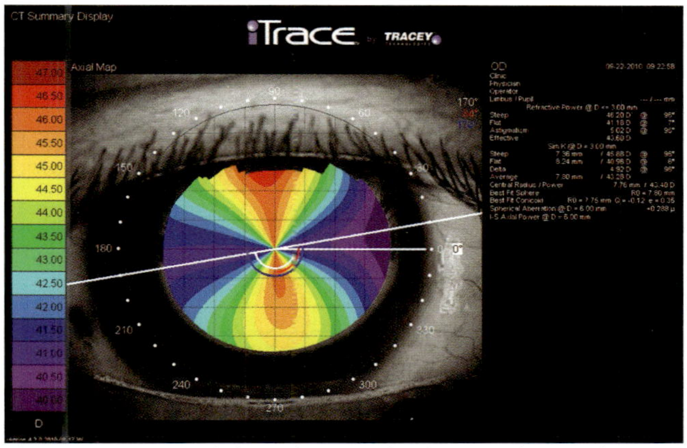


**Figure 7-14.** Use of the caliper tool. This may be used in surgery in patients with high astigmatism by marking the cornea, capturing the image, and locating the proper axis relative to the horizontal and vertical meridian. Alternatively, conjunctional landmarks are used.

# Aberrometry/Wavefront With the iTrace Ray Tracing Principle

Historically, the optical property of the eye has been described in terms of a single group as a simple refraction. Refraction can be measured with a variety of instruments: retinoscopy, refractometry, and autorefraction. However, these measurements represent only spherocylindrical measurements of the aberrations in the eye. To measure the spatially resolved optical properties of the eye, we must use another terminology to describe these properties. One method is by characterizing the wavefront or the total aberrations of the eye's optical system.

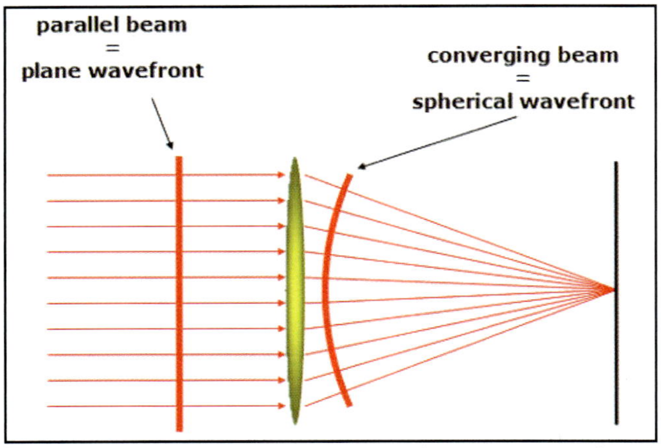


**Figure 7-15.** Plane and spherical wavefronts. (Reprinted with permission of Joe S. Wakil, MD.)

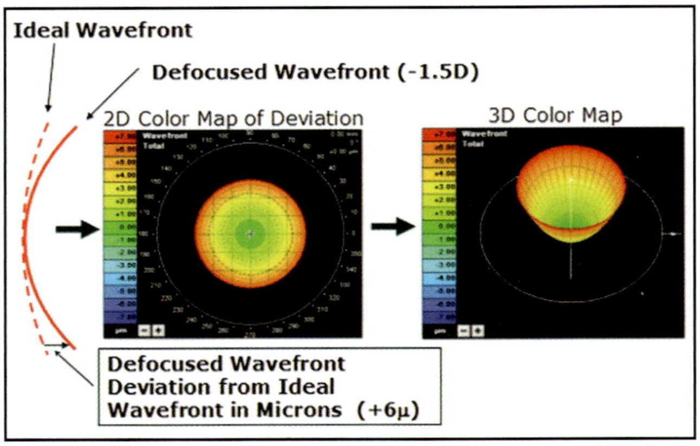


**Figure 7-17.** Representation of a defocused wavefront from the ideal.

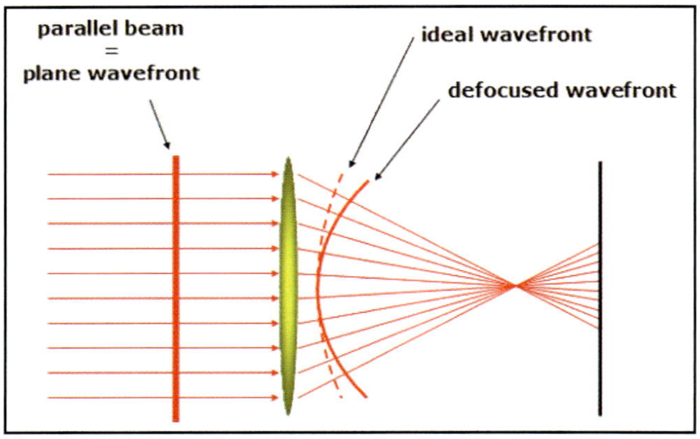


**Figure 7-16.** Wavefront for myopic optical system. (Reprinted with permission of Joe S. Wakil, MD.)

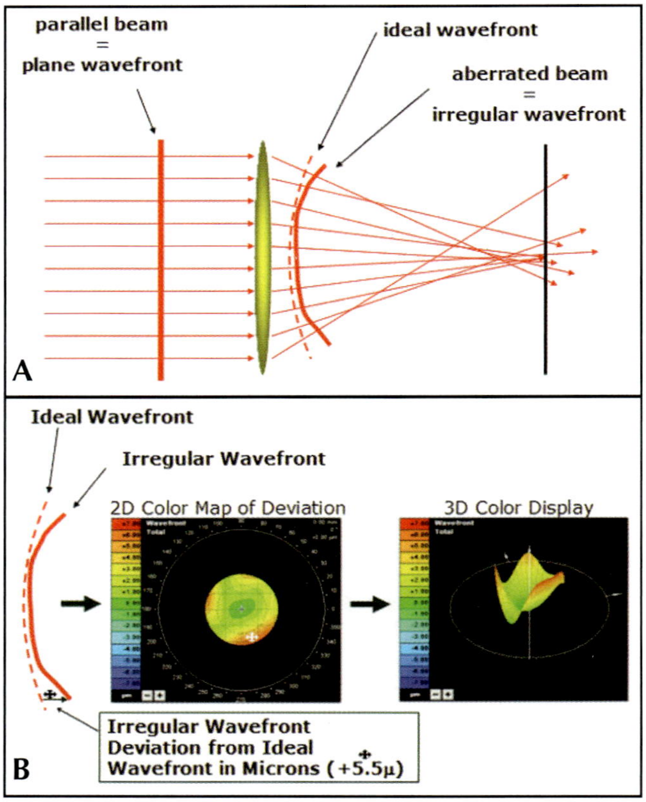


**Figure 7-18.** (A) Irregular wavefront results from the human eye because it is not purely spherical or aspheric. (B) Variations in refractive power at each point over the entrance pupil can also be demonstrated as an irregular wavefront of the eye in both 2- and 3-dimensional maps.

A wavefront is an imaginary surface joining all points in space that are reached at the same time by a lightwave propagating through a medium. The solid, vertical red line in Figure 7-15 depicts such a wavefront. Parallel light entering the eye would have a flat or plane wavefront. Each point in the lightwave arrives at the imaginary surface in front of the eye at the same time.

For the human emmetropic eye, the wavefront is curved. When light travels different distances through variable media at different speeds, the imaginary surface that represents the points reached at the same time is curved. For a myopic eye of identical length, the wavefront would be more curved secondary to the greater refractive power, as drawn in Figure 7-16.

The difference between an ideal wavefront and the actual wavefront over the entire surface of the optical system is calculated in terms of microns of deviation. When the actual wavefront is more advanced than the ideal wavefront, the error is described as a positive deviation in microns. If the actual wavefront were retarded, the deviation would have a negative value. This spatially resolved deviation of the measured wavefront from the ideal as a 2-dimensional color map and a 3-dimensional display is shown for the defocused wavefront in Figure 7-17.

The eye, however, is rarely described by a purely spherical or aspheric surface. The resulting wavefront error is irregular in deviation pattern as depicted in cross-section in Figure 7-18. Variations in refractive power at each point over the entrance pupil can also be demonstrated as an irregular wavefront of the eye in both 2- and 3-dimensional maps.

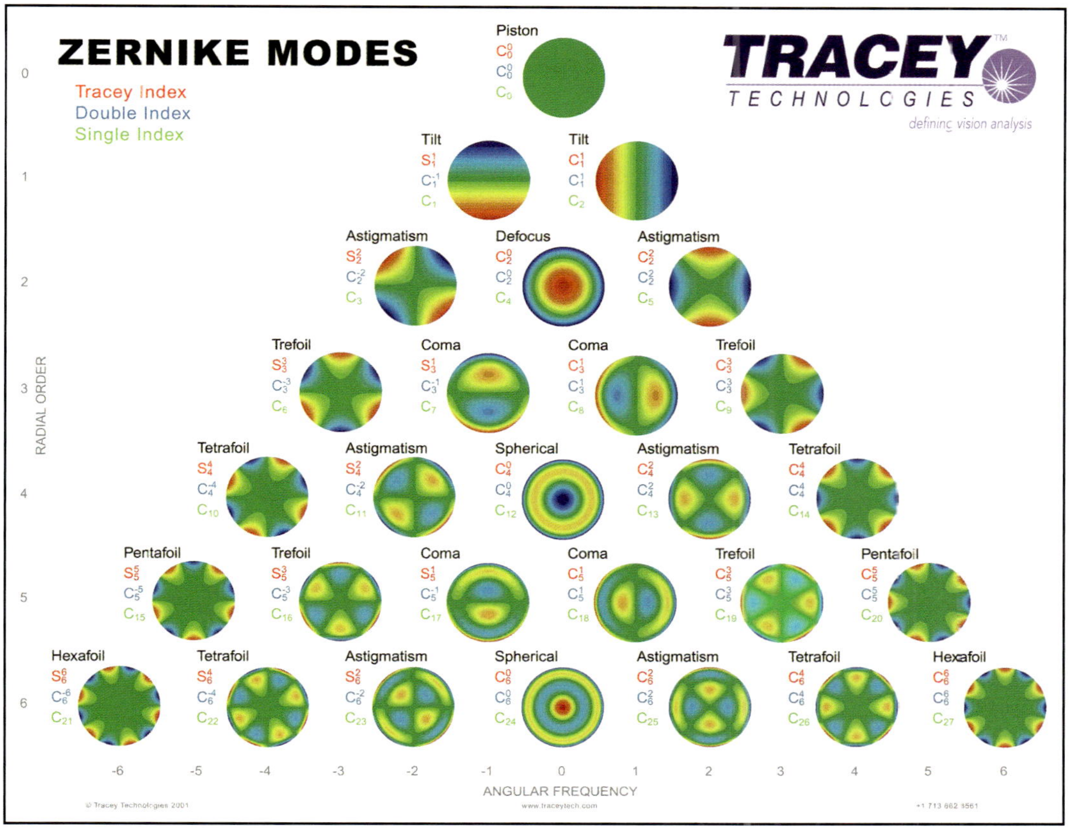


**Figure 7-19.** Visual representation of a Zernike polynomial. (Reprinted with permission of Sonya Dakin.)

The deviations between the actual wavefront and ideal wavefront are referred to as aberrations. In 1934, Fritz Zernike published a paper describing a set of polynomials that could be used to expand the aberration function. Each polynomial represents a particular type of optical aberration. Each wavefront can be described by mathematical coefficients that, when taken as a whole, reconstruct the wavefront map as shown in Figure 7-19, which shows the Zernike modes for an expansion through 6th order polynomials.

There are 4 technologies commercially available to measure aberrations in the eye. These include: Hartmann-Shack, Tscherning, differential skiascopy, and ray tracing. Tracey Technologies uses the ray tracing principle that projects a sequential series of thin laser beams through the entrance pupil parallel to the eye's line of sight. The location of each beam of light focused onto the retina is measured by capturing the exiting reflected light and focusing it onto position-sensing detectors. Ray tracing measures the forward aberration of light passing into the eye. The Hartmann-Shack principle assumes an ideal point source of light is generated from the retina, therefore measuring the reverse aberrations of light as it passes from the retina out the exit pupil of the eye. Measuring forward aberrations is more physiologic in analyzing vision as it follows the natural path of light into the eye.

Ray tracing has additional advantages over other technologies. First, the rapid sequential capture of data means that there is no confusion in the analysis between the origin

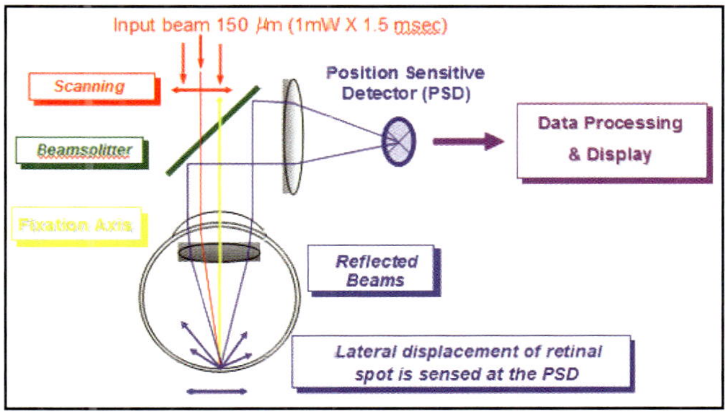


**Figure 7-20.** Schematic layout of ray tracing aberrometer. (Reprinted with permission of Joe S. Wakil, MD.)

location in the entrance pupil and the reflected location from the retina. This means that highly aberrated eyes can be easily measured with ray tracing. Second, because the pattern of laser spots projected through the entrance pupil is rapidly controlled with software, the system can track the pupil size and project all 256 points into a pupil as small as 2 mm or as large as 8 mm. Third, because each point is measured separately, the software's task of locating the center of each spot is much easier; therefore, processing is very fast, requiring only basic computer power, which helps allow for a cost-efficient system. Measurement has successfully been performed in children with amblyopia,

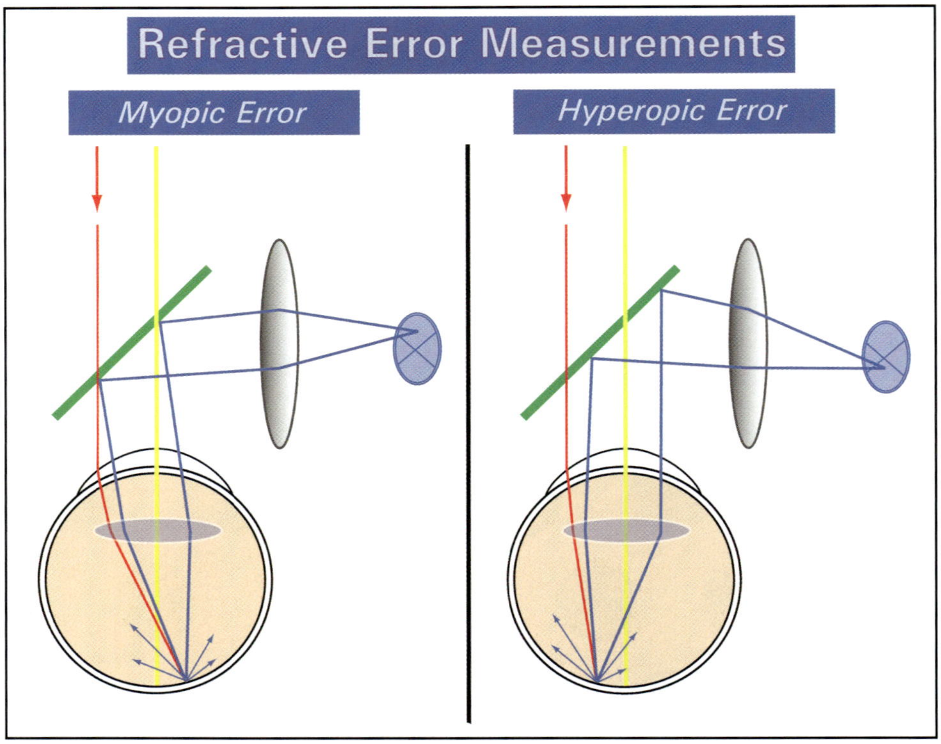


**Figure 7-21.** Shift of retinal spot location based on local aberrations of the eye. Myopia is described on the left; hyperopia on the right. (Reprinted with permission of Joe S. Wakil, MD.)

where higher order aberration (HOA) quantification aids diagnosis.[3]

Figure 7-20 is a schematic layout of the ray tracing technique developed by Tracey Technologies. Once the position of point 1 is determined, the laser beam is moved to a new position, and the location of the next point on the retina is then determined. This process continues until 256 separate points have been projected through the entrance pupil, which occurs in approximately 100 msec. If the eye were emmetropic, then all 256 points would fall on one spot in the center of the macula as shown in Figure 7-19. Generally, local aberrations at the beam's entry point on the cornea or the lens cause a shift in the location on the retina. Figure 7-21 illustrates a single measurement point for a myopic and hyperopic eye. After a series of points are projected sequentially through the entrance pupil, the retinal spot pattern is created (Figure 7-22).

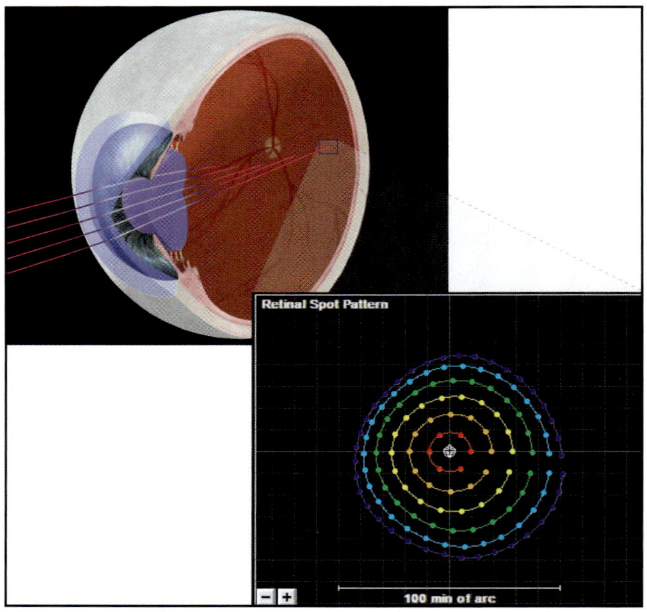


**Figure 7-22.** Schematic eye and retinal spot pattern illustrating the resulting spot pattern (256 points). (Reprinted with permission of Joe S. Wakil, MD.)

## Advantages of Combined Wavefront/Corneal Topography Display

The iTrace system measures total ocular aberrations of the eye (aberrometry) using ray tracing and calculates corneal anterior surface aberrations from the corneal topography data acquired through the Placido image. This calculation involves simply performing a Zernike polynomial computation on the data generated from the refractive map of the cornea using the classic Snell's Law of Refraction formula across the cornea's surface. By subtracting the corneal aberrations from the total ocular aberrations of the eye, the aberrations of the internal optics (primarily the lens) are generated. This is a good first approximation of aberrations attributed to the internal optics of the eye. This also provides clinical insight into the optical relationship between the crystalline lens and cornea.

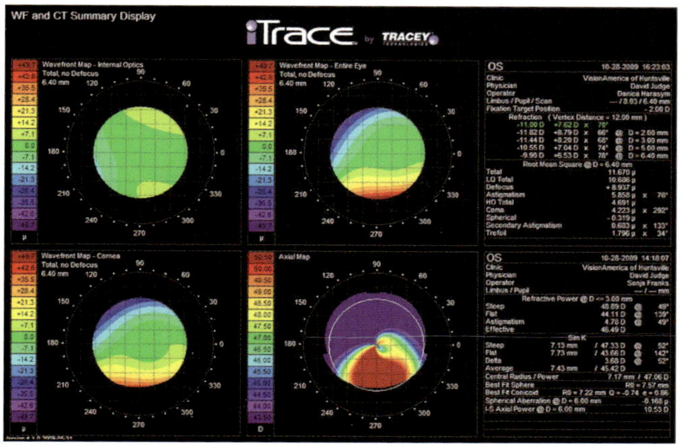


**Figure 7-23.** Case example of a keratoconic patient with irregular astigmatism. Note the wavefront pattern for the entire eye (upper right) closely resembles the pattern of the CW (lower left), suggesting the majority of the aberrations are due to the cornea.

Locating the sources of astigmatism is a prime example of the power of the combined Wavefront and Corneal Topography Display. In Figure 7-23, a keratoconic eye is shown. The upper right map provides the whole eye wavefront and clearly shows irregularity, which closely resembles the CW map (lower left). This indicates that the majority of the visual disturbance is found on the cornea.

Figure 7-24 depicts an eye with an iris cyst superiorly tilting the crystalline lens and inducing astigmatism. Here, the CW is green, indicating a regular cornea while the interior optics reveal coma secondary to lens tilt.

Figure 7-25 is an example from a patient who underwent implantation of a ReStor presbyopia-correcting lens (Alcon Laboratories, Fort Worth, TX) and suffered from glare and mild vision loss. The clinical picture at the slit lamp did not indicate a problem, and the surgeon was perplexed as to the etiology of the patient's complaint. The iTrace identified coma resulting from tilting of the ReStor lens.

Figure 7-26 illustrates the advantage of the iTrace with regard to refractive surgery candidacy. The combination of wavefront and topography identifies those with early ectasia who should not undergo LASIK. Coma on CW may indicate early keratoconus or, in this case, pellucid marginal degeneration. Clinical exam and pachymetry are used to rule out lens warpage and dry eye, which also manifest as inferior steepening.

The iTrace uniquely demonstrates changes in the lens during accommodation.[4,5] Using the open field window, the patient fixates on a distance target binocularly or monocularly. The measurement is then repeated while looking at a near point target, such as a reading card using an attached near-point reading rod. The difference map represents the accommodative change of the eye. Accommodation traditionally calls for a spherical change in the lens power across the pupil, but in many cases the iTrace demonstrates that cylinder as well as HOAs are induced by the lens, which provide an increased depth of field (pseudo-accommodation)

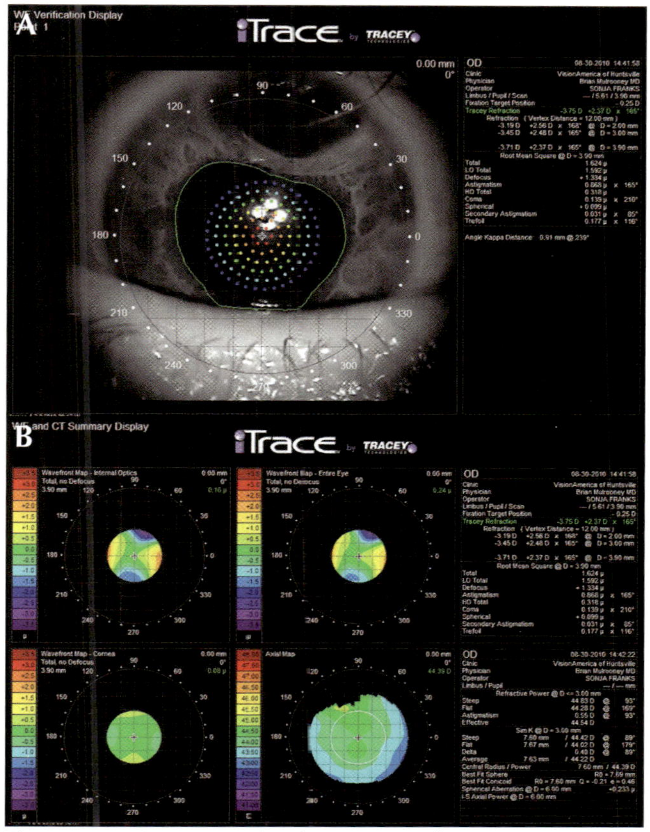


**Figure 7-24.** Case example of a patient with iris cysts causing a tilt of the crystalline lens, and refractive astigmatism. The cyst is easily seen on the eye image. The combination topography and wavefront display suggests the astigmatism is not on the cornea but rather due to the tilting of the lens secondary to the cyst. Note the green CW, indicating few aberrations generated on the cornea.

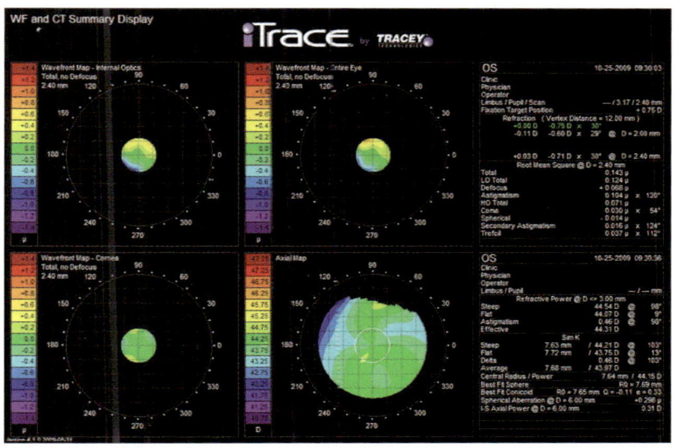


**Figure 7-25.** Lenticular coma resulting from a tilted ReStor lens (Alcon, Fort Worth, TX). (Reprinted with permission of Joe S. Wakil, MD.)

to assist the patient's visual processing to enhance near vision. New studies are being performed to understand these mechanisms in natural accommodation and accommodating IOL technology. Figure 7-27 shows the refractive

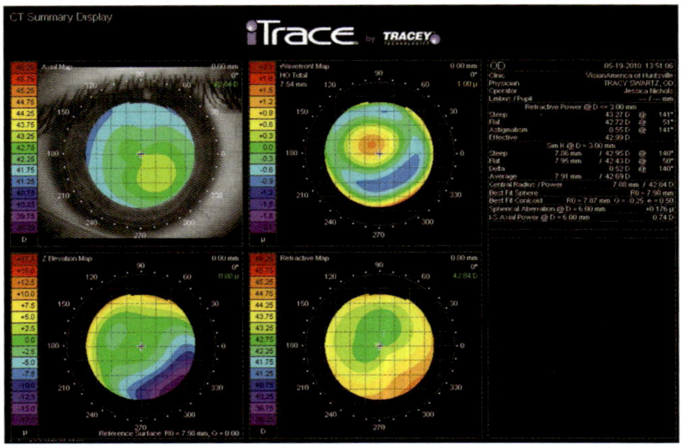


**Figure 7-26.** Moderate coma in a patient presenting for LASIK. Coma on CW may indicate early ectasia, and contact lens overwear dry eye should be treated prior to proceeding with LASIK. Should the asymmetry fail to resolve without treatment, LASIK may be ill advised.

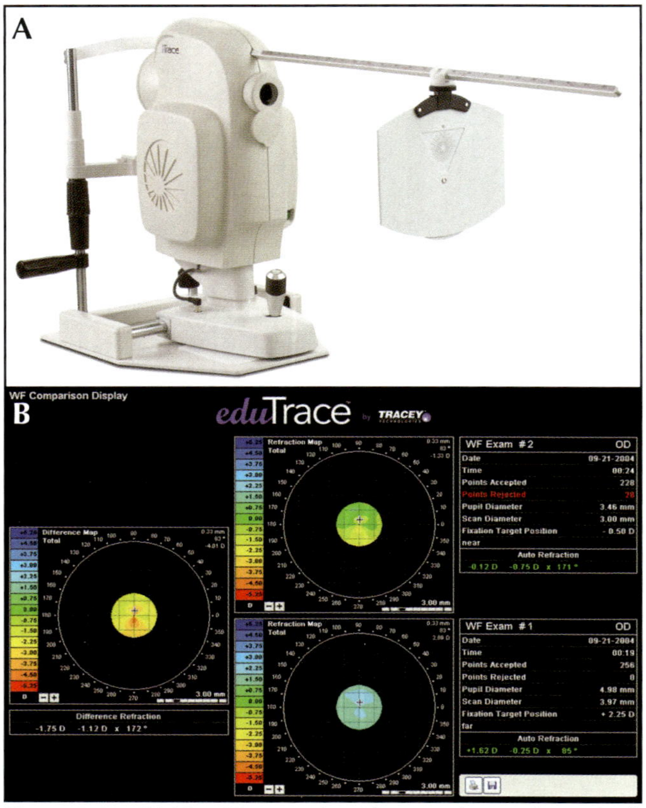


**Figure 7-27.** (A) The iTrace unit with a reading rod attached. (Reprinted with permission of Joe S. Wakil.) (B) Difference map of near and far measurements showing accommodative response.

change from far (A) and near point (B) measurements. Note the change in lenticular aberrations provides almost 2 D of accommodation for this hyperopic patient. While we expect changes in the lens aberrations during accommodation, the classic model of accommodation does not explain the dramatic shift of 90 degrees in the lens astigmatism observed in this patient during accommodation.

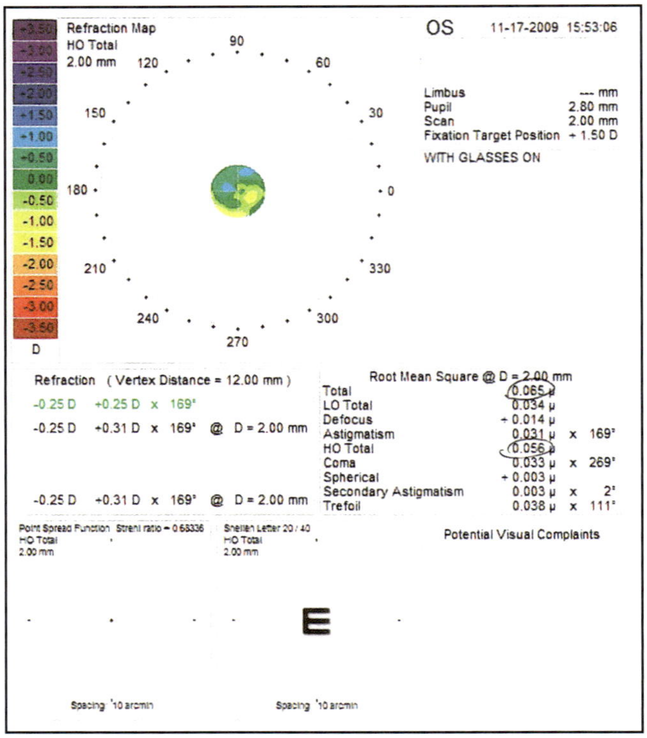


**Figure 7-28.** A nuance of the system is the ability to measure aberrometry through spectacles. This allows an objective evaluation of the glasses and is extremely helpful when patients with early cataracts complain about their spectacles being incorrect. This display may be used to educate the patient to the location of the visual problem.

The ability to reveal corneal aberrations separately from those of the lens combined with the ability to measure a patient's ocular aberrations at true far- and near-point fixation is providing a new level of diagnostic information on how the eye accommodates and how well we are able to return such function through either accommodating or multifocal implants.

An additional nuance unique to the iTrace is the ability to perform objective evaluation of the spectacle correction. This is valuable when patients present reporting dissatisfaction with the glasses. The Visual Function Display (Figure 7-28) can be used to educate patients that they are dissatisfied with their glasses due to lenticular changes that cannot be corrected with spectacles. In this example, the refractive error is negligible while the internal aberrations are significant. This patient was 20/20 in each eye, but mild cataracts reduced the vision subjectively. The patient presented upset about the quality of vision, but left with an understanding that only cataract surgery would improve the vision. Measurements can be obtained over gas-permeable lenses as well to demonstrate the benefit of this modality upon vision.[6]

The iTrace can also be used to fit contact lenses. Wavetouch hydrogel lenses are fitted, and then the patient is scanned to determine the over-aberrometry measurements (Figure 7-29). These are sent to the Wavetouch

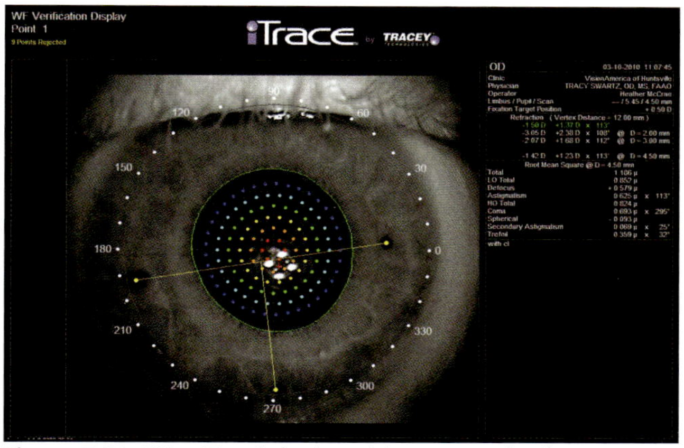


**Figure 7-29.** WaveTouch hydrogel lenses can be fit to correct aberrations measured over the lens and incorporated into the lens prescription. Lenses are traditionally fitted, and then the patient is measured using the iTrace to determine the appropriate prescription using aberrometry. These parameters are used to build a quarterly replacement lens.

manufacturer, and quarterly replacement lenses are created. These can be used to correct healthy corneas with 20/20 vision as well as those with reduced vision secondary to irregular astigmatism.

## Conclusion

The power of the iTrace to measure the refraction of the total eye through ray tracing aberrometry and integrating it with the corneal aberrations derived directly from the corneal topography measurement provides tremendous diagnostic information to enhance vision correction and disease diagnosis. The iTrace represents a new platform of refraction diagnosis to understand a patient's quality of vision and to pinpoint the source of aberrations in the eye.

# *The Nidek OPD Scan II: A Comprehensive Diagnostic and Planning Platform for Intraocular and Refractive Surgery*

Phillip M. Buscemi, OD; Harkaran S. Bains, BSc;
Murray McFadden, MD, FRCSC, DABO; and Katherine E. Paton, MD, FRCSC, DABO

Corneal topography was the first technology that objectively allowed ophthalmologists to perform pre- and postoperative assessment of the cornea, which contributes the greatest magnitude of HOAs to the eye. While this technique was an indirect assessment, clinical wavefront aberrometry enabled direct measurement of the optical effects of intraocular surgery and corneal surgery. Combining these 2 techniques allows greater analysis for preoperative planning and postoperative assessment of vision. For example, the separation of internal aberrations (mainly lenticular) from corneal aberrations allows the surgeon to determine whether lenticular or surface aberrations are the source of visual blur. Isolation of the source of the aberrations enhances surgical planning and provides greater diagnostic insight.

The Nidek OPD Scan II and the new OPD Scan III combine aberrometry and corneal topography to allow the separation of corneal front surface aberrations and internal aberrations. Corneal topography is measured using Placido disk technology. Measurement of ocular (whole eye) aberrations is performed with spatial dynamic skiascopy, a technique that allows a wide dynamic range of measurement of spherical refractive error ranging from -20 to +22 D and ±12 D of astigmatism, the ability to measure severely aberrated eyes, and refractive wavefront maps that separate corneal from lenticular aberrations.[7]

Additional software programs are available for use with the OPD Scan family of instruments that allow enhanced diagnostic ability, visual quality simulation, and IOL power calculations. For example, corneal disease screening software using the Corneal Navigator detects keratoconus, keratoconus suspect, pellucid marginal degeneration, and postsurgical corneas. Modulation transfer functions (MTFs) of the ocular, corneal, and internal and HOAs allow the evaluation of visual performance before and after surgery. The IOL Station software has recently been introduced for IOL power calculations and for selection of spherical and aspheric IOLs for virgin corneas and postrefractive surgery cases.

The combined use of the OPD SCAN II and OPD Station will be described here with attention to clinical examples that are commonly encountered. Explanation of the full clinical utility of the data and exam sets available would occupy several chapters. For example, the OPD Scan II plots 20 different maps; the OPD Station plots an additional 30 maps. We have therefore limited the examples to those that are clinically pertinent to a general ophthalmic practice.

TABLE 7-1.

## Specifications of the OPD-SCAN II

| | |
|---|---|
| Spherical power | -20 to +22 D |
| Cylinder power | ±12 D |
| Axis | 0 to 180 degrees |
| Wavefront data points | 1440 |
| Zernike order | 8th order (selectable) |
| Aberrometry maps | Distribution of refractive power due to wavefront (D)<br>Wavefront distortion based on Zernike functions (μm) |
| Pupil size | 6 mm |
| Corneal topography data points | >6800 points |
| Topography maps | Axial, instantaneous, refractive, elevation, difference maps |
| Accommodation control | Autofog using simulated scenery |
| Pupillometry | Photopic and mesopic diameters<br>Infrared light |
| Eye centration landmarks | Visual axis (coaxially sighted corneal light reflex)<br>Photopic and mesopic line of sight<br>Photopic angle kappa<br>Mesopic angle kappa |

## Features

The OPD Scan II is a combination aberrometer, corneal topographer, autorefractor, autokeratometer, and pupillometer. All measurements are performed on the same optical axis without moving the patient. This allows direct correlation of ocular, corneal, and internal aberrations of the eye. The technical specifications are presented in Table 7-1. Important features include the small footprint similar to a conventional autorefractor; a large cone Placido disk that is less sensitive to eye movement and has a larger range of focus than small cone Placidos; an internal eyetracker and autoshot function to reduce the effect of saccadic eye movements during measurement; infrared aberrometry measurements that reduce the need for dilation; and approximately 5 times more wavefront data points compared to most Hartmann Shack aberrometers. The measurement modes can be selected by the user to perform only one specific measurement, such as autorefraction, autokeratometry, or corneal topography based on the clinical workup. Physiologic dark-adapted pupil measurements are preferred, and if pupil dilation is required, we recommend the use of 2.5% phenylephrine to avoid any cycloplegic artifact in measuring wavefront data.

The OPD Scan III offers higher-resolution aberrometry and other improvements compared to the OPD Scan II. The OPD Scan III features higher-resolution topography with 33 rings and 11,880 data points versus 19 rings and 6840 data points currently available on the OPD Scan II. In addition, the mire illumination has been changed to blue, which dramatically reduces pupil artifacts due to constriction during measurement. The aberrometry functions have also been enhanced in the OPD Scan III. The wavefront measurements are currently performed for a 6-mm pupil diameter, which will be increased to 9 mm (user selectable) with the OPD Scan III. Additionally, the number of data points used for measuring and plotting wavefront maps has increased from 1440 currently to 2520 data points along with 20% faster acquisition times with the OPD Scan III. Other new features in the OPD Scan III specifically for cataract surgery include retroillumination image capture for lens opacity and average pupillary power (APP) for IOL calculations. Average pupillary power is the average power within the 4-mm central cornea calculated using 5 to 7 Placido mires that comprise approximately 2000 data points. Average pupillary power may serve as a more accurate reflection of corneal power for IOL calculations compared to averaging the 2 principle meridians of the cornea.

A host of other improvements including database management and ease of service have also been implemented on the OPD Scan III. As the OPD Scan III is a very new machine, the patient examples in this chapter have been acquired with the OPD Scan II.

## Refractive Wavefront Maps

The OPD Scan II plots refractive wavefront maps that are unique to this instrument and therefore require a detailed explanation of the interpretation and use in clinical practice. The raw data from the spatial dynamic skiascopy are converted to refractive wavefront maps. The OPD, Internal OPD, and OPD higher-order maps are refractive wavefront maps that plot the distribution of refractive power across the pupil created by ocular aberrations. Interpretation of the maps involves evaluation of the uniformity of color, the symmetry of the patterns, metrics such as root mean square, and refractive values. The difference in power from the warmest color to the coolest color (or vice versa) on the map determines the maximal difference in refractive power across the pupil.

A number of options are available for the selection of scale step size and color palette. Our preferred color palette and scale for refractive wavefront maps is the "adjustable common scale" setting with the autostep function on and the International Standards Organization (ISO) or the Smolek/Klyce color palette. While it is arguable that the normalized scale will provide the highest detail for any given exam (wavefront or corneal topography), when comparing changes from visit to visit, the adjustable common scale allows direct comparison due to the consistent color palette and step size between serial exams. Based on our clinical experience, both color palettes are adequate for clinical practice, although the Smolek/Klyce colors tend to provide greater contrast between scale steps, enhancing subtle changes in refractive power within the pupil. The scale for these maps is plotted in diopters where light green indicates no refractive power, warmer colors indicate myopic power, and cooler colors indicate hyperopic power.

The OPD map plots the distribution of refractive power across the pupil, incorporating the effects of all lower- and higher-order aberrations (Figure 7-30). In Figure 7-30A, the OPD map has a red asymmetric bow-tie pattern, indicating the combined effects of lower and higher aberrations on refraction. The difference in power across the pupil is approximately 1.26 D with the warmer (red) colors indicating myopic powers comprising the central pupil. The autorefraction (measured for a 2.30-mm pupil diameter), 3-mm wavefront refraction, and 5-mm wavefront refraction provide the effect on refractive power as the pupil dilates. Increasing hyperopia peripherally indicates increasing negative ocular spherical aberration, whereas increasing myopia indicates positive spherical aberration. Positive spherical

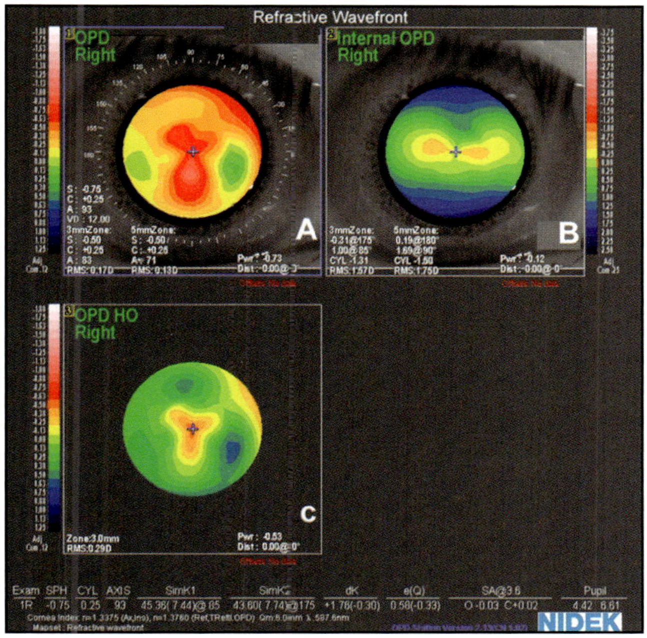


**Figure 7-30.** OPD SCAN II refractive wavefront maps of (A) the entire eye, (B) the internal (lenticular) aberrations, and (C) the HOAs of the entire eye.

aberration can occur due to increasing cataractous changes or excimer laser corneal ablation. Increasing cylinder values indicate high astigmatism or coma aberration. Postoperative causes of high astigmatism include decentered IOLs, tilted IOLs, IOLs placed at the incorrect axis, or a decentered refractive ablation. Multicolor OPD maps, with greater asymmetry and root mean square (RMS) values over 0.50 D, indicate that HOAs are likely playing a significant role in the distribution of refractive power across the pupil.

Figure 7-30B plots the internal OPD map. The internal OPD map subtracts the effects of the corneal surface and plots the remaining refractive wavefront. As only the corneal surface data are removed, the internal OPD map incorporates the effects of all structures behind the corneal tear film and epithelium. In eyes with posterior ectasia or severely distorted corneas, such as in severe pellucid marginal degeneration or postpenetrating keratoplasty, the aberrations of the back corneal surface will register and may predominate on this map. However, in normal eyes, the internal OPD map can be considered an accurate representation of the refractive wavefront due to the physiologic, pathologic, or pseudophakic lens. Figure 7-30B presents an example with a symmetric bowtie indicating lenticular astigmatism. In this case, corneal astigmatism (1.76 D, dk value on the bottom row of Figure 7-30) and lenticular astigmatism were compensating each other, indicated by the minimal refractive astigmatism on the OPD map (autorefraction cylinder value +0.25 D, Figure 7-30A).

Figure 7-30C presents the OPD HO map. The OPD HO map removes the effects of the lower-order aberrations such as sphere and cylinder, plotting the effects of the HOAs on refractive power distribution (see Figure 7-30C). The color changes across the map indicate that approximately 1 D of refractive change is caused by HOAs. Comparison with the OPD map determines whether HOAs are the source of the refractive difference within the pupil. In this case of a mild myope, the majority of refractive difference is due to HOAs (1 D due to HO aberrations versus 1.26 D total difference). This finding indicates that visual complaints from this patient cannot be addressed by reducing refractive error alone and will require reduction or elimination of wavefront error.

Traditional Zernike-based higher-order maps are plotted by conversion of data from the OPD maps. Convolution of the Zernike maps allows simulation of the MTF, point spread function (PSF), and visual acuity of the entire eye (ocular) or corneal and internal aberrations. Simulations based on each individual aberration within the Zernike table or combinations of aberrations are also possible.

# Clinical Use

Peer-review publications have reported the use of OPD Scan II in refractive surgery,[8] corneal disease screening,[9,10] alignment of toric IOL and implantable collamer lens,[11,12] and the study of aberration compensation after refractive surgery.[13] Comparison of OPD Scan II refractions to manifest refraction have shown differences less than 0.35 D in sphere and 0.25 D difference in cylinder.[14] Repeatability and reproducibility of the total, corneal higher-order and internal wavefront (IW) measurements easily surpass the tolerances required for clinical practice.[15] Bland-Altmann plots indicate that the dark-adapted mesopic pupillometry measurements with the OPD Scan II are consistent with the scotopic pupil diameter measured with the Procyon and Colvard pupillometers.[16] The data from these studies clearly indicate that the OPD Scan II can be used for a variety of diagnostic purposes with acceptable accuracy and reproducibility for routine clinical practice.

## Corneal Disease Screening

Corneal disease screening represents the major application of corneal topography. The OPD Scan II includes the axial, instantaneous, refractive, and elevation corneal topography maps. Additionally, the Corneal Navigator corneal disease screening module in the OPD Station software employs a neural network for comparison of corneal characteristics to a database of normal, diseased, and postsurgical corneal topographies. Based on the comparison, the cornea under measurement can be classified as normal, keratoconic, a keratoconus suspect, pellucid marginal degeneration, and postmyopic refractive surgery among other classifications.

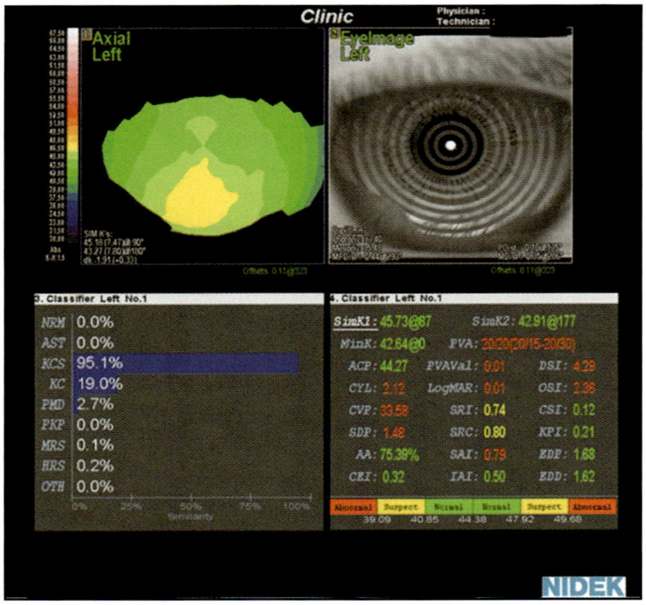


**Figure 7-31.** Corneal navigator analysis of a keratoconus suspect (KCS). Note the classification system (lower left). NRM denotes a normal cornea, AST denotes astigmatism, KC denotes keratoconus, PMD denotes pellucid marginal degeneration, PKP denotes penetrating keratoplasty, MRS denotes myopic refractive surgery, HRS denotes hyperopic refractive surgery, OTH denotes a classification other that the ones listed above.

Although the incidence of keratoconus is extremely low in the general population, keratoconus suspects and patients with frank keratoconus present at refractive surgery centers at a much higher rate for alleviation of their refractive error. Advanced cases of keratoconus and pellucid marginal degeneration have distinct corneal topographic features that enable quick diagnosis. However, cases with suspicious corneal topography not indicative of advanced corneal disease remain a clinical conundrum.

Figure 7-31 outlines a case of a patient who presented for a refractive evaluation with corneal features that were consistent with a keratoconus suspect classification. The features of this topography indicate that the left cornea is classified as a keratoconus suspect. The right eye of this patient was classified as normal. The lack of mirror image symmetry between corneas at presentation, clinical examination, serial corneal pachymetry, and long-term follow-up did confirm progression to keratoconus. The Corneal Navigator uses a color scheme where green is normal, yellow values warrant further investigation, and red indicates an abnormal value of the various indices based on neural network analysis. In this example of a keratoconus suspect, the surface asymmetry index (SAI) is high, which is often associated with keratoconus (see Figure 7-31).[9] The interested reader is directed to a comprehensive review by Klyce and colleagues[9] on the clinical interpretation of all the indices presented with the Corneal Navigator.

# Intraocular Surgery

## Preoperative Planning

Refractive surgery is rapidly incorporating IOL surgery (phakic and toric lens implantation). This shift in attitude is due to patient expectations, the increased accuracy of IOLs, and the introduction of wavefront IOLs. For example, aspheric IOLs are designed to compensate for corneal spherical aberration that addresses the loss in visual quality after spherical IOL implantation. Aspheric accommodating IOLs incorporate wavefront principles to allow better visual performance than standard accommodating lenses. Hence, the need for wavefront assessments is rapidly becoming a clinical necessity for many cataract surgeons and general ophthalmologists.

Aspheric IOLs are implanted based on the compensation of corneal and aspheric IOL spherical aberration. However, the selection of the correct aspheric IOL requires measurement of the corneal spherical aberration. The distribution of corneal spherical aberration across a population is widespread, following a bell-shaped curve.[17] Additionally, differences in HOAs across ethnic groups has been reported.[17] Hence, implanting one type of aspheric IOL in all patients is unrealistic. For example, significantly increasing negative ocular spherical aberration in a patient with preexisting negative corneal spherical aberration may result in a diminution of visual quality akin to keratoconic eyes or posthyperopic ablation, both of which can cause high negative spherical aberration. The aspheric IOL needs to be tailored to the individual's preoperative corneal spherical aberration. The OPD Scan II provides the corneal spherical aberration values for aspheric IOL selection calculated from the corneal topography.

Baby boomers are the largest subset of the population to undergo laser in situ keratomileusis (LASIK) or photorefractive keratectomy (PRK) worldwide. As this demographic ages, the need for accurate postrefractive surgery IOL calculations will increase, along with the need for a selection of specific aspheric monofocal IOLs or presbyopic IOLs. Hyperopic LASIK tends to induce negative spherical aberration, and myopic ablations tend to induce positive spherical aberration. The magnitude of induction varies based on aspheric or conventional ablation algorithms.[18] The distribution of residual postoperative corneal spherical aberration in refractive surgery patients will likely be abnormal, leading to the introduction of more aspheric IOLs. Corneal topography to measure corneal spherical aberration and postoperative keratometry will be instrumental in patients who have undergone LASIK and PRK. Additionally, postrefractive surgery IOL calculations are available on the Nidek IOL Station for such cases with the Camellin-Callosi formula.

Cataracts cause typical patterns on the internal OPD map. For example, the phakic eye of a young adult will present with emmetropia or mild myopia centrally surrounded by hyperopia (Figure 7-32). Cataractous eyes present with increasing myopia anywhere on the internal map along with flecks of power randomly distributed on the internal OPD map (see Figure 7-32). Progression of the cataract can be followed with serial measurements and comparison of the internal OPD maps.

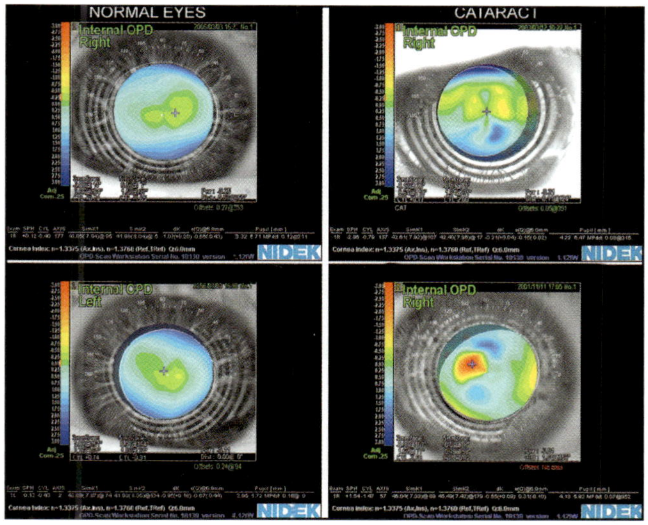


**Figure 7-32.** Internal OPD maps of the normal (top left) and cataractous eyes.

The axial corneal topography map, keratometry, and autorefraction from the OPD Scan II will assist the surgeon in planning the placement of the phaco incision, limbal relaxing incisions, and toric IOLs and toric phakic IOLs.

## Postoperative Evaluation

Postoperatively, the OPD Scan II can be used to evaluate toric IOL alignment, tilt, and torque. Serial corneal topography will allow the assessment of corneal wound healing and of the effect on corneal astigmatism over time.

In cases of refractive surprise or dysphotopsia post-implantation, the effect of an incorrectly placed limbal relaxing incision, phaco-incision, or IOL can be determined by comparing corneal topography, the OPD map, and the internal OPD. This enables the surgeon to determine surface versus internal sources and plan the appropriate retreatment. Figure 7-33 presents a case of a patient who complained of shadowing and ghosting after IOL implantation. Slit-lamp examination indicated a well-centered IOL in the capsular bag. OPD Scan II measurement shows the corneal topography was normal, yet the internal OPD maps show myopic and hyperopic areas bisecting the pupil, creating 2 focal planes on the retina resulting in ghosting. The 2 refractive planes were due to a subtle tilt of the IOL, resulting in coma, a common cause of ghosting and diplopia (see Figure 7-33).

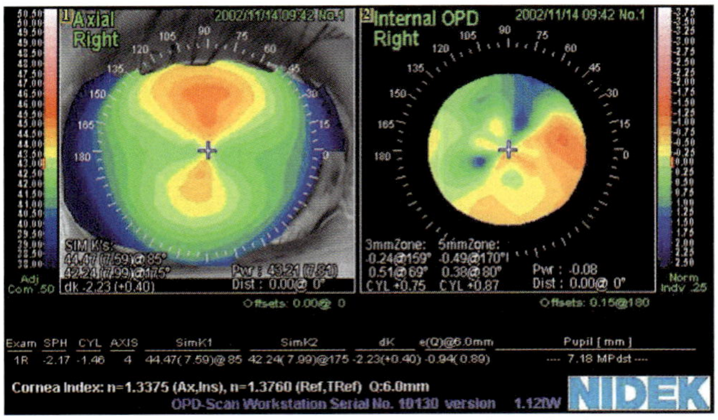


**Figure 7-33.** Measurement of a patient with a tilted IOL.

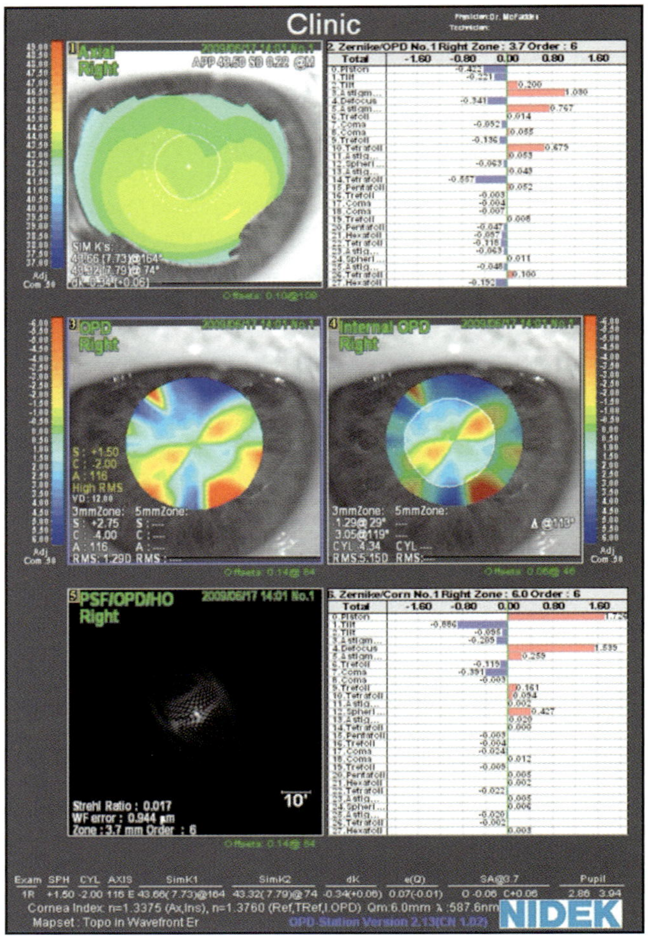


**Figure 7-34.** Preoperative OPD Station assessment of an 88-year-old patient with a cataract. Map on the top left is an axial corneal topography map. The figure on the top right lists Zernike wavefront aberration values for the whole eye. Aberration number 12 is ocular spherical aberration. The OPD map (middle row, left side) is a refractive wavefront map plotting the refractive distribution due to the lower- and higher-order aberrations of the whole eye. The internal OPD map (middle row, right side) is a refractive wavefront map plotting the refractive distribution due to the lower- and higher-order aberrations excluding the front corneal surface. In this case, aberrations are due to a cataract. The map on the bottom left is the PSF, which plots the retinal image quality of the ocular HOAs. The figure at the lower right lists Zernike values for corneal aberrations. Aberration number 12 is corneal spherical aberration. All Zernike aberrations are reported for the patient's mesopic pupil diameter of 3.7 mm out to the 6th Zernike order. Spherical Aberration correcting IOLs are calculated at a 6 mm lens diameter and the corneal mires are not compromised by a reduced pupil diameter.

Figure 7-34 presents a 1-page summary recommended for cataract surgery by one of the authors (MM). This 88-year-old male patient presented with 20/40 pinhole acuity and a 2+ nuclear sclerotic cataract. The cornea was classified as "normal" by the corneal navigator screening software. The axial topography was unremarkable with a difference in keratometry (dk value) of 0.34 D, indicating mild corneal astigmatism (see Figure 7-34). The preoperative dk astigmatic axis is useful intraoperatively as it is frequently easy to shift the incisional axis to reduce corneal astigmatism. Pre- and postoperative keratometry values are valuable during implantation of toric lenses and evaluation of both the keratometric and real total visual outcomes (see Figure 7-34).

The Zernike/OPD graph plots the magnitude of each ocular lower- and higher-order Zernike aberration in µm (see Figure 7-34). This value theoretically represents the deviation from an individual with perfect vision. We have elected to present this example with a real-world mesopic pupil diameter of 3.70 mm as pharmacologically dilated pupils are not representative of the conditions this patient functions under for daily living activities (see Figure 7-34). Furthermore, miotic pupils are often encountered in this segment of the population; hence, peripheral aberrations from an artificially dilated pupil are clinically irrelevant.

The OPD map is flagged "High RMS," indicating significant visual problems likely due to optical aberrations, with the differences in color indicating greater than 6 D difference across the pupil (see Figure 7-34). The internal OPD map shows a pattern similar to the OPD map and not the corneal topography, indicating an internal (lenticular) cause of the optical aberrations (see Figure 7-34). The high central myopic area and the high internal cylinder values (4.34 D) are commensurate with cataract formation. These data confirm that the primary visual problem is cataractous in origin. The internal OPD RMS is 5.15 D, indicating significant internal aberrations, which not surprisingly are affecting vision. The PSF simulates the retinal image quality with best-corrected vision. The corneal Zernike values indicate +0.427 µm of corneal spherical aberration, which aids in the selection of the best aspheric IOL for this patient (see Figure 7-34).

Figure 7-35 presents the postoperative OPD documenting the remarkable optical transformation from elective cataract surgery with implantation of a Tecnis ZCBOO aspheric IOL (Abbott Medical Optics, Santa Ana, CA). The axial topography map indicates the corneal astigmatism remained unchanged, despite a 2.75-mm temporal incision. The ocular Zernike graph plots a marked diminution of all

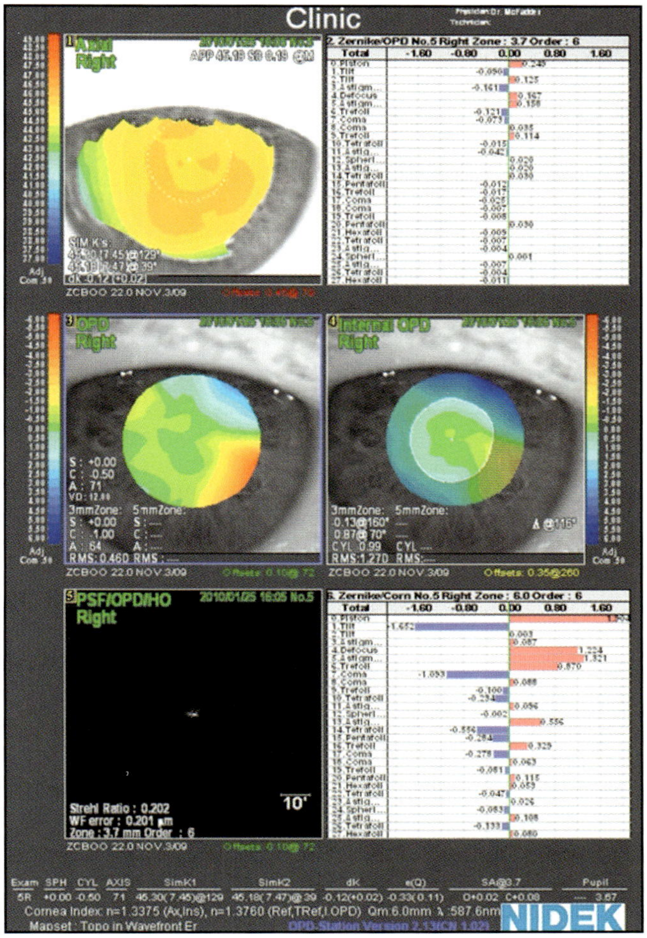


**Figure 7-35.** Postoperative OPD Station assessment of an eye that underwent aspheric IOL implantation. Map on the top left is an axial corneal topography map. The map on the top right is a Zernike graph of the ocular (whole eye) aberrations. Aberration number 12 is ocular spherical aberration. The OPD map (middle row, left side) is a refractive wavefront map plotting the refractive distribution due to the lower- and higher-order aberrations of the whole eye. The internal OPD map (middle row, right side) is a refractive wavefront map plotting the refractive distribution due to the lower- and higher-order aberrations excluding the front corneal surface. In this case, the visual complaint is due to the IOL. The map on the bottom left is the PSF, which plots the retinal image quality of the ocular HOAs. The map on the lower right is a Zernike graph of the corneal aberrations.

lower and higher optical aberrations including a change in spherical aberration from -0.063 μm preoperatively to +0.02 μm postoperatively (see Figure 7-35). The OPD map documents a postoperative autorefraction of 0.00 -0.50 x 71 and an RMS value of 0.46 D, indicating a significant reduction in aberrations across the pupil. The internal OPD indicates the optical power of the implanted IOL with this eye's new optics and an RMS deviation of 1.27 D versus 5.15 D, preoperatively (see Figure 7-35). The PSF indicates the excellent best-corrected retinal image quality postoperatively and a final ocular higher-order wavefront error of

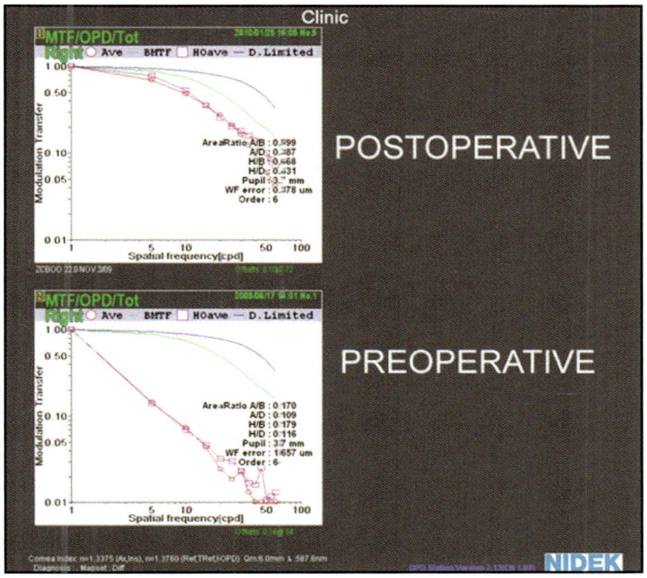


**Figure 7-36.** MTF/OPD/Tot difference plot. The area ratios on the graph represent the ratio between the curves; A/B is the ratio between the average curve and the best MTF curve; A/D indicates the relation of the average curve and the diffraction limit; H/B indicates the ratio of the HOAs and the best MTF curve; H/D indicates the ratio between HOAs curve and diffraction limit.

0.201 μm compared to a preoperative ocular higher-order wavefront error of 0.944 μm (see Figure 7-35).

Figure 7-36 plots the preoperative and postoperative MFT graphs, which allow an assessment of visual performance after IOL implantation. The H/B ratio indicates the area under the best-corrected curve of the patient compared to a subset of emmetropes with excellent visual quality (see Figure 7-36). In this case, the H/B ratio has increased from 17.9% preoperatively to 66.8% postoperatively, indicating the significant increase in visual performance after IOL implantation (see Figure 7-36). The patient's postoperative uncorrected Snellen acuity remains 20/25+ to date, and he is satisfied with the outcome of surgery.

The combination of corneal topography and aberrometry in the OPD Scan II allows thorough assessment, diagnosis, and management of elective lens surgery. Additionally, the outcomes of intraocular surgery can be superbly documented. It is anticipated that surgeons will be able to use the preoperative measurement of corneal spherical aberration and postoperative measurements of total aberration to develop individual nomograms that will allow them to deliver more accurate outcomes to patients.

## Refractive Surgery Screening

Wavefront measurements are commonplace during LASIK and PRK consultations. The OPD Scan II measures refraction, the pre-existing corneal and lenticular aberrations, and the preoperative retinal image quality and simulates potential visual performance after treatment of HOAs. Recent findings with different excimer platforms indicate patients with lower magnitudes of preoperative (0.30 µm or less) ocular HOAs tend to have greater induction of HOAs postoperatively after wavefront-guided ablation.[19,20] However, the interaction of aberrations is also a determinant of visual quality. Based on these findings, a prolate ablation or wavefront ablation can be planned based on the magnitude of HOAs preoperatively. Using the OPD Scan II, patients can be screened for corneal or lenticular contraindications. Additionally, selection of the correct laser algorithm is possible for candidates undergoing excimer surgery.

Wavefront-guided ablation has reignited the controversy regarding centration of the laser ablation. Initially considered a problem only in hyperopic patients due to angle kappa, the benefits of centration closer to the visual axis in myopes have been documented by 2 recent studies.[21,22] Better optical quality by centering on the "visual axis " in myopes has been reported.[21,22] Currently, the OPD Scan II is the only unit with an automated, repeatable method of measuring the difference between the line of sight (pupil center) and the "visual axis" (coaxially sighted corneal light reflex) and transferring these data to an excimer laser (Figure 7-37). The measurement of difference in pupil center (either mesopic or photopic) and visual axis is possible with this unit due to the combined corneal topography and aberrometry measurements on the same optical axis.

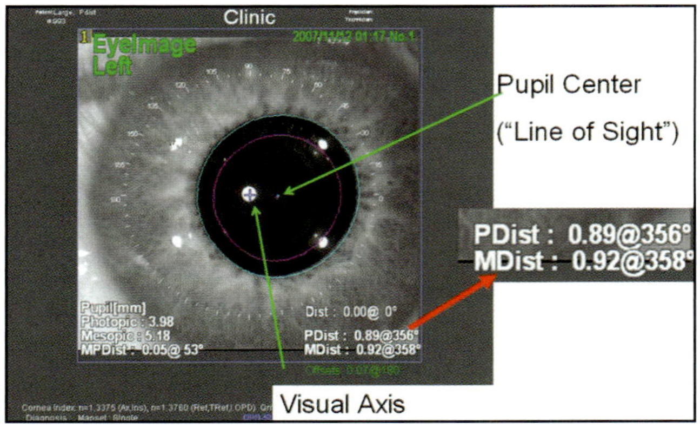


**Figure 7-37.** Pupillography with the OPD SCAN II presenting a hyperopic patient with a large angle kappa. The pink circle denotes the photopic pupil shape, PDist denotes the distance between photopic pupil center and the optical axis, MDist denotes the distance between the mesopic pupil center and the optical axis. The pink and blue crosses represent the photopic and mesopic pupil centers.

Custom ablation treatment of normal and postsurgical eyes requires meticulous measurement in order to negate spurious data that may be incorporated into treatment planning. One method to mitigate measurement errors is to repeat measurements and average all maps. The OPD Station incorporates an averaging function that averages up to 10 measurements to yield a composite map. The option to exclude maps of lower measurement quality is provided in order to reduce the effects of inordinately high or low values.

The field of excimer laser surgery continues to advance from treating solely refraction a decade ago to incorporating the treatment of HOAs of the cornea or the entire eye. Corneal topography data and ocular spherical aberration from the OPD Scan II are used in optimized prolate ablation algorithms (OPA) to create a physiologically prolate cornea over the entire mesopic pupil. The corneal surface data are used to create a compensation matrix that addresses the loss of excimer energy as the ablation moves peripherally. The ocular spherical aberration is used to create a target spherical aberration value postoperatively while maintaining physiologic corneal asphericity. Without topographic data, an accurate asphericity target cannot be calculated. In a prospective, contralateral, randomized study of 32 myopes who underwent LASIK with OPA in one eye and conventional ablation in the fellow eye, the refractive outcomes were similar between groups. However, the best-corrected visual acuity, postoperative HOAs, spherical aberrations, and contrast sensitivity favored the OPA group.[23] The authors attribute these outcomes to the postoperative prolate corneas and the inclusion of corneal topography and OW data.[23]

In conclusion, the combined use of corneal topography and wavefront data aids surgeons to achieve excellent refractive outcomes following cataract surgery, phakic IOL implantation, and LASIK. The OPD Scan II is a unique combination corneal topographer and aberrometer that aids the clinical assessment, surgical planning, and postoperative assessment of surface and intraocular surgery.

## TOPO-ABERROMETRY WITH KERATRON ONDA

Renzo Mattioli, PhD; Massimo Camellin, MD; and Nancy K. Tripoli, MA

The Keratron Onda (Figure 7-38) is a combined instrument, developed and produced by Optikon 2000 SpA (Rome, Italy) to measure corneal topography (CT) and aberrations of the total OW contemporarily. The instrument also tracks and measures the pupil in photopic and scotopic or mesopic conditions and performs dynamic

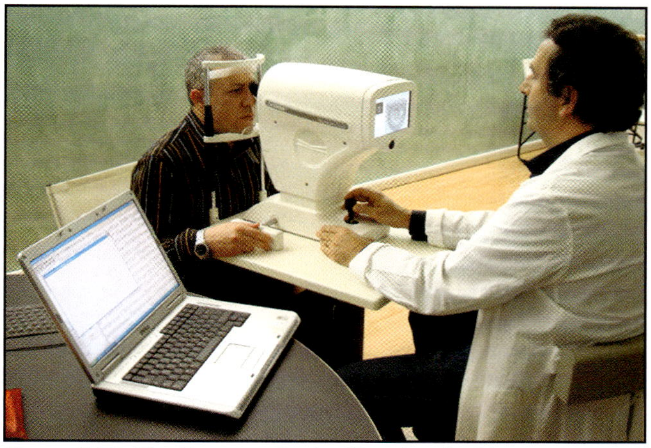

**Figure 7-38.** The Keratron Onda. (Reprinted with permission of Renzo Mattioli, PhD.)

pupillometry. It is able to evaluate patients' residual capability to accommodate by measuring the OW in different conditions of accommodation.[24] The name "Onda" means "wave" in both Italian and Spanish.

The Onda is the latest in the successful line of Keratron instruments. The Keratron has been the first reflection-type corneal topographer that is not spherically biased to introduce color-coded maps of the instantaneous (ie, local or tangential) curvature (1993)[25,26] "spherical offset" height maps and the "move axis" feature (1994)[27] and CW analysis (2001)[28,29]—all of which are rigorously underpinned by an arc-step algorithm that guarantees submicron accuracy measurements[30,31] and high spatial resolution maps even of irregular corneas (see Chapter 5, "The Keratron Corneal Topographers" section).

The IW, produced by refraction through internal ocular structures, can be calculated as the difference between the OW, captured by aberrometry, and CW, derived from corneal topography. All of these wavefronts can be represented by all of the analysis tools available in the Keratron Scout software, including Zernike terms (RMS, skyline, histogram, and aberrations summary) and visual simulations (Visus, PSF, MTF; see Chapter 5, "The Keratron Corneal Topographers" section).

## Basic Features

As a corneal topographer, the Keratron Onda shares similar features with other Keratrons: accuracy, corneal coverage up to 80% to 90%, and a wide range of curvature measurement (from 0 to 130 D).[32,33]

The aberrometry acquisition system includes a high-resolution motorized system to compensate for defocus from higher than +6 D to lower than -11 D. This allows measurement of myopic and hyperopic patients from -20 to +10 D (at vertex distance of 14 mm), although there is a proportional reduction of the maximum measurable pupil at extreme values. The OW is measured in the image space. The sensor is a Microlens Array (MLA) designed by Optikon, with a spatial resolution at the cornea of 128 µm. It can measure wavefront over a pupil area up to 7 x 7 mm, within a sensor area about 7.9 x 10.5 mm. The light source for the retinal reflex is a low-coherence, low-power collimated beam (<30uW at $\lambda$ = 840 nm), well within safety limits.

The instrument embeds a PC of ETX type with WinXPe and is equipped with a 7" wide screen color display with touch-screen user interface. It can process both CT and OW sensor images immediately following acquisition and/or transfer them to the Keratron Scout software. This allows tests to be printed, saved, edited, and analyzed using all the features previously developed for Keratrons. For example, tests can be compared over time, test repeatability checked, images edited, contact lenses designed and fit, and lasers linked. All information about corneal topography implemented on previously developed Keratron models is available, including the Maloney and CLMI indices.

## Corneal Topography and Wavefront Aberrometry in a Single Instrument: Technical Solutions

### Retro-Mires

To combine topography and aberrometry in a single instrument presents several challenges. First, there must be a compromise between corneal coverage and the range of measurable aberrations. A good arc-step analysis of reflective topography requires that mires are equally spaced. The central hole in the Dekking cone or Placido disk must be very small and distant so that its reflection does not leave a gap in the center. In *Keratrons*, this hole diameter is around 6 mm at 70 mm distance from the cornea. However, aberrometry requires a visual field larger than the maximum pupil and optics closer to the eye so that all rays of the wavefront coming back from the pupil are collected by the measuring optics. For this reason, topo-aberrometers usually sacrifice central coverage in their corneal topography, as in the pattern on the bottom left of Figure 7-39. Furthermore, CT requires visible light ($\lambda = 550 \div 650$ nm) to optimize the reflected mire's contrast with the iris background, whereas aberrometry requires near infrared ($\lambda = 780 \div 900$ nm) so as not to induce pupil constriction, which restricts the size of the acquired image.

Optikon handled this problem by adopting a proprietary system of "retro-mires" as shown in Figure 7-39. The retro-mires (204, Figure 7-39) are positioned behind a mirror (207, Figure 7-39) that splits the optical path by their different wavelengths, so they can fill the CT pattern in the center (Figure 7-39, bottom right). Thus, the Keratron Onda's mire pattern is the same as in the other Keratrons, with a uniform step beginning in the cone center, without compromise.[34]

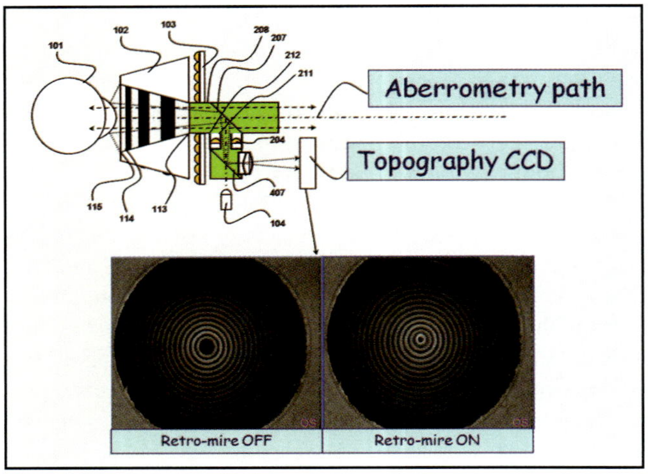


**Figure 7-39.** Optikon's proprietary retro-mire method allows combining Keratron topography with other measures of the eye that can be made at the same time without compromising the efficacy of the Keratron arc-step reconstruction. (Reprinted with permission of Renzo Mattioli, PhD.)

Following the path behind the mirror, the OW can thus be measured through a central hole much wider and closer (Ø>12 mm, at about 40 mm from the cornea) than in a standard Keratron.

## Eye Position Control System With Analog-to-Digital Conversion Compensation

All Keratrons use a proprietary technique involving 2 photocells called the Eye Position Control system (EPCS; see Chapter 5)[35] that allows acquisition only at a preset distance. In the Keratron Onda, the acquisition of topography, wavefront, and also pupillometry imaging may require a longer time and may induce patient movement. Therefore, the Keratron Onda has larger cells to widen the "OK range" during which an image can be acquired by a factor of 6. An analog-to-digital conversion (ADC) measurement in the "Z axis" (Figure 7-40) has been added. The resulting configuration compensates for eye movements within about 0.55 mm, resulting in an error less than ±0.1 D when imaging a standard 43.5-D sphere. This is illustrated by Figure 7-41, in which the violet curve shows ADC compensation, compared to the yellow curve, which shows no compensation. The Z displacement measured by the ADC is recorded within each image, and if the patients move more than the allowable 0.55 mm, the operator is warned to discard the test.

## Short Bivalent Cone

Because of the retro-mire solution described above, the Keratron Onda cone is one-third shorter, and its hole is twice as wide as other Keratrons. Also, unlike other Keratrons, which offer 2 cones that can be physically exchanged, the Keratron Onda has 2 pairs of photocells in its EPCS that allow measurement at 2 different distances as selected by the operator from the touch-screen (Figure 7-42). One distance allows greater corneal coverage, while the other is a less invasive approach that is especially useful when imaging deep-set eyes.

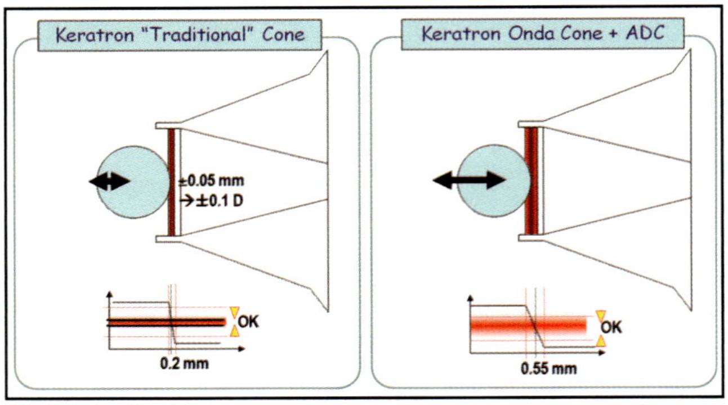


**Figure 7-40.** Keratron Onda measurements on a sphere at several Z distances, with and without ADC compensation. (Reprinted with permission of Renzo Mattioli, PhD.)

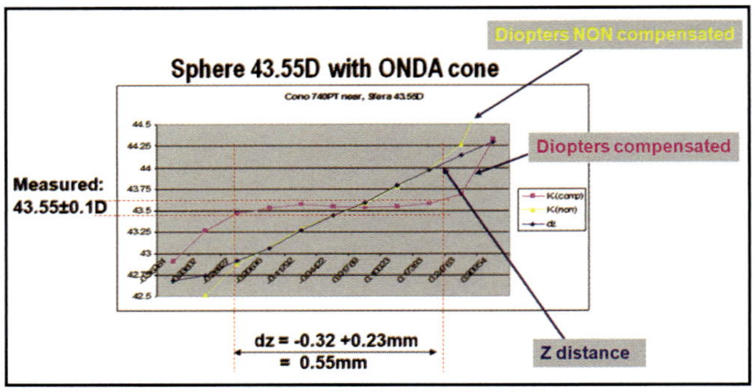


**Figure 7-41.** The short "bivalent cone" of the Keratron Onda allows the operator to choose quickly between "near" and "far," to get either greater corneal coverage or a less invasive approach for deep-set eyes, without needing to remove the cone and recalibrate.

## Aberrometry Measurement: Frequency Demodulation Method Versus Centroids

As in all OW measurements in "object space," a light source beam ($\lambda$ = 840 nm) is projected into the eye to produce a retinal point reflection, which is then projected back to a lenslet array. In the classic Shack Hartman method, the displacement ($\Delta x$, $\Delta y$) of the centroids on the sensor from their ideal position yields a measure of the X and Y gradients, and, from the gradients, one can reconstruct the wavefront aberration map (Figure 7-43).

The limit of this method is that the centroids are measurable only while they stay within their cells as in Figure 7-43A, and a more highly distorted pattern might not be measurable, as in Figure 7-43B.

The Keratron Onda employs another method, using frequency demodulation in the FFT domain (Figure 7-44). Methods of this type have been devised by several authors for use with different sensors,[36-39] one of which was

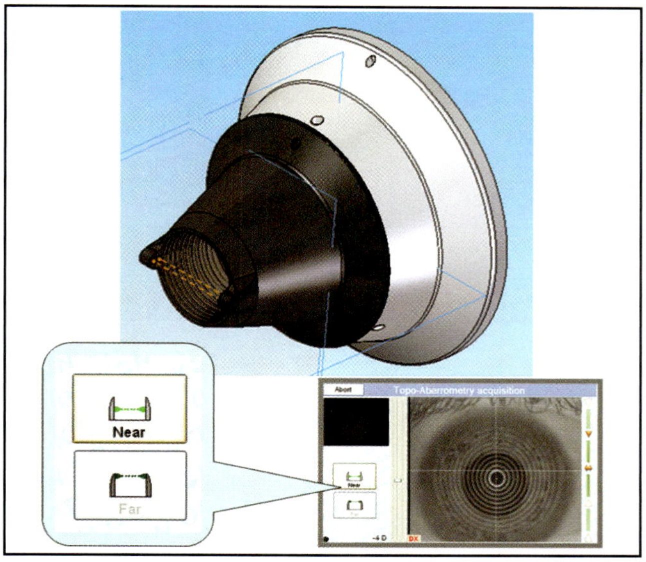


**Figure 7-42.** The new Keratron Onda cone with ADC compared to a Keratron traditional cone.

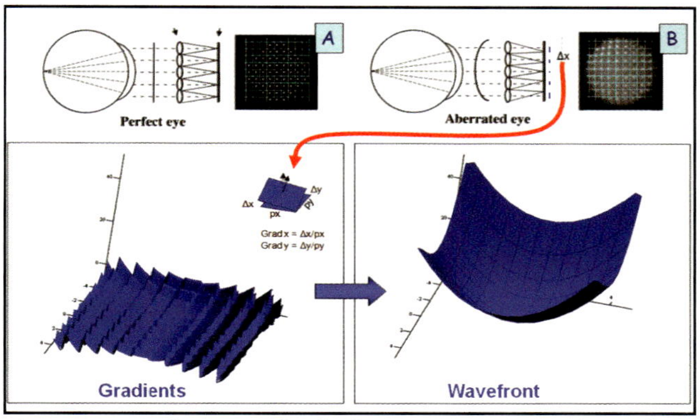


**Figure 7-43.** Classic method of measuring x,y gradients from the centroids displacement and then extracting the wavefront from the gradients (or from the Zernike gradients best-fit to the wavefront gradients). **(Reprinted with permission of Renzo Mattioli, PhD.)**

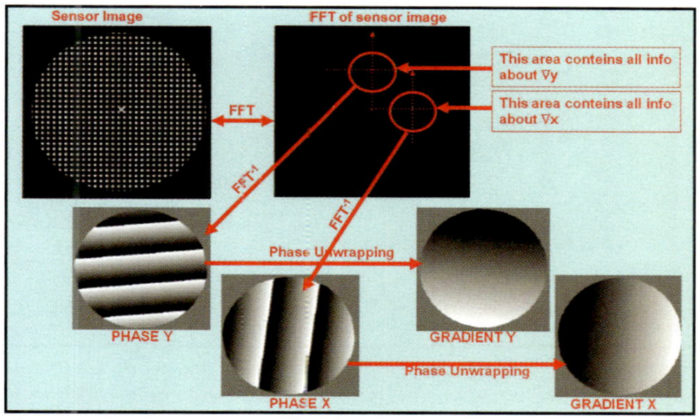


**Figure 7-44.** Keratron Onda's frequency demodulation method to get gradients from the wavefront sensor image.

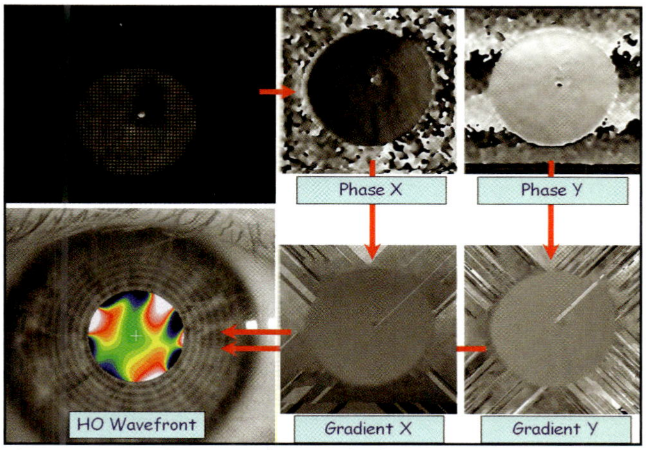


**Figure 7-45.** In this case, due to a bad sensor image, the reconstruction of gradients and the OW map are affected by "phase jump" artifacts.

well described by Dr. Edwin Sarver at the International Wavefront Congress in 2006.[40] In the FFT transform of the sensor image, the 2 small areas circled in red in Figure 7-44 contain all the information we need about the X and Y displacement of a regular orthogonal lenslet projection. Then, by anti-transforming the FFT, centered and masked at these points, we get maps of the phases (Figure 7-44, bottom left), and then a so-called "phase unwrapping" procedure[41] reconstructs the gradients X and Y (Figure 7-44, bottom right). The abrupt phase jump from black to white (Figure 7-44, bottom left) shows that, in the sensor image, the centroids have shifted to an adjacent "cell." The next phase jump from white to black indicates that they have shifted "2 cells away," and so on.

In practice, this method offers the advantages of a larger dynamic because the centroids are not constrained in their cells, and the Keratron Onda can measure wider aberrations, robustness in calculations, and fidelity in reconstruction of the aberrations.[42] The limits of the method are that calculations are somewhat slower and some "phase jumps" are not corrected by phase unwrapping as discussed below.

## Phase Jump Artifacts and Their Detection

Due to an opacity in the subject's crystalline lens and cornea reflections in a poor sensor image, phase unwrapping created a "phase jump," making the map in Figure 7-45 unreliable. Such a situation is analogous to a "ring jump" in Placido corneal topography. In this situation, double-clicking on the sensor image, as in Figure 7-46, will show maps of the X and Y gradients. The user can accept the acquisition and fix the artifact later or redo the acquisition at once.

In Figure 7-47, the same eye has been acquired again with better centering. The reflections are reduced, and we can see correct reconstruction of the gradients and the resulting correct OW map, in spite of some crystalline lens opacity.

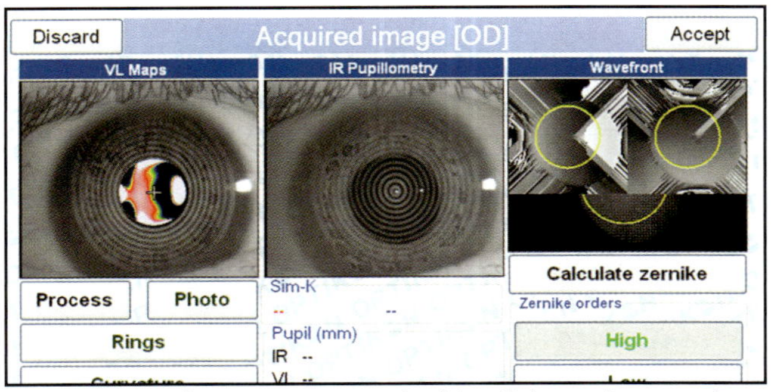


**Figure 7-46.** The operator can double-click on the wavefront sensor image to detect phase-jump artifacts on a topo-aberrometry test just after acquisition.

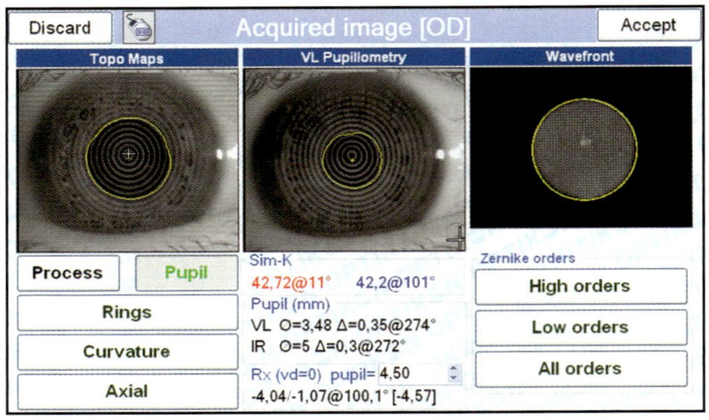


**Figure 7-48.** Mesopic-scotopic (IR=infrared) and photopic (VL=visible light) pupil images and sizes are shown just after topo-aberrometry acquisition.

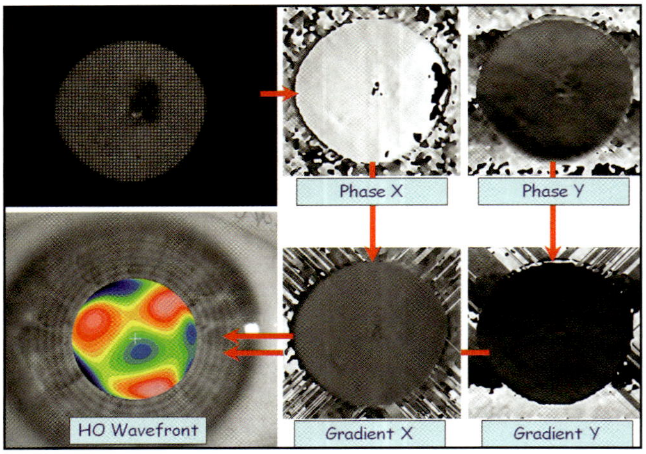


**Figure 7-47.** The operator acquired the same case as in Figure 7-45 again. This time, in spite of opacities in the crystalline lens, the reconstruction of gradients and the OW map are correct.

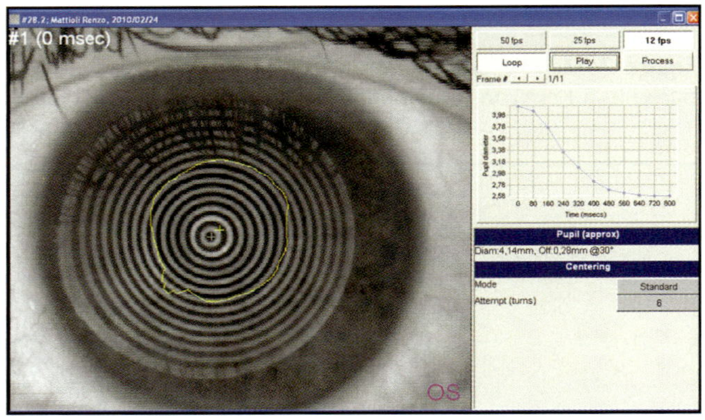


**Figure 7-49.** Dynamic pupillometry can be shown as a slow-motion movie. Here, one of the author's pupils changes from scotopic to photopic conditions over 800 ms. The changes have been transferred to the Scout software. Pupil size versus time response to visible light is plotted on the right.

## Pupillometry

In addition to corneal topography and wavefront aberrometry, the Keratron Onda acquires and measures the patient's pupil in 2 extreme conditions: "scotopic," which is taken in infrared light under mesopic conditions, and "photopic," taken about 1 second after turning on the LEDs (Figure 7-48). Actually, the instrument captures an entire movie sequence of images under these changing conditions, an example of which is shown in Figure 7-49. After turning the LEDs on, we can see that it takes about 800 milliseconds for the pupil to go into miosis. This sequence can be recorded at up to 50 fps and saved in the PC for further analyses.

## Acquiring Topo-Aberrometry

When "Topo-Aberrometry" (corneal topography + wavefront aberrometry) is selected with the Keratron Onda display touch screen, the "Acquisition" screen appears (Figure 7-50).

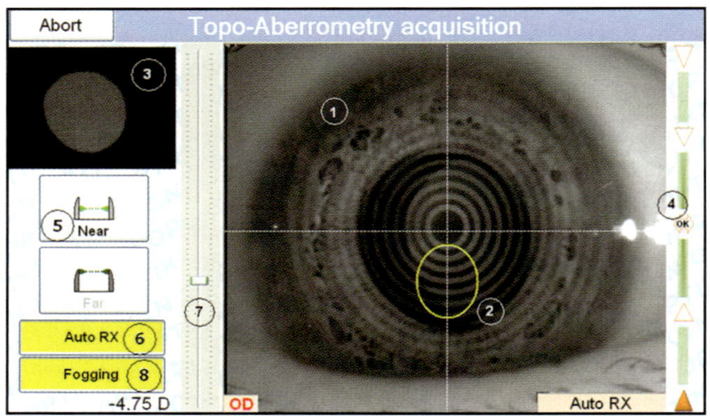


**Figure 7-50.** Acquisition of a topo-aberrometry test. The operator can align the patient's eye and view: the live image of the topography CCD (1) and of the wavefront sensor (3), the position of the light beam on the entrance pupil (2), and the Z distance of the eye according to the EPCS (4). He can select the near/far distance cone detectors (5) and the defocus compensation (7) and can activate or deactivate "Auto-RX" (6) and "fogging" (7) functions.

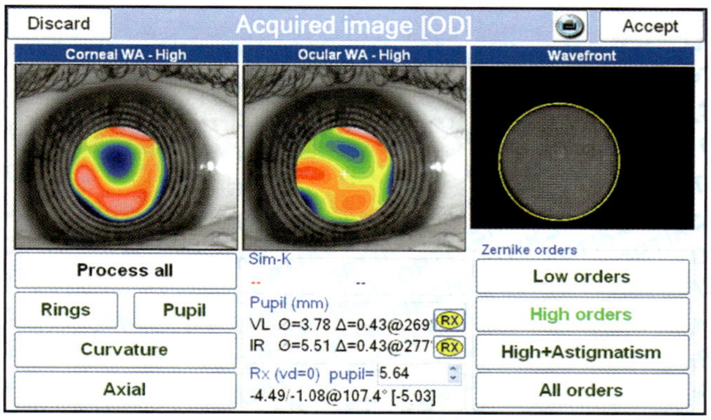


**Figure 7-51.** The corneal and OWs are shown side by side. The Rx refractive data at the bottom-center can be calculated at either a selected, photopic (VL), or scotopic (IR) pupil, with a single click.

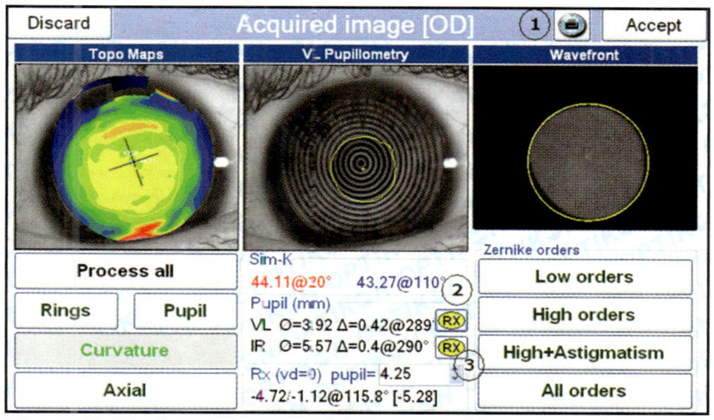


**Figure 7-52.** Curvature or axial maps and Sim-K can be shown on the Keratron Onda display before transferring the topo-aberrometry to the external PC with the Scout software.

The operator can choose the type of cone (see Figure 7-50, 1). Wavefront optics compensation for defocus can be selected manually by sliding a cursor from +6 to -11 D (see Figure 7-50, 7) or automatically by activating the "Auto Rx" button (see Figure 7-50, 6). Activating the "Fogging" button (see Figure 7-50, 8), presets the acquisition to show a fogging target in 3 or more steps, from virtual "close" (-1 D) to "far" distance (+1 D beyond the max defocus that he or she can objectively accommodate). Note that fogging is obviously unnecessary with presbyopic or pseudophakic patients.

The operator can monitor the acquisition while simultaneously centering the keratoscopic image of the eye (see Figure 7-50, 1) and paying attention to the wavefront sensor image (see Figure 7-50, 3). A yellow circle (see Figure 7-50, 2) shows where the beam is projected into the eye. The beam should fall within the pupil in order to have a valid retinal reflection in the screen (see Figure 7-50, 3) but at a distance from the corneal vertex to avoid corneal parasitic reflections (as also described in Figure 7-44). The EPCS visual feedback (see Figure 7-50, 4) and its characteristic varying intensity sound tells the operator when he or she is at the proper Z distance from the eye.

Pressing the button at the distance of "OK" starts the "Auto RX" and/or the patient's "Fogging" phases, depending on which buttons were previously activated. The images then freeze if the EPCS detects an acceptable Z distance. Then, the visible LEDs turn on and, after a minimum of 800 ms, an additional image is acquired for pupillometry with visible light. Finally, the "Preview" screen appears (see Figure 7-48).

At this point, the operator may decide whether to discard the image and proceed with another acquisition, send the topo-aberrometric test to an external PC for further processing and storage, or process the test immediately (Figures 7-51 and 7-52). Immediate processing allows the operator to examine the maps and data such as Sim-K (see Figure 7-52) and refraction without necessarily saving the entire examination.

The patient's refraction taken from the OW is shown as "Rx" (see Figure 7-52). This refraction can vary according to the selected vertex distance (VD), cylinder type (positive, negative, or automatic), and dioptric resolution (0.01, 0.12, or 0.25 D). Most important, the refraction can be greatly affected by pupil size, which can be manually selected between as small as 3 mm and up to a maximum of the size measured by the wavefront sensor. Alternatively, the operator can click either of the 2 little round "Rx" buttons to calculate pupil size at photopic (VL) or scotopic (IR) conditions as measured by the Keratron Onda's topographic pupillometry feature. Eventually, it will be possible to input the refraction (Rx) measured by topo-aberrometry as a "manifest refraction" in the test database for any Scout software applications (CW, CL, and laser links).

# Clinical Cases

## Case 1: A 51-Year-Old Patient Who Underwent Radial Keratotomy in 1989

The topographic map (Figure 7-53B) shows a small optical zone, which is usual after radial keratotomy (RK) treatment of moderate myopia, and the irregularities in the midperiphery that resulted from the 6 incisions. The OW map (Figure 7-53C) has been set to exclude the low orders (astigmatism and defocus) because it is important to understand the influence of the incisions and the resulting small optical zone on spherical aberration. Coma is also frequent in RK patients because the asymmetrical bulging of the radials is usually enhanced in the inferior sector. In this case, the amount of spherical aberration (0.42 μm) and coma (0.69 μm) are greater than normal, considering that this analysis was made at a pupil size of 4.75 mm. Most of the aberration in this case originates in the anterior cornea (Figure 7-53D), but the IW (Figure 7-53E) is affected by the posterior corneal surface, whose distortions match the incisions. The precise position and number of the incisions is clearly visible in Figure 7-53A.

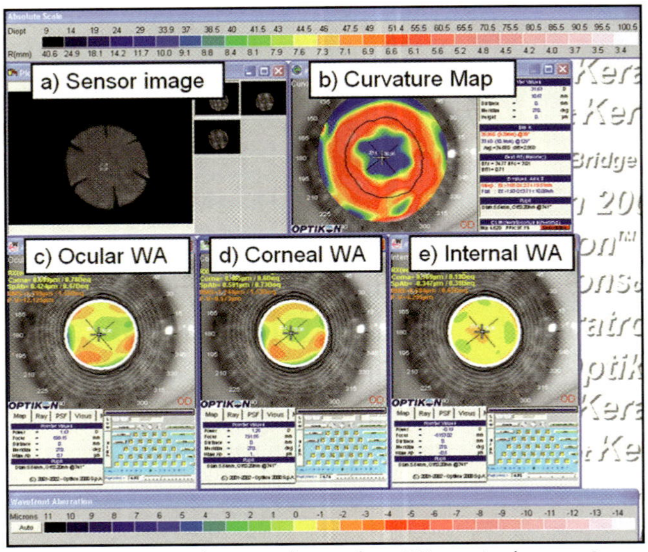


**Figure 7-53.** Wavefront analysis of an RK surgical case. Some internal aberrations are a result of posterior corneal surface deformation that corresponds to the radial incisions. (Reprinted with permission of Massimo Camellin, MD.)

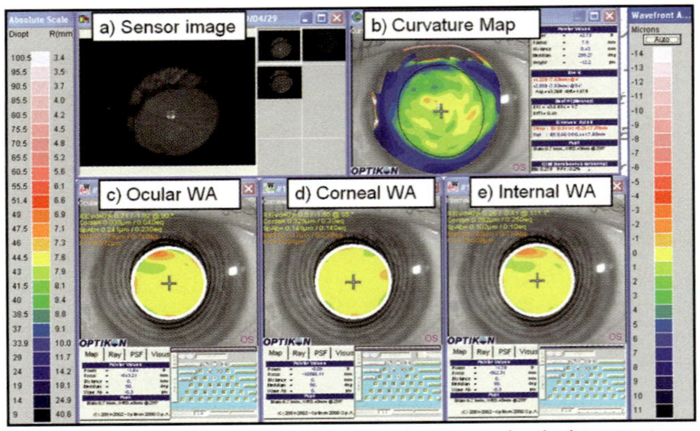


**Figure 7-54.** Wavefront analysis of a pseudophakic patient. An HOA due to fibrosis of the anterior capsule can be seen in the superior sector. (Reprinted with permission of Massimo Camellin, MD.)

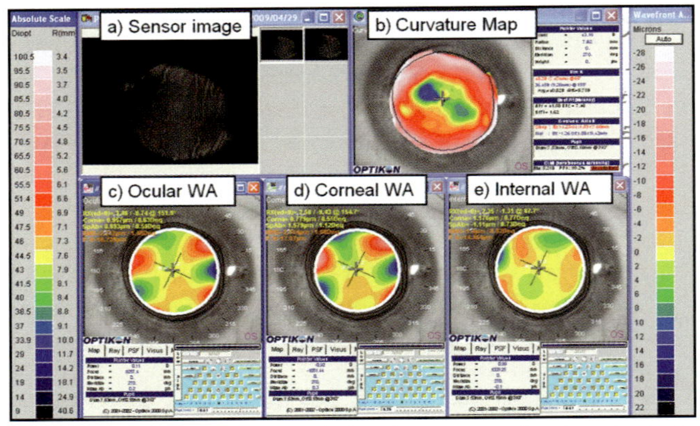


**Figure 7-55.** Wavefront analysis of a penetrating keratoplasty for a keratoconus. Some internal aberrations are due to the deep folds inside the transplant. (Reprinted with permission of Massimo Camellin, MD.)

## Case 2: A 70-Year-Old Pseudophakic Patient Who Complained of Night Glare

Clinically, the implanted IOL was spherical and appears to be well-centered with respect to the pupil. The corneal topography (Figure 7-54B) is unremarkable, but the wavefront sensor image (Figure 7-54A) shows an anterior capsular phimosis with reactive fibrosis in the upper left. While the total ocular component of coma (0.038 μm) and spherical aberration (0.24 μm) indicate perfect centering of the lens, some higher-order irregularities in the superior sector (Figure 7-54C) upon further analysis appear to be due to internal aberration (Figure 7-54E).

Thus, the patient's complaint of night glare is supported objectively, and one can attribute responsibility to the superior sector of the anterior capsule.

## Case 3: A 43-Year-Old Patient Who Underwent Penetrating Keratoplasty for Keratoconus in His Left Eye

The patient has high residual astigmatism that results in poor visual acuity (VA = 5/10) with spectacle correction (OS -4 sph +6.25 cyl at 65 degrees). Topographic analysis (Figure 7-55B) shows substantial regular astigmatism (Figure 7-55C). Ocular aberrometry is set to show higher orders, except coma and spherical aberration, which are deselected (Figure 7-55C-E). The remaining components have highly disturbing microirregularities. The OW (Figure 7-55C) is quite similar to the CW (Figure 7-55D). Few components of the IW have opposite signs from the CW, so the internal aberrations clearly stem from the posterior surface of the cornea. Therefore, the patient has stromal traction forces that distort both the front and the rear surface of the cornea. Because the refractive index of the air/stroma interface is much greater than that of the stroma/water interface, then obviously the posterior corneal distortions contribute less aberration. However, their contribution is still evident in Figure 7-55E. Figure 7-55A shows the wavefront sensor grid on which the vertical striae are due to folds of the donor cornea.

# Conclusion

The Keratron Onda measures corneal topography and aberrations of the total OW contemporarily; tracks and measures the pupil in photopic and scotopic or mesopic conditions; and performs dynamic pupillometry. Combining these functions in a single instrument required redesigning the cone architecture and developing an alternative for centroid displacement, as well as other adjustments for increased acquisition time. The Scout software that runs all Keratron operations coordinates the multiple functions of the Keratron Onda while offering the operator great flexibility. Examples of preliminary clinical applications demonstrated the remarkable advantage of the combined instrument.

# Topcon KR-1W

Naoyuki Maeda, MD

With the advancements in refractive surgery, cataract surgery, and contact lenses, there is a huge demand to evaluate the quality of vision objectively. Corneal topographic analysis is very useful to show the optical quality of the corneas following refractive surgery or with corneal diseases such as keratoconus.[43-45] Interpretation of color-coded maps reveals the corneal irregular astigmatism qualitatively.[46] Topographic indices such as SRI[47] or the results of Fourier analysis[48] and Zernike analysis[45] can show the effects of corneal irregular astigmatism on vision quantitatively.

Recently, the compensational association between cornea and internal optics became obvious not only for regular astigmatism but also for irregular astigmatism or HOAs.[49] For this reason, instruments that measure both corneal and ocular HOAs may be useful for the comprehensive evaluation of the optical system of the eye.

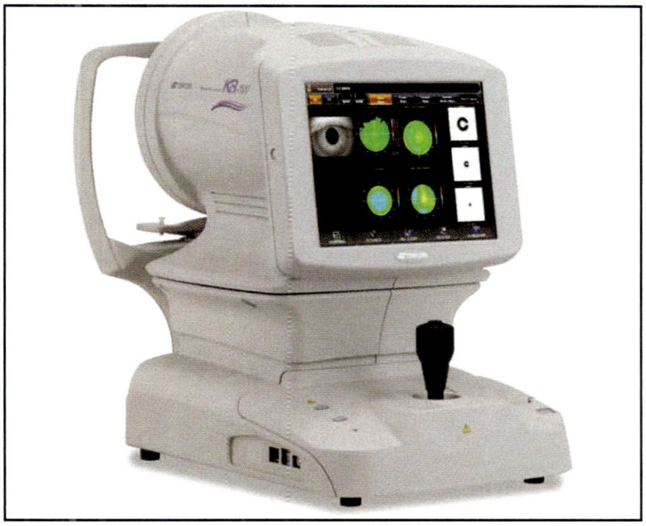

Figure 7-56. The Topcon unit provides 4 functions: autokeratometry, autorefractometry, videokeratography, and wavefront sensing.

## Main Features

The Topcon KR-1W (Figure 7-56) provides 4 functions: autokeratometry, autorefractometry, videokeratography, and wavefront sensing, sequentially in a session. Table 7-2 indicates the specifications of the machine. Many original articles and reviews have already been published with the previous machine (KR-9000PW) or prototype of this instrument.[50-77] The machine is capable of fully-automated measurement including autofocus and X-Y alignment, enabling measurements for both eyes by just touching the center of the pupil on the instrument's touch screen.

### Keratometry and Refractometry

Keratometry and refractometry are performed like conventional autorefractometers or autokeratometers. In addition to this conventional autorefractometry, this machine may provide better objective refractions than conventional ones with the aid of wavefront technology, especially following refractive surgery or corneal surgeries.[78] Although conventional autorefraction obtains sphere and cylinder values based on paracentral values (from 1.4- to 3.0-mm diameter), this wavefront sensor can calculate sphere and cylinder using the whole data inside the defined pupil: from inside 2 mm (minimum) to 8 mm (maximum) diameter and default 4 mm for day vision and 6 mm for night vision. The difference between these 2 methods may be small in normal eyes but increases dramatically in cases following refractive surgery with optical zone abnormality or in post-keratoplasty cases.

### Topography

This machine uses Placido rings for corneal topography. Infrared illumination is used to project the Placido rings, improving the patient's fixation during measurements by reducing the luminance and minimizing miosis of the pupil during the wavefront sensing.

Output display for corneal topography consists of a mire image, corneal power map, and corneal HOA map (Figure 7-57). The axial power and instantaneous power map with the Smolek/Klyce scale[79] are set as the default. An absolute scale with 1.5-D steps best illustrates clinically significant abnormality in corneal shape, while screening for clinically insignificant differences in topography.[80] Conventional videokeratoscope users easily perform visual inspection of topographic maps using a standard scale.

In addition to the conventional display of corneal power distribution, the KR-1W enables assessment of corneal HOAs both qualitatively and quantitatively. Figure 7-57 illustrates the color-coded map of corneal HOAs in addition to the corneal indices and corneal HOAs for 4 mm, 6 mm, and actual pupil size. The absolute scale is used for the display of the corneal HOA map to show the clinically significant HOAs or irregular corneal astigmatism with the rapid pattern recognition. Different from the conventional power maps, irregular astigmatism is easily differentiated from sphere and cylinder with the corneal HOA map. By comparing the corneal HOA map and the ocular HOA map, the origin of irregular astigmatism can be identified.

TABLE 7-2.

**Specifications of KR-1W**

| | |
|---|---|
| Auto-refractometry | Spherical refractive power: -25 to +22 D<br>Cylindrical refractive power: 0 to 10 D<br>Measured minimum pupil diameter: 2 mm |
| Auto-keratometry | Corneal curvature radius: 5.00 to 10.00 mm<br>Corneal refractive power: 67.50 to 33.75 D<br>Corneal astigmatic power: 0 to 10 D |
| Ocular HOAs | Hartmann-Shack wavefront aberrometer<br>HOA: Zernike polynomial up to 10th or 4th order<br>Aberration display: Total aberration, HOA<br>Measuring range: -25 to +22 D<br>Measuring area: 8.0 mm |
| Corneal topography/corneal HOAs | Numbers of Placido rings: 19<br>Corneal curvature radius: 5.00 to 10.00 mm<br>Corneal refractive power: 67.50 to 33.75 D<br>Cornea shape measurement area: 0.8 mm to 9.2 mm<br>Axial power map, Instantaneous power map<br>HOA: Zernike polynomial up to 10th or 4th order |
| Range of pupil distance measurement | 20 to 85 mm |
| External connection terminal | USB (input/output, output), RS-232C (output),<br>LAN (input/output) |

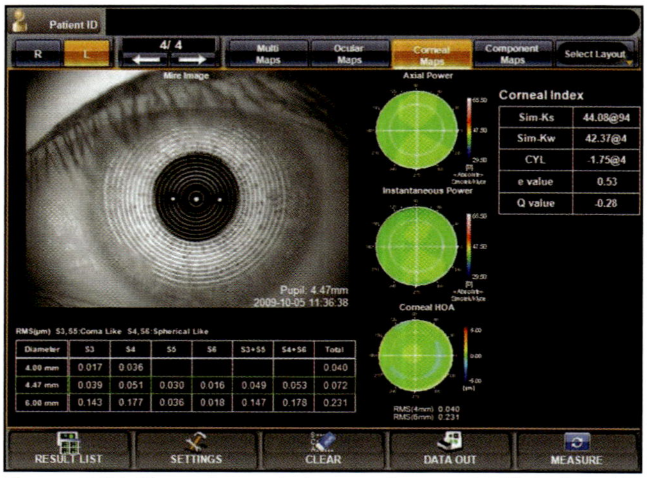


**Figure 7-57.** The color-coded map of corneal HOAs in addition to the corneal indices and corneal HOAs for 4-mm and actual pupil size (4.47-mm).

## Aberrometry

The purpose of aberrometry is to evaluate the optical quality of the eye by analyzing the shape of its wavefront.[50,51] This machine uses Hartmann-Shack sensors, and wavefront aberrations are calculated by expanding the wavefront into sets of Zernike polynomials.

The total aberration map represents the aberrations of the eye including defocus (sphere), regular astigmatism (cylinder), and irregular astigmatism (Figure 7-58; lower center). The ocular total aberration map relates to the uncorrected visual acuity (UCVA), allowing estimation of UCVA using the total aberration map.

The ocular HOA map (Figure 7-58; lower right) eliminates lower-order aberrations and isolates only the HOAs, highlighting irregular astigmatism. As HOAs relate to the best spectacle-corrected visual acuity (BSCVA), BSCVA may be estimated using the HOA map. In addition to the ocular total and HOA maps, PSF, MTF, and simulated retinal images of Landolt rings may also be displayed (Figure 7-59).

# Representative Cases

The result from a typical emmetropic eye is displayed in Figure 7-60. Mire image (upper left) consists of a smooth concentric circle, and axial power map (upper center) indicates no astigmatism. Corneal HOA map (upper right) shows the relatively flat wavefront without clinically significant irregular astigmatism at the anterior corneal surface.

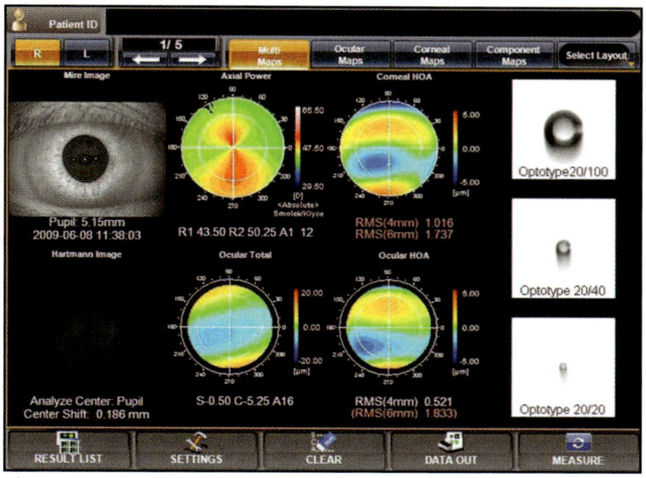


**Figure 7-58.** Comparison of the topography with corneal and whole eye aberrations aids in diagnosis. The ocular HOA map (lower right) eliminates lower-order aberrations and isolates HOAs, highlighting irregular astigmatism. BSCVA may be estimated using the HOA map.

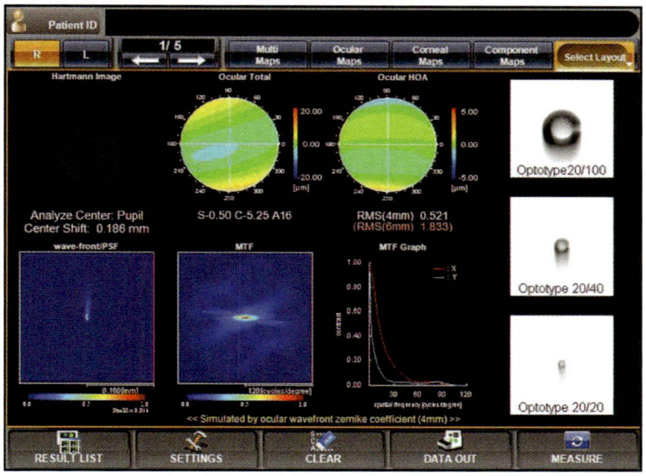


**Figure 7-59.** PSF, MTF, and simulated retinal images of Landolt rings. Point spread function (PSF, lower left), 2-dimensional modulation transfer function (MTF, lower center), MTF graph for X and Y axis (lower right), and simulated retinal images of Landolt rings (right) are shown.

The Hartmann image (lower left) shows the regular grid pattern. A uniform pattern is seen in the ocular total aberration map (lower center) indicating emmetropia, with minimal irregularity in the HOA map (lower right).

Figure 7-61 illustrates myopic astigmatism. Vertical bow-tie pattern that indicates regular astigmatism with prolate asphericity is seen in the corneal axial power map. Ocular total aberration shows a slow oval wavefront in the center characteristic of severe myopia with regular astigmatism. The flat wavefront in both corneal and ocular HOA maps indicate lack of irregularity.

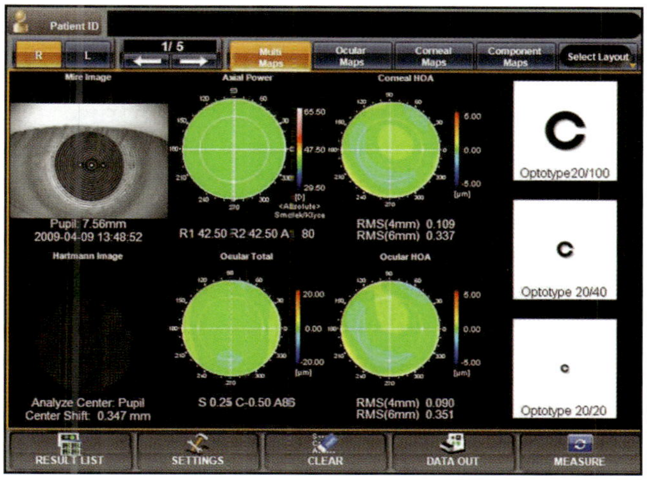


**Figure 7-60.** A typical emmetropic eye is displayed. Mire image (upper left) consists of a smooth concentric circle, and axial power map (upper center) indicates no astigmatism. Corneal HOA map (upper right) shows the relatively flat wavefront without clinically significant irregular astigmatism at the anterior corneal surface. The Hartmann image (lower left) shows the regular grid pattern. A uniform pattern is seen in the ocular total aberration map (lower center) indicating emmetropia, with minimal irregularity in the HOA map (lower right).

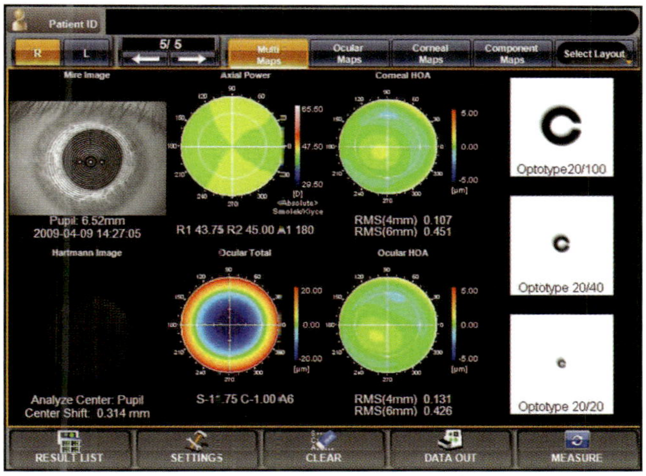


**Figure 7-61.** Myopic astigmatism. Vertical bowtie indicating regular astigmatism with prolate asphericity is seen on the corneal axial power map. Ocular total aberration shows a slow oval wavefront in the center characteristic of severe myopia with regular astigmatism. The flat wavefront in both corneal and ocular HOA maps indicates mild irregularity.

Distorted mires and localized abnormal steepening are typical of a keratoconic eye (see Figure 7-58). Ocular total aberration map illustrates myopic astigmatism, while the corneal HOA map reveals coma—the combination of advanced wavefront superiorly and delayed wavefront inferiorly.[68] The corneal HOA map reveals that the irregular astigmatism is attributed to the cornea. The simulated retinal images are characteristic of coma aberration.

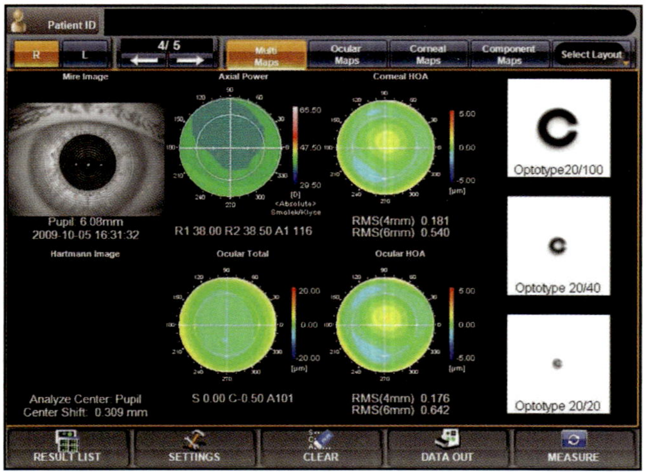


**Figure 7-62.** An eye after conventional myopic LASIK. The flat area seen in the center of the axial power map (top left) and flat wavefront seen in the ocular total aberration map (lower left) are the result of myopic correction. In the corneal and ocular HOA maps, advanced wavefront in the center indicates mild increase of spherical aberration.

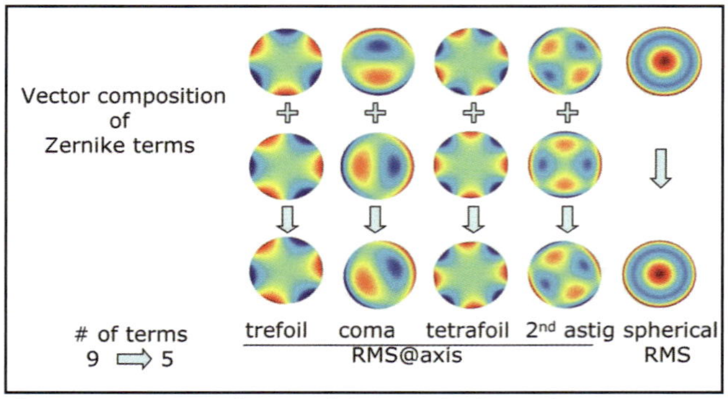


**Figure 7-63.** For each pair of the standard Zernike terms, a single magnitude and axis value are calculated using Campbell's simplified Zernike functions

An example of an eye following conventional myopic LASIK is shown in Figure 7-62. The flat area seen in the center of the axial power map and flat wavefront seen in the ocular total aberration map are the result of myopic correction. In the corneal and ocular HOA maps, advanced wavefront in the center indicates mild increase of spherical aberration.

## Zernike Vector Map

HOA maps are a combination of several Zernike terms. It is sometimes difficult to perform visual inspection of wavefront maps. Pairs in the Zernike terms (Figure 7-63) such as in *trefoil* and *coma* make it difficult to analyze the characteristics of ocular HOAs quantitatively. Describing the Zernike terms as vector components with a magnitude and orientation similar to the cylinder power and axis may be helpful. For each pair of the standard Zernike terms, a single magnitude and axis value are calculated using Campbell's simplified Zernike functions[81] as shown in Figure 7-63.

In the Zernike vector map, the magnitudes and orientations of coma, trefoil, secondary astigmatism, and tetrafoil in addition to the spherical aberration were shown. At a glance of the map, the character of the HOA in each clinical case can be easily understood. In a myopic patient (Figure 7-64), the map for total HOA (top, left) shows mild but complex patterns. On the other hand, Zernike vector maps (bottom) clearly show that the pattern is due to the combination of a small amount of coma and a small amount of spherical aberration. Figure 7-65 reveals the Zernike vector analysis in a patient with keratoconus. The output of Zernike vector maps indicates the magnitudes and angles for each term.

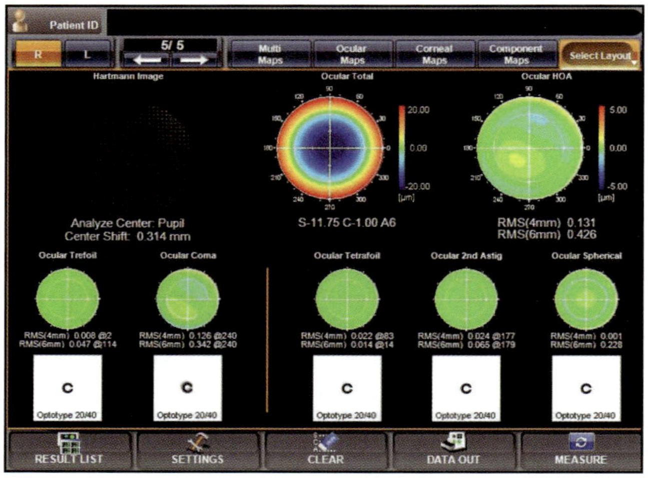


**Figure 7-64.** In a myopic patient, the map for total HOA (top) shows mild but complex patterns. Zernike vector maps (bottom row) clearly show that the pattern is due to the combination of a small amount of coma and spherical aberration.

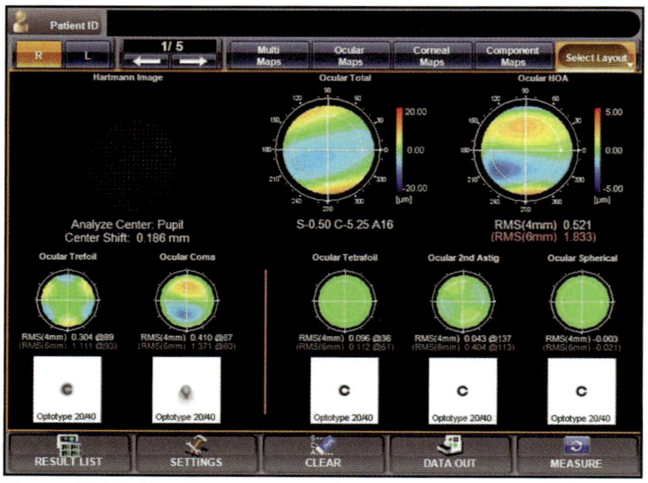


**Figure 7-65.** Zernike vector analysis in a patient with keratoconus. Zernike vector maps indicate magnitudes and angles for each term. Coma is the dominant aberration, followed by trefoil and secondary astigmatism.

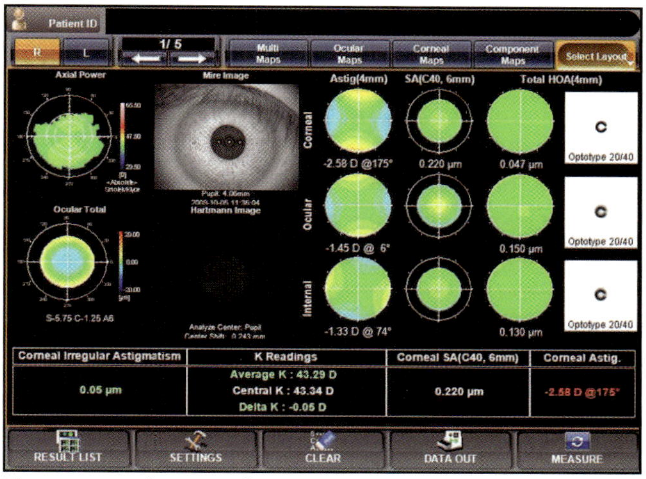

**Figure 7-66.** The IOL selection map can be used as a screening tool for premium IOL candidates. It highlights corneal irregular astigmatism, regular astigmatism, and spherical aberration.

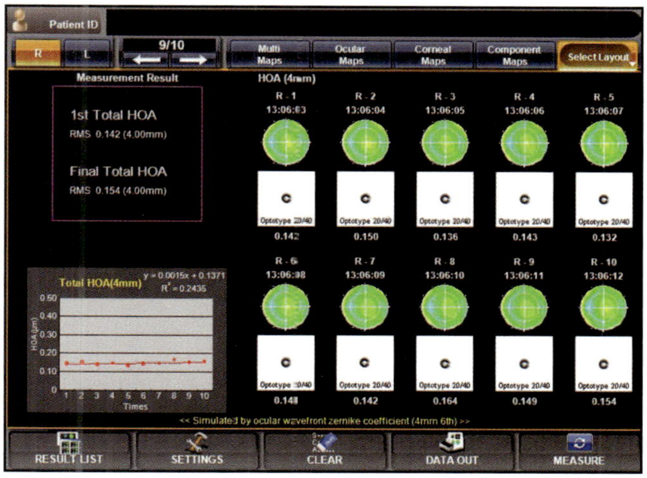

**Figure 7-67.** Sequential HOA measurements were obtained as subjects were asked to inhibit blink for 10 seconds and maps were captured every second.

It is obvious that coma aberration is dominant followed by trefoil and secondary astigmatism in this eye.[68]

## Intraocular Lens Selection

With the development of new technology, aspheric, toric, and multifocal IOLs are currently available. To ensure successful implantation of these newer IOLs, the optical properties of the cornea must be evaluated prior to cataract surgery.

The IOL selection map (Figure 7-66) can be used as a screening tool for candidates of new-technology IOLs. In this program, the screening process consists of 4 steps. First, evaluate the amount of corneal irregular astigmatism as the total corneal HOA (Figure 7-67; bottom left). If there is a clinically significant amount of corneal irregular astigmatism, it will be important to exclude such a candidate from multifocal IOLs. Also, surgeons can educate the patient about the possibility of a limited outcome postoperatively due to irregular astigmatism when total corneal HOA is beyond the clinically significant range.

The second step involves the IOL power calculation. By comparing the corneal power between center and paracentral areas, surgeons estimate the need for special IOL power calculation. This will be especially important for cataract following LASIK or keratoplasty.

The third step is to assess corneal spherical aberration when considering aspherical IOLs. There is a wide range of variation of corneal spherical aberration even in the normal population, and aspherical IOLs for the eyes with negative corneal spherical aberration or spherical IOLs for the eyes with extremely positive corneal spherical aberration should be avoided.

Last, evaluate the amount of corneal cylinder (Figure 7-66; bottom right). Surgical correction of regular astigmatism using toric IOL, touch-up with excimer laser, or limbal relaxing incisions should be considered for the cases with high corneal cylinder.

## Serial Measurements of Ocular Wavefront Aberration

It is well-known that the ocular refraction is dynamic due to the changes in accommodation, pupil size, and tear film. On the other hand, most of the autorefractometers and aberrometers measure the refraction with static fashion. KR-1W enables us to measure HOA sequentially for 10 seconds.

During the measurements of sequential HOA, subjects were asked to inhibit blink for 10 seconds to obtain maps every second (Figure 7-67). Serial measurements of HOAs in healthy eyes[69] showed variations even in clinically normal subjects (classified into 4 groups by pattern: stable, small fluctuation, saw tooth, and others). The sequential changes of HOAs in dry eye[70,71] soft contact lens wear,[72] or after punctal plug insertion[73] were shown using the prototype machine.

## Conclusion

Using the combination of Placido disk-based corneal topographer and Hartmann-Shack wavefront sensor, the detailed information about corneal and ocular HOAs can be obtained in the clinic.

# References


1. Molebny VV, Panagopoulou SI, Molebny SV, Wakil JS, Pallikaris IG. Principles of ray tracing aberrometry. *J Refract Surg*. 2000;16:S570-S575.
2. Holladay JT, Lynn MJ, Waring GO, et al. The relationship of visual acuity, refractive error, and pupil size after radial keratotomy. *Arch Ophthalmol*. 1991;109:70-76.
3. Kirwan C, O'Keefe M. Higher order aberrations in children with amblyopia. *J Pediatr Ophthalmol Strabismus*. 2008;45(2):92-96.
4. Iida Y, Shimizu K, Ito M, Suzuki M. Influence of age on ocular wavefront aberration changes with accommodation. *J Refract Surg*. 2008;24(7):696-701.
5. Win-Hall DM, Glasser A. Objective accommodation measurements in pseudophakic subjects using an autorefractor and an aberrometer. *J Cataract Refract Surg*. 2009;35(2):282-290.
6. Gemoules G, Morris KM. Rigid gas-permeable contact lenses and severe higher-order aberrations in postsurgical corneas. *Eye Contact Lens*. 2007;33(6 Pt 1):304-307.
7. MacRae S, Fujieda M. Slit skiascopic-guided ablation using the Nidek laser. *J Refract Surg*. 2000;16:S576-S580.
8. McAlinden C, Moore JE. Comparison of higher order aberrations after LASIK and LASEK for myopia. *J Refract Surg*. 2010;26:45-51.
9. Klyce SD, Karon MD, Smolek MK. Screening patients with the corneal navigator. *J Refract Surg*. 2005;21:S617-S622.
10. Holladay JT. Keratoconus detection using corneal topography. *J Refract Surg*. 2009;25:S958-S962.
11. Gatinel D, Hoang-Xuan T. Objective assessment of the quality of vision before and after repositioning of a dislocated iris-fixated aphakic anterior chamber lens. *J Refract Surg*. 2007;23:S1005-S1010.
12. Carey PJ, Leccisotti A, McGilligan VE, Goodall EA, Moore CB. Assessment of toric intraocular lens alignment by a refractive power/corneal analyzer system and slitlamp observation. *J Cataract Refract Surg*. 2010;36:222-229.
13. Gatinel D, Adam PA, Chaabouni S, et al. Comparison of corneal and total ocular aberrations before and after myopic LASIK. *J Refract Surg*. 2010;26(5):333-340.
14. Nissman SA, Tractenberg RE, Saba CM, Douglas JC, Lustbader JM. Accuracy, repeatability, and clinical application of spherocylindrical automated refraction using time-based wavefront aberrometry measurements. *Ophthalmology*. 2006;113:577.
15. Barreto J Jr, Netto MV, Cigna A, Bechara S, Kara-José N. Precision of higher order aberration repeatability with NIDEK OPD-SCAN retinoscopic aberrometry. *J Refract Surg*. 2006;22:S1037-S1040.
16. McDonnell C, Rolincova M, Venter J. Comparison of measurement of pupil sizes among the colvard pupillometer, procyon pupillometer, and NIDEK OPD-SCAN. *J Refract Surg*. 2006;22:S1027-S1030.
17. Lim KL, Fam HB. Ethnic differences in higher-order aberrations: spherical aberration in the South East Asian Chinese eye. *J Cataract Refract Surg*. 2009;35:2144-2148.
18. Hori-Komai Y, Toda I, Asano-Kato N, Ito M, Yamamoto T, Tsubota K. Comparison of LASIK using the NIDEK EC-5000 optimized aspheric transition zone (OATz) and conventional ablation profile. *J Refract Surg*. 2006;22:546-555.
19. Venter J. Wavefront-guided custom ablation for myopia using the NIDEK NAVEX laser system. *J Refract Surg*. 2008;24:487-493.
20. Subbaram MV, MacRae SM. Customized LASIK treatment for myopia based on preoperative manifest refraction and higher order aberrometry: the Rochester nomogram. *J Refract Surg*. 2007;23:435-441.
21. Okamoto S, Kimura K, Funakura M, Ikeda N, Hiramatsu H, Bains HS. Comparison of myopic LASIK centered on the coaxially sighted corneal light reflex or line of sight. *J Refract Surg*. 2009;25:S944-S950.
22. Wu L, Zhou X, Chu R, Wang Q. Photoablation centration on the corneal optical center in myopic LASIK using AOV excimer laser. *Eur J Ophthalmol*. 2009;19(6):923-929.
23. El Danasoury AM. NIDEK optimized prolate ablation for the treatment of myopia with and without astigmatism. *J Refract Surg*. 2009;25:S136-S141.
24. Mattioli R. Topo-aberrometry with Keratron Onda. Congress: "Refractive on line," ICH-Milano, Italy, Sept. 2009. http://www.refractiveonline.com/2009/eng/52mattioli/player.html.
25. Carones F, Gobbi PG, Brancato R, Venturi E. Comparison between two computer-assisted keratoscopes in measuring aspheric surfaces. *Invest Ophtalmol Vis Sci (suppl)*. 1994:3748.
26. Brancato R, Carones F. Topografia corneale computerizzata. Fogliazza, Milano (Italy), 1994.
27. Mattioli R, Carones F, Cantera E. New algorithms to improve the reconstruction of corneal geometry on the Keratrontm videokeratographer. *Invest Ophthalmol Vis Sci*. 1995;36(suppl):1400.
28. Mattioli R. Rappresentazione della wavefront corneale della topografia. Congress: "Refractive on Line," ICH-Milano, Italy, Sept. 2001. http://www.refractiveonline.com/eng/pages/edition.aspx?anno=2001.
29. Mattioli R. Corneal topography and wavefront analysis. In: Caimi F, Brancato R, eds. *The Aberrometers*. Canelli, Italy: Fabiano; 2003:113-132.
30. Tripoli NK, Cohen KL, Holmgren DE, Coggins JM. Assessment of radial aspheres by the *Keratron* keratoscope using an arc-step algorithm. *Am J Ophthalmol*. 1995;120:658-664.
31. Cohen KL, Tripoli NK, Holmgren DE, Coggins JM. Assessment of the power and height of radial aspheres reported by a computer-assisted keratoscope. *Am J Ophthalmol*. 1995;119:723-732.
32. Mattioli R, Tripoli NK. Corneal geometry reconstruction with the *Keratron* videokeratographer. *Optom Vis Sci*. 1997;74:881-894.
33. Mattioli R, Frondizi S, Rubeo A, Saldutti M. The *Keratron Scout* and wavefront analysis. In: Caimi F, Brancato R, eds. *The Aberrometers*. Canelli, Italy: Fabiano; 2003:243-257.
34. Mattioli R, Frondizi S, inventors; Optikon 2000 S.p.A., assignee. Multi-purpose ophtalmological apparatus, US patent 7878654; February 1, 2011.
35. Mattioli R, inventor; Optikon Oftalmologia S.p.A., assignee. An apparatus for topographical analysis of anatomical surfaces in particular of cornea, US patent 5,526,073; March 30, 1994.
36. Takeda M, Ina H, Kobayashi S. Fourier-transform method of fringe-pattern analysis for computer-based topography and interferometry. *JOSA*. 1982;72(1):156-160.
37. Carmon Y, Ribak EN. Phase retrieval by demodulation of a Hartmann-Shack sensor. *Optics Comm*. 2003;215:285-288.
38. Ribak EN, Carmon Y, Talmi A, Glazer O, Srour O, Zon N. Full wave front reconstruction in the Fourier domain. *Proc. SPIE*. 2006;6272(54):1-9.
39. Horwitz LS. Wavefront sensor using near-field diffraction effects. 5th International Congress on Wavefront Sensing and Optimized Refractive Correction; February 21-23, 2004; Whistler, Canada.
40. Sarver EJ. Extracting wavefront error from S/H images using spatial demodulation. 7th International Congress on Wavefront Sensing and Optimized Refraction Correction; January 26-29 2006; Nassau, Bahamas.

41. Ghiglia DC, Pritt MD. *Two-Dimensional Phase Unwrapping: Theory, Algorithms and Software*. New York, NY: Wiley; 1998:1-57.
42. Ribak EN, Canovas C. Comparison of Hartmann analysis methods. *Applied Optics*. 2007;46(10):1830-1835.
43. Klyce SD, Maeda N, Byrd TJ. Corneal topography. In: Kaufman HE, Barron BA, McDonald MB, eds. *The Cornea*. 2nd ed. Boston, MA: Butterworth-Heinemann; 1998:1055-1075.
44. Applegate RA, Hilmantel G, Howland HC, et al. Corneal first surface optical aberrations and visual performance. *J Refract Surg*. 2000;16:507-514.
45. Naoyuki M. Evaluation of optical quality of corneas using corneal topographers. *Cornea*. 2002;21:S75-S78.
46. Maguire LJ, Singer DE, Klyce SD. Graphic presentation of computer-analyzed keratoscope photographs. *Arch Ophthalmol*. 1987;105:223-230.
47. Wilson SE, Klyce SD. Quantitative descriptors of corneal topography. A clinical study. *Arch Ophthalmol*. 1991;109:349-353.
48. Oshika T, Tomidokoro A, Maruo K, Tokunaga T, Miyata N. Quantitative evaluation of irregular astigmatism by Fourier series harmonic analysis of videokeratography data. *Invest Ophthalmol Vis Sci*. 1998;39:705-709.
49. Artal P, Guirao A, Berrio E, Williams DR. Compensation of corneal aberrations by the internal optics in the human eye. *J Vis*. 2001;1:1-8.
50. Maeda N. Wavefront technology in ophthalmology. *Current Opin Ophthalmol*. 2001;12:294-299.
51. Maeda N. Wavefront technology and LASIK application. In: Azar DT, Koch DD, eds. *LASIK: Fundamentals, Surgical Techniques, and Complications*. New York, NY: Marcel Dekker, Inc; 2002:139-151.
52. Kuroda T, Fujikado T, Maeda N, Oshika T, Hirohara Y, Himashi T. Wavefront analysis in eyes with nuclear or cortical cataract. *Am J Ophthalmol*. 2002;134:1-9.
53. Koh S, Maeda N, Kuroda T, et al. Effect of tear film break-up on higher-order aberrations measured with wavefront sensor. *Am J Ophthalmol*. 2002;134:115-117.
54. Kuroda T, Fujikado T, Maeda N, Oshika T, Hirohara Y, Mihashi T. Wavefront analysis of higher-order aberrations in patients with cataract. *J Cataract Refract Surg*. 2002;28:438-444.
55. Kuroda T, Fujikado T, Ninomiya S, Maeda N, Hirohara Y, Mihashi T. Effect of aging on ocular light scatter and higher order aberrations. *J Refract Surg*. 2002;18:S598-S602.
56. Ninomiya S, Fujikado T, Kuroda T, et al. Changes of ocular aberration with accommodation. *Am J Ophthalmol*. 2002;134:924-926.
57. Ninomiya S, Maeda N, Kuroda T, et al. Evaluation of lenticular irregular astigmatism using wavefront analysis in patients with lenticonus. Arch Ophthalmol. 2002;120:1388-1393.
58. Maeda N, Fujikado T, Kuroda T, et al. Wavefront aberrations measured with Hartmann-Shack sensor in patients with keratoconus. *Ophthalmology*. 2002;109:1996-2003.
59. Ninomiya S, Fujikado T, Kuroda T, et al. Wavefront analysis in eyes with accommodative spasm. *Am J Ophthalmol*. 2003;136:1161-1163.
60. Kelly JE, Mihashi T, Howland HC. Compensation of corneal horizontal/vertical astigmatism, lateral coma, and spherical aberration by internal optics of the eye. *J Vis*. 2004;4:262-271.
61. Fujikado T, Kuroda T, Maeda N, et al. Wavefront analysis of an eye with monocular triplopia and nuclear cataract. *Am J Ophthalmol*. 2004;137:361-363.
62. Fujikado T, Kuroda T, Maeda N, et al. Light scattering and optical aberrations as objective parameters to predict visual deterioration in eyes with cataracts. *J Cataract Refract Surg*. 2004;30:1198-1208.
63. Amano S, Amano Y, Yamagami S, et al. Age-related changes in corneal and ocular higher-order wavefront aberrations. *Am J Ophthalmol*. 2004;137:988-992.
64. Tanabe T, Miyata K, Samejima T, Hirohara Y, Mihashi T, Oshika T. Influence of wavefront aberration and corneal subepithelial haze on low-contrast visual acuity after photorefractive keratectomy. *Am J Ophthalmol*. 2004;138:620-624.
65. Yamane N, Miyata K, Samejima T, et al. Ocular higher-order aberrations and contrast sensitivity after conventional laser in situ keratomileusis. *Invest Ophthalmol Vis Sci*. 2004;45:3986-3990.
66. Fujikado T, Kuroda T, Ninomiya S, et al. Age-related changes in ocular and corneal aberrations. *Am J Ophthalmol*. 2004;138:143-146.
67. Bellucci R, Morselli S, Piers P. Comparison of wavefront aberrations and optical quality of eyes implanted with five different intraocular lenses. *J Refract Surg*. 2004;20:297-306.
68. Kosaki R, Maeda N, Bessho K, et al. Magnitude and orientation of Zernike terms in patients with keratoconus. *Invest Ophthalmol Vis Sci*. 2007;48:3062-3068.
69. Koh S, Maeda N, Hirohara Y, et al. Serial measurements of higher-order aberrations after blinking in normal subjects. *Invest Ophthalmol Vis Sci*. 2006;47:3318-3324.
70. Koh S, Maeda N, Hirohara Y, et al. Serial measurements of higher-order aberrations after blinking in patients with dry eye. *Invest Ophthalmol Vis Sci*. 2008;49:133-138.
71. Koh S, Maeda N, Hori Y, et al. Effects of suppression of blinking on quality of vision in borderline cases of evaporating dry eye. *Cornea*. 2008;27:275-278.
72. Koh S, Maeda N, Hamano T, et al. Effects of internal lubricating agents of disposable soft contact lenses on higher-order aberrations after blinking. *Eye & Contact Lens*. 2008;34:100-105.
73. Koh S, Maeda N, Ninomiya S, et al. Paradoxical increase of visual impairment with punctal occlusion in a patient with mild dry eye. *J Cataract Refract Surg*. 2006;32:689-691.
74. Fujikado T, Shimojyo S, Hosohata J, et al. Wavefront analysis of eye with monocular diplopia and cortical cataract. *Am J Ophthalmol*. 2006;141:1138-1140.
75. Mihashi T, Hirohara Y, Koh S, Ninomiya S, Maeda N, Fijikado T. Tear film break-up time evaluated by real-time Hartmann-Shack wavefront sensing. *Jpn J Ophthalmol*. 2006;50:85-89.
76. Oie Y, Maeda N, Kosaki R, et al. Characteristics of ocular higher-order aberrations in patients with pellucid marginal corneal degeneration. *J Cataract Refract Surg*. 2008;34:1928-1934.
77. Maeda N. Clinical application of wavefront aberrometry—A review. *Clinical & Experimental Ophthalmology*. 2009;37:118-129.
78. Thibos LN, Hong X, Bradley A, Applegate RA. Accuracy and precision of objective refraction from wavefront aberrations. *J Vis*. 2004;4:329-351.
79. Smolek MK, Klyce SD, Hovis JK. The Universal Standard Scale: proposed improvements to the American National Standards Institute (ANSI) scale for corneal topography. *Ophthalmology*. 2002;109:361-369.
80. Wilson SE, Klyce SD, Husseini ZM. Standardized color-coded maps for corneal topography. *Ophthalmology*. 1993;100:1723-1727.
81. Campbell CE. A new method for describing the aberrations of the eye using Zernike polynomials. *Optom Vis Sci*. 2003;80:79-83.

# SECTION III

# TOPOGRAPHIC APPLICATIONS

Chapter 8

# Topography in Corneal Diseases

Gaurav Prakash, MD and Amar Agarwal, MS, FRCS, FRCOphth

Corneal topography is a vital tool in the assessment of the diseased cornea. Many disorders of the cornea, such as keratoconus, are identified by subtle changes in the topography before there are visual symptoms or clinically visible signs in slit-lamp biomicroscopy. As topography looks at the central as well as the peripheral cornea, many disorders that can be missed on central evaluation by the keratometry can instead be diagnosed by an astute clinician using a topography device.[1-7]

However, measurement technique, diurnal variation of the corneal hydration, calibration of the device, positioning of the patient's head, post-LASIK status, and use of anesthetic drops can influence topographic evaluation, and therefore it is essential to reduce these factors to a minimum.[8-12] In the case of subclinical disease, there is a narrow zone of high sensitivity and low specificity necessitating consistent and precise measurements. Recent topography devices, such as the Pentacam, have been found to be more accurate than Orbscan when measuring corneas with certain conditions.[13-15] The most classical corneal disorders identified by topography are corneal ectasias: keratoconus, pellucid marginal degeneration, or post-LASIK ectasia. In addition, the irregular astigmatism resulting from corneal dystrophies, degenerations, scarring, inflammatory conditions, pterygium, or dry eye can also be quantified with the help of topography.

## KERATOCONUS

Keratoconus is a bilateral, noninflammatory disorder of the cornea that, despite years of study, is not completely understood. Early researchers focused on the optical and clinical signs, morphology, and rehabilitation by the means of glasses, contact lenses, and keratoplasty.[15,16] With increasing application of corneal topography, multiple indices have been described to diagnose cases with early or forme fruste keratoconus, ranging from simple grading scores to advanced algorithms to monitor progression.[17-25] It is important to be comfortable with a grading system and use it in sequential follow-ups in the patients. The indications of topography are not limited to diagnosis and monitoring pre-intervention progression. With the advent of intrastromal ring implantation and collagen cross-linking, postoperative follow-up with topography can provide vital information in collecting more information on the disease process.

Keratoconus is generally associated with adolescents and young adults and has been historically known to stabilize in older age groups, probably because of increased cross-linkage in the cornea with growing age.[26] It can occur both sporadically or inherited as a genetic disorder. Keratoconus may be associated with atopy, corneal dystrophies, cataracts, Lebers', as well as systemic disorders such as Pierre Robins' sequence, congenital adrenal hyperplasia, Turner's syndrome, and Noonen syndrome.[27-47] Syndromic associations, although rare, should be ruled out in all cases.



Wang M. *Corneal Topography: A Guide for Clinical Application in the Wavefront Era, Second Edition (pp. 201-214)*

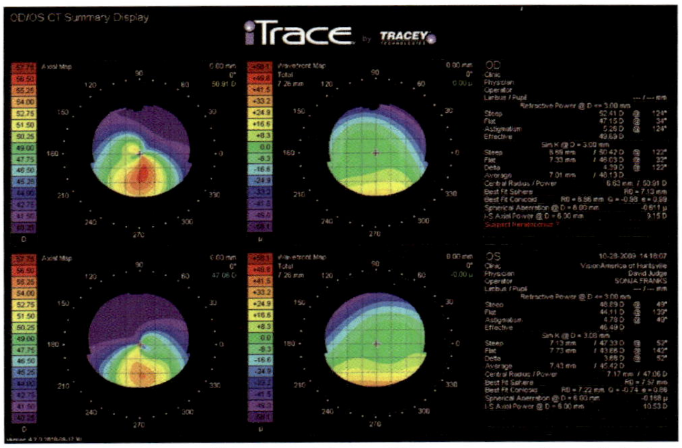


**Figure 8-1.** The earliest suspicion of keratoconus is an inferior or central steepening, with or without a difference between the keratometry of the fellow eye. (Reprinted with permission of Tracy Schroeder Swartz, OD, MS, FAAO.)

Recently, interest in biomechanics and long-term outcomes in the fellow eye in keratoconus has increased. Bilaterality of keratoconus remains a debatable topic. Certain large studies concluded that unilateral keratoconus is a rare entity and up to 50% of fellow eyes of a keratoconic eye eventually develop keratoconus, with the greatest risk of development in the first 6 years of diagnosis.[48-54]

The earliest suspicion of keratoconus is an inferior or central steepening, with or without a difference between the keratometry of fellow eyes (Figure 8-1). There may be mild astigmatism, with or without any corneal thinning. Classic signs of keratoconus, such as Munson's sign, Rizzuti's sign, and Fleischer ring, may not be present. According to a classification proposed by Rabinowitz, this presentation is known as keratoconus suspect.[55] Several indices have been used to differentiate these patients from normal eyes, particularly in patients presenting for elective refractive procedures. However, "keratoconus suspect" is a diagnosis with high sensitivity and therefore holds a high rate of false-positives. Some of these patients will not develop keratoconus and are simply on the tail end of the normal population distribution.

Forme fruste keratoconus (FFKC) presents with topographic changes not causing any visual symptoms and no ocular morbidity other than mild spherocylinder refractive error (Figure 8-2A). These patients are at a higher risk of developing keratoconus. The fellow eyes in cases of FFKC (Figure 8-2B) may have normal topography or a mildly steep cornea, and are also at a higher-than-normal risk for keratoconus. These eyes are also at risk of developing post-LASIK ectasia, so excimer laser ablation should be avoided. *Early keratoconus* is another term used to describe patients who have no slit-lamp findings but have subtle signs like early scissoring on retinoscopy in addition to topographic deviations seen in "forme fruste" keratoconus.[55]

As keratoconus advances, the topographic features associated with keratoconus manifest. These include refractive

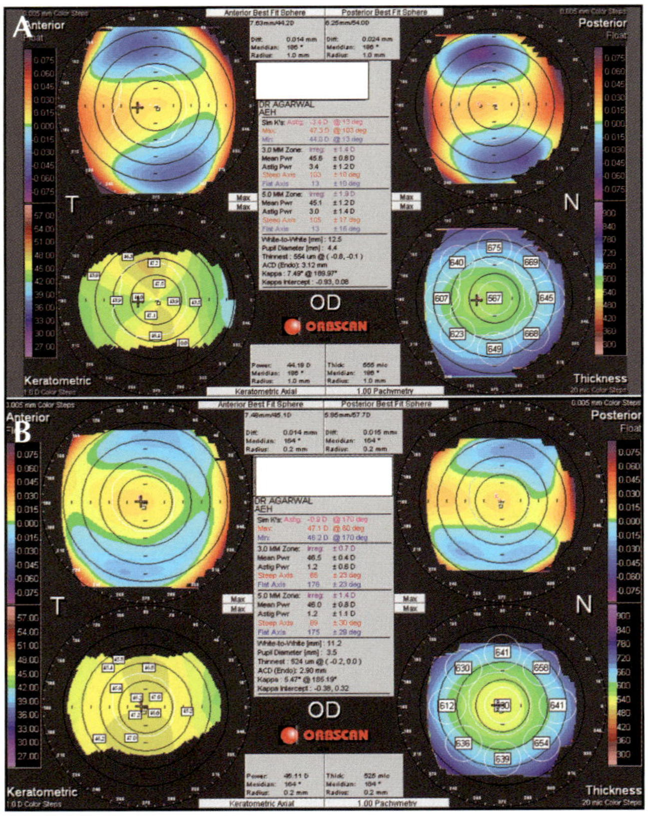


**Figure 8-2.** (A) A case of forme fruste keratoconus. Note the steepest keratometric value of 47.7 and 47.5, the astigmatism of 3.4 D, and the asymmetric bow-tie. The patient has a normal corneal thickness and posterior elevation as of now. (B) A case with steep corneal curvature, low astigmatism, normal posterior float, and low pachymetry. This patient had a fellow-eye forme fruste keratoconus.

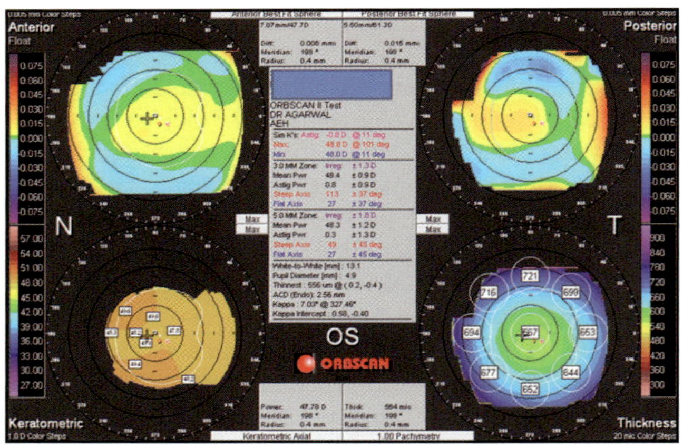


**Figure 8-3.** A case of suspected early keratoconus, with keratometry values <50 D. Even though the pachymetry seems relatively normal and the astigmatism is low, this patient should not undergo LASIK.

islands (Figures 8-3 through 8-5). An island of dioptric power results from increased corneal curvature surrounded by concentric annuluses of decreasing power.[7,16,24,56] This island may be in either of the 2 inferior quadrants

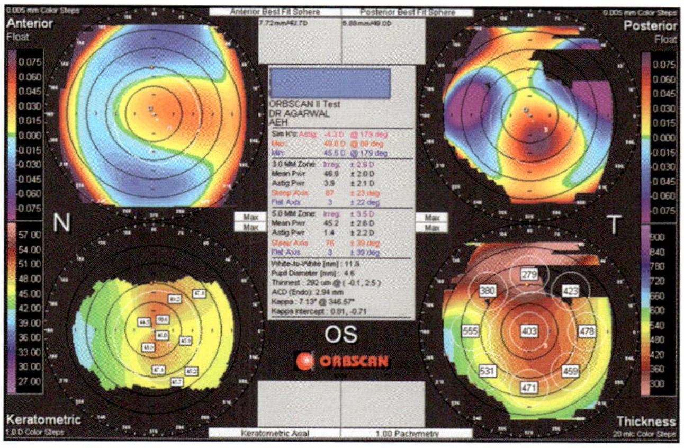


**Figure 8-4.** A case of moderate keratoconus. Note the asymmetric bowtie, high posterior elevations, and low central corneal thickness. The extremely low pachymetry readings in the superior cornea are artifactual, due to a superior corneal nebulomacular haze.

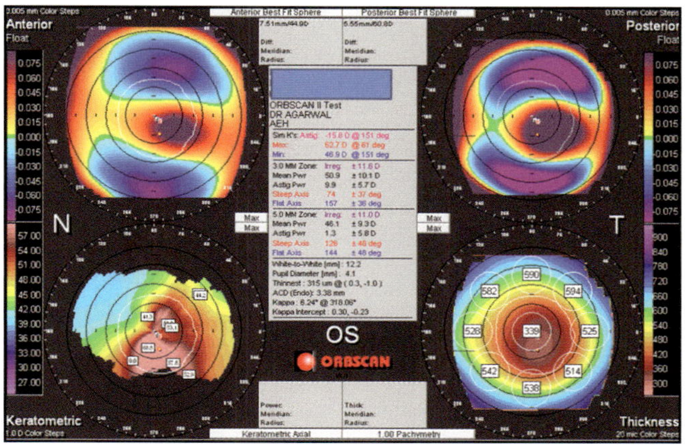


**Figure 8-5.** A case of advanced keratoconus. Note the very high astigmatism (15 D), corneal thinning, and high posterior as well as anterior elevation.

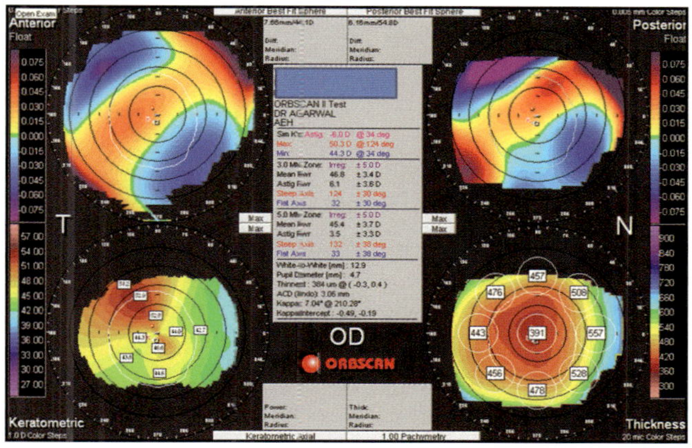


**Figure 8-6.** A case of atypical keratoconus with superior meridians being steeper than the inferior. Note that other signs of keratoconus, such as asymmetric bowtie, thin cornea, and high posterior elevation, are present.

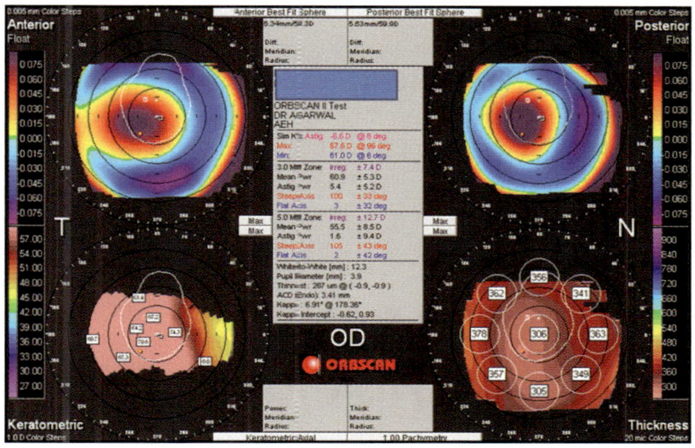


**Figure 8-7.** A case of keratoglobus. Note the generalized high keratometry (>60 D) with astigmatism, low pachymetry values extending from limbus to limbus, and very high posterior and anterior elevations.

(in primary keratoconus) or central (in secondary keratoconus); however, the steepening involves more than one quadrant as the disease progresses. A difference in the powers of the interior and superior cornea is called inferosuperior power asymmetry. Skewing of the steepest radial axes above and below the horizontal meridian may also occur. Increased posterior elevation may be noted on tomography, where the area of maximum steepening corresponds with the area of reduced corneal pachymetry. In pellucid marginal degeneration, the maximal thinning is just below the area of maximum dioptric power. An asymmetric bow-tie, or "kissing bird" appearance, may be seen in some patients, while others will demonstrate a globus type of cone or, rarely, superior keratoconus where steeper values may be found superiorly rather than inferiorly (Figure 8-6).

In addition to topographic signs, higher-order aberration (HOA) profiles in early keratoconus are being investigated.[57-60] Alio and Shabayek have suggested grading criteria for the same.[60] Topography following intrastromal ring implantation and collagen cross-linking topography can be used to monitor treatment efficacy, stability, and improvement in the keratometric power of the anterior corneal surface.[61-64]

# Keratoglobus

Unlike keratoconus, keratoglobus characterizes a more diffuse involvement of the cornea.[65,66] Generalized thinning is seen extending from limbus to limbus (Figure 8-7). Features suggestive of keratoconus, keratoglobus, or pellucid marginal degeneration can be found in the fellow eyes, suggesting a similar etiology for the 3.[67,68] Clinical findings in keratoglobus include the lack of a specific bowtie or similar pattern but rather a diffusely steep cornea with irregular keratometry values, a high posterior elevation, and reduced pachymetry Keratoglobus has been associated

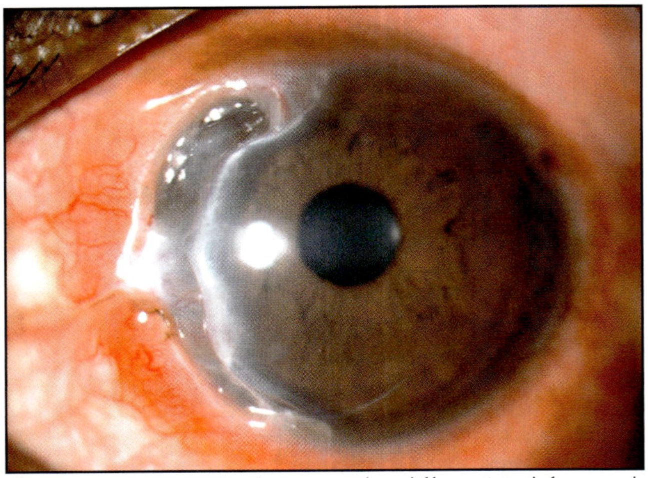

**Figure 8-8.** Mooren's ulcer must be differentiated from pellucid marginal degeneration.

with other disorders like posterior polymorphous dystrophy, Lebers congenital amaurosis, subcapsular cataracts, and Rubinstein-Taybi syndrome.[68-73] There are sporadic reports of hydrops in a case of keratoglobus, which is managed using hyperosmotics with or without intracameral gas injections.[74-76]

# PELLUCID MARGINAL DEGENERATION

A cousin to keratoconus is pellucid marginal degeneration (PMD), which should be differentiated from Mooren's ulcer (Figure 8-8). The term *pellucid* means "clear" and is used to differentiate PMD from Terrien's marginal degeneration. PMD demonstrates peripheral thinning, which is opacified or translucent. PMD can present as progressive astigmatism with difficulty in contact lens wear, frequent change of glasses, or an incidental fellow eye of a "normal eye" with 20/20 acuity.

PMD differs from keratoconus because the area of thinning most often occurs inferiorly to the area of increased dioptric power (Figure 8-9). The midperipheral cornea may decrease in power above the inferior oblique meridians. Literature describes flattening of the central cornea along a vertical axis and steepening of the inferior corneal periphery, which may extend into midperipheral inferior oblique corneal meridians.[77] The "claw sign," which was previously thought to be strongly associated with PMD, has recently been shown to be nonspecific and may be associated with keratoconus.[78] The HOA profiles and Gaussian fitting patterns for corneal topographic maps have been found to be different for keratoconus and PMD, perhaps because of the difference in the location of the apex and resulting power distribution.[79,80]

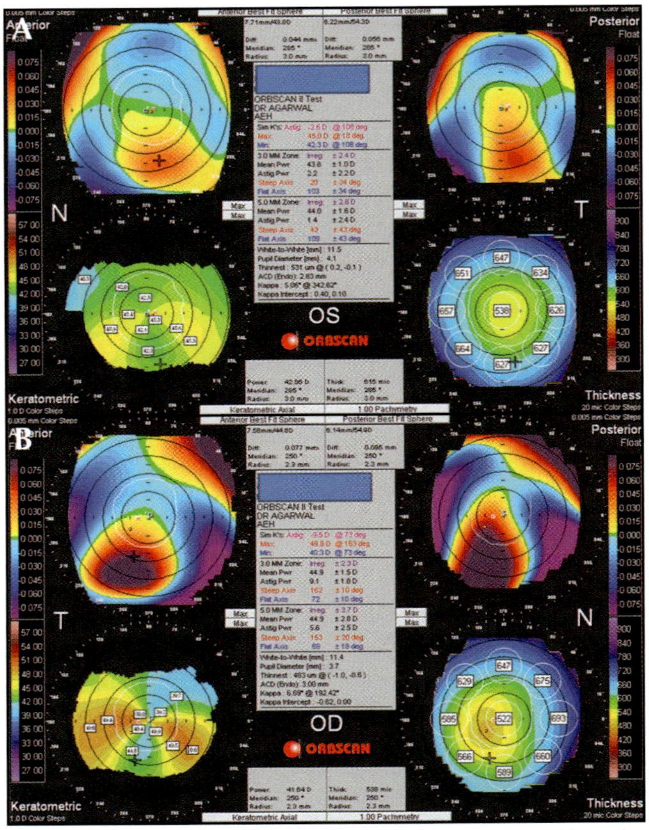


**Figure 8-9.** (A) Early pellucid marginal degeneration. Note the "crab claw sign," also called the "bow-tie sign." The thinnest point does not coincide with the steepest one, and, more markedly, the point with the highest posterior elevation is displaced inferiorly. (B) An advanced case of pellucid marginal degeneration. Note that the area of steepening (the claw area on the topography map) lies above the thinnest area on the pachymetry map. The points of highest posterior and anterior elevation are displaced inferiorly. The thinnest point has a relatively normal keratometry.

# KERATOECTASIA

Keratoectasia, or ectasia following corneal refractive surgery, is one of the most dreaded and challenging complications for refractive surgeons. It is important to understand that all subtractive methods where the excimer laser is used (LASIK, epi-LASIK, LASEK, and PRK) and incisional methods (radial keratotomy or astigmatic keratotomy) predispose the cornea to varying levels of biomechanical weakening. The common presenting sign in most of these patients is increasing astigmatism months to years after refractive surgery. Disturbance of strong peripheral and anterior corneal collagen fibers following RK may induce ectasia, but because excimer is presently the predominant method of elective surgical correction, the subsequent discussion is based on the biomechanics of excimer procedures.

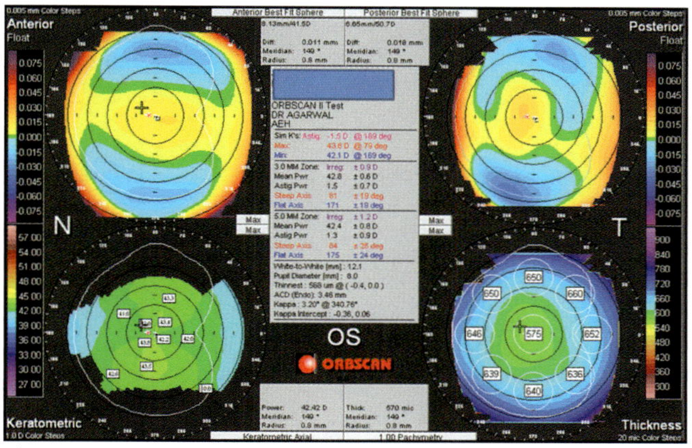


**Figure 8-10.** A topographically normal LASIK candidate with moderate astigmatism, normal keratometry values, good corneal thickness, and low posterior elevation. The refractive error was stable at -4 D sphere and -1.75 D cylinder for 3 years. Based on topography and refraction, he is a good candidate for LASIK.

A limit of 250 μm of unablated cornea or residual bed thickness (RBT) was assumed adequate for corneal biomechanical strength.[81,82] However, as cases with ectasia occurred in patients with RBT greater than 250 μm, this numerical limit was found to be inadequate. As understanding of corneal hysteresis, elasticity, and other biomechanical properties increased, it was realized that a simple numerical limit may not be safe.[83]

Multiple parameters and ectasia scoring schemes have been used in the literature.[84-106] Randleman's Ectasia Risk Score System is one such recent index based on topography, age, preoperative corneal thickness, RBT, and spherical equivalent.[85,92,94] This scoring system was subsequently validated in a follow-up study.[94] However, another study found using the score would have put the patients at a higher risk warning as these patients eventually did not develop ectasia on follow-up.[95] Conversely, cases with low risk scores using the Randleman criteria and cases with RBT more than 300 μm have also been demonstrated to develop post-LASIK ectasias.[96,97] This suggests that other biomechanical evaluations and accurate predictions of variable tissue behavior as a function of time may be required to provide an improved risk assessment for keratoectasia.

When evaluating patients for elective surgical correction, it is important to select cases with low topographic risk for ectasia using topography (Figure 8-10). It is normal to have a mild amount of topographic astigmatism post-LASIK with other parameters being stable (Figure 8-11). Progressive astigmatism, increased irregularity, increasing posterior float, and a progressive decrease in pachymetry are highly suggestive of keratoectasia (Figures 8-12 through 8-14). Cases with even mild interface or surface haze may result in a falsely low value upon optical pachymetry measurement using slit-scanning technology, and diagnosis must not be made on this isolated criterion.[98,99]

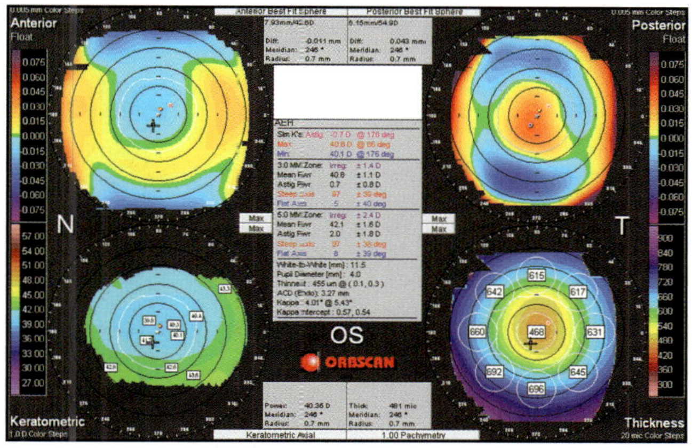


**Figure 8-11.** Note the low amount of astigmatism and slightly decentered ablation in this post-LASIK patient. The clinical picture is stable for 2 years without progression of astigmatism, change in uncorrected or best-corrected vision, increase in posterior elevation, or reduction in pachymetry.

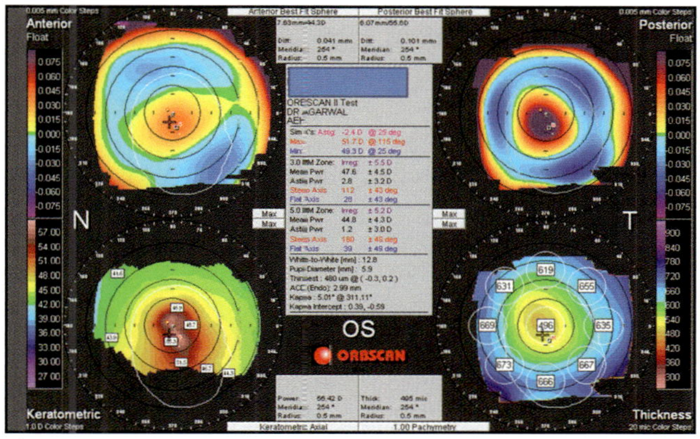


**Figure 8-12.** Post-LASIK ectasia. Note the high keratometry, astigmatism, and elevated posterior float. There has been a progressive deterioration over a period of the last 7 months, after an initial stability of 1 year in this patient.

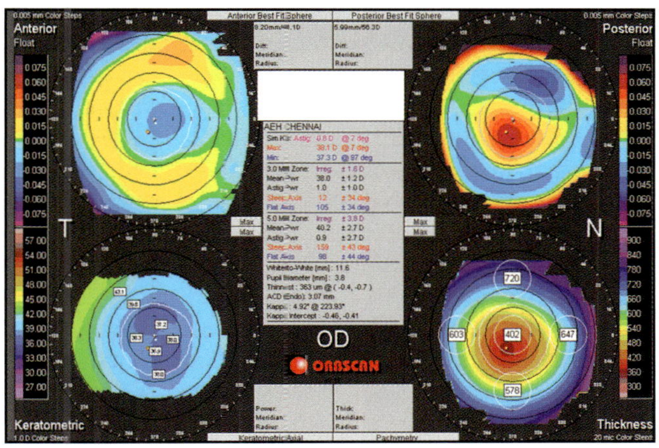


**Figure 8-13.** Suspicious case of post-LASIK ectasia: Note the asymmetric bowtie pattern, high posterior elevation, and low pachymetry readings in this 8-months-postoperative patient. The astigmatism and keratometry are still numerically normal and thus were not denoted as "red" on the color scale.

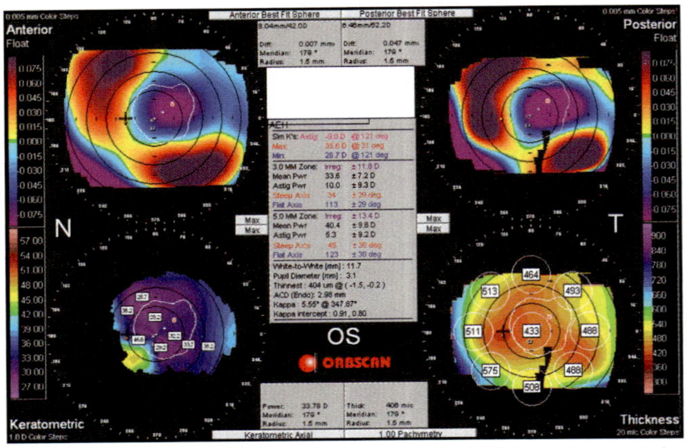


**Figure 8-14.** Post-radial keratotomy ectasia. Note the peripheral data loss, high irregular astigmatism, multiple areas of high posterior elevation, and a trifocal distribution of corneal thinning. These cases can be rehabilitated using contact lenses and/or keratoplasty.

In such cases, ultrasound pachymetry validates measurement. Furthermore, all cases of post-LASIK astigmatism should not be automatically linked to keratoectasia. Flap contraction, surface irregularity, and severe dry eyes may result in topographic findings that incorrectly suggest keratoectasias.

## Dry Eyes

Dry eye disease comprises a constellation of symptoms and signs resulting from primary or secondary reduction in the amount or quality of the tear film or problems with the ocular surface. Inferior steepening in the absence of thinning pachymetry is often seen (Figure 8-15). A review study noted the prevalence ranged from 7% in the United States to 33% in Taiwan and Japan and summarized risk factors as advanced age, female gender, smoking, extreme heat or cold weather conditions, low relative humidity, use of video display terminals, history of refractive surgery, contact lens wear, and certain medications.[100] The features of dry eye range from nonspecific difficulty in reading and near work and tired eyes to paradoxically increased tearing.

Topography using Placido imaging is a noninvasive method to assess the tear break-up time (TBUT), a test that requires a smooth anterior corneal-tear film-air complex. Cases of unstable tear film can be screened using topography. In a study comparing noninvasive and invasive TBUT, short average tear break-up values are associated with small differences between these 2 methods, whereas long average tear break-up values are associated with large differences between the methods.[101] High-speed videokeratoscopy has been used as an investigational tool in the evaluation of dry eyes.[102] A new tear film stability analysis system (TSAS) based on the phenomenon that topographic maps are subject

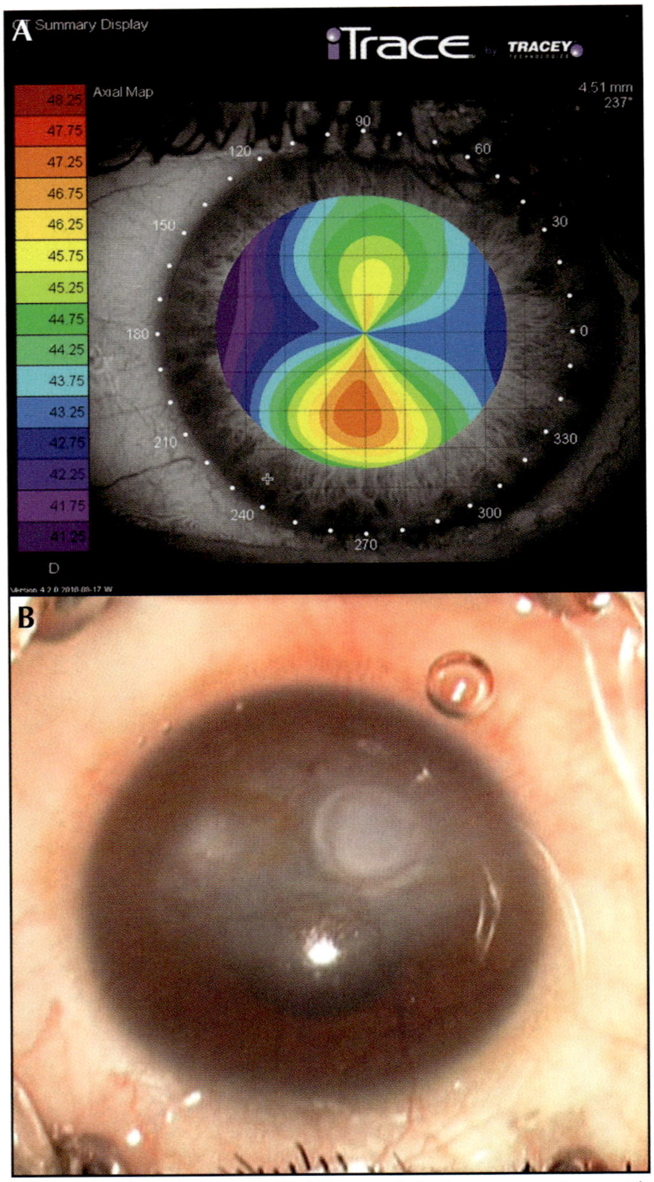


**Figure 8-15.** (A) Dry eye disease. Inferior steepening with normal pachymetry is a common sign. (Reprinted with permission of Tracy Schroeder Swartz, OD, MS, FAAO.) (B) In severe cases of dry eye, melts, scarring, and neovascularization occur.

to change because of fluctuation of tear film stability has previously been used.[103-105]

## Contact Lens Warpage

The phenomenon where habitual contact lens wear alters corneal topography is called "corneal warpage." Warpage has been reported with all lens types: PMMA, gas permeable, and hydrogel. Clinical signs include reduced vision, irregular keratometry mires, and irregular topography.

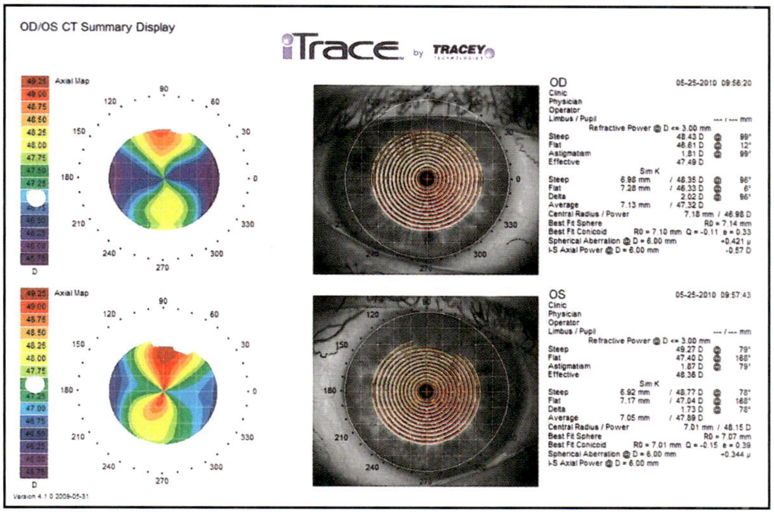


**Figure 8-16.** Contact lens warpage is often seen in patients with a history of gas-permeable lens wear but can occur with hydrogel lens wear as well. (Reprinted with permission of Tracy Schroeder Swartz, OD, MS, FAAO.)

Often, there is an absence of slit-lamp findings. Topographic patterns may resemble keratoconus or PMD, or they may be irregular with no particular pattern (Figure 8-16). CL warpage is often identified in patients seeking elective vision correction. When preparing for keratorefractive surgery or intraocular lens implantation, resolution of topographic irregularities is required. Resolution of contact lens warpage should be closely monitored using refractive error and corneal curvature. Irregularity typically improves after lens wear is discontinued, but, in some cases, does not completely resolve. The amount of time required for resolution varies widely. Mobillia and Kenyon[105] reported that, when chronic lens wearers discontinue contact lens wear, the refractive error changes quickly, and astigmatism increases. The change reaches a maximum approximately 3 days after lens removal. These corneal contour and physiologic changes require time to resolve.

While long-term gas-permeable wear is commonly thought to cause more warpage, Wang et al[106] found that soft extended wearers required 11.6 weeks, more than the 8.8 weeks required by gas-permeable lens wearers. Resolution of topographic abnormality averaged nearly 8 weeks with an incidence of 12%.

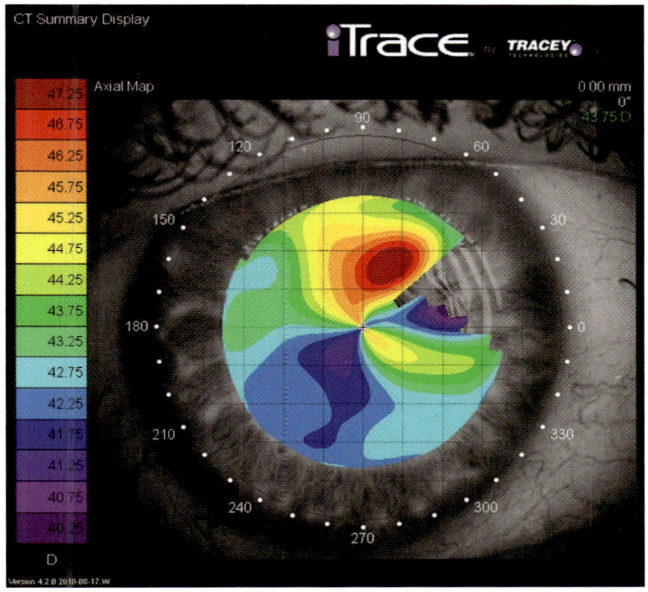


**Figure 8-17.** Irregular astigmatism secondary to severe EBMD. (Reprinted with permission of Tracy Schroeder Swartz, OD, MS, FAAO.)

## Corneal Dystrophies

Anterior corneal dystrophies affecting the epithelium, Bowman's membrane, and anterior stroma may alter the cornea's topographical landscape. The 3 main epithelial dystrophies include epithelial basement membrane dystrophy (EBMD), Reiss-Buckler dystrophy, and Meesman's dystrophy, with EBMD being the most common (Figure 8-17). Stromal dystrophies may have more severe effects on vision due to loss of transparency, but may also cause RCE and dry eye. These include granular, lattice, Schnyder's, and macular dystrophies.

## Corneal Degenerations

Several corneal degenerations may alter corneal topography. Most commonly known to affect topography are Mooren's ulcer, Terrien's ulcer, band keratopathy, and Slazmann's nodules. Mooren's ulcer, a peripheral ulcerative condition typically presenting in patients older than 40, is often rapidly progressive. Terrien's ulcer, another peripheral ulcerative condition, occurs more in men and at a younger age than Mooren's ulceration.

Band keratopathy results from calcium salts in Bowman's layer causing opacification of the anterior cornea. It can cause severely irregular topography and poor tear film distribution.

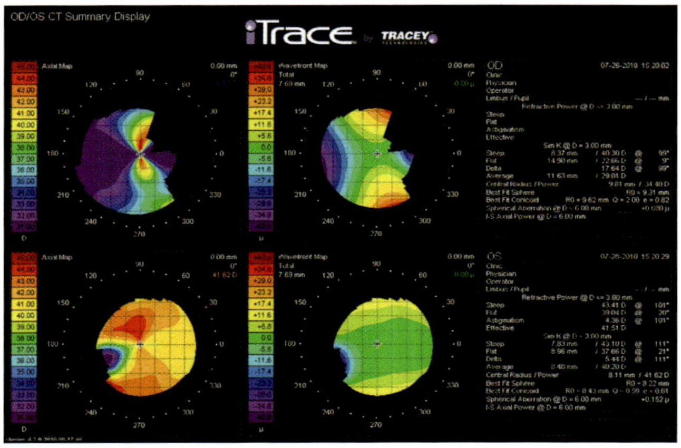


**Figure 8-18.** Salzmann's nodules may cause severe corneal irregularity and vision loss. (Reprinted with permission of Tracy Schroeder Swartz, OD, MS, FAAO.)

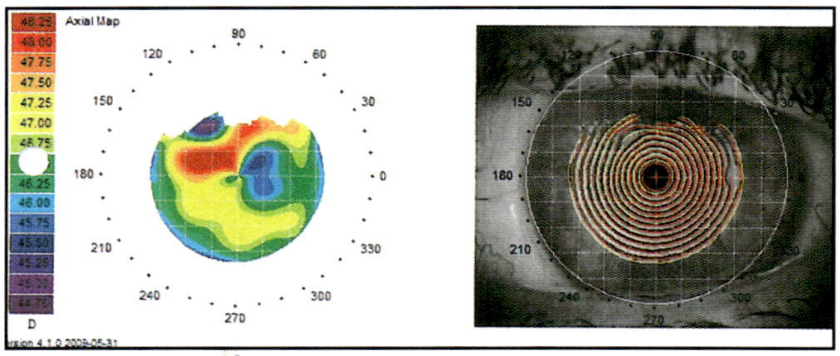


**Figure 8-19.** Corneal scarring, in this case from a corneal ulcer corresponding to the flat blue area, may cause irregular astigmatism. (Reprinted with permission of Tracy Schroeder Swartz, OD, MS, FAAO.)

Salzmann's nodular degeneration may cause irregular astigmatism (Figure 8-18) and scarring and may require surgical removal.

# Corneal Scarring

Opacification of the cornea may result from infection, trauma, chronic inflammation, and surgery. Infectious keratitis can cause severe corneal scarring with severe corneal irregularity (Figure 8-19). Particularly devastating infections include Acanthamoeba keratitis, bacterial keratitis, fungal keratitis, and sclerokeratitis.

Herpes keratitis, caused by the herpes simplex virus (HSV), is a leading cause of corneal blindness in industrialized nations. A single severe infection, or repeated infections, may result in scarring and irregular astigmatism (Figure 8-20). Prior to surgical correction, irregular astigmatism should be addressed cautiously with a gas-permeable contact lens and frequent lubrication. In some cases, corneal opacification limits visual prognosis, and corneal thinning may limit laser treatment options. Penetrating keratoplasty

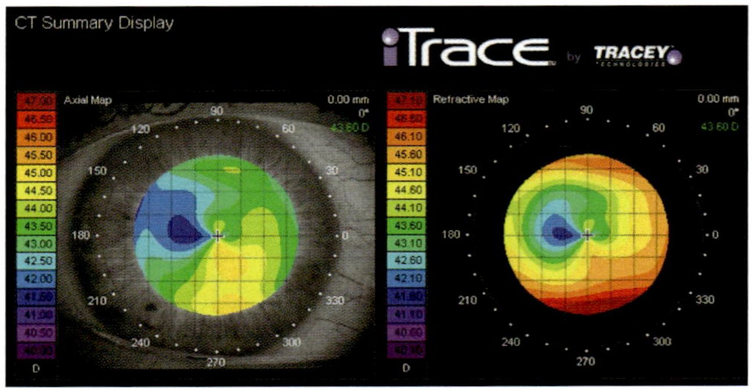


**Figure 8-20.** Herpetic keratitis resulted in scarring and irregular astigmatism. The effect on vision is illustrated in the refractive map, and vision was limited to 20/30 in spectacles.

becomes the only alternative in such cases, providing the eye is quiet and anatomy is normal.

# Immune-Mediated Disorders

Immune-mediated disorders often cause corneal pathology and irregular astigmatism. Diseases range from the very mild to devastatingly severe and include atopic keratoconjunctivitis, marginal corneal infiltrates associated with blepharoconjunctivitis (Figure 8-21), nonulcerative keratitis, ocular mucous membrane pemphigoid, peripheral keratitis, and peripheral ulcerative keratitis associated with systemic immune-mediated diseases, including rheumatoid arthritis, Wegener granulomatosis, systemic lupus erythematosus, and inflammatory bowel disease. Treatment includes topical steroids and systemic immunosuppressive agents, but clinical findings may progress despite aggressive treatment.

# Pterygium

Pterygium (Figure 8-22) is an elastotic disorder of the cornea, occurring more frequently in the nasal area of the bulbar conjunctiva than the temporal. UV light may induce corneal invasion of matrix metalloproteinases, expressing altered limbal epithelial basal cells.[107,108] Without the advent of topography, the indications for pterygium removal included cosmetic complaint, encroachment on the pupillary axis, or increasing cylindrical power. With topography, early changes such as increasing irregularity within the central 5-mm zone prior to it affecting the refraction indicate surgical intervention. Correction can occur earlier, preventing a dissection affecting the pupillary axis. Both topographic profile and manifest astigmatism have been shown to improve after removal of the pterygium.[109,110]

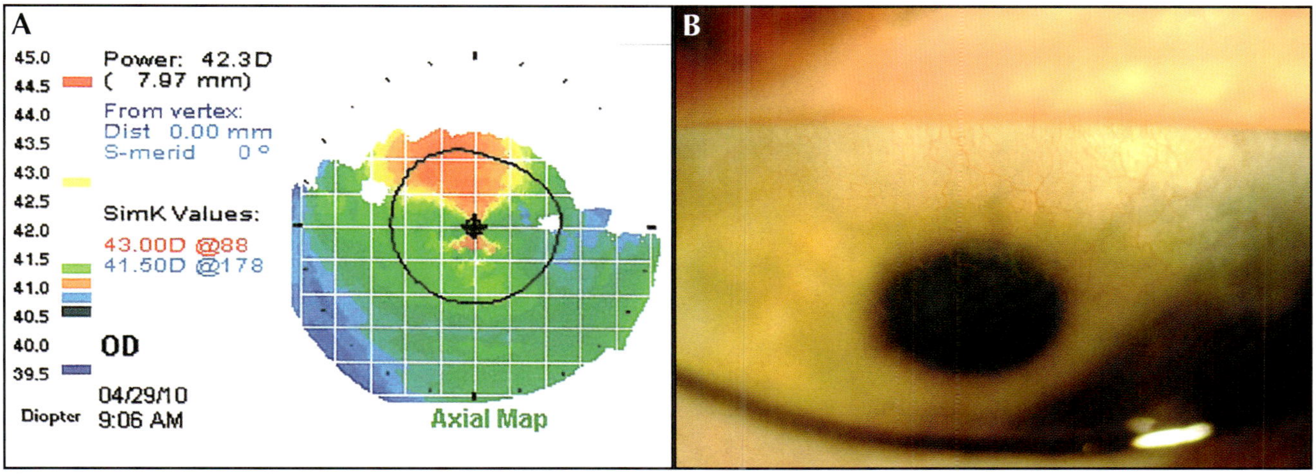


**Figure 8-21.** (A) Marginal keratitis causing superior data loss and irregular astigmatism. (B) Slit-lamp view of the superior cornea.

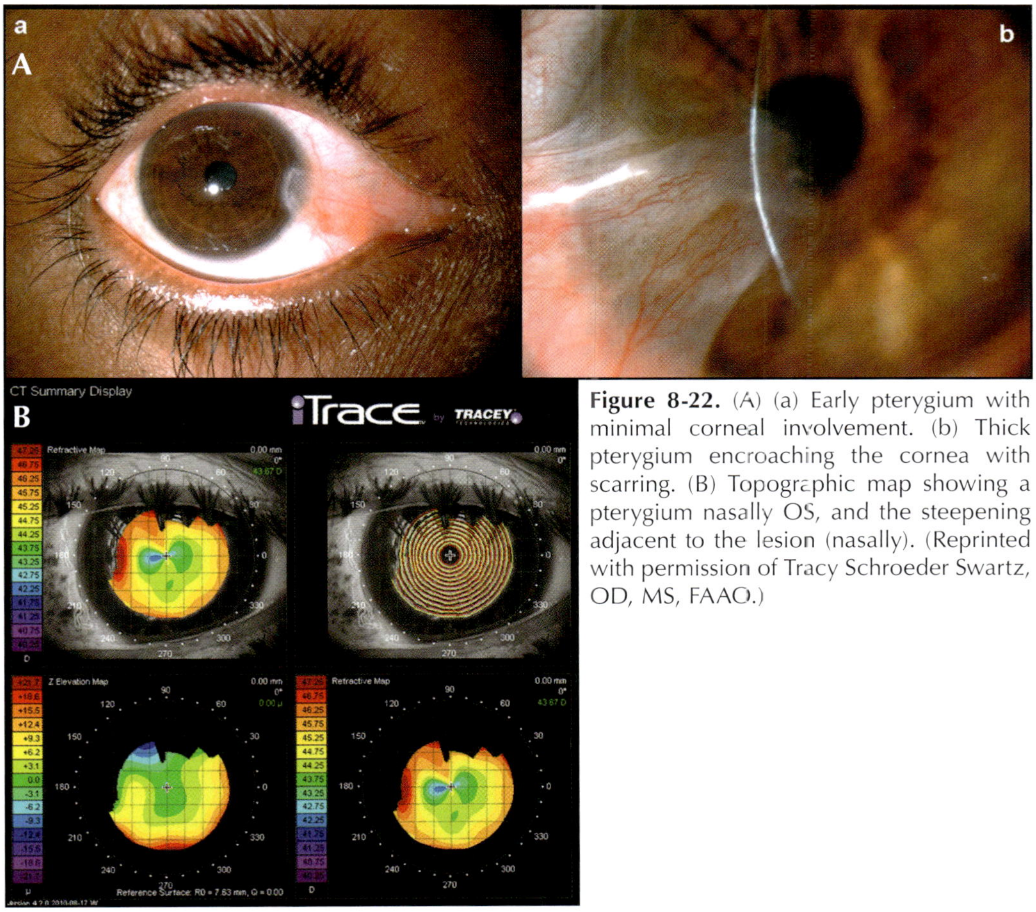


**Figure 8-22.** (A) (a) Early pterygium with minimal corneal involvement. (b) Thick pterygium encroaching the cornea with scarring. (B) Topographic map showing a pterygium nasally OS, and the steepening adjacent to the lesion (nasally). (Reprinted with permission of Tracy Schroeder Swartz, OD, MS, FAAO.)

## POSTKERATOPLASTY

Topography plays a vital role in the postoperative management and optical rehabilitation of cases that have undergone keratoplasty (Figures 8-23 through 8-25). Selective suture removal based on the topography may be very useful in improvement of uncorrected visual acuity by reducing the postoperative astigmatism.[111,112] Intraoperative topography devices have been shown to reduce postoperative cylinder.[113] In cases of postkeratoplasty astigmatism persistent after suture removal, arcuate keratotomy or excimer laser ablation may be performed based on the topography findings.[114-117]

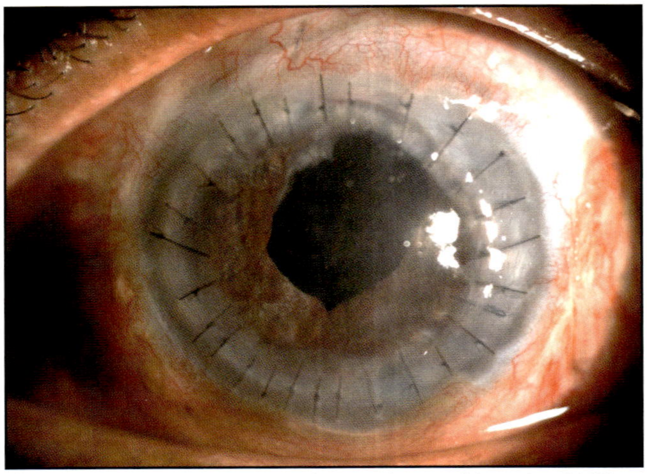

**Figure 8-23.** Post-penetrating keratoplasty with a glued IOL.

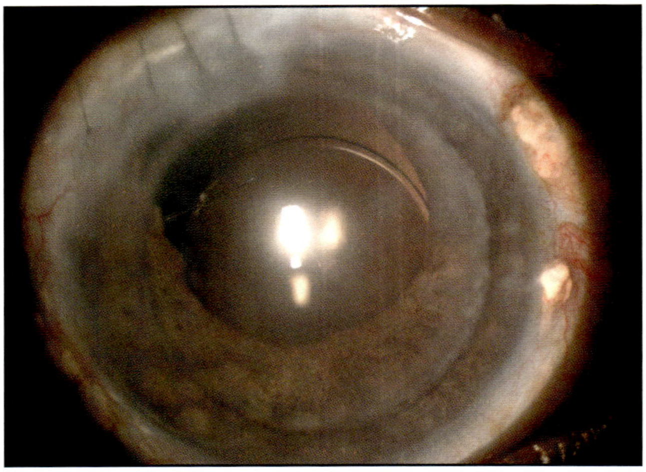

**Figure 8-24.** Intralase endothelial keratoplasty with a glued IOL—1-year postoperatively.

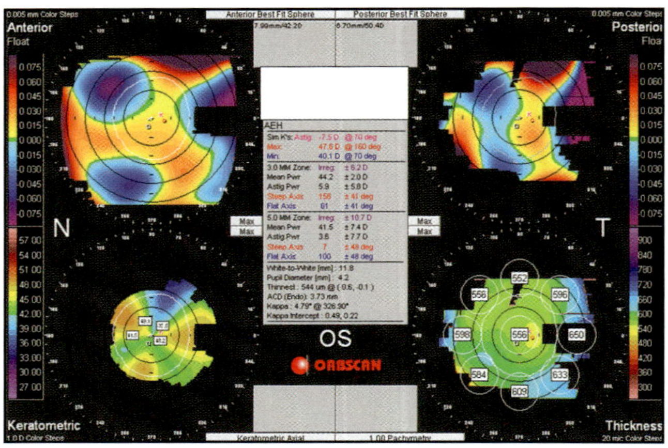


**Figure 8-25.** Postkeratoplasty astigmatism. Note the high irregular astigmatism due to tight sutures and the abrupt shift in the pachymetry due to graft-host size disparity.

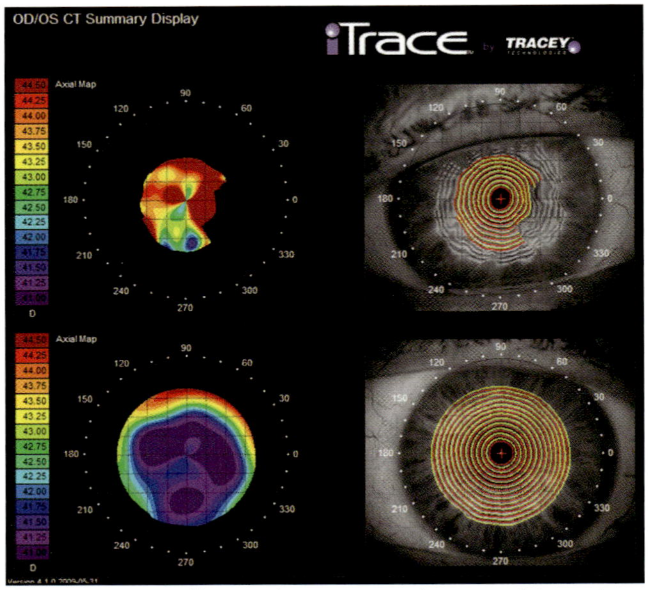


**Figure 8-26.** Small central zones are often noted in patients with a history of radial keratotomy). (Reprinted with permission of Tracy Schroeder Swartz, OD, MS, FAAO.) The small irregular zone seen on the axial map OD (top row) corresponds to the easily noted irregularity seen on the Placido image. The left eye (bottom row) was 20/20 and asymptomatic.

## Radial Keratotomy

Incisional procedures alter corneal curvature resulting in a change in the refractive error. Unfortunately, it is not uncommon for astigmatism to increase in magnitude and irregularity. Patients with a history of RK often demonstrate excessively small optical zones and severe central flattening with a loss of best-corrected vision (Figure 8-26).

## Keratorefractive Surgery

Excimer procedures ablate tissue, altering corneal shape to reduce the refractive error and allow the patient lens independence upon refractive correction. Resulting topographical patterns should be easily recognizable. Normal myopic treatments ablate centrally, resulting in central thinning corresponding to the ablation area and a central plateau. This creates positive spherical aberration (Figure 8-27). Hyperopic treatments result in central steepening and negative spherical aberration (Figure 8-28). Decentered myopic and hyperopic ablations, when significant, result in polyplopia (Figure 8-29).

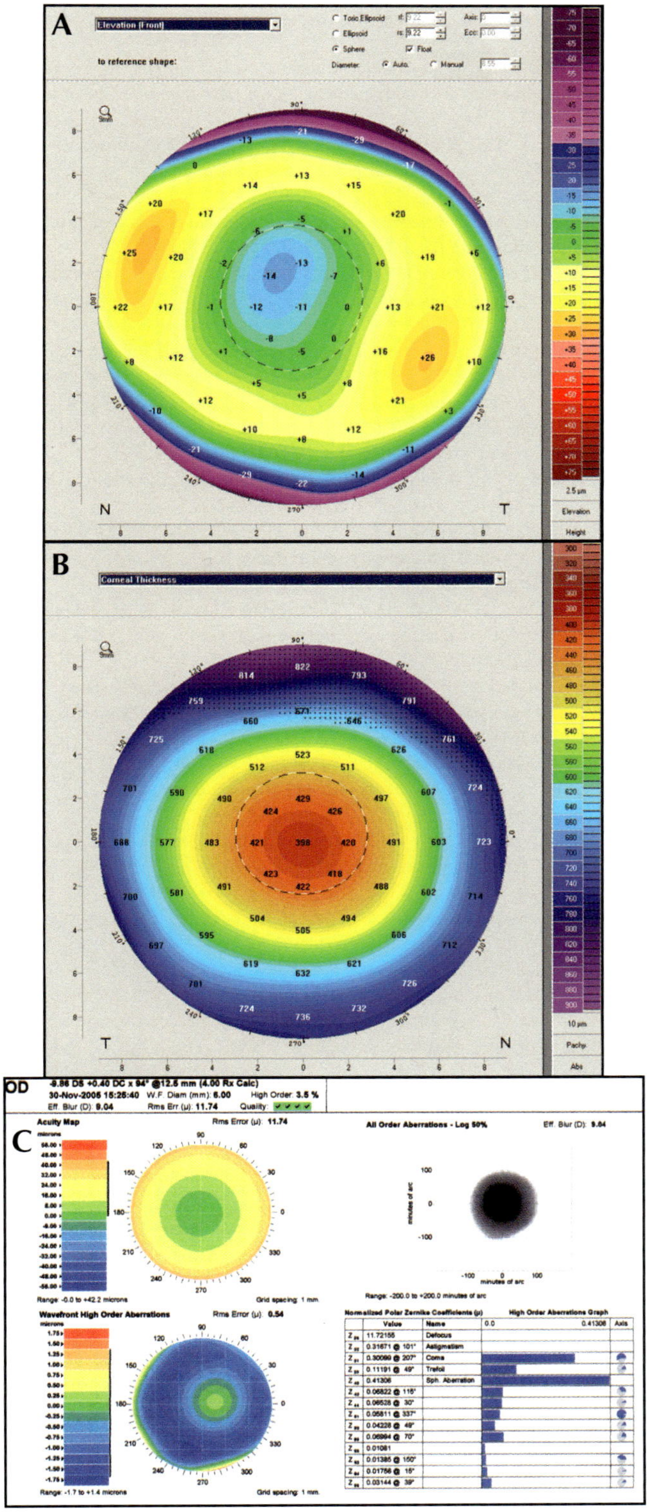


**Figure 8-27.** (A) Myopic excimer treatments cause central flattening seen on the elevation map. (B) Myopic excimer treatments cause central thinning. (C) Myopic excimer treatments cause a more oblate cornea and positive spherical aberration. (Reprinted with permission from Trattler WB, Majmudar PA, Luchs JI, Swartz TS. *Corneal Handbook*. Thorofare, NJ: SLACK Incorporated; 2009.)

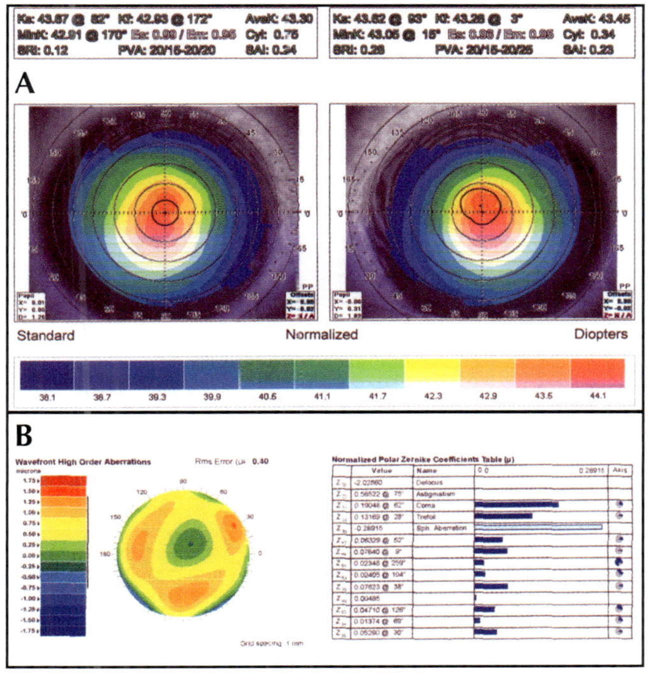


**Figure 8-28.** (A) Hyperopic excimer treatments cause central steepening. (B) Hyperopic excimer treatments cause negative spherical aberration. (Reprinted with permission from Trattler WB, Majmudar PA, Luchs JI, Swartz TS. *Corneal Handbook*. Thorofare, NJ: SLACK Incorporated; 2009.)

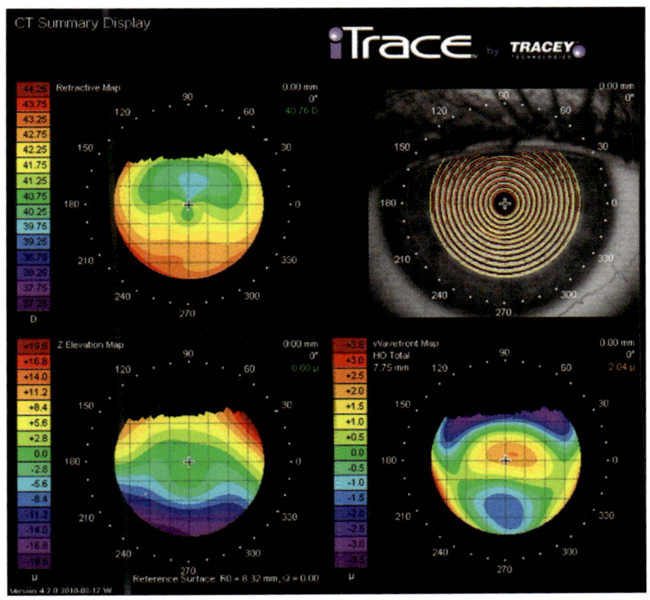


**Figure 8-29.** Decentered myopic ablation. Note the coma on the wavefront map corresponds to the asymmetry noted on the axial and elevation maps. This can be differentiated from ectasia by questioning if the visual disturbance was noted immediately after surgery (suggesting decentration) or developed over time (suggesting ectasia). (Reprinted with permission of Tracy Schroeder Swartz, OD, MS, FAAO.)

# Conclusion

To conclude, judicious use of corneal topography can be useful for the clinician in cases that are likely to be missed on clinical examination only. There is a unique role of topography in cases with corneal ectasias and other pathology, which can be well-supplemented by the use of wavefront aberrometry in these cases. As combined platforms will evolve and topography devices will become more sensitive and specific, accurate predictions on cases like post-LASIK ectasia or keratoconus suspects will improve.

# References


1. Swartz T, Marten L, Wang M. Measuring the cornea: the latest developments in corneal topography. *Curr Opin Ophthalmol.* 2007;18(4):325-333.
2. Wilson SE, Ambrosio R. Computerized corneal topography and its importance to wavefront technology. *Cornea.* 2001;20(5):441-454.
3. Naseri A, McLeod SD, Lietman T. Evaluating the human optical system: corneal topography and wavefront analysis. *Ophthalmol Clin North Am.* 2001;14(2):269-273, vii.
4. Mejía-Barbosa Y, Malacara-Hernández D. A review of methods for measuring corneal topography. *Optom Vis Sci.* 2001;78(4):240-253.
5. Herrmann C, Ludwig U, Duncker G. Corneal topography. Analysis of the corneal surface. *Ophthalmologe.* 2008;105(2):193-204.
6. Cairns G, McGhee CN. Orbscan computerized topography: attributes, applications, and limitations. *J Cataract Refract Surg.* 2005;31(1):205-220.
7. Rao SN, Raviv T, Majmudar PA, Epstein RJ. Role of Orbscan II in screening keratoconus suspects before refractive corneal surgery. *Ophthalmology.* 2002;109(9):1642-1646.
8. Giráldez-Fernández MJ, Díaz-Rey A, García-Resua C, Yebra-Pimentel-Vilar E. Diurnal variations of central and paracentral corneal thickness and curvature. *Arch Soc Esp Oftalmol.* 2008;83(3):183-191.
9. Martin R, de Juan V, Rodríguez G, Cuadrado R, Fernandez I. Measurement of corneal swelling variations without removal of the contact lens during extended wear. *Invest Ophthalmol Vis Sci.* 2007;48(7):3043-3050.
10. Asano-Kato N, Toda I, Sakai C, et al. Pupil decentration and iris tilting detected by Orbscan: anatomic variations among healthy subjects and influence on outcomes of laser refractive surgeries. *J Cataract Refract Surg.* 2005;31(10):1938-1942.
11. Asensio I, Rahhal SM, Alonso L, Palanca-Sanfrancisco JM, Sanchis-Gimeno JA. Corneal thickness values before and after oxybuprocaine 0.4% eye drops. *Cornea.* 2003;22(6):527-532.
12. Maldonado MJ, López-Miguel A, Nieto JC, Cano-Parra J, Calvo B, Alió JL. Reliability of noncontact pachymetry after laser in situ keratomileusis. *Invest Ophthalmol Vis Sci.* 2009;50(9):4135-4141.
13. Read SA, Collins MJ. Diurnal variation of corneal shape and thickness. *Optom Vis Sci.* 2009;86(3):170-180.
14. Nilforoushan MR, Speaker M, Marmor M, et al. Comparative evaluation of refractive surgery candidates with Placido topography, Orbscan II, Pentacam, and wavefront analysis. *J Cataract Refract Surg.* 2008;34(4):623-631.
15. Krachmer JH, Feder RS, Belin MW. Keratoconus and related noninflammatory corneal thinning disorders. *Surv Ophthalmol.* 1984;28(4):293-322.
16. Rabinowitz YS. Keratoconus. *Surv Ophthalmol.* 1998;42(4):297-319.
17. Sherwin T, Brookes NH. Morphological changes in keratoconus: pathology or pathogenesis. *Clin Experiment Ophthalmol.* 2004;32(2):211-217.
18. Parker J, Ko WW, Pavlopoulos G, Wolfe PJ, Rabinowitz YS, Feldman ST. Videokeratography of keratoconus in monozygotic twins. *J Refract Surg.* 1996;12(1):180-183.
19. Rabinowitz YS. Videokeratographic indices to aid in screening for keratoconus. *J Refract Surg.* 1995;11(5):371-379.
20. Maeda N, Klyce SD, Smolek MK. Comparison of methods for detecting keratoconus using videokeratography. *Arch Ophthalmol.* 1995;113(7):870-874.
21. Rabinowitz YS, McDonnell PJ. Computer-assisted corneal topography in keratoconus. *Refract Corneal Surg.* 1989;5(6):400-408.
22. Twa MD, Parthasarathy S, Roberts C, Mahmoud AM, Raasch TW, Bullimore MA. Automated decision tree classification of corneal shape. *Optom Vis Sci.* 2005;82(12):1038-1046.
23. Li X, Yang H, Rabinowitz YS. Longitudinal study of keratoconus progression. *Exp Eye Res.* 2007;85(4):502-507.
24. Li X, Yang H, Rabinowitz YS. Keratoconus: classification scheme based on videokeratography and clinical signs. *J Cataract Refract Surg.* 2009;35(9):1597-1603.
25. Karimian F, Aramesh S, Rabei HM, Javadi MA, Rafati N. Topographic evaluation of relatives of patients with keratoconus. *Cornea.* 2008;27(8):874-878.
26. Li X, Rabinowitz YS, Rasheed K, Yang H. Longitudinal study of the normal eyes in unilateral keratoconus patients. *Ophthalmology.* 2004;111(3):440-446.
27. Rabinowitz YS. Tangential vs sagittal videokeratographs in the "early" detection of keratoconus. *Am J Ophthalmol.* 1996;122(6):887-889.
28. Rabinowitz YS, Yang H, Brickman Y, et al. Videokeratography database of normal human corneas. *Br J Ophthalmol.* 1996;80(7):610-616.
29. Bron AJ, Rabinowitz YS. Corneal dystrophies and keratoconus. *Curr Opin Ophthalmol.* 1996;7(4):71-82.
30. Lin ML, Jhanji V, Vajpayee RB. Keratoconus associated with the Pierre Robin sequence. *Cont Lens Anterior Eye.* 2010;33(1):41-42.
31. Cremona FA, Ghosheh FR, Rapuano CJ, et al. Keratoconus associated with other corneal dystrophies. *Cornea.* 2009;28(2):127-135.
32. Sherwin JC, Hewitt AW, Ruddle JB, Mackey DA. Genetic isolates in ophthalmic diseases. *Ophthalmic Genet.* 2008;29(4):149-161.
33. Simon GJ, Grinbaum A. Anhidrotic ectodermal dysplasia with spontaneous corneal perforation and keratoconus. *Ophthalmic Surg Lasers Imaging.* 2004;35(6):495-498.
34. Georgiou T, Funnell CL, Cassels-Brown A, O'Conor R. Influence of ethnic origin on the incidence of keratoconus and associated atopic disease in Asians and white patients. *Eye (Lond).* 2004;18(4):379-383.
35. Kim J, Netto MV. Keratoconus associated with hyperimmunoglobulin E syndrome. *Cornea.* 2004;23(1):93-96.
36. Hughes AE, Dash DP, Jackson AJ, Frazer DG, Silvestri G. Familial keratoconus with cataract: linkage to the long arm of chromosome 15 and exclusion of andidate genes. *Invest Ophthalmol Vis Sci.* 2003;44(12):5063-5066.
37. Iqbal A, Jan S, Babar TF, Khan MD. Corneal complications of vernal catarrh. *J Coll Physicians Surg Pak.* 2003;13(7):394-397.
38. Incorvaia C, Parmeggiani F, Costagliola C, Perri P, Tittoni M, Sebastiani A. Congenital adrenal hyperplasia due to 21-hydroxylase deficiency associated with bilateral keratoconus. *Am J Ophthalmol.* 2003;135(4):557-559.
39. Igarashi S, Makita Y, Hikichi T, Mori F, Hanada K, Yoshida A. Association of keratoconus and Avellino corneal dystrophy. *Br J Ophthalmol.* 2003;87(3):367-368.
40. Gusek-Schneider GC, Langenbucher A, Seitz B. Association of keratoconus and Möbius' syndrome. *J Pediatr Ophthalmol Strabismus.* 2001;38(1):47-48.

41. Lichter H, Loya N, Sagie A, et al. Keratoconus and mitral valve prolapse. *Am J Ophthalmol.* 2000;129(5):667-668.
42. Koçak Altintas AG, Gül U, Duman S. Bilateral keratoconus associated with Hashimoto's disease, alopecia areata and atopic keratoconjunctivitis. *Eur J Ophthalmol.* 1999;9(2):130-133.
43. Macsai M, Maguen E, Nucci P. Keratoconus and Turner's syndrome. *Cornea.* 1997;16(5):534-536.
44. Wilhelmus KR. Keratoconus and progressive cone dystrophy. *Ophthalmologica.* 1995;209(5):278-279.
45. Elder MJ. Leber congenital amaurosis and its association with keratoconus and keratoglobus. *J Pediatr Ophthalmol Strabismus.* 1994;31(1):38-40.
46. Ascaso FJ, Del Buey MA, Huerva V, Latre B, Palomar A. Noonan's syndrome with keratoconus and optic disc coloboma. *Eur J Ophthalmol.* 1993;3(2):101-103.
47. Stokes DW, Parrish CM. Axenfeld's anomaly associated with Down's syndrome. *Cornea.* 1992;11(2):163-164.
48. Fontes BM, Ambrósio R Jr, Salomão M, Velarde GC, Nosé W. Biomechanical and tomographic analysis of unilateral keratoconus. *J Refract Surg.* 2009;24:1-5.
49. Schweitzer C, Roberts CJ, Mahmoud AM, Colin J, Maurice-Tison S, Kerautret J. Screening of forme fruste keratoconus with the ocular response analyzer. *Invest Ophthalmol Vis Sci.* 2010;51(5):2403-2410.
50. Yildiz EH, Diehl GF, Cohen EJ, Hammersmith KM, Laibson PR, Rapuano CJ. Demographics of patients older than 50 years with keratoconus. *Eye Contact Lens.* 2009;35(6):309-311.
51. Lema I, Suárez AI, Díez-Feijoo E. Unilateral keratoconus: videokeratography and Orbscan study—optical correction. *Eye Contact Lens.* 2009;35(1):15-19.
52. Lema I, Romero P, Mato JL, Feijóo ED. Corneal descriptive indices in the fellow eye of unilateral keratoconus. *Eye Contact Lens.* 2009;35(2):65-68.
53. Li X, Rabinowitz YS, Rasheed K, Yang H. Longitudinal study of the normal eyes in unilateral keratoconus patients. *Ophthalmology.* 2004;111(3):440-446.
54. Holland DR, Maeda N, Hannush SB, et al. Unilateral keratoconus. Incidence and quantitative topographic analysis. *Ophthalmology.* 1997;104(9):1409-1413.
55. Rabinowitz YS. Diagnosing keratoconus and patients at risk. *Cat Refract Surg Today.* May 2007. Accessed on 15th May 2010 from http://bmctoday.net/crstoday/2007/05/article.asp?f=CRST0507_15.php
56. Lim L, Wei RH, Chan WK, Tan DT. Evaluation of keratoconus in Asians: role of Orbscan II and Tomey TMS-2 corneal topography. *Am J Ophthalmol.* 2007;143(3):390-400.
57. Schlegel Z, Lteif Y, Bains HS, Gatinel D. Total, corneal, and internal ocular optical aberrations in patients with keratoconus. *J Refract Surg.* 2009;25(10 Suppl):S951-S957.
58. Sabesan R, Yoon G. Visual performance after correcting higher order aberrations in keratoconic eyes. *J Vis.* 2009;9(5):6.1-6.10.
59. Nakagawa T, Maeda N, Kosaki R, et al. Higher-order aberrations due to the posterior corneal surface in patients with keratoconus. *Invest Ophthalmol Vis Sci.* 2009;50(6):2660-2665.
60. Alió JL, Shabayek MH. Corneal higher order aberrations: a method to grade keratoconus. *J Refract Surg.* 2006;22(6):539-545.
61. Vinciguerra P, Albè E, Trazza S, et al. Refractive, topographic, tomographic, and aberrometric analysis of keratoconic eyes undergoing corneal cross-linking. *Ophthalmology.* 2009;116(3):369-378.
62. Piñero DP, Alió JL, El Kady B, Pascual I. Corneal aberrometric and refractive performance of 2 intrastromal corneal ring segment models in early and moderate ectatic disease. *J Cataract Refract Surg.* 2010;36(1):102-109.
63. Piñero DP, Alio JL, El Kady B, et al. Refractive and aberrometric outcomes of intracorneal ring segments for keratoconus: mechanical versus femtosecond-assisted procedures. *Ophthalmology.* 2009;116(9):1675-1687.
64. Ertan A, Karacal H, Kamburoğlu G. Refractive and topographic results of transepithelial cross-linking treatment in eyes with intacs. *Cornea.* 2009;28(7):719-723.
65. Baillif S, Garweg JG, Grange JD, Burillon C, Kodjikian L. Keratoglobus: review of the literature. *J Fr Ophtalmol.* 2005;28(10):1145-1149.
66. Cameron JA. Keratoglobus. *Cornea.* 1993;12(2):124-130.
67. Karabatsas CH, Cook SD. Topographic analysis in pellucid marginal corneal degeneration and keratoglobus. *Eye (Lond).* 1996;10(Pt 4):451-455.
68. Rumelt S, Rehany U. Surgically induced keratoglobus in pellucid marginal degeneration. *Eye (Lond).* 1998;12(Pt 1):156-158.
69. Patel SP, Sajnani MM, Pineda R. Posterior polymorphous dystrophy and keratoglobus in a child. *J Pediatr Ophthalmol Strabismus.* 2010;8:1-3.
70. Harissi-Dagher M, Dana MR, Jurkunas UV. Keratoglobus in association with posterior polymorphous dystrophy. *Cornea.* 2007;26(10):1288-1291.
71. Ku JY, Grupcheva CN, Fisk MJ, McGhee CN. Keratoglobus and posterior subcapsular cataract: surgical considerations and in vivo microstructural analysis. *J Cataract Refract Surg.* 2004;30(1):237-242.
72. Elder MJ. Leber congenital amaurosis and its association with keratoconus and keratoglobus. *J Pediatr Ophthalmol Strabismus.* 1994;31(1):38-40.
73. Nelson ME, Talbot JF. Keratoglobus in the Rubinstein-Taybi syndrome. *Br J Ophthalmol.* 1989;73(5):385-387.
74. McClellan KA, Billson FA. Acute hydrops in keratoglobus. *Arch Ophthalmol.* 1987;105(10):1432-1433.
75. Gupta VP, Jain RK, Angra SK. Acute hydrops in keratoglobus with vernal keratoconjunctivitis. *Indian J Ophthalmol.* 1985;33(2):121-123.
76. Kiire C, Srinivasan S. Management of bilateral acute hydrops secondary to keratoglobus with perfluoroethane (C2F6) pneumodescemetopexy. *Clin Experiment Ophthalmol.* 2009;37(9):892-894.
77. Maguire LJ, Klyce SD, McDonald MB, Kaufman HE. Corneal topography of pellucid marginal degeneration. *Ophthalmology.* 1987;94(5):519-524.
78. Lee BW, Jurkunas UV, Harissi-Dagher M, Poothullil AM, Tobaigy FM, Azar DT. Ectatic disorders associated with a claw-shaped pattern on corneal topography. *Am J Ophthalmol.* 2007;144(1):154-156.
79. Oie Y, Maeda N, Kosaki R, et al. Characteristics of ocular higher-order aberrations in patients with pellucid marginal corneal degeneration. *J Cataract Refract Surg.* 2008;34(11):1928-1934.
80. Tang M, Shekhar R, Miranda D, Huang D. Characteristics of keratoconus and pellucid marginal degeneration in mean curvature maps. *Am J Ophthalmol.* 2005;140(6) 993-1001.
81. Seiler T, Koufala K, Richter G. Iatrogenic keratectasia after laser in situ keratomileusis. *J Refract Surg.* 1998;14(3):312-317.
82. Probst LE, Machat JJ. Mathematics of laser in situ keratomileusis for high myopia. *J Cataract Refract Surg.* 1998;24(2):190-195.
83. Guirao A. Theoretical elastic response of the cornea to refractive surgery: risk factors for keratectasia. *J Refract Surg.* 2005;21(2):176-185.
84. Randleman JB, Woodward M, Lynn MJ, Stulting RD. Risk assessment for ectasia after corneal refractive surgery. *Ophthalmology.* 2008;115:37-50.
85. Randleman JB, Russell B, Ward MA, Thompson KP, Stulting RD. Risk factors and prognosis for corneal ectasia after LASIK. *Ophthalmology.* 2003;110:267-275.
86. Amoils SP, Deist MB, Gous P, Amoils PM. Iatrogenic keratectasia after laser in situ keratomileusis for less than -4.0 to -7.0 diopters of myopia. *J Cataract Refract Surg.* 2000;26:967-977.
87. Klein SR, Epstein RJ, Randleman JB, Stulting RD. Corneal ectasia after laser in situ keratomileusis in patients without apparent preoperative risk factors. *Cornea.* 2006;25:388-403.

88. Randleman JB, Banning CS, Stulting RD. Corneal ectasia after hyperopic LASIK. *J Refract Surg.* 2007;23:98-102.
89. Caster AI, Friess DW, Potvin RJ. Absence of keratectasia after LASIK in eyes with preoperative central corneal thickness of 450 to 500 microns. *J Refract Surg.* 2007;23:782-788.
90. Binder PS. Analysis of ectasia after laser in situ keratomileusis: risk factors. *J Cataract Refract Surg.* 2007;33:1530-1538.
91. Condon PI, O'Keefe M, Binder PS. Long-term results of laser in situ keratomileusis for high myopia: risk for ectasia. *J Cataract Refract Surg.* 2007;33:583-590.
92. Randleman JB. Post-laser in-situ keratomileusis ectasia: current understanding and future directions. *Curr Opin Ophthalmol.* 2006;17(4):406-412.
93. Rao SN, Epstein RJ. Early onset ectasia following laser in situ keratomileusis: case report and literature review. *J Refract Surg.* 2002;18(2):177-184.
94. Randleman JB, Trattler WB, Stulting RD. Validation of the Ectasia Risk Score System for preoperative laser in situ keratomileusis screening. *Am J Ophthalmol.* 2008;145(5):813-818.
95. Binder PS, Trattler WB. Evaluation of a risk factor scoring system for corneal ectasia after LASIK in eyes with normal topography. *J Refract Surg.* 2010;26(4):241-250.
96. Ambrósio R Jr, Dawson DG, Salomão M, Guerra FP, Caiado AL, Belin MW. Corneal ectasia after LASIK despite low preoperative risk: Tomographic and biomechanical findings in the unoperated, stable, fellow eye. *J Refract Surg.* 2010;19:1-6.
97. Tuli SS, Iyer S. Delayed ectasia following LASIK with no risk factors: is a 300-microm stromal bed enough? *J Refract Surg.* 2007;23(6):620-622.
98. Altan-Yaycioglu R, Pelit A, Akova YA. Comparison of ultrasonic pachymetry with Orbscan in corneal haze. *Graefes Arch Clin Exp Ophthalmol.* 2007;245(12):1759-1763.
99. Boscia F, La Tegola MG, Alessio G, Sborgia C. Accuracy of Orbscan optical pachymetry in corneas with haze. *J Cataract Refract Surg.* 2002;28(2):253-258.
100. Gayton JL. Etiology, prevalence, and treatment of dry eye disease. *Clin Ophthalmol.* 2009;3:405-412.
101. Cho P, Douthwaite W. The relation between invasive and noninvasive tear break-up time. *Optom Vis Sci.* 1995;72(1):17-22.
102. Iskander DR, Collins MJ. Applications of high-speed videokeratoscopy. *Clin Exp Optom.* 2005;88(4):223-231.
103. Goto T, Zheng X, Okamoto S, Ohashi Y. Tear film stability analysis system: introducing a new application for videokeratography. *Cornea.* 2004;23(8 Suppl):S65-S70.
104. Goto T, Zheng X, Klyce SD, et al. Evaluation of the tear film stability after laser in situ keratomileusis using the tear film stability analysis system. *Am J Ophthalmol.* 2004;137(1):116-120.
105. Mobillia EF, Kenyon KR. Contact lens-induced corneal warpage. *Int Ophthalmol Clin.* 1986;26:43-53.
106. Wang X, McCulley JP, Bowman RW, Cavanagh HD. Time to resolution of contact lens-induced corneal warpage prior to refractive surgery. *The CLAO Journal.* 2002;28(4):169-171.
107. Di Girolamo N, Coroneo MT, Wakefield D. UVB-elicited induction of MMP-1 expression in human ocular surface epithelial cells is mediated through the ERK1/2 MAPK-dependent pathway. *Invest Ophthalmol Vis Sci.* 2003;44(11):4705-4714.
108. Dushku N, John MK, Schultz GS, Reid TW. Pterygia pathogenesis: corneal invasion by matrix metalloproteinase expressing altered limbal epithelial basal cells. *Arch Ophthalmol.* 2001;119(5):695-706.
109. Oh JY, Wee WR. The effect of pterygium surgery on contrast sensitivity and corneal topographic changes. *Clin Ophthalmol.* 2010;4:315-319.
110. Maheshwari S. Pterygium-induced corneal refractive changes. *Indian J Ophthalmol.* 2007;55(5):383-386.
111. Avisar R, Loya N, Yassur Y, Weinberger D. Pterygium-induced corneal astigmatism. *Isr Med Assoc J.* 2000;2(1):14-15.
112. Shimazaki J, Tsubota K. Analysis of videokeratography after penetrating keratoplasty: topographic characteristics and effects of removing running sutures. *Ophthalmology.* 1997;104(12):2077-2084.
113. Sarhan AR, Dua HS, Beach M. Effect of disagreement between refractive, keratometric, and topographic determination of astigmatic axis on suture removal after penetrating keratoplasty. *Br J Ophthalmol.* 2000;84(8):837-841.
114. Vinciguerra P, Epstein D, Albè E, et al. Corneal topography-guided penetrating keratoplasty and suture adjustment: new approach for astigmatism control. *Cornea.* 2007;26(6):675-682.
115. Geggel HS. Arcuate relaxing incisions guided by corneal topography for postkeratoplasty astigmatism: vector and topographic analysis. *Cornea.* 2006;25(5):545-557.
116. Kovoor TA, Mohamed E, Cavanagh HD, Bowman RW. Outcomes of LASIK and PRK in previous penetrating corneal transplant recipients. *Eye Contact Lens.* 2009;35(5):242-245.
117. Vajpayee RB, Sharma N, Sinha R, Bhartiya P, Titiyal JS, Tandon R. Laser in-situ keratomileusis after penetrating keratoplasty. *Surv Ophthalmol.* 2003;48(5):503-514.

Chapter 9

# Topography-Guided Contact Lens Fitting

Shawna Hill Vanderhoof, OD, FAAO; Randy Kojima, OD, FAAO, FOAA; Jason Jedlicka, OD, FAAO; Matthew Lampa, OD, FAAO; and Tracy Schroeder Swartz, OD, MS, FAAO

The topographer has become an indispensable tool to understand the anterior surface shape of the cornea and give much information about corneal power, curvature, elevation, and disease. It is also an incredible asset to our contact lens practice for the fitting of specialty contact lenses. Traditionally, topography gave us a starting point in choosing the initial diagnostic lens. Now, using topography and its contact lens fitting software, we can actually design a gas-permeable (GP) lens more efficiently. A software-generated GP lens can be created to compare with an actual trial on the eye of the same parameters. These programs can help in the initial lens design selection and aid in the efficiency of choosing the optimal parameters for each individual eye. This is infinitely beneficial when dealing with diseased or asymmetrical eyes, which are challenging to start.

The software is not limited to topographers or GPs alone; we will also discuss specialty soft and GP contact lens design cases from aberrometers to tomographers.

## Raw Images to Analyzing Maps

For this instrument to provide the practitioner with valuable information, a good capture is required. Train your staff comprehensively on the need to take good photos. This means slow, steady movements with the instrument, a comfortably seated patient, wide fissure size, and an even tear film. Always check the Placido rings prior to finishing the mapping process to be sure a good image has been taken. Take multiple images when building GP contact lenses so there are many to choose from if 1 or 2 captures should be less than ideal.

Most cameras require light to bounce off the object, and this reflection is recorded as an image. A corneal topographer bounces its own light (the Placido rings) off the hydraulic fluid layer on the corneal surface and records the image of the Placido reflection on the tear film.[1] Considering that we must capture a photo reflected from the corneal surface, it becomes imperative that the fluid covering the surface is smooth, even, and devoid of tear break-up or dryness.[2,3] Figure 9-1 exhibits these imperfections caused by tear film break-up, dryness, or inconsistencies in the fluid layer in the Placido reflection. The instrument determines the shape and elevation of the eye by analyzing the ring reflection off the corneal surface. If any number of these rings should distort, break, or collapse on one another, the accuracy of the instrument will be hindered.

When analyzing the maps, use an axial interpretation to understand corneal power or astigmatism and tangential to measure shape or curve at a particular point. To appreciate the acuity that is derived from the anterior surface, a



Wang M. *Corneal Topography: A Guide for Clinical Application in the Wavefront Era, Second Edition (pp. 215-230)*

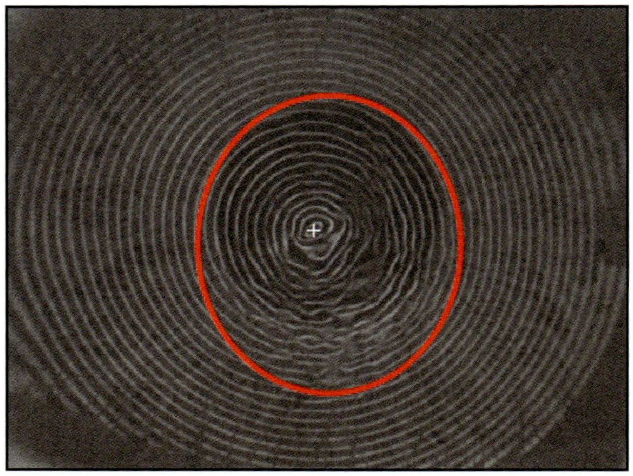

**Figure 9-1.** Note the distorted rings inside the red circle. This would result in analysis error (extrapolation error). A quality topography capture should exhibit rings that look even and parallel, as most appear outside the red circle.

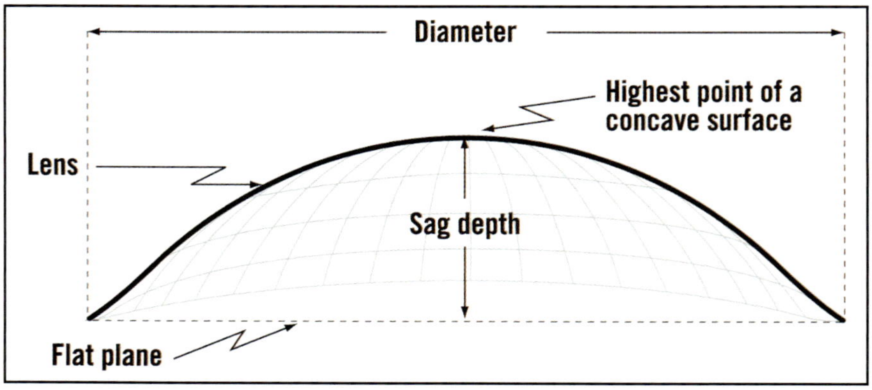


**Figure 9-2.** Sagittal depth.

refractive power map can be helpful to understand asymmetries within the virtual pupil. Last, an elevation map is the best way to discern where the peaks and depressions in the cornea exist. Topographers use the elevation display to calculate the height differences across the cornea by placing a reference sphere and then displaying the elevation of the cornea above or below the reference surface across the entire map display. The reference sphere is the curve that aligns with the most number of points on the cornea. Each instrument has built into it the parameters of many contact lenses and then takes the difference between the known surface of the contact lens (based on the individual parameters for that lens) and the elevation display.

Some topographers also have sagittal depth information. Corneal sagittal depth (z-value) is defined as a measurement in mm or µm of the distance between the geometric center of the cornea and the intersection of a specified chord length (y-value)[4] as seen in Figure 9-2. Scleral lens fitting is based on the sagittal depth as the sclera cannot be described in curvature or shape factors as the cornea can. Van der Worp and colleagues found the shape of the limbus and anterior sclera to be tangential in shape, showing that the sclera is nonspherical and nonrotationally symmetric in nature.[5] Factors that affect the sagittal depth for the lens and cornea, respectively, include base curve radius/keratometry (K) values, peripheral curves/peripheral corneal asphericity, and lens diameter/corneal diameter.[6] Scleral contact lenses completely vault the cornea and rest upon the bulbar conjunctiva. The difference in sagittal depth between the contact lens and the eye determines this relationship. Using anterior segment OCT at the Pacific University College of Optometry, the corneal-scleral tangential angle between 10.00 mm and 15.00 mm (the limbal angle) was measured as well as the angle from 15.00 mm to 20.00 mm (the scleral angle).[5] This would suggest that toric and/or quadrant-specific scleral designs could lead to better fitting characteristics and possibly better lens comfort. While keratometry values might be the same between patients, a smaller eye will result in significantly less sagittal depth and marked difference in the limbal/scleral angles. This is in contrast to corneal GP lenses for which you determine the fit by the base curve-to-keratometry measurement because they are fit to align with the cornea.

## THE "RULES" OF GAS-PERMEABLE LENS FITTING

The following set of rules to guide the fitting of GP lenses will facilitate fitting and minimize the time required[7]:

- *Diameter selection*: The optimum diameter should be large enough to stabilize the lens along the horizontal meridian while smaller than the visible iris diameter to allow for 1 mm of movement vertically.
- *Apical clearance (base curvature)*: The central base curve should be steep enough to clear the corneal apex. The base curve radii you choose should create an apical clearance of between 20 and 30 µm. Apical clearances larger than 40 µm may produce apical steepening and spectacle blur. When this occurs, the pattern will exhibit the appearance of excessive central clearance.
- *Horizontal alignment*: The GP lens should be steep enough to land midperipherally along the horizontal meridian.
- *Vertical channel of tears*: The lens should exhibit unobstructed movement along the vertical meridian (Figure 9-3).

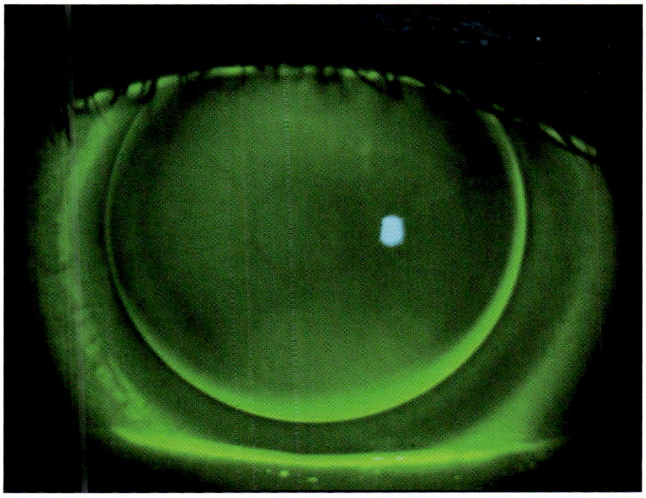

**Figure 9-3.** An ideal GP fit with apical clearance, landing at 3 and 9 o'clock and a channel of tear layer along the vertical meridian.

# Topography-Guided Fitting

## Wave Contact Lens System

The Keratron Scout (Optikon 2000, Rome, Italy) and Medmont E300 (Medmont International Pty Ltd, Vermont, Melbourne, Australia) corneal topographers use the Wave contact lens design software program. The Wave design program uses the topography output from the Keratron/Medmont topographer to design virtually any type of lens desired. The lens designs are broken down into 3 categories: rotationally symmetric (RSym), geometrically symmetric (GSym), or free form (FForm). Using these categories, it is possible to design soft or GP single vision, multifocal (center near, center distance, or segmented), aspheric toric, and aspheric bitoric lenses, as well as reverse geometry GP designs.

The lens design software is powerful enough to combine elements of design to create virtually any lens design imaginable. GP lens diameters can be made up to 15.0 mm, while soft lens designs range from 13.0 to 15.0 mm. Preset controls allow for auto designs of standard lenses, myopic ortho-k lenses, or hyperopic ortho-k lenses.

Once topography has been obtained, the user chooses the type of lens to be designed (soft or GP) and the WAVE program begins to design the lens. As the lens is being designed, the lens design screen will appear (Figure 9-4).

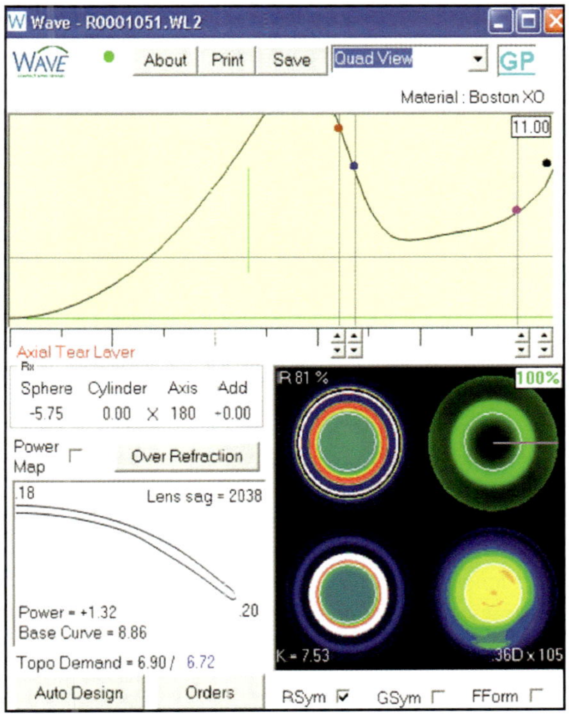


**Figure 9-4.** WAVE design box.

Once the initial design is complete, the program will ask for the spectacle prescription to be entered. This will allow the software to create the lens with the correct power, whether it be spherical or toric. In addition, a power map can create an asymmetric correction to enhance vision in eyes with higher-order aberrations (HOAs) or asymmetric astigmatism. At this point, the initial lens design will be complete.

The lens design box has various aspects that can be accessed. The upper region of the box includes the lens material, the lens diameter, and the lens clearance profile. These are all customizable. This profile is set up so as to allow the user to increase or decrease lens clearance in any area of the lens, as well as to change the widths of any of the respective curves.

The midregion of the lens design box is where the patient's prescription is listed, as well as the option for a power map for asymmetric power to be cut into the lens, and the box to click to enter any over-refraction found over a current design. The bottom third of the design box has an area that describes the lens thickness in the center and edge (either of which can be altered by the designer), the lens power, the actual base curve at the region selected by the user, and the various lens views available, which include a simulated fluorescein pattern, the back or front of the lens surface viewed from an axial or curvature perspective, as well as other options. A quad view option allows for multiple views to be seen all at one time.

The initial lens design may be an RSym, GSym, or FForm design, chosen by the program based upon the type of corneal shape. The user can alter the type of lens after the initial design. For fairly regular, spherical, or low astigmatic corneas, an RSym design is usually acceptable. For highly toric corneas, it may be desirable to have the lens in a GSym design, which allows for "normal" toricity correction. In cases of irregular corneas, or where other highly specific characteristics are desired (such as a spherical base curve with toric peripheral curves), an FForm design may be preferred. The FForm design allows for asymmetric lens designs to be achieved using the flexibility of 24 zones of curve modification.

From there, further adjustments to the lens can be made using one of the many modification tools. There are drop-down menus that allow for steepening or flattening the base curve, midperiphery, or peripheral curves; changing the diameter; or adding an over-refraction. If a lens design needs modifying after dispensing, the lens design box can be reopened, modifications can be made to the lens design, and a new lens can be ordered with the modifications made. All lens designs are transmitted via e-mail to the main lab, where they are fed directly into the lathe for production.

The Wave design system, while effective for many types of lens fits, is particularly helpful in difficult cases where standard lens fitting sets are less effective, such as reverse geometry lens designs, orthokeratology, or for post-surgical eyes.

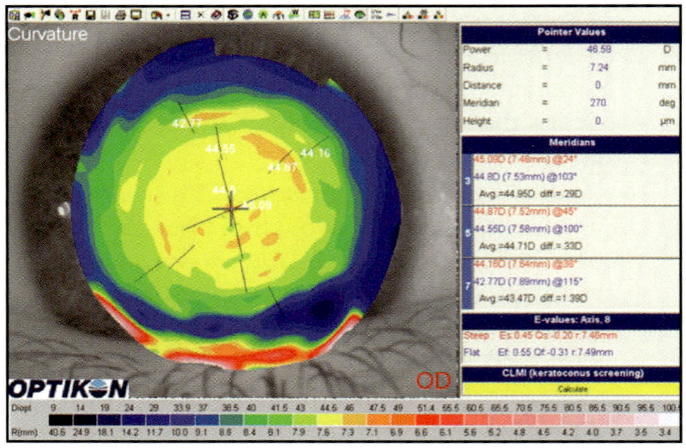


**Figure 9-5.** Topography for DS, preorthokeratology OD.

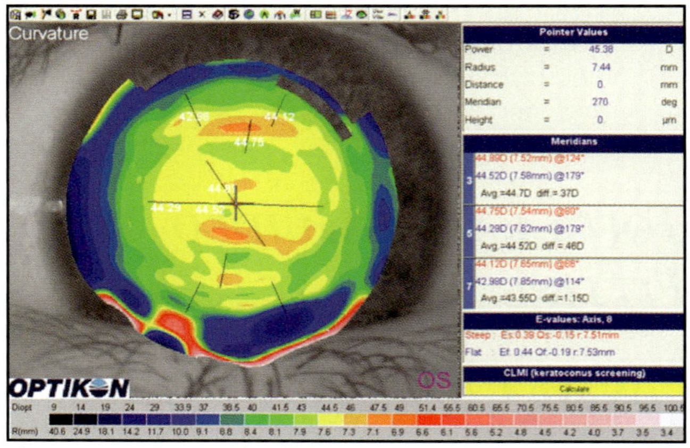


**Figure 9-6.** Topography for DS, preorthokeratology OS.

## Orthokeratology Application

One of the most useful applications of the Wave system is the designing of lenses for orthokeratology or corneal reshaping. Because you have the ability to control all lens parameters, you can sometimes fit patients who would otherwise get less-than-optimal results with one of the many lens design systems for orthokeratology available commercially. This was the case for DS, a 12-year-old patient who was already exhibiting significant myopia at this early age. DS presented for examination in May 2004 with an interest in corneal reshaping. After a complete examination, we determined a prescription of:

OD: -5.50-0.25 x 20 20/20
OS: -5.00-0.25 x 180 20/20

His corneal topography in each eye (Figures 9-5 and 9-6) showed enough curvature for orthokeratology, but with his correction being roughly -5.00, the patient and his mother were cautioned that full correction may not be attainable. Because of the higher correction and the potential for the correction to increase due to his young age, flexibility of planning to optimize parameters and change diameter and optic zone sizes as needed in the future was desired. Rather than fit him in a standard orthokeratology lens design, a Wave designed lens was chosen.

Because he had little astigmatism, an RSym design was an acceptable lens design. A larger lens diameter (11.0 mm) was chosen to accommodate his larger pupil size and to try to increase the treatment zone as much as possible. The lens designs for each eye are shown in Figures 9-7 and 9-8. Using this design, he was able to obtain uncorrected vision of 20/20 in each eye. His topographies at 1-year post-initiation of treatment are shown in Figures 9-9 and 9-10. The topographies demonstrate excellent centration of correction and minimal astigmatic correction. DS continues in orthokeratology now 6 years later. His correction has increased by less than 1 D in each eye during the past 6 years with maintenance of 20/20 BCVA.

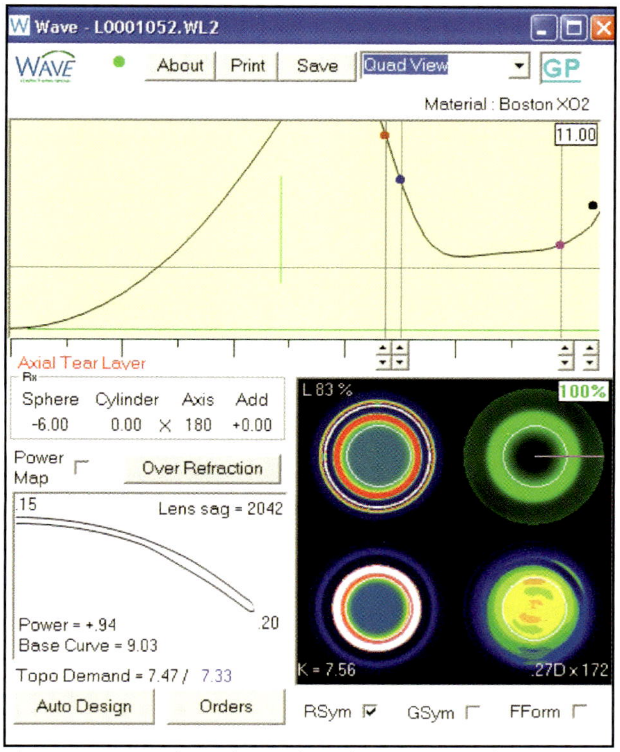


**Figure 9-7.** OD lens design box for DS. Note lens parameters.

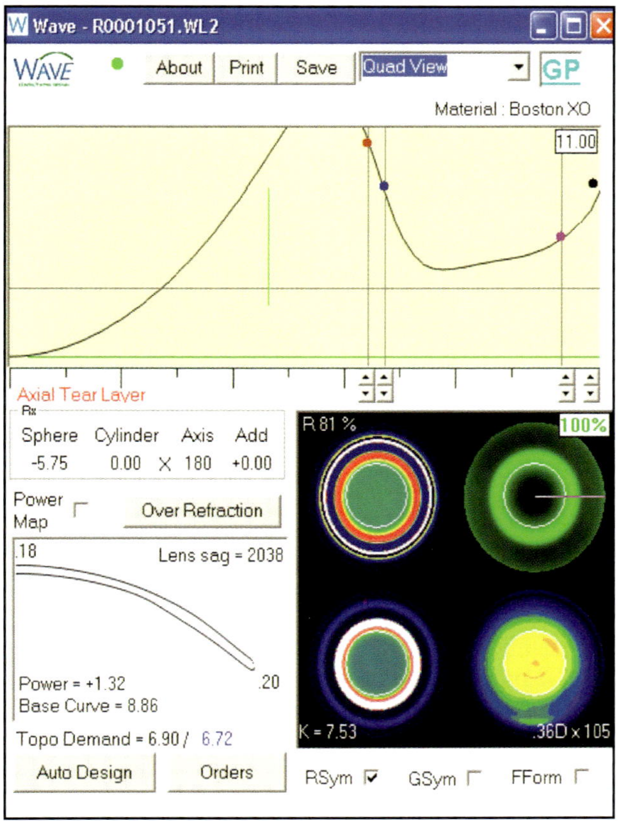


**Figure 9-8.** OS lens design box for DS. Note lens parameters.

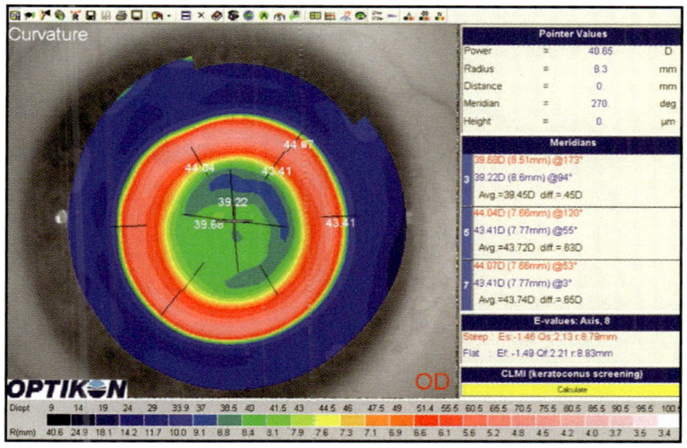


**Figure 9-9.** OD topography for DS, 1-year post-initiation of orthokeratology.

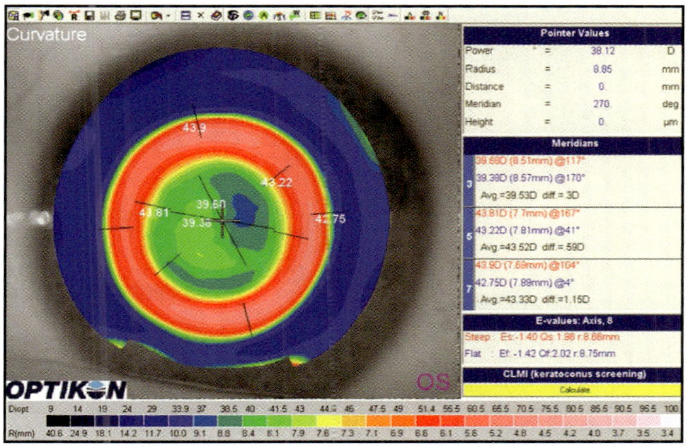


**Figure 9-10.** OS topography for DS, 1-year post-initiation of orthokeratology.

## Reverse Geometry Lenses

The postsurgical eye that is steep centrally but even steeper in the midperiphery is a challenging fit. This is most common in those eyes that are post-penetrating keratoplasty for keratoconus. ZB is a 54-year-old man who had a history of keratoconus and corneal transplants in 1991 in the right eye and 1993 in the left eye. He subsequently wore soft toric lenses for several years, but found the vision to be deteriorating.

His vision with soft toric lens correction was 20/50 in the right eye and 20/40 in the left. Pinhole did not improve the vision. His refraction was

R: -9.00 +5.50 x 125 20/50
L: -8.75 +4.50 x 55 20/40

His grafts were clear in each eye and were free of signs of rejection. Corneal topography demonstrated a highly astigmatic central area with significant steepening in the midperiphery (Figures 9-11 and 9-12).

After explaining the status of his prescription, vision, and corneal shape, it was decided that trying a GP lens

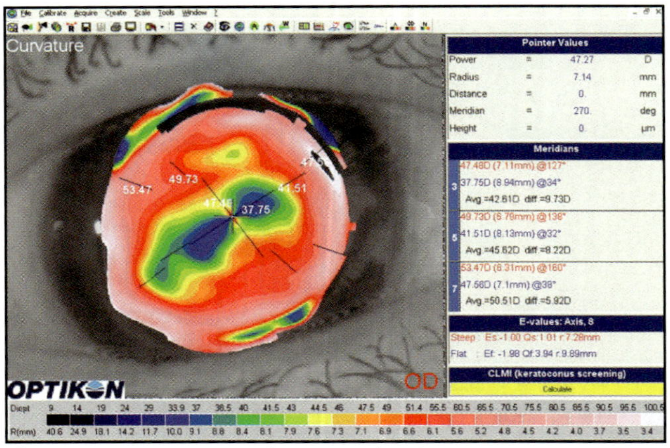


**Figure 9-11.** ZB's corneal topography OD.

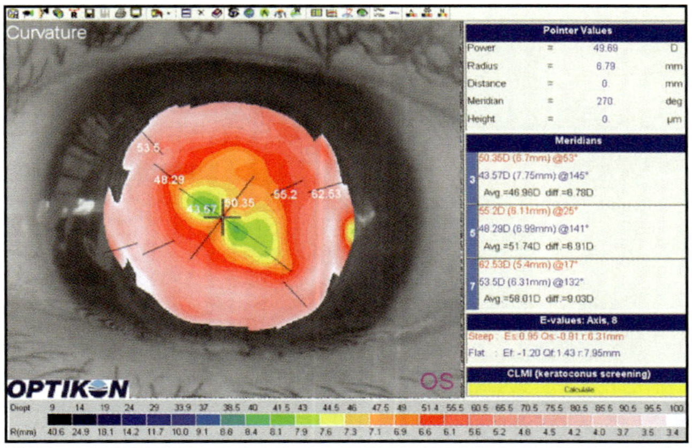


**Figure 9-12.** ZB's corneal topography OS.

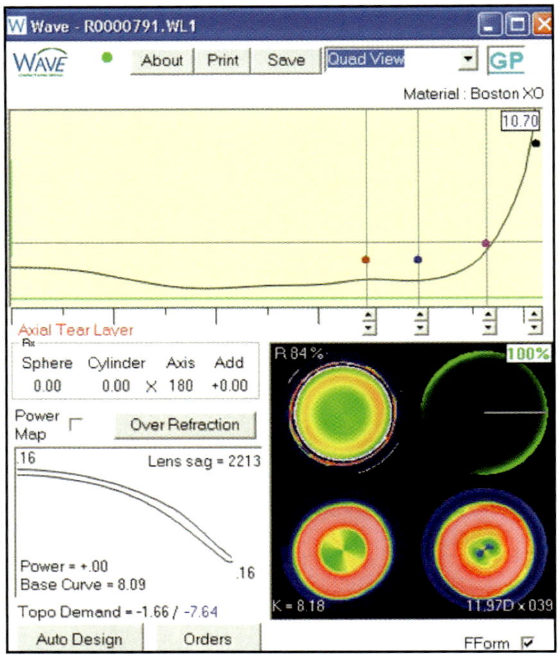


**Figure 9-13.** ZB's WAVE lens design OD.

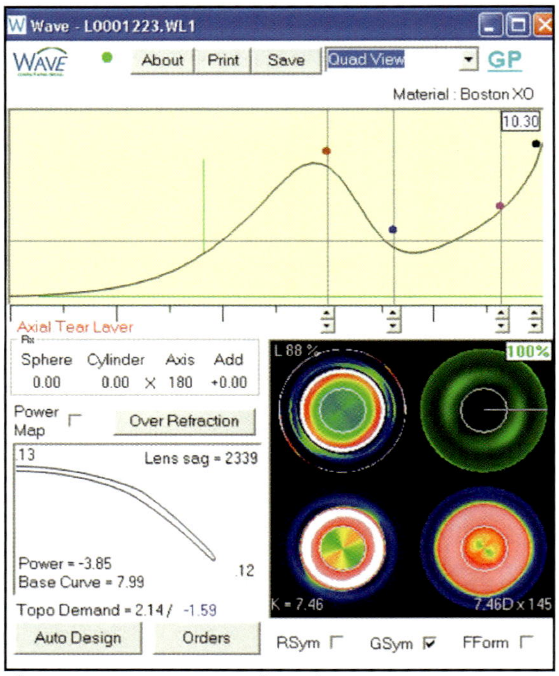


**Figure 9-14.** ZB's WAVE lens design OS.

might offer better vision than the soft lenses he had been using. A GP lens fitting was undertaken, which produced visual acuities approaching 20/20, but with an unstable fit. What was needed was a reverse geometry lens design, but one with a smaller optic zone and steeper base curves than most commercially available reverse geometry lens design options. To achieve the desired fit, an FForm Wave lens was designed for each eye.

The Wave lens design for each eye is shown in Figures 9-13 and 9-14. For the right eye, a lens diameter of 10.7 was chosen, while the left eye, due to the steeper midperiphery, was fitted in a 10.3 diameter. The lenses were dispensed, and ZB was able to adapt to the lenses and achieve 20/20-2 vision in each eye. Minor adjustments were made to the peripheral curves in each eye to facilitate tear exchange, but the end result was an acceptable fit and vision in each eye. The actual lenses on the eye are shown in Figures 9-15 and 9-16.

Another lens fitting challenge is the post-radial keratotomy (RK) patient. These patients often have somewhat sensitive corneas as well as a small, very flat area centrally with a steeper midperiphery. LJ is a 42-year-old man with a history of RK in 1993. He had done well for several years, but recently felt his vision deteriorating. He had seen several eye care providers seeking improved vision, and though the lenses he had tried had provided better visual acuity, he could not tolerate those lenses. His entering acuity uncorrected was 20/60-2 in each eye. All entrance tests were normal. His refraction was:

| | |
|---|---|
| OD: | +2.00 +3.25 x 90 20/25-2 |
| OS: | -1.75 +1.75 x 75 20/30 |

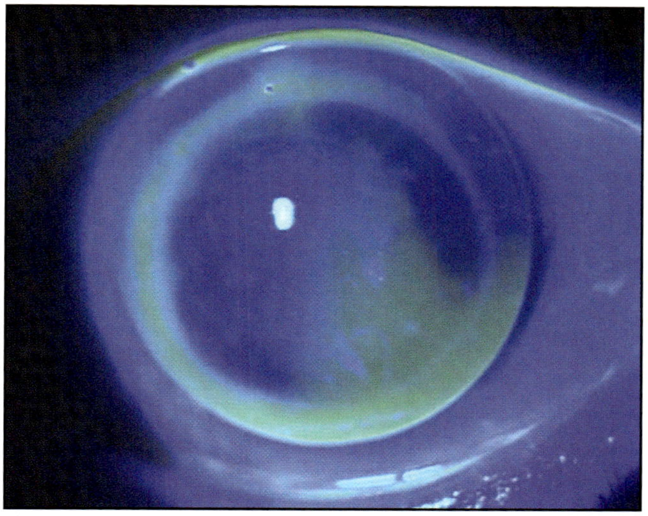

**Figure 9-15.** ZB's WAVE lens OD.

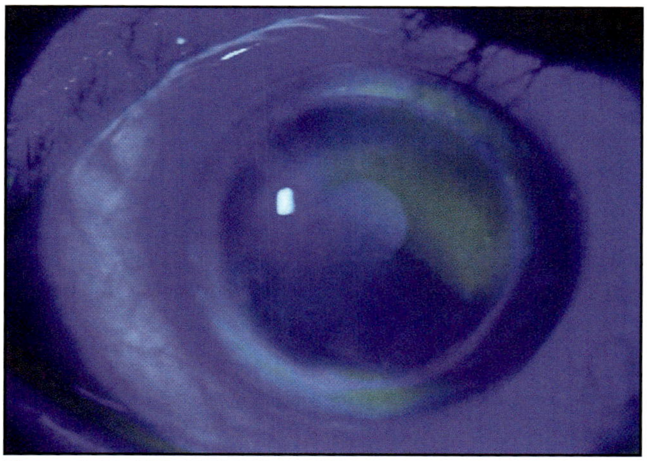

**Figure 9-16.** ZB's WAVE lens OS.

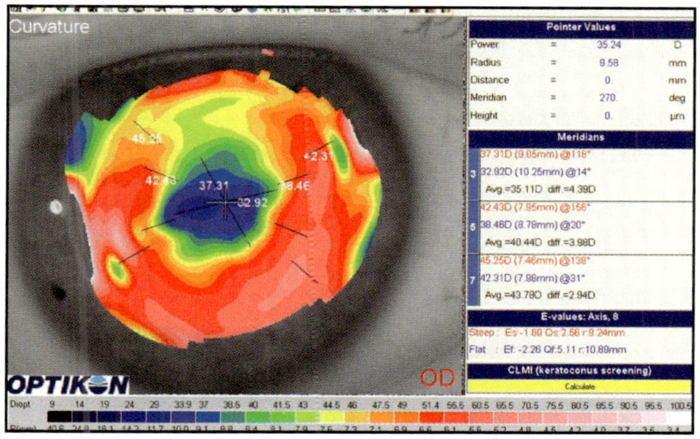


**Figure 9-17.** LJ's corneal topography OD.

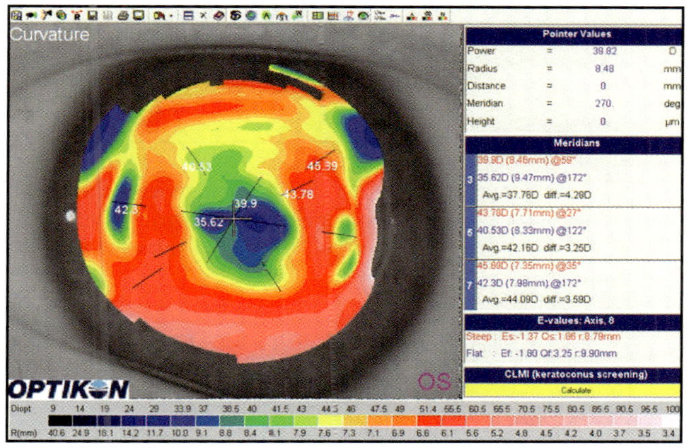


**Figure 9-18.** LJ's corneal topography OS.

Slit-lamp examination revealed 8 radial scars from his previous RK, as well as 2 arcuate scars in each eye from an astigmatic keratectomy. The temporal aspect of the right cornea was significant for mild evidence of wound gape between the arcuate cut and one of the radial cuts. All other ocular findings were normal. Corneal topography demonstrated a fairly typical post-RK map in each eye, with a small flat central area surrounded by a steeper midperiphery (Figures 9-17 and 9-18).

His contact lens history included previous fittings in hybrid lenses, semi-scleral GPs, as well as various corneal GP lenses. His main problem with all previous lenses was the development of photosensitivity with lens wear. He had not worn any lenses prior to his initial visit in more than 2 years. After discussing his options, which included reconsideration of surgical options as well as various contact lens designs, we decided to proceed with an RSym OD and GSym OS Wave lens design. The lenses were designed based upon his corneal maps and his spectacle prescription. A diameter of 11.5 was chosen for each eye for stability of lens fit. The lens design boxes are shown in Figures 9-19 and 9-20.

The lenses were dispensed, and the visual acuity with correction was recorded at 20/25+1 in each eye and 20/20-1 in both eyes. The lenses fit well and the patient's initial comfort was acceptable. The lens fit is shown in Figures 9-21 and 9-22. The patient adapted to the lenses, was happy with the quality of vision, and was able to tolerate lens wear 10 hours daily, which was acceptable to LJ.

## Medmont E300

The Medmont E300 corneal topographer uses a simulated fluorescein display for evaluating the fit of GP contact lenses. The software allows the selection of many generic and specific manufacturers' lens designs, and the parameters are calculated based on the captured topography. The manifest refraction will also be specified here in order for the software to calculate the required contact lens power. It can predict residual astigmatism by comparing the corneal and manifest refractive astigmatism.

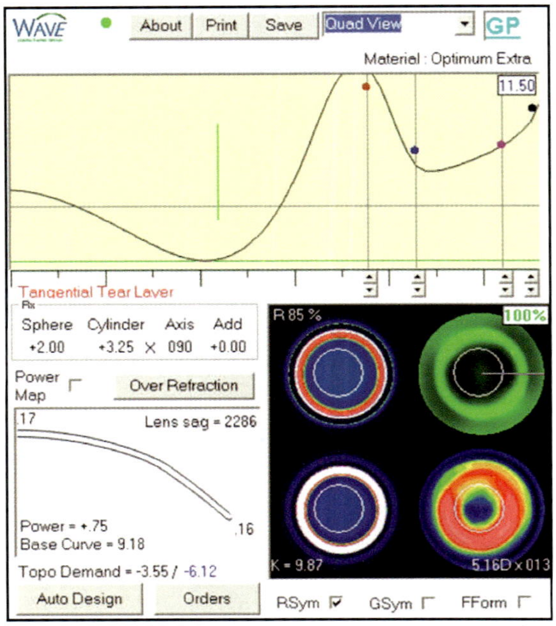


**Figure 9-19.** LJ's Wave lens design OD. Note that the lens is an RSym design, and the lens view in the lower right area of the lens design box demonstrates a spherical base curve lens, with a resulting toric fluorescein pattern.

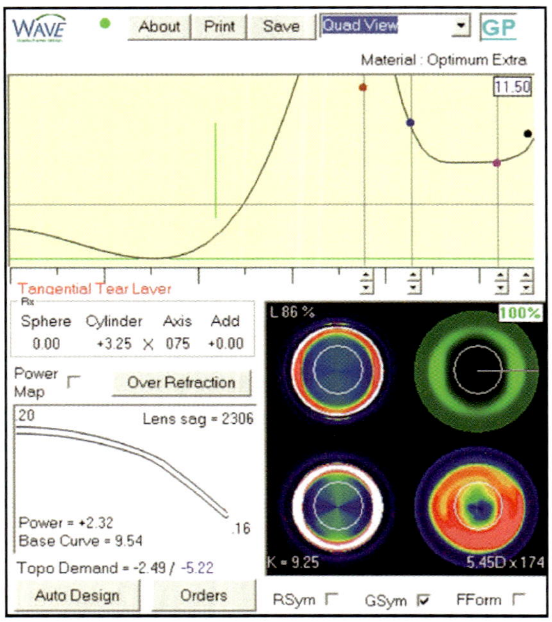


**Figure 9-20.** LJ's Wave lens design OS. Note that the lens is a GSym design, and the lens view in the lower right area of the lens design box demonstrates a toric base curve lens, with a resulting spherical fluorescein pattern.

Lens diameter, base curvature, and peripheral curvatures are customizable. The changing of some values will automatically cause other values to be recalculated. Changing them manually and unchecking the auto-update option can override this function.

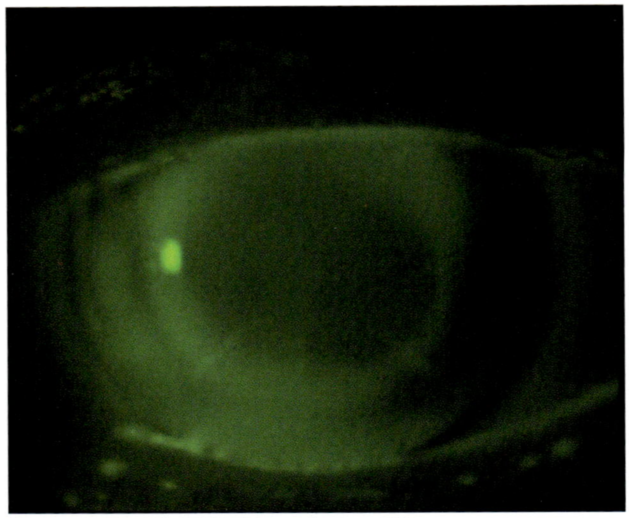

**Figure 9-21.** LJ's WAVE lens design OD.

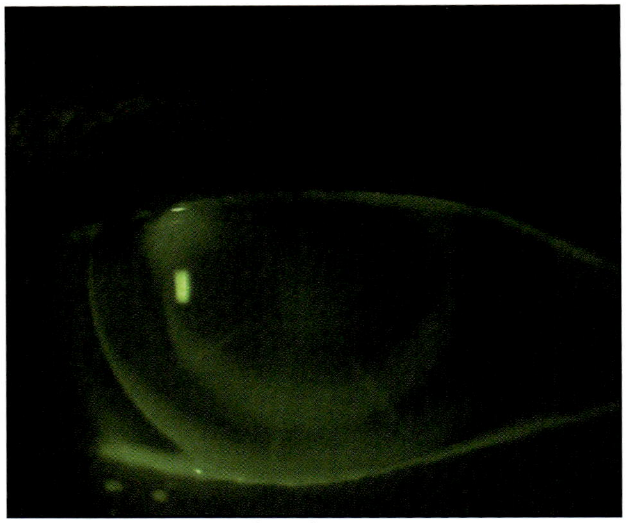

**Figure 9-22.** LJ's WAVE lens design OS.

In the fluorescein display, the simulated contact lens can be moved over the cornea to determine how the fit varies as the lens repositions. The N and T on the sides denote the nasal (N) or temporal (T) orientation. Dragging the lens with the mouse to reposition the lens is left at that location and a new simulated fluorescein pattern is generated.

RM, a 24-year-old male graduate student, presented to the office complaining of blurry vision in both eyes at distance. He was interested in contact lenses as he had only worn spectacles in the past. His last eye exam was 1 year ago. His medical and ocular history is unremarkable except for seasonal allergies. After a complete examination, we determined the refraction and keratometry as listed in Table 9-1. His corneal topography in each eye (Figures 9-23 and 9-24) showed high regular with-the-rule astigmatism, making him a good candidate for a bitoric GP contact lens. We educated the patient on the options, and the patient decided to proceed.

TABLE 9-1.

## Bitoric Gas Permeable Fitting Clinical Data

| | OD | OS |
|---|---|---|
| Refraction | Plano-3.75x014, 20/20 | +0.25-4.75x169, 20/20 |
| Keratometry | 41.50 @ 012 / 45.00 @ 102 | 41.25 @ 179 / 45.50 @ 089 |
| Initial lens parameters | 40.75/44.50D<br>8.30/7.60<br>+0.50/-3.00<br>9.5mm | 40.75/44.50D<br>8.30/7.60<br>+0.75/-3.00<br>9.5mm |
| Adjusted lens parameters | 41.50/44.25<br>8.13/7.63<br>-0.25/-3.00<br>9.5mm | 41.25/45.00<br>8.18/7.50<br>+0.25/-3.75<br>9.5mm |

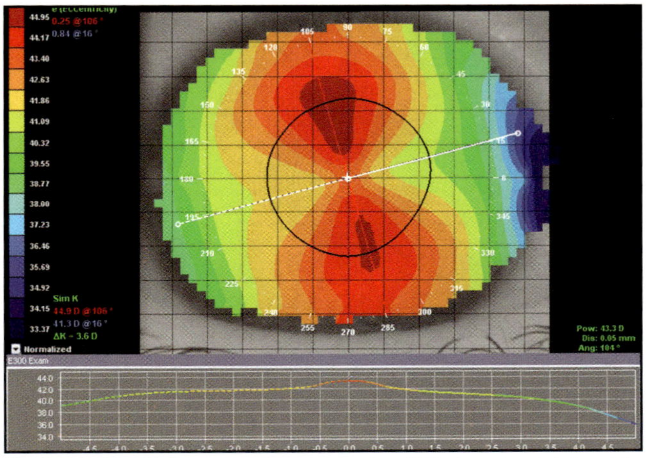

**Figure 9-23.** RM's corneal topography OD showing high with-the-rule astigmatism.

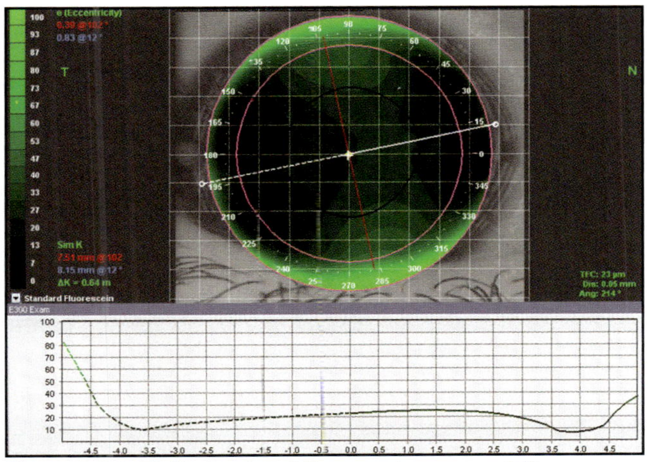

**Figure 9-25.** RM's simulated fluorescein pattern OD.

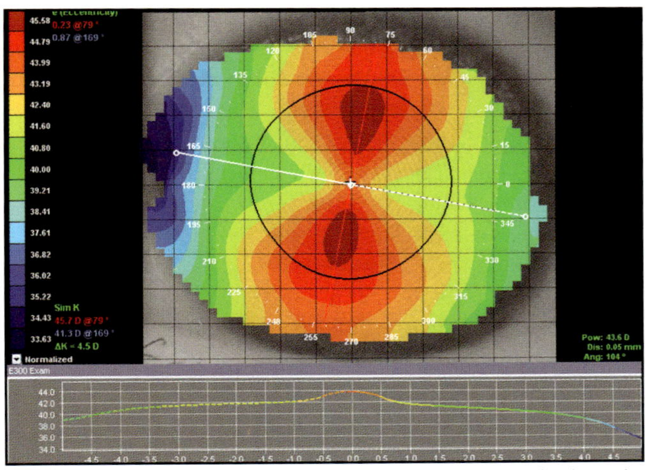

**Figure 9-24.** RM's corneal topography OS showing high with-the-rule astigmatism.

Computer software suggested the parameters listed in Table 9-1 based on topography. The simulated fluorescein patterns of these lenses can be seen in Figures 9-25 and 9-26. Note that the flat meridians in both eyes have less than 20 to 30 µm of clearance. Therefore, we steepened the flat meridian of each eye, causing a change in the lens power. More minus was added to each lens, -0.25 for every 0.25 of curvature change. The steep meridian was steepened by 0.50 in the left eye to improve apical clearance. There was no residual astigmatism calculated in this case. The adjusted lens parameters are listed in Table 9-1.

The contact lenses were dispensed to the patient (Figures 9-27 and 9-28). The patient was able to achieve 20/20 vision with the bitoric GPs and was able to adapt to the lenses after building up his wear time over 2 weeks.

BW, a 31-year-old male contractor, presented to the office complaining of blurred distance vision, in the left eye more than the right eye, especially while driving. He is

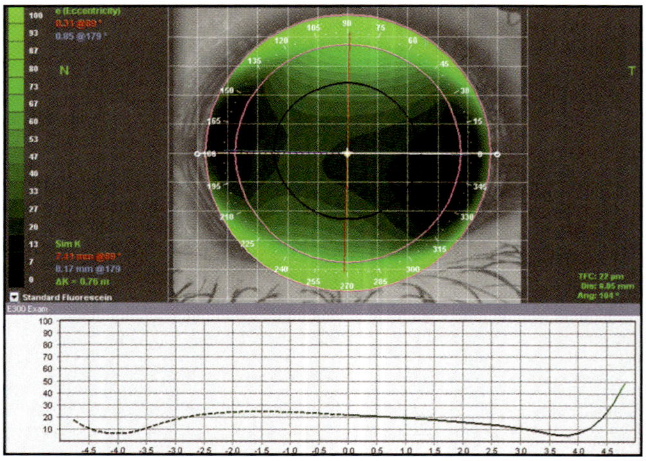

Figure 9-26. RM's simulated fluorescein pattern OS.

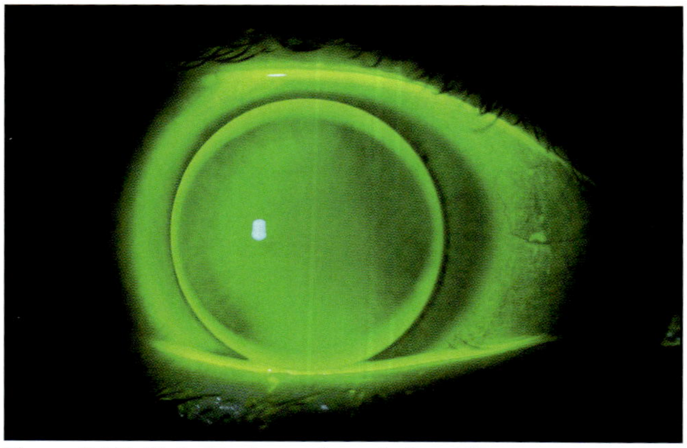
Figure 9-27. RM's Medmont lens design OD.

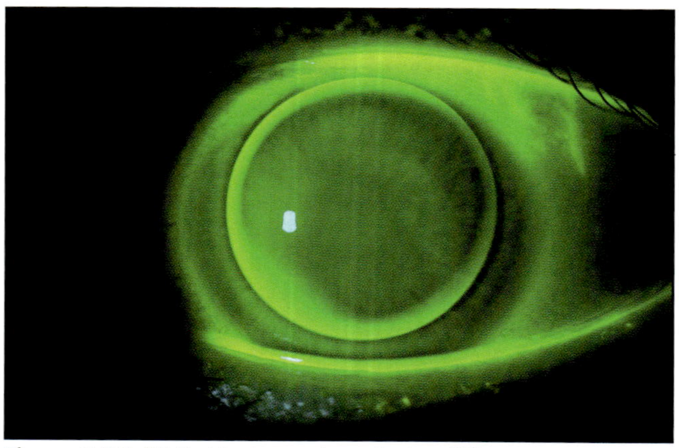
Figure 9-28. RM's Medmont lens design OS.

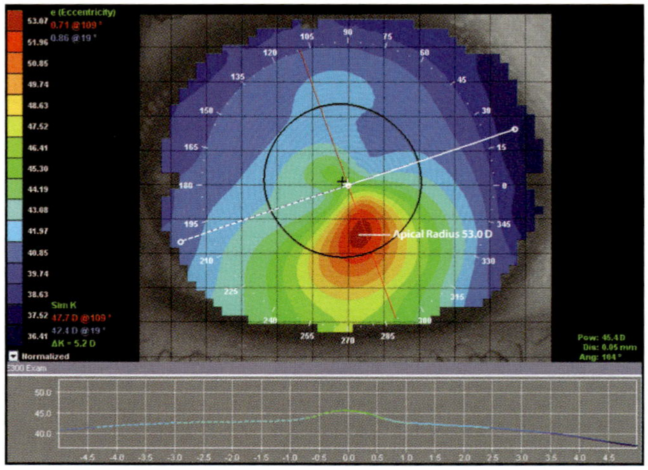

Figure 9-29. BW's corneal topography OD showing keratoconus. Apical radius is 53.00 D (6.35).

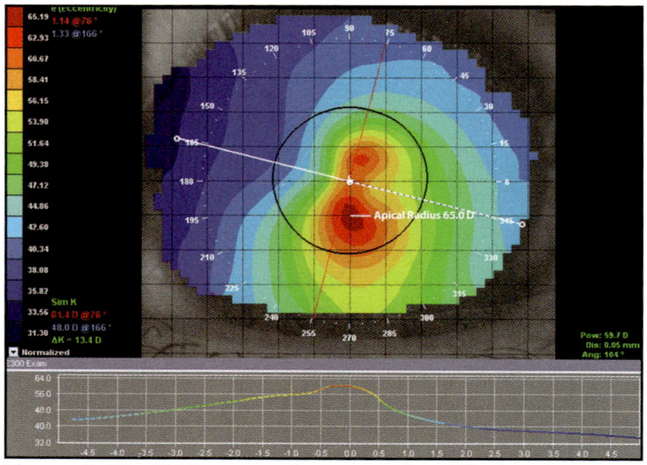

Figure 9-30. BW's corneal topography OS showing more advanced keratoconus. Apical radius is 65.00 (5.20).

interested in contact lenses and was diagnosed with keratoconus at his last eye exam 2 months ago. BW's uncorrected vision was 20/25 in the right eye and 20/50 in the left eye. Slit-lamp examination showed clear corneas in both eyes. His corneal topography in each eye (Figures 9-29 and 9-30) showed keratoconus, more in the left eye than the right eye. After educating BW on his options, we decided that GPs were his best option.

Computer software suggested the parameters listed in Table 9-2 based on topography. The simulated fluorescein patterns of these lenses can be seen in Figures 9-31 and 9-32. The keratoconus bi-aspheric (KBA) lens from Essilor Contact Lens is a 10.2-mm diameter GP design with a 9.2-mm back surface optic zone. The large optic zone combined with a custom aspheric back surface allows for centration over the pupil and, thus, reduced flare and glare.[8] Also, the KBA enables you to match its eccentricity (e-value) to that of the cornea. Aspheric lenses have a varying base curve defined by the back optic zone eccentricity.

Corneas that flatten at a significant rate from their geometric center outward have high e-values, and those that flatten mildly from the geometric center have low e-values.[6]

TABLE 9-2.

## Keratoconus Bi-Aspheric (KBA) Fitting Clinical Data

| | OD | OS |
|---|---|---|
| Refraction | +1.00-3.00x043, 20/25 | Plano-3.00x142, 20/50 |
| Keratometry | 42.50 @ 019 / 47.75 @ 109 | 48.00 @ 166 / 61.50 @ 076 |
| Initial lens parameters | KBA /45.63 (7.40) / 10.2 / 1.0 ecc | KBA / 50.38 (6.70) / 10.2 / 1.2 ecc |
| Adjusted lens parameters | KBA / 45.63 (7.40) / -4.25 / 10.2 / 1.0 ecc | KBA / 52.00 (6.50) / -10.50 / 10.2 / 1.3 ecc |

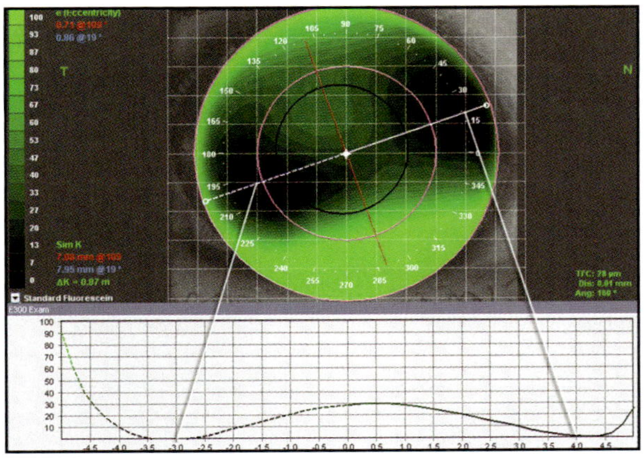

**Figure 9-31.** BW's simulated fluorescein pattern OD. Note the GP is approximately resting at 3 and 9 o'clock.

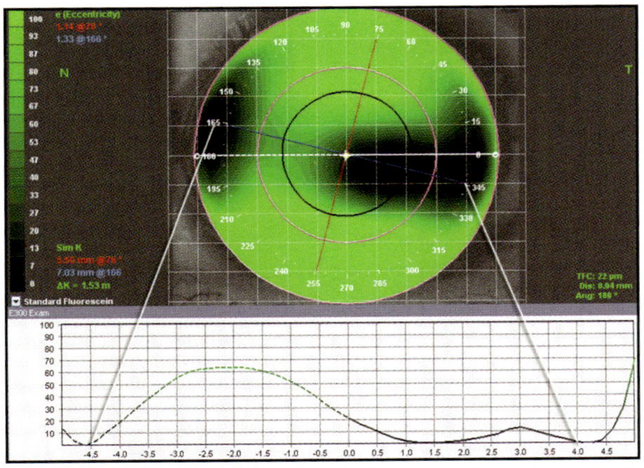

**Figure 9-32.** BW's simulated fluorescein pattern OS. Note the GP is approximately resting at 3 and 9 o'clock.

The right lens (see Figure 9-31) shows 30 μm of apical clearance and a good peripheral fit as well. The left lens (see Figure 9-32) shows approximately 20 μm of apical clearance, which rapidly decreases to touch, only 1 mm temporal. Therefore, we steepened the base curve, thereby increasing eccentricity as shown in Table 9-2.

The contact lenses of the actual lenses ordered were dispensed to the patient (Figures 9-33 and 9-34). The patient

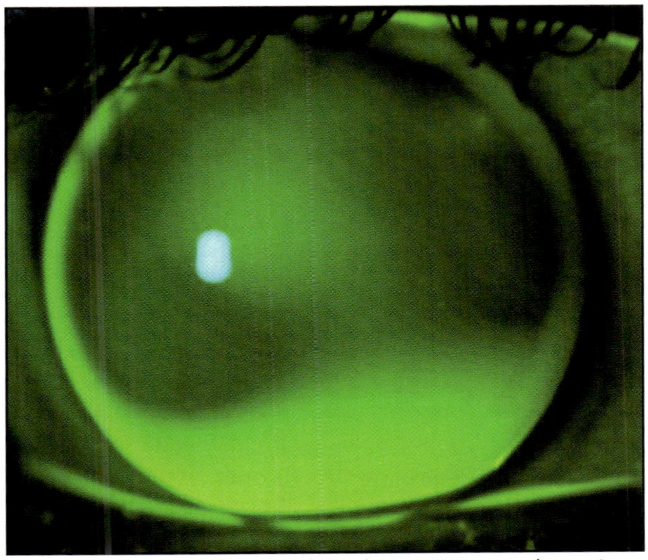

**Figure 9-33.** BW's Medmont lens design OD, exactly as simulated in Figure 9-31.

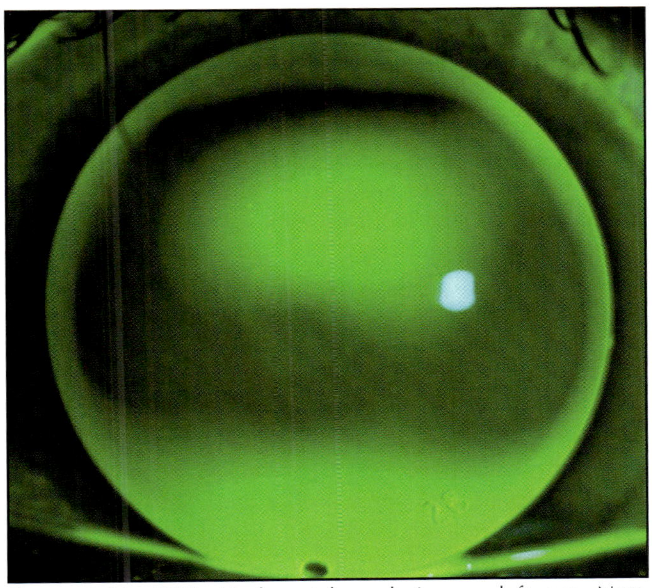

**Figure 9-34.** BW's Medmont lens design on left eye. Note the improved fluorescein pattern centrally and increased tear profile inferiorly.

TABLE 9-3.

**Atlas Topography With the MasterFit Software**

| | OD | OS |
|---|---|---|
| Refraction | -5.00 -1.50 x 009; 20/20 | -3.00 -2.50 x 174; 20/20 |
| Keratometry | 41.75 @ 010 / 43.50 @ 100 | 43.00 @ 175 / 46.00 @ 085 |
| Initial lens parameters | 42.25 / -4.50 / 9.5 mm | 43.25 / -3.00 / 9.8 mm |
| Adjusted lens parameters | 42.50 / -4.50 / 9.5 mm | 43.50 / -3.00 / 9.5 mm |

was able to achieve 20/20 vision with the aspheric GPs and was able to adapt to the lenses after building up his wear time over the first 2 weeks. He also understands that refitting will be necessary if the keratoconus progresses.

## Zeiss Atlas 9000 and MasterFit II Software

The Atlas 9000 topographer (Carl Zeiss Meditec, Jena, Germany) and optional MasterFit II Contact Lens Software enable the user to design GP contact lenses and to simulate the resulting fluorescein pattern on the cornea.[9] MasterFit II features both topographic and keratometric-based lens-fitting methods. Based on customizable fitting preferences, MasterFit II will recommend the most appropriate lens type (including spherical, aspheric, front toric, back toric, and bitoric designs) and will design a custom lens that best achieves the desired fitting preferences. MasterFit II also features region-specific databases of stock (finished) lenses that may be used as an alternative to creating custom lens designs.

The user may create multiple lens designs per topography exam to simulate the effect of adjusting the available lens parameters on the fluorescein pattern. After finalizing the lens design, the user may print the lens design using the order form templates provided, or the order form may be saved as a PDF and sent by e-mail to the preferred laboratory.

The MasterFit II software also displays tear film thickness profile graphs. To the right of the fluorescein map is the vertical (90 degrees) tear film thickness profile graph, which plots the tear layer thickness (µm; solid green area) along the corneal surface. Below the fluorescein map are the horizontal (180 degrees) tear film thickness profile graph, which plots the tear layer thickness (µm) along the corneal surface, and white profile meridian (white graph) on the fluorescein map.

This case demonstrates the software in a patient having with-the-rule astigmatism. A 36-year-old woman presented to the office complaining of blur at distance in both eyes.

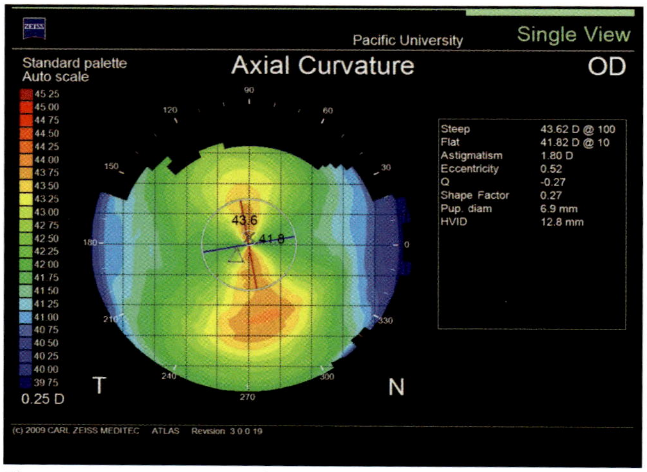


**Figure 9-35.** FC's corneal topography OD showing with-the-rule astigmatism.

Her last eye exam was 2 years ago. Her ocular and medical history is unremarkable. After a complete examination, we determined her refraction as described in Table 9-3.

Her corneal topography in each eye (Figures 9-35 and 9-36) showed with-the-rule astigmatism, greater in the left eye. Computer software suggested the parameters based on topography, which are listed in Table 9-3. The simulated fluorescein patterns of these lenses can be seen in Figures 9-37 and 9-38. A Computer Aided Design (CAD) GP lens from Valley Contax (Springfield, OR) was selected due to her low to moderate with-the-rule astigmatism. This lens has a spherical optical zone and an aspheric periphery.

The right eye shows a lens 0.50 D steeper than flat K, and the apical clearance is right under the 20-µm mark so the final lens is steepened by 0.25 (see Figure 9-37). The left eye shows a lens virtually on flat K with the horizontal and vertical tear film thickness less than adequate (see Figure 9-38). The left lens was also steepened. Actual lens parameters are listed in Table 9-3. The contact lenses of the actual lenses ordered were dispensed to the patient (Figures 9-39 and 9-40). The patient was able to see 20/20 with her GPs. If there was residual with-the-rule astigmatism in either eye, a bitoric could be ordered.

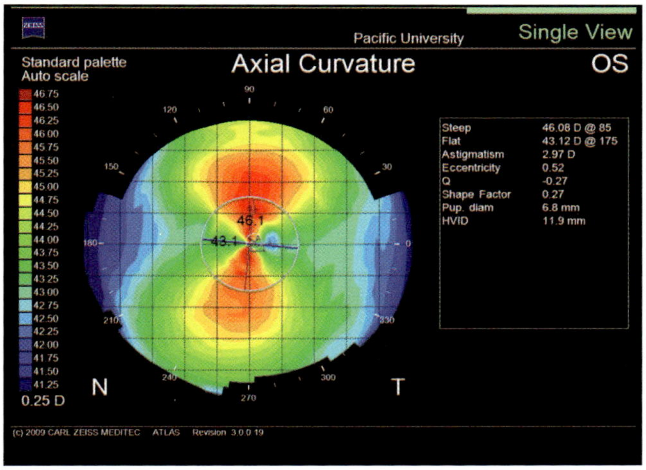


**Figure 9-36.** FC's corneal topography OS showing with-the-rule astigmatism.

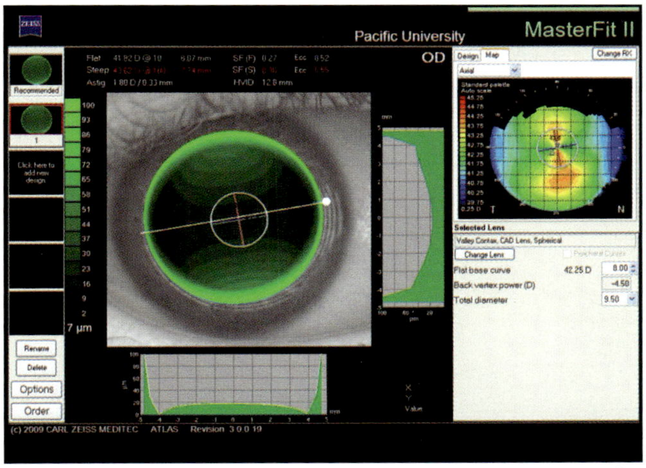


**Figure 9-37.** FC's simulated fluorescein pattern OD. Note the Flat K is 41.87 D.

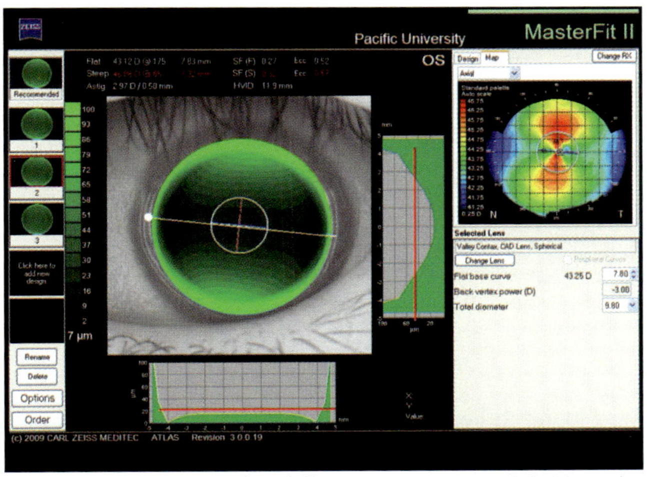


**Figure 9-38.** FC's simulated fluorescein pattern OS. Note the Flat K is 43.12 D.

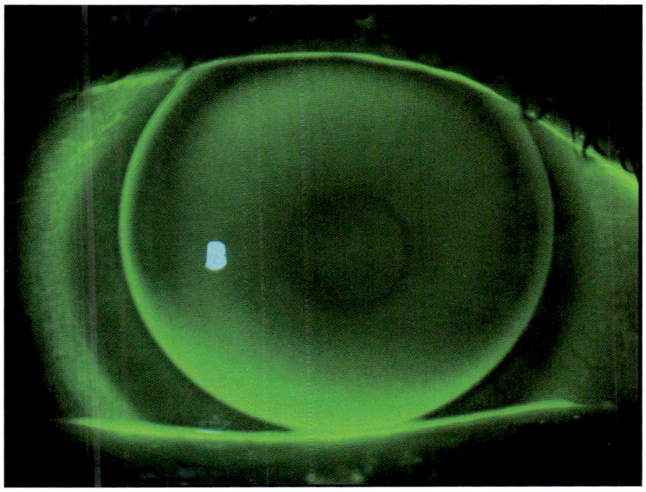

**Figure 9-39.** FC's MasterFit CAD lens design OD.

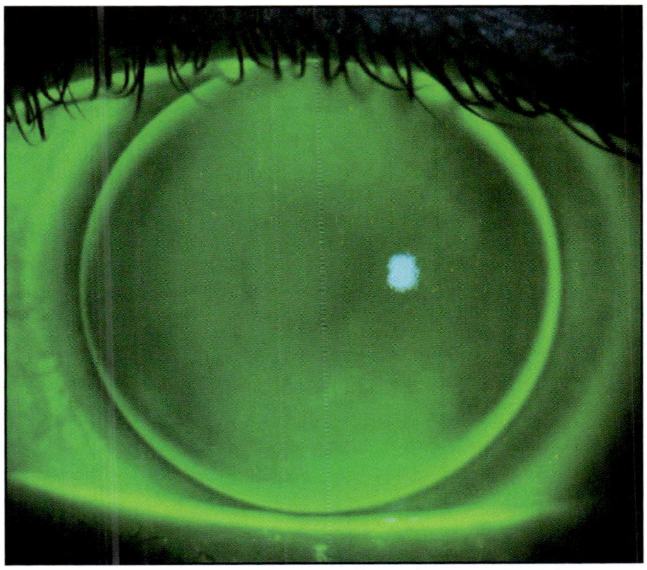

**Figure 9-40.** FC's MasterFit CAD lens design OS with appropriate amount of tears in the vertical channel.

Finally, some systems incorporate aberrometry with topography to guide contact lens fitting. An irregular topography results in irregular aberrations. Correction of the aberrations may yield improvement in vision.

# Aberration Correction Contact Lenses

## Wavetouch Hydrogel Contact Lenses

Wavetouch hydrogel lenses use wavefront aberrometry to correct for both refraction and optical aberration as measured by a certified aberrometer, such as the iTrace Visual Function Analyzer (Tracey Technologies, Houston, TX).

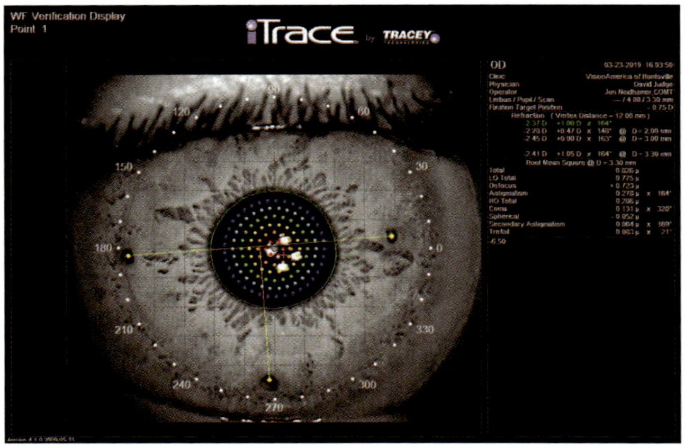

**Figure 9-41.** Aberrometry measurement is performed over the contact lens. The system uses the dots to determine where the visual center should be placed on the lens.

TABLE 9-4.

**Wavetouch Hydrogel Lens Parameters**

| | |
|---|---|
| Base curve supplied in the WaveTouch Acquisition set* | MDN (median)<br>STP (steep) |
| Diameter | 14.7mm |
| Material | Methafilcon A, 55% water content |
| Daily wear schedule | Supplied for the patient as quarterly replacement lens after the initial fit is finalized |

*Practitioners can get a "made to order" BC with additional information, through the Consultation Department

Wavefront custom contact lenses may provide superior quality of vision compared to standard contact lenses, particularly for those patients with RMS values greater than 0.3 μm. Because aberrometry measurement is sensitive to ocular surface disease and corneal instability, contact lenses (soft and GP) should be discontinued, and ocular surface disease should be addressed prior to fitting.

These lenses are manufactured from patient information gathered from aberrometry readings to correct both lower- and higher-order aberrations. This is accomplished by performing the measurements prior to fitting and then again with the lens on the eye (Figure 9-41). This allows the prescription to include the aberrations induced by the lens and incorporates the change the lens creates. Data are forwarded to WaveTouch Technologies, where individualized lenses are manufactured and returned to the practitioner. Lens parameters are described in Table 9-4. The lenses are dispensed and evaluated similar to traditional lenses. Minor adjustments are made using customary spherical changes to improve the vision.

The following case illustrates the fitting process. A 40-year-old man with a history of keratoconus greater in the right eye and difficulty wearing GP lenses presented for evaluation. He wore contact lenses to the initial visit despite severe discomfort in his right eye, and results are listed in Table 9-5. We discussed management options, and he desired Intacs implantation. Unfortunately, we learned his insurance would not cover this procedure. He discontinued the lenses due to comfort issues and returned the following month for fitting with Wavetouch lenses.

Topography and aberrometry were obtained for both eyes (Figure 9-42 and 9-43). The aberrometry refraction was checked by traditional refraction, and his vision improved to 20/50 OD, 20/25 OS from 20/100 OD, 20/30 OS. Steep trial contact lenses with a power of -6.50 D OD and -5.50 D OS were chosen based on his keratometry readings and refractive status. These lenses were worn for 20 minutes. The movement and centration of the trial lenses

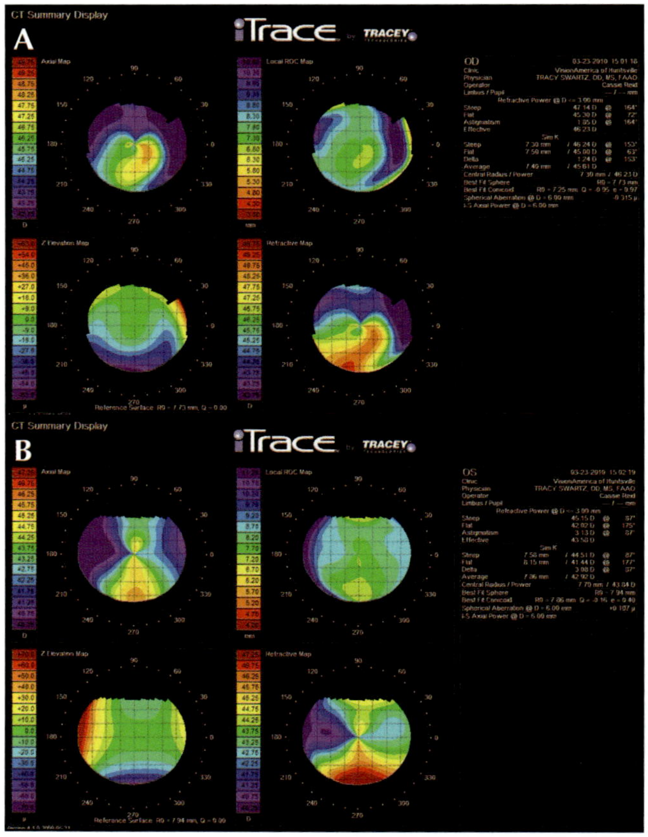

**Figure 9-42.** (A) Corneal topography OD. (B) Corneal topography OS.

were found to be satisfactory. After this, aberrometry was performed twice for each eye over the trial lenses.

Lenses were ordered and dispensed. The patient reported exceptional comfort with the new lenses and good vision. Vision upon dispensing was 20/50 in the right eye and 20/25 in the left eye, and the patient was released for 1 week. After 1 week, the vision was 20/50 with an

TABLE 9-5.

**Patient's Clinical Information**

| | OD | OS |
|---|---|---|
| Vision with GP lens | 20/50 | 20/40- |
| Refraction March 2010 | -8.00, 20/100 | -8.00 +4.25 x 89, 20/30+ |
| iTrace refraction April 2010 | -8.50 +0.50 x 124 | -8.12+4.00 x 85 |
| **Prefitting** | | |
| HOA Value | 0.786 | 0.253 |
| Coma | 0.678 | 0.178 |
| Astigmatism | 0.352 | 1.345 |
| Spherical | +0.087 | -0.042 |
| **With Contact Lens** | | |
| Vision at 1 week: | 20/70 | 20/25 |
| HOA Value | 0.460 | 0.173 |
| Coma | 0.139 | 0.053 |
| Astigmatism | 0.548 | 0.318 |
| Spherical | -0.098 | -0.020 |

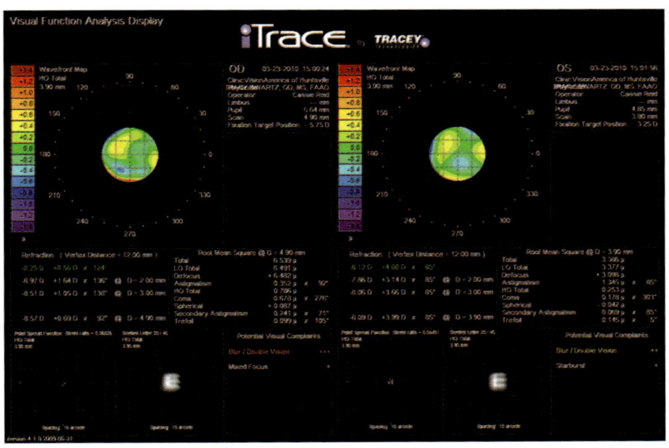


**Figure 9-43.** Visual function analysis for each eye prior to lens fitting.

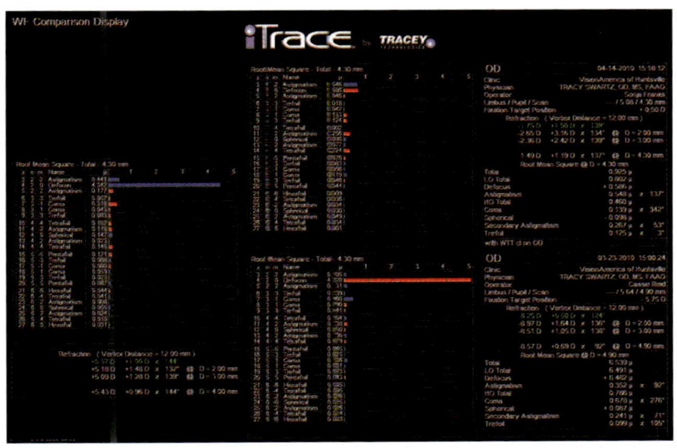


**Figure 9-44.** Visual function analysis for each eye with the lens in each eye.

over-refraction of +0.50 in the right eye and 20/25 in the left eye. The patient reported significant improvement in vision, illustrated by Figures 9-44 and 9-45. The lenses were adjusted by +0.50 in the right eye, and the patient is doing well with 10 to 12 hours of daily wear long-term.

## CONCLUSION

If your aberrometer, topographer, and/or tomographer are accurate, the theoretical fitting and actual fitting will closely agree in a high percentage of cases. If this is true, diagnostic lens fitting may not be necessary on normal corneas. Instead, the practitioner can design lenses with the best possible tear layer profile from the GP (or soft) fitting software and custom order. However, if the theoretical and actual do not consistently agree, then the instrument still serves to offer a diagnostic lens starting point and will reduce the number of modifications or remakes and, therefore, the number of office visits and lost chair time.

Software can be used to design the most simple as well as the most complex lens designs. Quality of the topographical image is crucial to success with the lens design

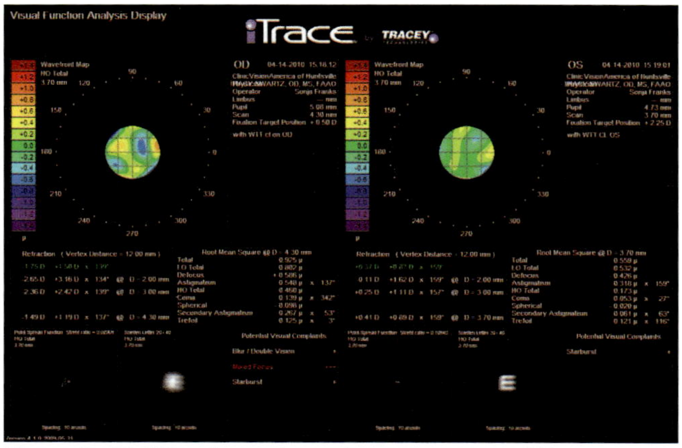


**Figure 9-45.** Wavefront aberration comparison OD.

software. For the user who wishes to make full use of this sophisticated lens design system, time is required to study lens design videos and programs, as well as some trial and error in the early stages.

## References


1. Maeda N. Topcon KR-9000PW. In: Wang M, ed. *Corneal Topography in the Wavefront Era: A Guide for Clinical Application*. Thorofare, NJ: SLACK Incorporated; 2006:259-268.
2. Kojima R. Validating corneal topography maps. *Contact Lens Spectrum*. July 2007. http://www.clspectrum.com/article.aspx?article=100638. Accessed July 20, 2011.
3. Erdélyi B, Csákány B, Németh J. Spontaneous alterations of the corneal topographic pattern. *J Cataract Refract Surg*. 2005;31(5):973-978.
4. Anderson D. Map out your lens fitting. *Optometric Management*. October 2008. http://www.optometric.com/article.aspx?article=102235. Accessed July 20, 2011.
5. Van der Worp E, Graf T, Caroline P. Exploring beyond the corneal borders. *Contact Lens Spectrum*. June 2010. http://www.clspectrum.com/article.aspx?article=104343. Accessed July 20, 2011.
6. Sindt C. Basic scleral lens fitting and design. *Contact Lens Spectrum*. October 2008. http://www.clspectrum.com/article.aspx?article=102163. Accessed July 20, 2011.
7. Kojima R, Caroline P. Designing GPs from corneal topography. *Contact Lens Spectrum*. October 2009. http://www.clspectrum.com/article.aspx?article=103490. Accessed July 20, 2011.
8. Anderson D, Kojima R. "Eccentricity" is in against thin. *Optometric Management*. November 2008. http://www.optometric.com/article.aspx?article=102288. Accessed July 20, 2011.
9. *Atlas Corneal Topography System User Manual System Software Version 3.0*. Dublin, CA: Carl Zeiss Meditec, Inc.

Chapter 10

# Pre-refractive Surgery Topographic Evaluation

J. Bradley Randleman, MD

Evaluation of corneal curvature and biomechanical integrity is critical in preoperative patient evaluation for a variety of surgeries, including keratorefractive and intraocular lens-based refractive procedures. Operating on irregular corneal curvatures can produce unpredictable and unstable refractive outcomes, while operating on biomechanically weak corneas can have untoward results, including unstable refractions, induced irregular astigmatism, and postoperative ectasia.[1]

As we have seen in previous chapters, there are a variety of different techniques and technologies for obtaining unique information about the cornea that prove useful in producing a thorough picture of preoperative corneal characteristics. These include corneal topography, corneal tomography, and ocular hysteresis measurements. Corneal topography is essential to evaluate anterior corneal curvature. Corneal tomography (with scanning slit beam or Scheimpflug systems and high-resolution anterior segment optical corneal tomography) provides regional corneal epithelial and stromal thickness profiles and elevation data. Corneal hysteresis measurement may provide direct measurements of corneal "strength" via hysteresis measures obtained with the ocular response analyzer.

Corneal topography is essential for keratorefractive evaluation and remains the primary technology used in screening. However, in some cases, additional testing may provide important supplementary details on overall cornea shape and strength; in these patients, a combination of technologies may be needed to generate a thorough overall evaluation.

## Corneal Topography

Corneal topographic images are generated from Placido ring reflections from the corneal surface; the distance between these rings indicates focal curvature changes. This ring pattern is then converted into color-coded maps (Figure 10-1). Appropriate topographic evaluation requires a systematic approach to the scans produced (Tables 10-1 and 10-2).

When evaluating a topographic image, it is first essential to determine the color scale used. Most surgeons use a 0.5-D to 1.0-D color scale for keratorefractive surgical evaluations, although a 1.5-D scale has been advocated for consistency.[2] Color step identification is critical because identical topographies can look significantly different based on the color step used (Figure 10-2).

Once the color step is identified, the topographic pattern can be evaluated. There are a variety of established patterns[3] (Figure 10-3) that can be grouped into 4 major patterns in an otherwise healthy cornea (Figures 10-4 through 10-11)[4]:



Wang M. *Corneal Topography: A Guide for Clinical Application in the Wavefront Era, Second Edition (pp. 231-242)*

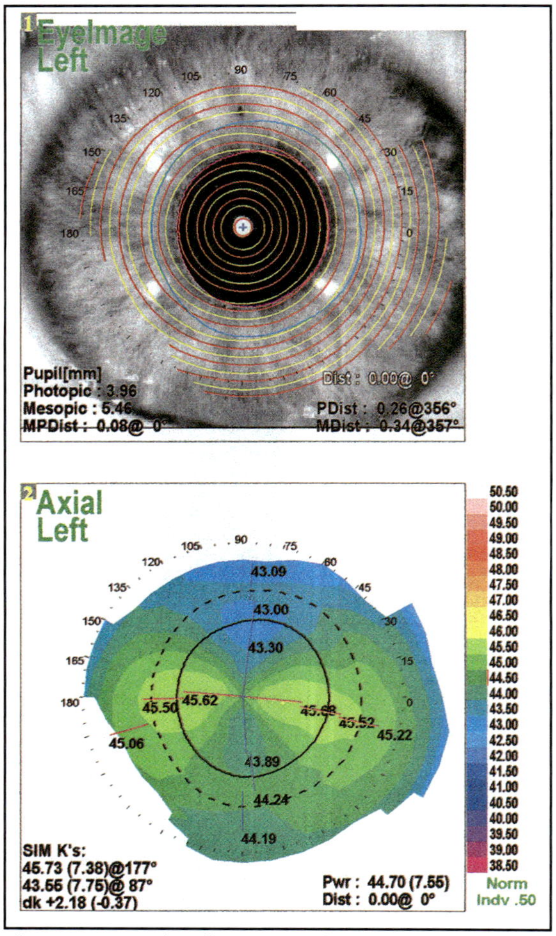


**Figure 10-1.** Placido image showing Placido rings reflected off the corneal surface (top) with the resultant color-coded generated image (bottom).

1. Normal (including round, oval, or regular bowtie patterns)
2. Asymmetric bowtie
3. Focal steep or skewed radial axis patterns
4. Abnormal patterns, including keratoconus, forme fruste keratoconus (FFKC), or pellucid marginal corneal degeneration.

Normal patterns include round or oval patterns and those with symmetric bowtie patterns. Asymmetric bowtie patterns include asymmetric steepening between 0.5 D and 1.0 D in any meridian. Focal steep patterns are those with asymmetric steepening of 1.0 D or more in any meridian (that do not meet published criteria for FFKC). Forme fruste patterns are those that meet published FFKC criteria.[5] Traditional pellucid corneal marginal degeneration (PCMD) patterns are those that demonstrate a crab-claw pattern or those with steepening in the far inferior periphery between the 4 and 8 o'clock meridian.[6] The traditional crab-claw pattern can be found in either keratoconus or PCMD eyes.[7]

TABLE 10-1.

**Corneal Topographic Evaluation: Step-By-Step Approach**

1. Identify color scale
2. Assess image quality
3. Identify topographic pattern
4. Additional considerations for topographic pattern evaluation
   a. Age
   b. Between-eye symmetry
   c. Dry Eye
   d. Corneal Scars
   e. Contact lens corneal warpage
   f. Unusual pattern location

TABLE 10-2.

**Corneal Tomographic Evaluation: Step-By-Step Approach**

1. Identify color scales/units of measurement
2. Assess image quality
3. Evaluate regional corneal thickness profiles
4. Evaluate focal anterior and posterior elevation changes

Most practitioners are comfortable identifying clearly normal and abnormal patterns. However, the challenge lies in discriminating between the subtle patterns that exist on a continuum between "normal" (acceptable for surgery) and "abnormal" (not acceptable for surgery). Some level of topographic asymmetry can be found in at least one-third of individuals presenting for refractive surgical evaluation.[8] In these cases, the following information can provide clues in the analysis: patient age, between-eye pattern symmetry, against-the-rule topographic patterns, unusual pattern location, contact lens history, and corneal health.

## Patient Age

Young patient age is a risk factor for the development of ectasia.[4,9,10] This is likely due to the fact that eyes predisposed to naturally occurring corneal ectasia will have evolving topographic patterns that advance over time.[11,12] Thus, when young patients are evaluated, their "final" naturally occurring topographic pattern may not yet have become manifest. Extra caution is therefore necessary when evaluating topographic patterns in these individuals, and more weight is given to subtle patterns.

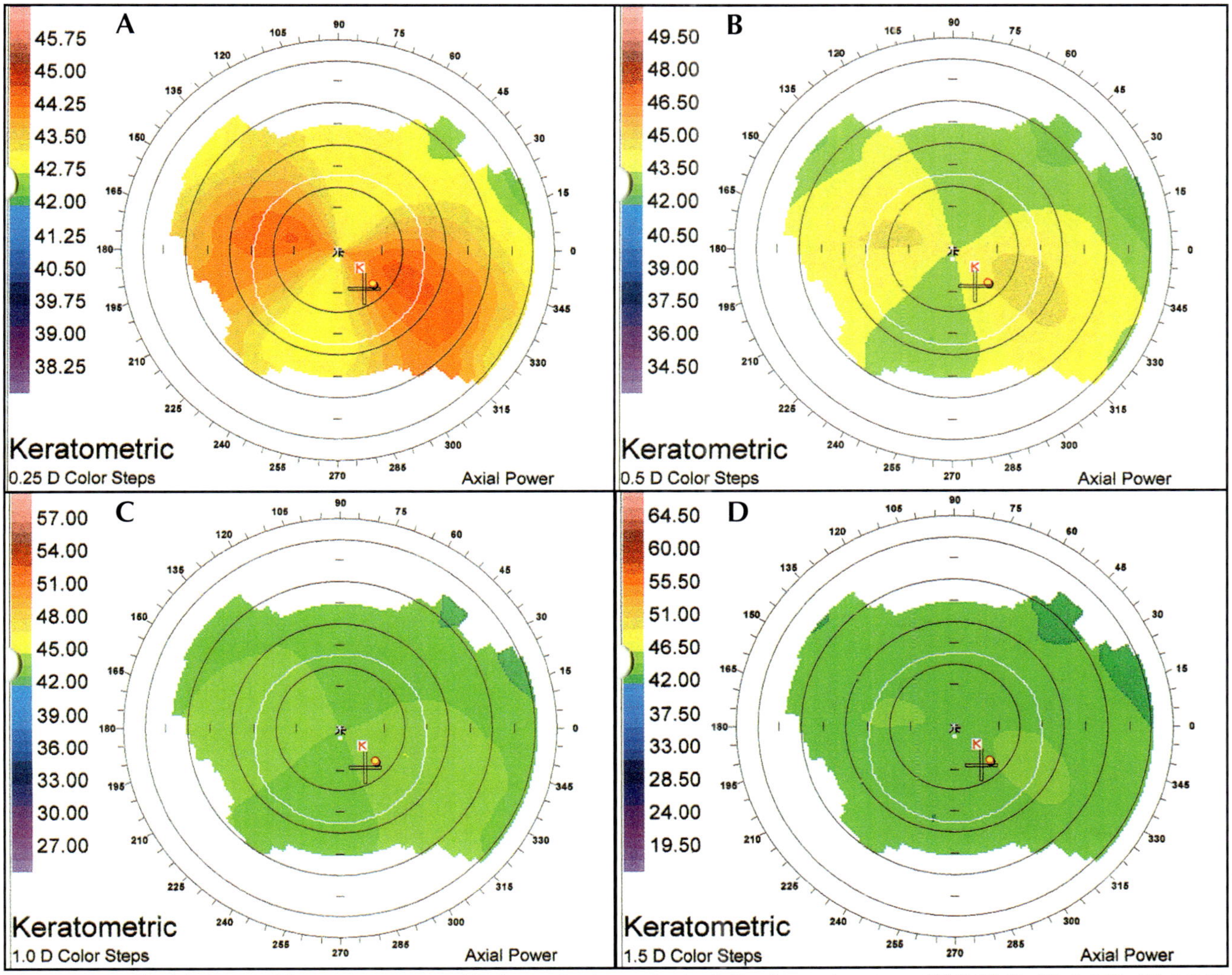


**Figure 10-2.** Placido image. The same topographic image is shown in the following color steps: (A) 0.25 D, (B) 0.5 D, (C) 1.0 D, and (D) 1.5 D. Note the apparent difference in pattern based on the color step used.

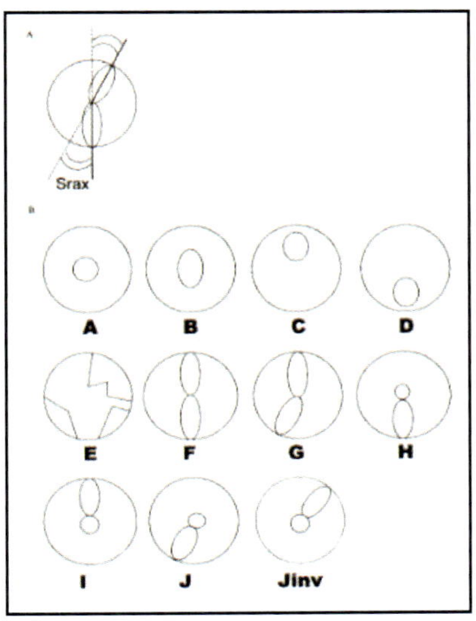


**Figure 10-3.** Patterns of steepening, with an Srax over 21 degrees and an Abs(I-S) value over 0.8 D, may correspond to FFKC. (Reprinted with permission from Wang M, ed. *Corneal Topography in the Wavefront Era: A Guide for Clinical Application.* Thorofare, NJ: SLACK Incorporated; 2006).

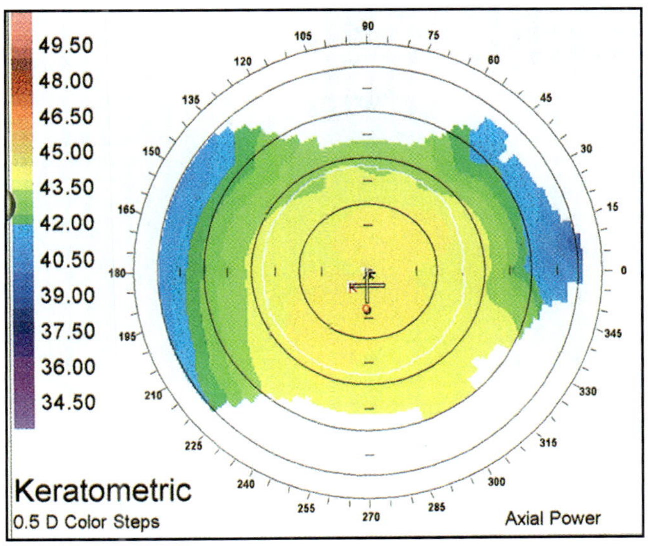


**Figure 10-4.** Placido image: normal pattern.

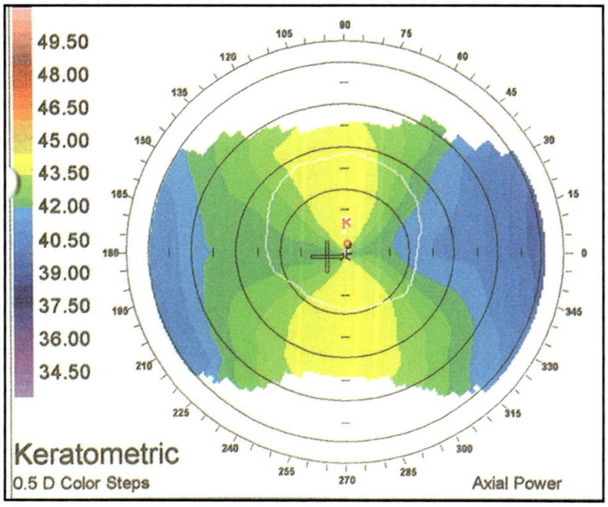


**Figure 10-5.** Placido image: symmetric bowtie pattern.

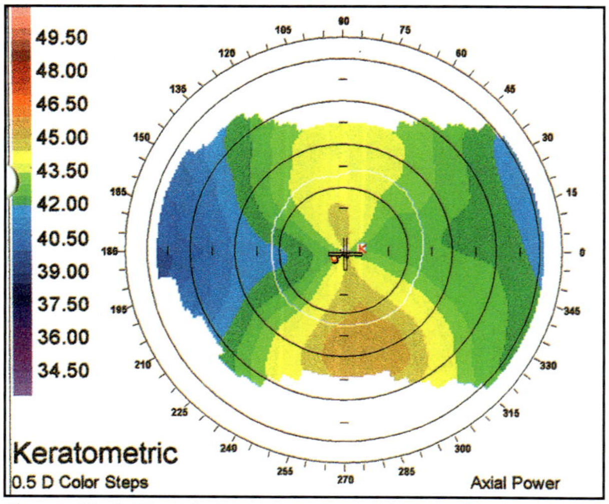


**Figure 10-6.** Placido image: asymmetric bowtie pattern.

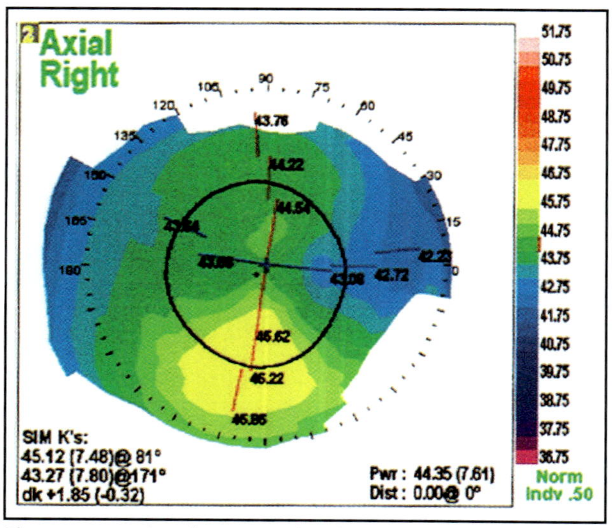


**Figure 10-7.** Placido image: focal steep pattern.

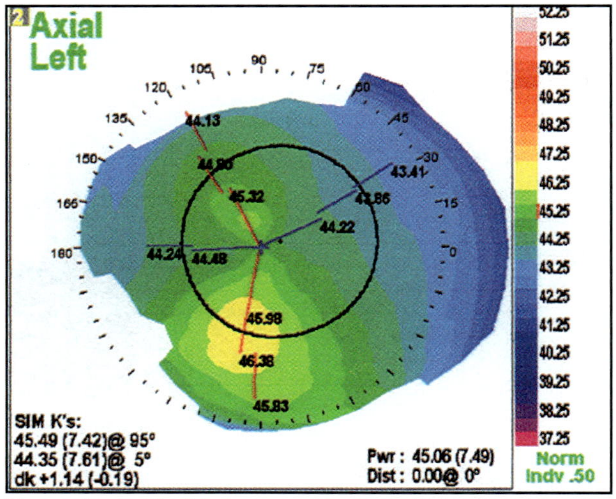


**Figure 10-8.** Placido image: skewed radial axis pattern.

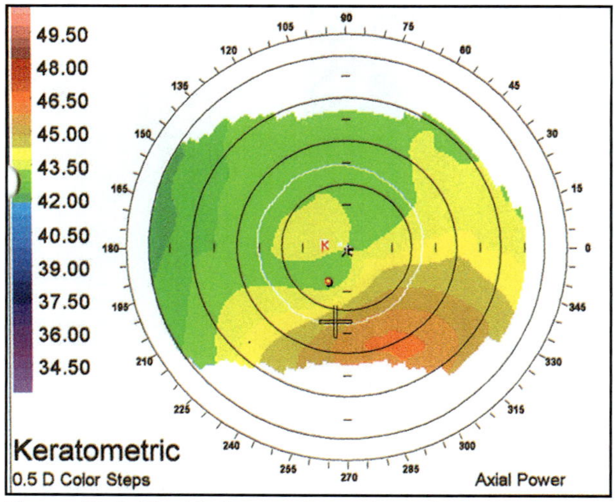


**Figure 10-9.** Placido image: forme fruste keratoconus.

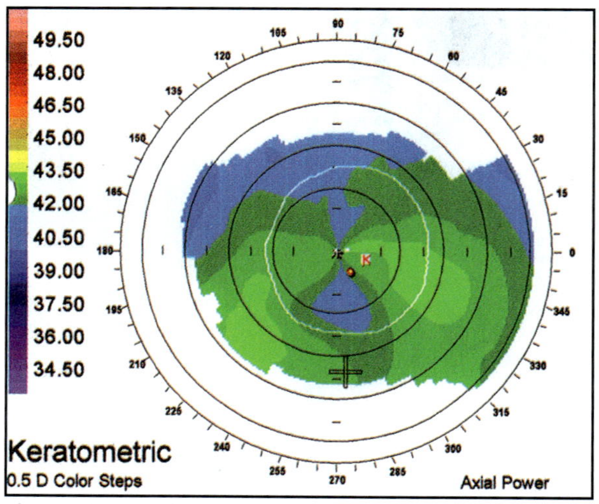


**Figure 10-10.** Placido image: pellucid marginal corneal degeneration suspect pattern.

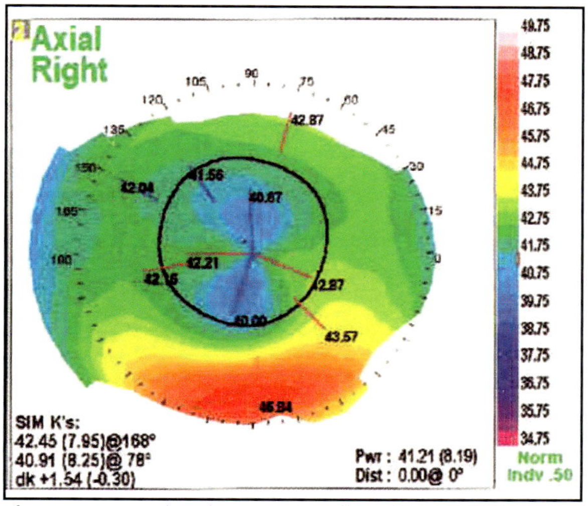


**Figure 10-11.** Placido image: pellucid marginal corneal degeneration pattern.

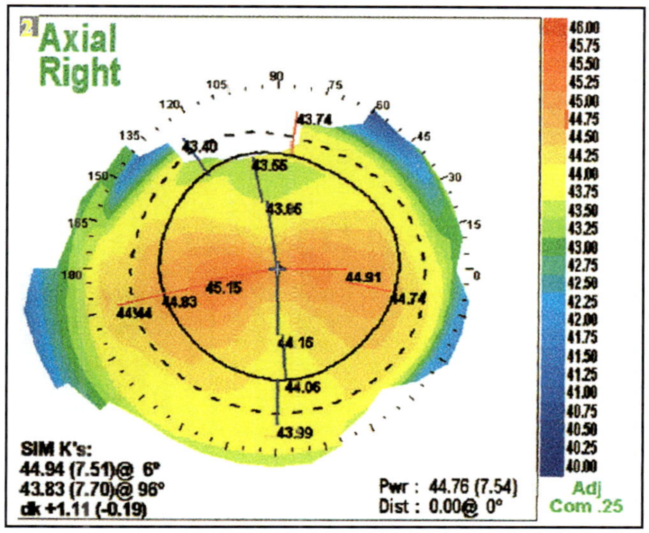


**Figure 10-12.** Placido image: against-the-rule astigmatism pattern. Note that the bow-tie pattern is displaced inferiorly toward the periphery (also known as "sagging"). This is consistent with an early crab-claw type pattern.

## Between-Eye Pattern Asymmetry

Topographic patterns are usually symmetric in normal corneas, and significant between-eye asymmetry should raise suspicion in the clinician. Further, keratoconus should be considered a bilateral disease for the purposes of keratorefractive surgical evaluation, and if either eye has a highly suspicious topographic pattern, then both eyes should be considered abnormal and should be excluded from surgery.

## Against-the-Rule Topographic Patterns

Against-the-rule patterns should also raise suspicion in the clinician (Figure 10-12). While these patterns can be a normal variant, they may also be the initial signs of an evolving PCMD "suspect" topography.[7,13,14] Special attention should be paid to the far periphery of the image to make sure that the pattern does not begin to "droop" downward, indicating the early stages of a crab-claw type pattern.

## Unusual Pattern Locations

Traditional patterns suspicious for ectatic disorders, including keratoconus and PCMD suspects, have inferior steepening to varying degrees; however, superior keratoconus and PCMD can occur (Figure 10-13).[15-21] Focal steepening in *any* meridian should be considered abnormal unless other causes for this steepening can be elucidated, such as significant corneal pannus or corneal scars (Figure 10-14).[13,22-24]

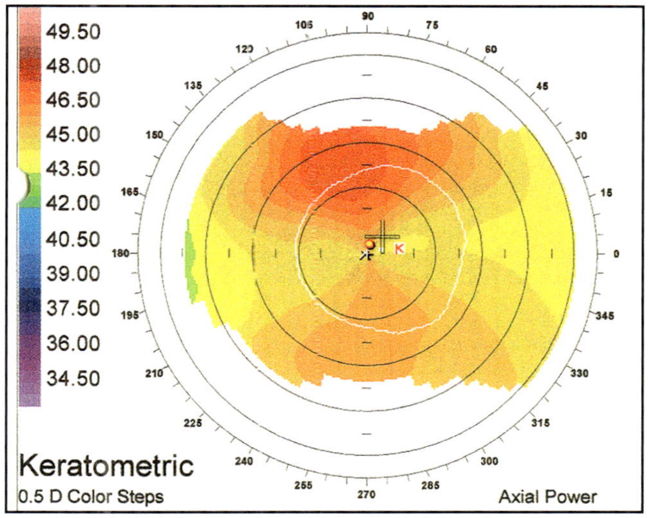


**Figure 10-13.** Placido image: superior steepening pattern.

## Other Considerations and Topographic Artifacts

Many other situations may generate irregular corneal topographies. These include corneal scars and opacities from previous corneal ulcers or epithelial basement membrane dystrophy (EBMD; Figure 10-15). In these situations, it is generally reasonable to proceed with keratorefractive surgery if all other parameters are within range; however, for most scars, opacities, and EBMD, surface ablation is preferable to LASIK.

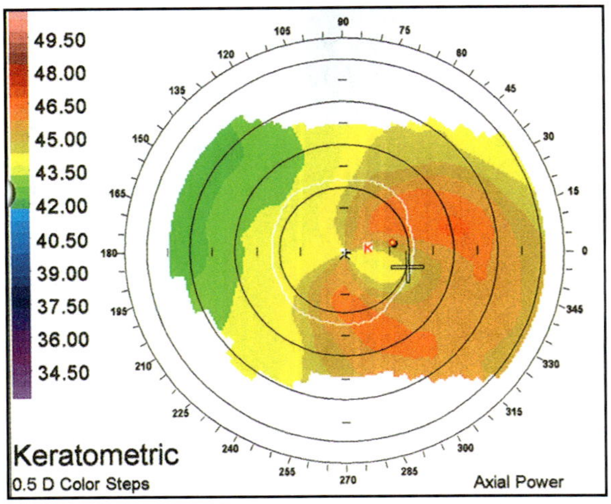


**Figure 10-14.** Placido image: Lateral steepening pattern (also called a "vertical D" pattern).

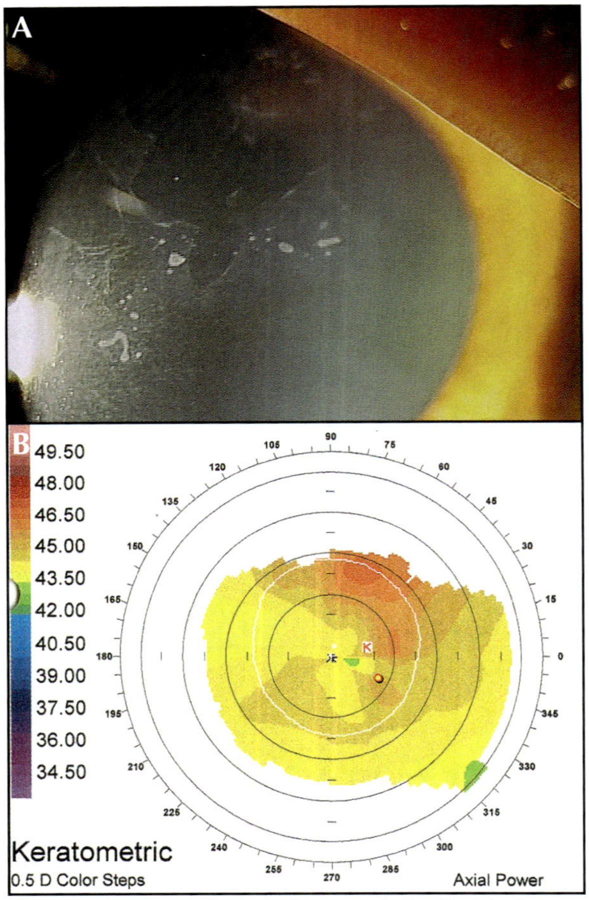


**Figure 10-15.** (A) Clinical photo and (B) Placido image: irregular astigmatism pattern associated with EBMD.

Extensive contact lens wear, including years of wear, number of hours/day, and overnight wear, can affect topographic patterns long after the contact lenses have been removed.[25] Soft toric and rigid gas-permeable contact lenses may have even more effect on topographic pattern,

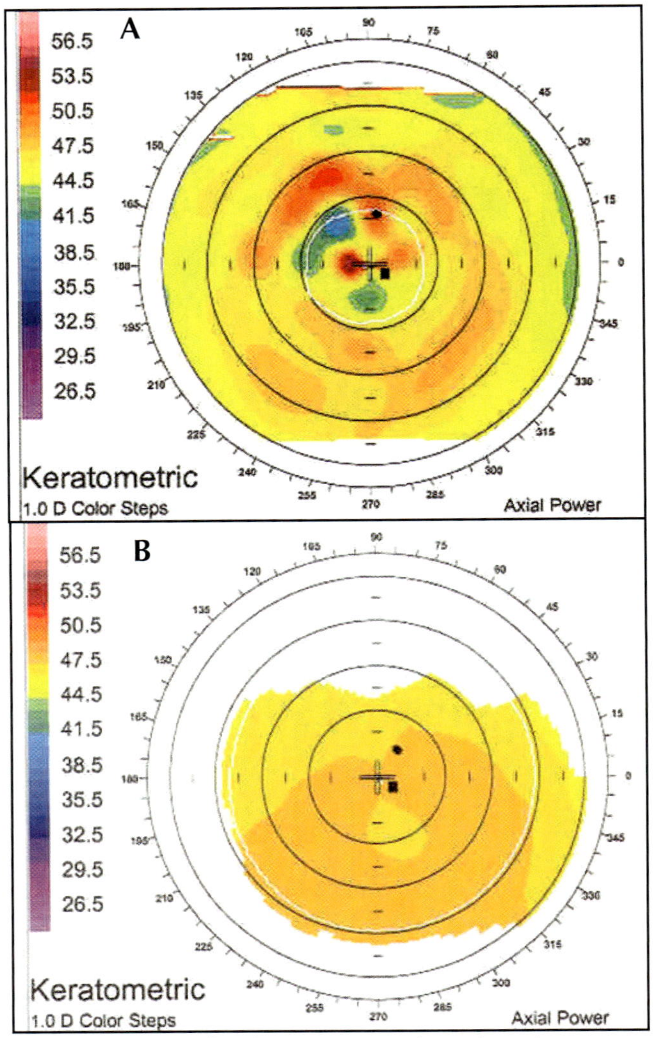


**Figure 10-16.** (A) Placido image: irregular astigmatism pattern secondary to dry eye (B) that appears more normalized following aggressive lubrication and repeat topographies.

and if an irregular pattern is found in a contact lens wearer, lenses should be discontinued for a longer period.

Dry eyes and blepharitis can also significantly impact topographic pattern.[26-28] These conditions should be evaluated, and in many instances the patient will benefit from treatment prior to repeat topographies (Figure 10-16). Effective treatment strategies include topical artificial tear use, topical cyclosporine to increase tear production, and topical azithromycin or oral tetracycline antibiotic use for blepharitis management.

Finally, while it may seem intuitively obvious, the quality of the scan will directly affect the pattern, and this should not be overlooked. Technicians should be properly trained not only to obtain quality scans but also to recognize poor-quality scans and automatically repeat these to give the practitioner high-quality data to evaluate. The most common causes of poor quality scans include patient-topographer misalignment, small images generated from

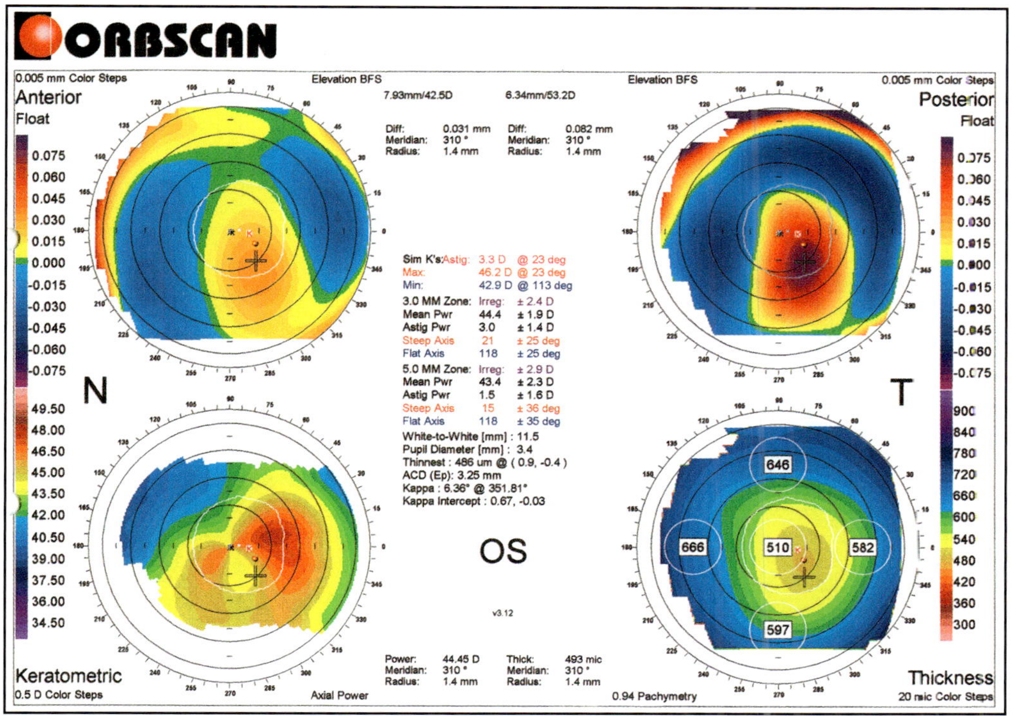


**Figure 10-17.** Scanning slit beam image (Orbscan II): Note the abnormal Placido pattern (lower left). There are focal areas of anterior and posterior elevations inferotemporally (upper left and upper right, respectively). There is also a corresponding area of focal corneal thickness inferotemporally (lower right) that is thinner than the central corneal thickness.

poor corneal exposure, data drop-out from debris in the tear film or eyelashes, and tear lake irregularities.

## Corneal Tomography

In addition to anterior curvature data generated by topography, technologies that generate corneal tomographic data may be useful for preoperative screening. There are numerous machines available clinically today that measure the cornea using slightly different techniques, including scanning slit beam (Orbscan II, Bausch & Lomb, Rochester, NY), Scheimpflug imaging (Pentacam, OCULUS, Inc, Wetzlar, Germany and Galilei, Ziemer Ophthalmics, Port, Switzerland), and high-resolution ocular coherence tomography (OCT). With scanning slit beam and Scheimpflug technologies, both corneal thickness profiles and corneal elevations as compared to best-fit spheres are generated in an attempt to better characterize overall corneal shape.

The Orbscan II device incorporates both Placido imaging and scanning slit beam-based imaging to generate both standard topographic and tomographic data. Overall, corneal thickness profiles are measured, and from these anterior and posterior elevation data are generated. These are measured against a "best-fit sphere" to give an overall impression of focal elevations (Figure 10-17). There have been reports discussing the value of these individual parameters, especially posterior float metrics[29-32]; however, these remain to be validated clinically. Another useful metric is the relationship between central and peripheral corneal thickness. While no absolute ratio between peripheral corneal thickness has been determined, in one study, population average inferior corneal thickness measurements were more than 60 μm thicker than central corneal measurements in a normal population.[33] A reduction in the peripheral/central corneal thickness ratio may be an early indicator of an abnormal cornea.[34] Ambrosio and colleagues reported significant differences in corneal thickness spatial profiles and corneal volume distribution between keratoconic and normal corneas,[35,36] and these metrics may be useful in screening, especially in eyes with borderline topographies.

Corneal thickness profiles and elevation data can also be generated by Scheimpflug imaging technology (Figure 10-18).[37-39] The Pentacam generates corneal thickness spatial profiles that may indicate early corneal pathology (Figure 10-19).

Corneal thickness profiles can also be generated by high-resolution ultrasound[40-42] and ocular coherence tomography (Figure 10-20).[43,44] Subtle changes in epithelial and stromal thickness may have implications for screening, as compensatory epithelial thinning overlying an ectatic region may be an early sign of a corneal ectatic disorder.[45-47]

The relative weight given to tomographic data versus topographic data is still hotly debated; however, the 2 together are likely additive. Anterior curvature changes with concomitant elevation abnormalities and abnormal corneal thickness profiles increases the odds that a cornea is biomechanically weaker and should be excluded for keratorefractive surgery.

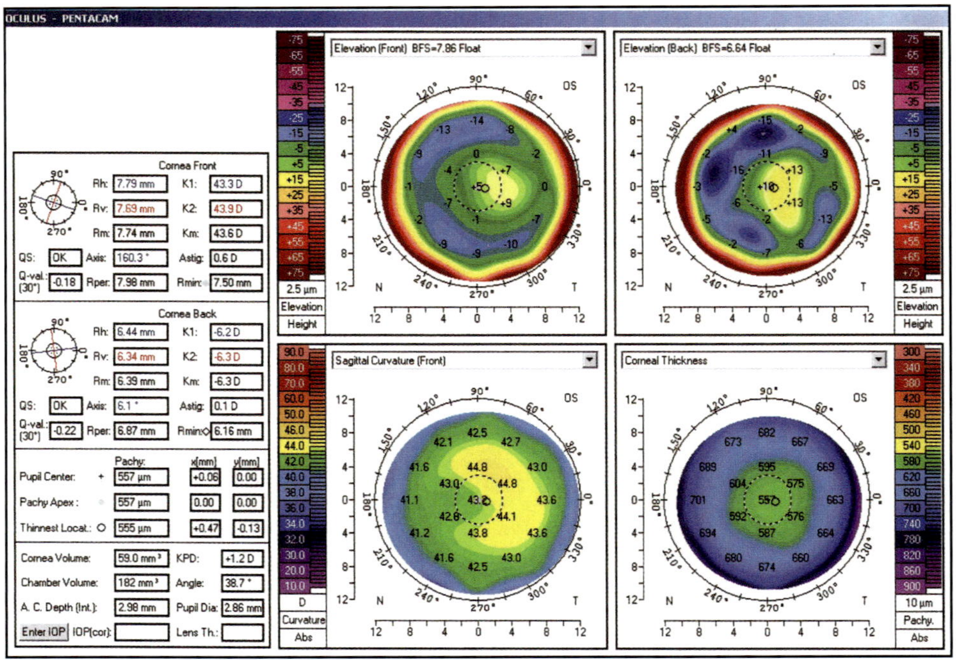


**Figure 10-18.** Scheimpflug image (Pentacam). Note the abnormal sagittal curvature pattern, with focal steepness laterally (lower left). There are focal areas of front and back elevations laterally (upper left and upper right, respectively).

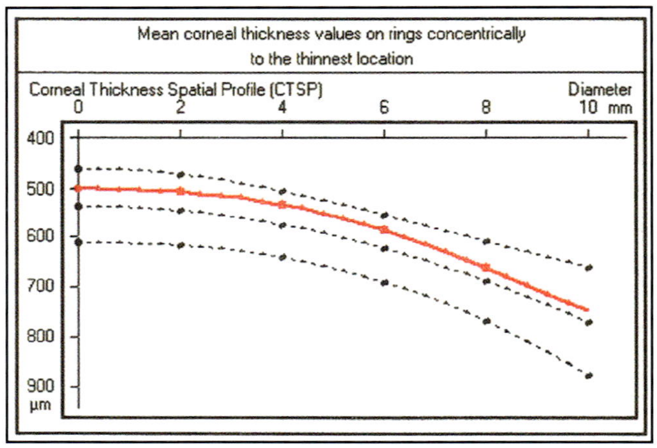


**Figure 10-19.** Corneal thickness spatial profile from the Scheimpflug image (Pentacam). Note the drop-off in values in the corneal peripheral diameter.

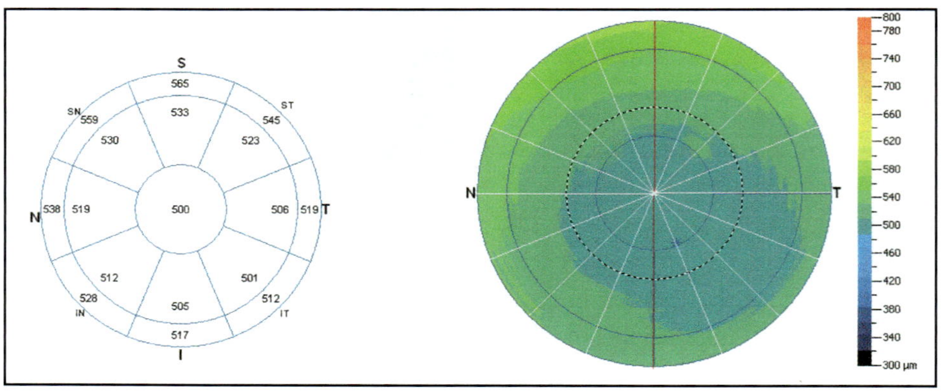


**Figure 10-20.** High-resolution anterior segment OCT image. Note the numerical values (left) and the corresponding color-coded mapping (right).

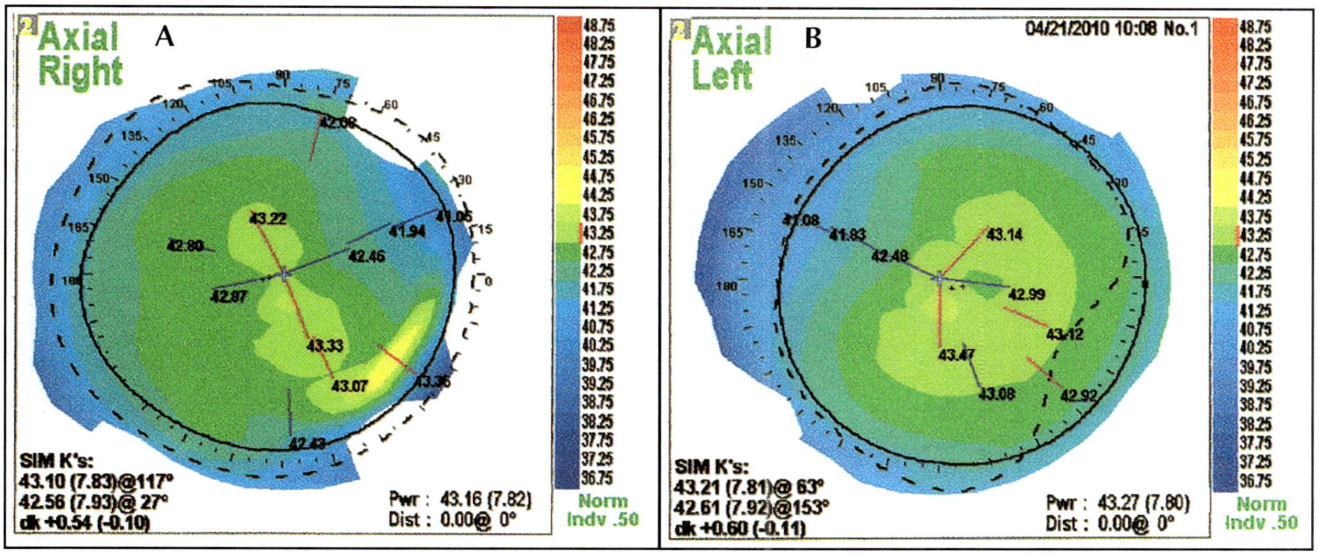


**Figure 10-21.** Placido image of (A) right and (B) left eyes. In the right eye, note the symmetric bowtie pattern oriented along the 110-degree meridian in the right eye combined with the moderate asymmetry oriented along the 30-degree meridian. In the left eye, note the focal steepening inferotemporally.

## Evaluating Topographic and Tomographic Data Independently From Other Patient Factors

While a complete surgical evaluation requires the clinician to evaluate and consider a variety of information in addition to topographic pattern, including refraction, corneal thickness, overall ocular health, and patient age, it is critical that topographic pattern evaluation initially be done independently. This statement is essential and bears repeating: First evaluate topographic patterns independent of other patient information. Abnormal topographic patterns can occur in any age group, with any refraction or corrected visual acuity, and with any corneal thickness. Some clinicians may be tempted to devalue subtle abnormalities if the patient has a low myopic or hyperopic refraction, their correctable acuity is "excellent," or the cornea is "thick enough"; however, abnormal topography can occur in any eye and is an independent risk factor for ectasia. Ectasia has occurred in hyperopic eyes, thick corneas, and eyes that otherwise appeared "normal" but that could have been excluded by close topographic pattern analysis alone.[13,14,34,48,49]

## Patient Evaluation: Case Example

A 22-year-old man presented for refractive surgery evaluation. His manifest refraction was -3.25 sphere and -4.00 +1.00 x 055 in the right and left eyes, respectively, with best spectacle-corrected visual acuities of 20/20 in both eyes. Central corneal thickness was 560 µm in the right eye and 570 µm in the left eye. The anterior segment and dilated fundus exam was unremarkable in both eyes. Topographies are shown (Figure 10-21). Additional images of the left eye are shown (Figures 10-22 through 10-24).

Topographic evaluation of the right eye Placido image (in 0.5 D color scale) demonstrates what initially appears to be a symmetric bowtie pattern (with some inferior artifact, likely from tear film) oriented in the 110-degree meridian. However, on further inspection, there is subtle asymmetry oriented along the 30-degree meridian, with the inferior temporal cornea approximately 0.8 D steeper in some areas than the corresponding superior nasal area. Topographic evaluation of the left eye Placido image (in 0.5 D color scale) demonstrates more pronounced asymmetry oriented along the 150-degree meridian, with the inferior temporal cornea approximately 1.5 D steeper in some areas than the corresponding superior nasal area. In comparing the 2 eyes, there is some between-eye asymmetry between the patterns.

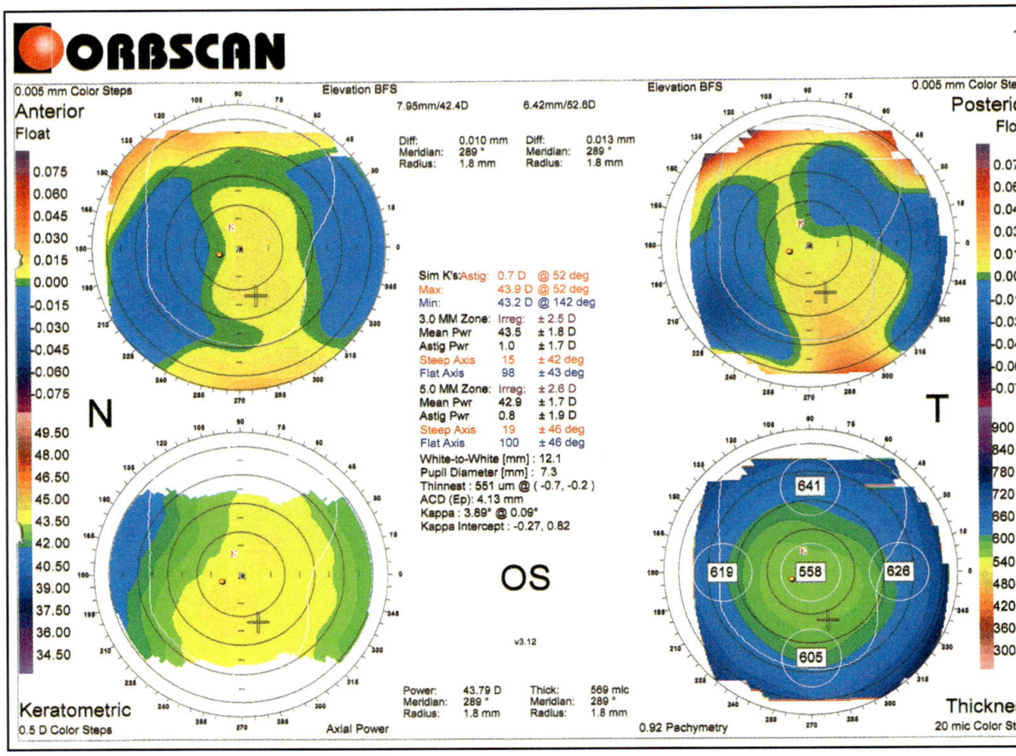


**Figure 10-22.** Scanning slit beam image (Orbscan II). Note the Placido pattern that is quite similar to the Placido pattern from Figure 10-21. Also note the focal increased anterior and posterior elevations inferiorly in the far periphery (upper left and right images, respectively).

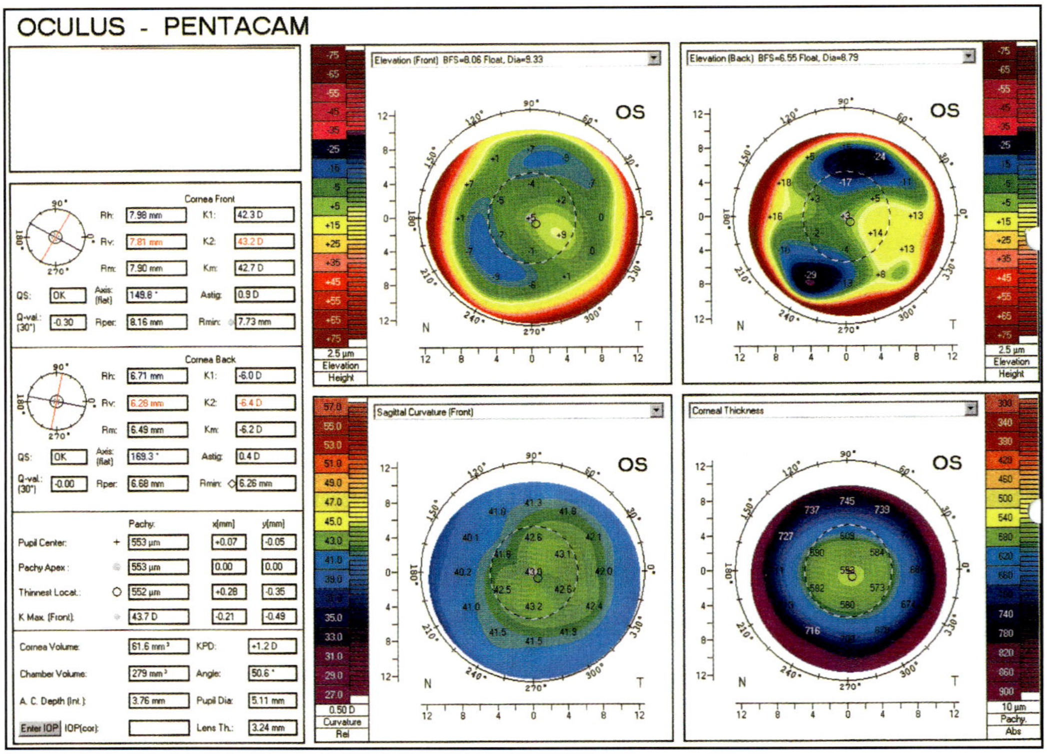


**Figure 10-23.** Scheimpflug image (Pentacam). Note the sagittal curvature map (lower left) that corresponds in pattern to the Placido images from Figures 10-21 and 10-22. There is more pronounced focal steepening in both the front and back elevation maps (upper left and right images, respectively).

Further evaluation of the left eye with scanning slit beam technology (Orbscan II) confirms the Placido pattern (see Figure 10-22, lower left, also in 0.5 D color scale). The corneal thickness profile (see Figure 10-22, lower right) appears normal, with the thinnest portion of the cornea in the center and appropriate peripheral thickening in relation to the central thickness. Neither anterior nor posterior elevations are overly remarkable (see Figure 10-22, upper left and right, respectively); however, there is some increased elevation in the far inferior periphery that warrants further evaluation.

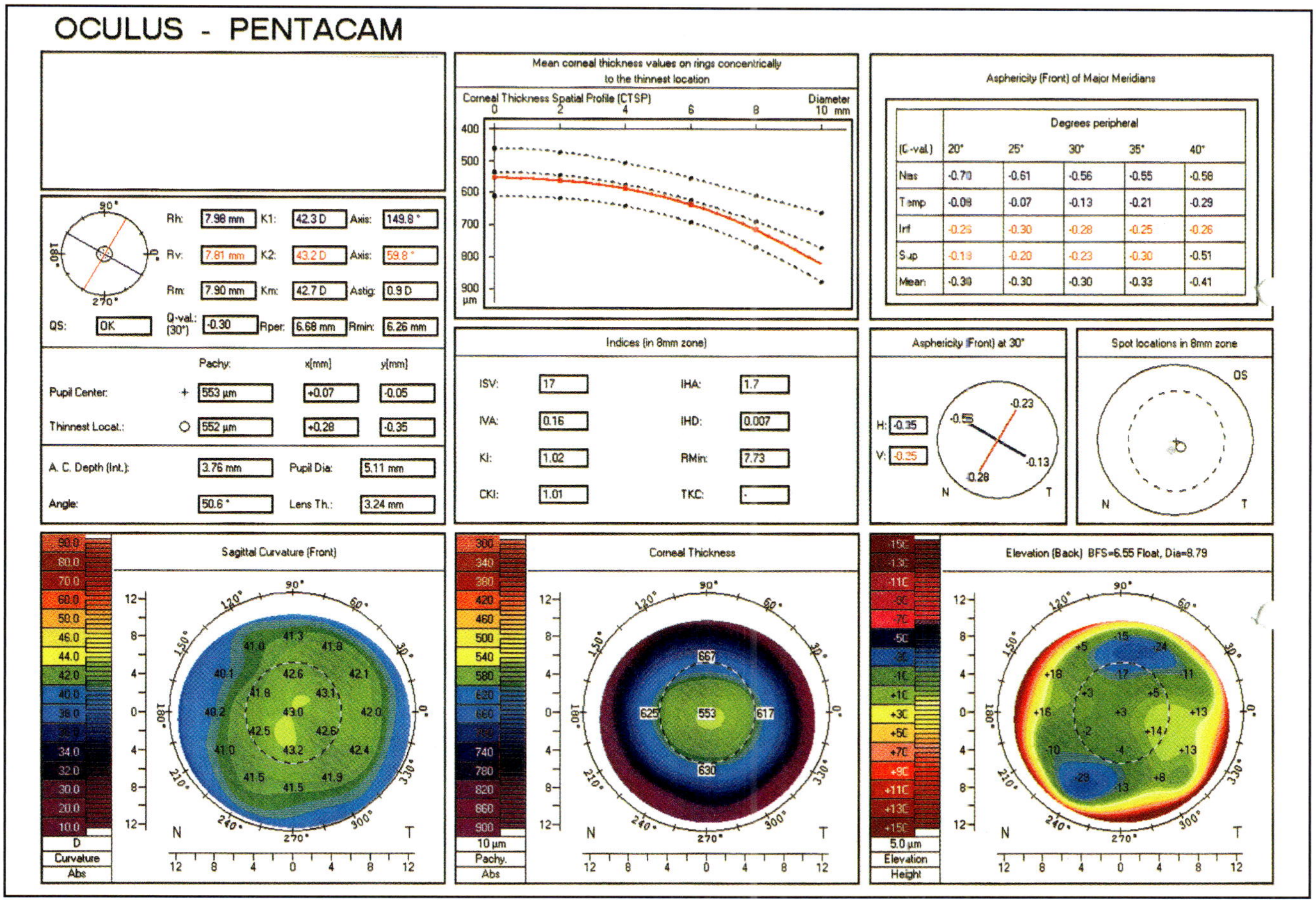


**Figure 10-24.** Scheimpflug image (Pentacam): The corneal thickness spatial profile (upper middle image) exhibits a gradual relative reduction toward the periphery.

Scheimpflug imaging technology (Pentacam) demonstrates a sagittal curvature pattern (see Figure 10-23, lower left) that correlates well with the Placido patterns. The corneal thickness profile (see Figure 10-23, lower right) appears normal, with the thinnest portion of the cornea in the center and apparently normal peripheral thickening in relation to the central thickness. There is a more focal area of elevation visible on both the front and back elevation maps (see Figure 10-23, upper left and upper right, respectively). Further, mean corneal thickness values (see Figure 10-24, upper middle box) demonstrate a gradual relative reduction toward the periphery.

So, the overall topographic and tomographic evaluation for this patient reveals an asymmetric pattern with between-eye asymmetry, borderline corneal thickness spatial profiles, and subtle increased anterior and posterior elevations more notable in the left eye. The patient's young age makes this pattern highly suspicious; therefore, LASIK is not recommended, and a reasonable approach would be to delay surgery for 1 to 2 years to re-evaluate the topographic and tomographic data before considering surface ablation.

## Conclusion

There are a variety of technologies available for patient tomographic and topographic screening. Careful evaluation of these modalities, sometimes in combination for suspect topographic patterns, can improve the refractive screening process and thereby improve the safety and efficacy of keratorefractive surgery.

## References

1. Randleman JB, Russell B, Ward MA, et al. Risk factors and prognosis for corneal ectasia after LASIK. *Ophthalmology*. 2003;110(2):267-275.
2. Smolek MK, Klyce SD, Hovis JK. The Universal Standard Scale: proposed improvements to the American National Standards Institute (ANSI) scale for corneal topography. *Ophthalmology*. 2002;109(2):361-369.
3. Rabinowitz YS, Yang H, Brickman Y, et al. Videokeratography database of normal human corneas. *Br J Ophthalmol*. 1996;80(7):610-616.

4. Randleman JB, Woodward M, Lynn MJ, Stulting RD. Risk assessment for ectasia after corneal refractive surgery. *Ophthalmology.* 2008;115(1):37-50.
5. Rabinowitz YS, McDonnell PJ. Computer-assisted corneal topography in keratoconus. *Refract Corneal Surg.* 1989;5(6):400-408.
6. Maguire LJ, Klyce SD, McDonald MB, Kaufman HE. Corneal topography of pellucid marginal degeneration. *Ophthalmology.* 1987;94(5):519-524.
7. Lee BW, Jurkunas UV, Harissi-Dagher M, et al. Ectatic disorders associated with a claw-shaped pattern on corneal topography. *Am J Ophthalmol.* 2007;144(1):154-156.
8. Varssano D, Kaiserman I, Hazarbassanov R. Topographic patterns in refractive surgery candidates. *Cornea.* 2004;23(6):602-607.
9. Klein SR, Epstein RJ, Randleman JB, Stulting RD. Corneal ectasia after laser in situ keratomileusis in patients without apparent preoperative risk factors. *Cornea.* 2006;25(4):388-403.
10. Randleman JB, Trattler WB, Stulting RD. Validation of the Ectasia Risk Score System for preoperative laser in situ keratomileusis screening. *Am J Ophthalmol.* 2008;145(5):813-818.
11. Fogla R, Padmanabhan P. Bilateral keratectasia after unilateral laser in situ keratomileusis. *J Cataract Refract Surg.* 2004;30(10):2033-2034.
12. Wang JC, Hufnagel TJ, Buxton DF. Bilateral keratectasia after unilateral laser in situ keratomileusis: a retrospective diagnosis of ectatic corneal disorder. *J Cataract Refract Surg.* 2003;29(10):2015-2018.
13. Ambrosio R Jr, Wilson SE. Early pellucid marginal corneal degeneration: case reports of two refractive surgery candidates. *Cornea.* 2002;21(1):114-117.
14. Fogla R, Rao SK, Padmanabhan P. Keratectasia in 2 cases with pellucid marginal corneal degeneration after laser in situ keratomileusis. *J Cataract Refract Surg.* 2003;29(4):788-791.
15. Sridhar MS, Mahesh S, Bansal AK, Rao GN. Superior pellucid marginal corneal degeneration. *Eye (Lond).* 2004;18(4):393-399.
16. Bower KS, Dhaliwal DK, Barnhorst DA Jr, Warnicke J. Pellucid marginal degeneration with superior corneal thinning. *Cornea.* 1997;16(4):483-485.
17. Cameron JA, Mahmood MA. Superior corneal thinning with pellucid marginal corneal degeneration. *Am J Ophthalmol.* 1990;109(4):486-487.
18. Chiang CC, Lin JM, Tsai YY. Superior keratoconus with inferior paracentral corneal thinning and inferior peripheral pellucid marginal degeneration. *Eye (Lond).* 2007;21(2):266-268.
19. Weed KH, McGhee CN, MacEwen CJ. Atypical unilateral superior keratoconus in young males. *Cont Lens Anterior Eye.* 2005;28(4):177-179.
20. Prisant O, Legeais JM, Renard G. Superior keratoconus. *Cornea.* 1997;16(6):693-694.
21. Eiferman RA, Lane L, Law M, Fields Y. Superior keratoconus. *Refract Corneal Surg.* 1993;9(5):394-395.
22. Bansal AS, Randleman JB. Corneal ectasia after LASIK in a patient with superior pellucid marginal degeneration. *J Refract Surg.* 2009;25(2):172-174.
23. Rao SK, Fogla R, Padmanabhan P, Sitalakshmi G. Corneal topography in atypical pellucid marginal degeneration. *Cornea.* 1999;18(3):265-272.
24. Abad JC, Rubinfeld RS, Del Valle M, et al. Vertical D: a novel topographic pattern in some keratoconus suspects. *Ophthalmology.* 2007;114(5):1020-1026.
25. Wilson SE, Lin DT, Klyce SD, et al. Topographic changes in contact lens-induced corneal warpage. *Ophthalmology.* 1990;97(6):734-744.
26. De Paiva CS, Harris LD, Pflugfelder SC. Keratoconus-like topographic changes in keratoconjunctivitis sicca. *Cornea.* 2003;22(1):22-24.
27. Dursun D, Piniella AM, Pflugfelder SC. Pseudokeratoconus caused by rosacea. *Cornea.* 2001;20(6):668-669.
28. de Paiva CS, Lindsey JL, Pflugfelder SC. Assessing the severity of keratitis sicca with videokeratoscopic indices. *Ophthalmology.* 2003;110(6):1102-1109.
29. Quisling S, Sjoberg S, Zimmerman B, et al. Comparison of Pentacam and Orbscan IIz on posterior curvature topography measurements in keratoconus eyes. *Ophthalmology.* 2006;113(9):1629-1632.
30. Rao SN, Raviv T, Majmudar PA, Epstein RJ. Role of Orbscan II in screening keratoconus suspects before refractive corneal surgery. *Ophthalmology.* 2002;109(9):1642-1646.
31. Sonmez B, Doan MP, Hamilton DR. Identification of scanning slit-beam topographic parameters important in distinguishing normal from keratoconic corneal morphologic features. *Am J Ophthalmol.* 2007;143(3):401-408.
32. Tabbara KF, Kotb AA. Risk factors for corneal ectasia after LASIK. *Ophthalmology.* 2006;113(9):1618-1622.
33. Liu Z, Huang AJ, Pflugfelder SC. Evaluation of corneal thickness and topography in normal eyes using the Orbscan corneal topography system. *Br J Ophthalmol.* 1999;83(7):774-778.
34. Randleman JB, Banning CS, Stulting RD. Corneal ectasia after hyperopic LASIK. *J Refract Surg.* 2007;23(1):98-102.
35. Ambrosio R Jr, Alonso RS, Luz A, Coca Velarde LG. Corneal-thickness spatial profile and corneal-volume distribution: tomographic indices to detect keratoconus. *J Cataract Refract Surg.* 2006;32(11):1851-1859.
36. Ambrosio R Jr, Klyce SD, Wilson SE. Corneal topographic and pachymetric screening of keratorefractive patients. *J Refract Surg.* 2003;19(1):24-29.
37. Khachikian SS, Belin MW. Posterior elevation in keratoconus. *Ophthalmology.* 2009;116(4):816, e1; author reply -7.
38. Belin MW, Khachikian SS. An introduction to understanding elevation-based topography: how elevation data are displayed—a review. *Clin Experiment Ophthalmol.* 2009;37(1):14-29.
39. Ciolino JB, Khachikian SS, Belin MW. Comparison of corneal thickness measurements by ultrasound and Scheimpflug photography in eyes that have undergone laser in situ keratomileusis. *Am J Ophthalmol.* 2008;145(1):75-80.
40. Reinstein DZ, Archer TJ, Gobbe M, et al. Epithelial thickness in the normal cornea: three-dimensional display with Artemis very high-frequency digital ultrasound. *J Refract Surg.* 2008;24(6):571-581.
41. Reinstein DZ, Couch DG, Archer T. Direct residual stromal thickness measurement for assessing suitability for LASIK enhancement by Artemis 3D very high-frequency digital ultrasound arc scanning. *J Cataract Refract Surg.* 2006;32(11):1884-1888.
42. Reinstein DZ, Archer TJ, Silverman RH, Coleman DJ. Accuracy, repeatability, and reproducibility of Artemis very high-frequency digital ultrasound arc-scan lateral dimension measurements. *J Cataract Refract Surg.* 2006;32(11):1799-1802.
43. Li Y, Meisler DM, Tang M, et al. Keratoconus diagnosis with optical coherence tomography pachymetry mapping. *Ophthalmology.* 2008;115(12):2159-2166.
44. Li Y, Shekhar R, Huang D. Corneal pachymetry mapping with high-speed optical coherence tomography. *Ophthalmology.* 2006;113(5):792-799, e2.
45. Reinstein DZ, Gobbe M, Archer TJ, et al. Epithelial, stromal, and total corneal thickness in keratoconus: three-dimensional display with Artemis very-high frequency digital ultrasound. *J Refract Surg.* 2010;26(4):259-271.
46. Reinstein DZ, Archer TJ, Gobbe M. Corneal epithelial thickness profile in the diagnosis of keratoconus. *J Refract Surg.* 2009;25(7):604-610.
47. Reinstein DZ, Archer TJ, Gobbe M. Stability of LASIK in topographically suspect keratoconus confirmed non-keratoconic by Artemis VHF digital ultrasound epithelial thickness mapping: 1-year follow-up. *J Refract Surg.* 2009;25(7):569-577.
48. Malecaze F, Coullet J, Calvas P, et al. Corneal ectasia after photorefractive keratectomy for low myopia. *Ophthalmology.* 2006;113(5):742-746.
49. Randleman JB, Caster AI, Banning CS, Stulting RD. Corneal ectasia after photorefractive keratectomy. *J Cataract Refract Surg.* 2006;32(8):1395-1398.

Chapter 11

# Topography-Guided Custom Ablation

Tracy Schroeder Swartz, OD, MS, FAAO

There are a variety of etiologies for irregular astigmatism, directly measured as irregularity on topographical maps and manifesting as increased higher-order aberrations (HOAs) using wavefront analysis. Mild ocular surface changes such as dry eye and contact lens warpage are usually correctable by treating the dry eye and discontinuing the lenses. More severe ocular surface changes such as scarring, corneal dystrophies, and degenerations such as anterior basement membrane dystrophy and pterygium may require surgery to remove the scarring, address the dystrophy, or remove the pterygium. Refractive procedures including radial keratotomy, excimer ablation, and conductive keratoplasty can also create irregular astigmatism.

Correcting irregular astigmatism caused by refractive procedures is complex, as most devices used to perform refractive procedures are unable to correct the problems they may cause. These problems include a small optical zone, decentered ablation, severely prolate or oblate corneas, and irregularly irregular astigmatism induced by laser-assisted in situ keratomileusis (LASIK), photorefractive keratectomy (PRK), radial keratotomy, conductive keratoplasty, cataract surgery, and deep lamellar keratoplasty. Several systems have been used to correct these problems.[1-5] The following sections illustrate how several systems surgically address correction of irregular astigmatism.

## LaserSight AstraPro

David D. Liu, PhD; Zhengjun Fan, MD; Junhua Xiao, MD; and Bing Liu, MD

Even with the advancement of technologies and clinical applications, difficult corneal cases do occasionally prove to be a challenge in laser refractive surgery. To address such a challenge, LaserSight Technologies, Inc, has developed a 3-dimensional topography-based custom ablation product, AstraPro 2.2Z, to repair problems, such as decentered ablations and other irregular corneas. AstraPro 2.2Z uses precise 3-dimensional elevation data obtained from AstraMax, a 3-dimensional topographer, and subjective refraction data to calculate an ablation pattern that allows the restoration of both the desired shape of the postenhancement cornea and the desired visual axis of



Wang M. *Corneal Topography: A Guide for Clinical Application in the Wavefront Era, Second Edition* (pp. 243-252)

a problem cornea, resulting in tissue-saving ablation that creates an effective refractive optical zone on the most applicable optical axis.

In problem corneas, such as those with a decentered ablation, the corneal elevation is asymmetrical. When using a topographer to obtain the elevation measurement, the acquired data are misaligned with the visual axis of the eye (for normal cornea, the topography center is a good approximation to the visual axis center). If we design an ablation profile based on the misaligned axis, any attempts to fix the problem cornea will not only be ineffective, but also wasteful in cornea tissues. The new ablation algorithm used in AstraPro 2.2Z is based on this observation and understanding. The algorithm involves an optimized ellipsoidal model that targets a prolate postoperative surface (for better visual acuity) and at the same time also allows the axis of the postoperative ellipsoid of the corneal surface to be optimized with respect to the preoperative visual axis of the cornea. In the case of an asymmetrical cornea, its corneal topography-indicated visual axis is biased and therefore should not be used as the target axis for the postoperative corneal surface. The optimization criterion is to find a new axis that minimizes the tissue ablated while achieving the refractive correction needed using a prolate ablation model.

The optimized ablation profile is a point-by-point ablation pattern based on asymmetrical elevation data and can only be achieved with a point-by-point scanning refractive laser. LaserSight AstraScan XL is equipped with a high-speed eye tracker and high-speed micro spot scanning system, ideally suited for executing this type of precise, point-by-point, 3-dimensional asymmetrical ablation profile. The following case reports demonstrate the system's applications.

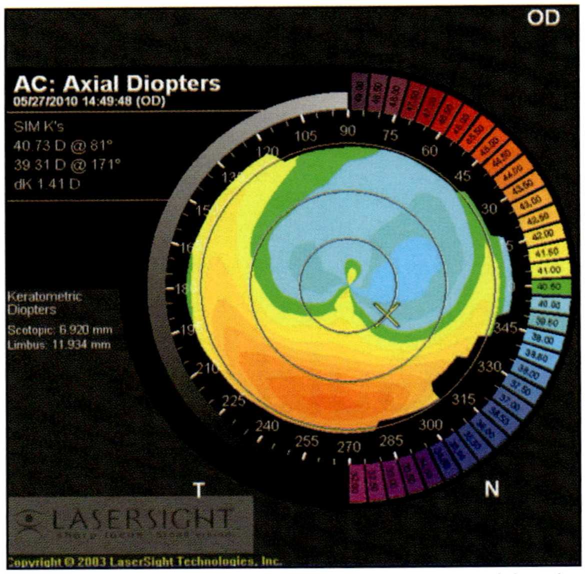


**Figure 11-1.** Decentered ablation as measured by the AstraMax 3-D topographer. It is important to properly adjust the patient's head and eye position prior to measurement of topography. The patient must properly fixate on the fixation target.

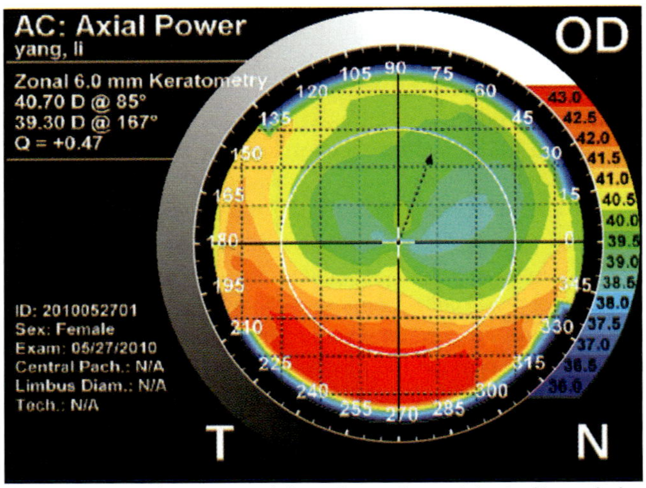


**Figure 11-2.** The arrowed line from the origin indicated the shift direction of the predicted post-enhancement visual axis. The shift amount is very small, typically well below 0.1 mm by 0.1 mm, and never exceeds 0.2 mm by 0.2 mm. The shift is always in the direction of the flat area of the pre-enhancement cornea, indicating that the measurement bias for the problem cornea is toward the steep axis.

## Case 1

A 24-year-old female patient underwent LASIK in May 2009 in a different hospital on the right eye. The patient complained of poor vision with ghost images. Uncorrected visual acuity was 40/100. The patient was referred to our hospital in May 2010. Upon examination with the AstraMax and manifest refraction, it was observed that a significantly decentered ablation existed, as shown in Figure 11-1. We evaluated the patient's cornea and decided to use LaserSight's AstraPro 2.2Z to plan an enhancement on the cornea. LaserSight AstraPro 2.2Z allows significant tissue saving over a standard algorithm. More importantly, it is effective in optimally choosing the post-enhancement target corneal visual axis, typically along the direction of the flat portion of the cornea, as indicated in Figure 11-2. The relatively small change of predicted postoperative visual axis allows for significant tissue saving and dramatically improved enhancement effectiveness. After the enhancement, the major complaint of double vision was resolved, and the patient achieved 20/20 uncorrected visual acuity. The corrected topography map and the difference map of the pre-enhancement and post-enhancement are displayed in Figure 11-3. As can be seen, the enhancement ablation was custom designed to just compensate for the ablation deficiency caused by the decentration.

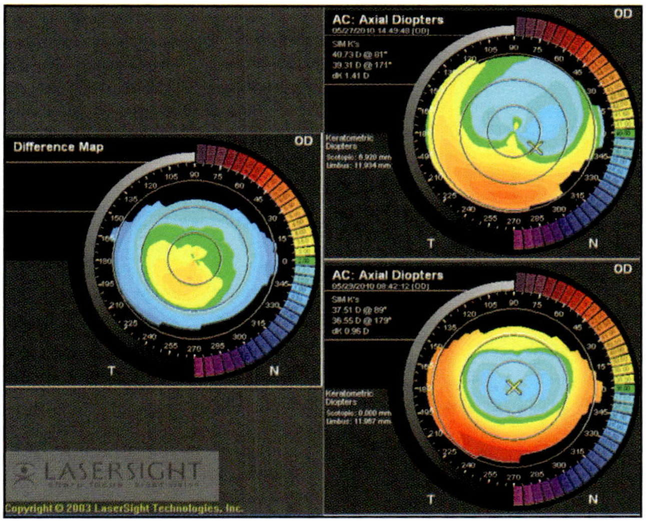


**Figure 11-3.** The upper right is the pre-enhancement and the lower right is the post-enhancement topography map. The left is the difference of the two. The post-enhancement map illustrates the restored center optical zone, and the difference map indicates approximately the amount of refractive power correction achieved for this problem cornea.

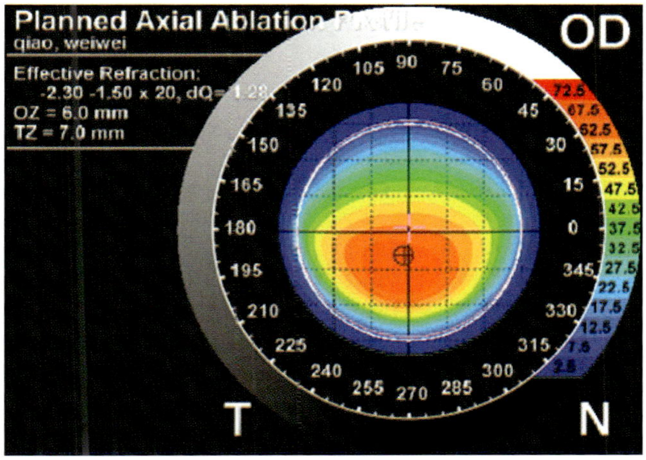


**Figure 11-5.** In this 3-d mens onal ablation profile, the ablation volume distribution is calculated precisely from the measured 3-dimensional corneal elevation data. The planned ablation profile is optimized to correct the missed ablation tissues to achieve a symmetrical and smooth postoperative corneal surface.

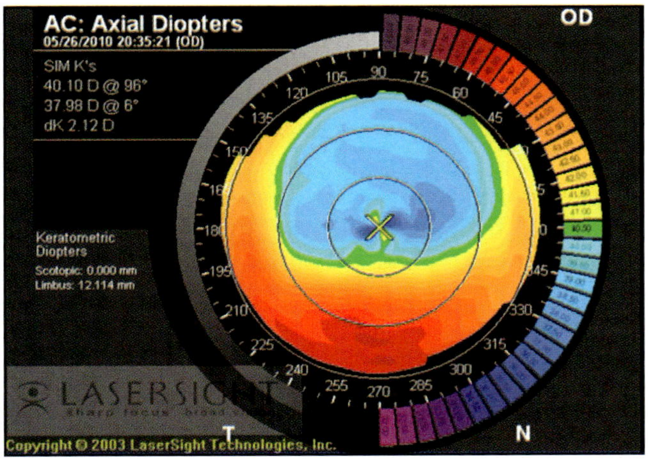


**Figure 11-4.** A significantly decentered ablation.

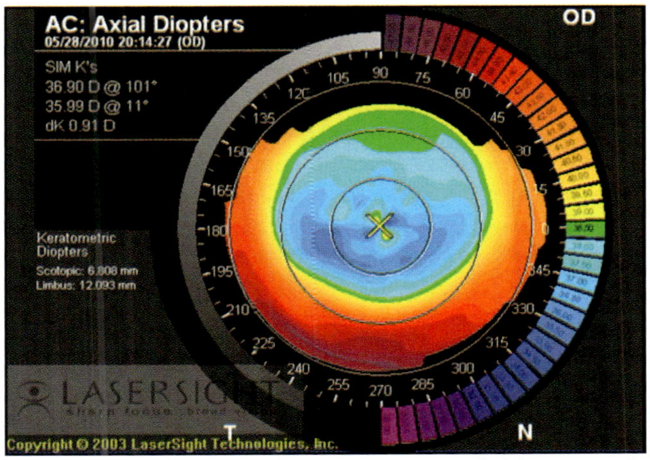


**Figure 11-6.** The post-enhancement map of this cornea is smooth and symmetrica', with resolution of the ghost image and poor visual acuity comp aint while saving unnecessary and excessive ablation. The topography-guided ablation technique, due to the high precision of the elevation data (on the order of 1 μm) and the advanced ellipsoidal model in free space, with optimization in both radius, shape factor, and axis, was able to repair severe irregularity of the cornea, achieving high confidence for the patients as well as for the surgeons.

## Case 2

This patient presented with a pre-enhancement UCVA 20/100. The decentered ablation is shown in Figure 11-4. AstraPro was used to create the ablation profile from the 3-dimensional corneal elevation data (Figure 11-5). Due to the high precision of the anterior corneal elevation data, the predicted postoperative target surface can be achieved with high precision with a smooth and precision micro-scanning ablation laser. As can be seen, the planned ablation profile is optimized to touch up on the missed ablation tissues to achieve a symmetrical and smooth postoperative corneal surface. Figure 11-6 shows that the post-enhancement map of this cornea is smooth and symmetrical, resolving the ghost image and poor visual acuity complaint while saving unnecessary and excessive ablation. After applying AstraPro 2.2Z, the decentration was corrected, and the post-enhancement UCVA was 20/20.

A topography data-guided ablation technique, due to the high precision of the elevation data and advanced ellipsoidal model in free space, with optimization in radius, shape factor, and axis, was successfully able to repair the severe irregularity of the cornea.

# Topography-Guided Custom Ablation With iVIS Suite

Aleksandar Stojanovic, MD and Xiangjun Chen, MD, MS

iVIS Technologies (Taranto, Italy) has pioneered topography-guided custom ablation since the mid-1990s by introducing Corneal Interactive Programmed Topographic Ablation (CIPTA) software. The software was used for custom ablation planning based on Orbscan topography (Bausch & Lomb, Rochester, NY) and for treatment on LaserSight 100-Hz, small-flying-spot laser (LaserSight Technologies Inc, Orlando, FL). Since then, the company developed its own Scheimpflug-based topographer, the Precisio, as well as a dynamic pupillometer (pMetrics) and a 1000-Hz, 0.6-mm flying-spot excimer laser (iRES), completing the "iVIS Suite" topography-guided custom ablation system.

In the iVIS Suite, corneal anterior and posterior elevation, pachymetry, pupil as well as iris and scleral vessel registration-data from the Precisio, pupillometry-data from the pMetrics, and the patient's refraction are fed to the CIPTA software. CIPTA then compiles a custom ablation plan with the aim of transforming the actual corneal shape into a regular aspheric shape of desired curvature, within the treatment zone suggested by pupillometry. The volume of the ablation is defined by the intersection between the corneal anterior surface as detected by Precisio and the targeted aspheric surface, determined by CIPTA. The curvature of the targeted surface is determined by subtracting the amount of desired dioptric change from the preoperative curvature. Hence, the corneal topography and the subjective refraction are used as bases for treatment of higher- and lower-order aberrations, respectively (the former is limited to the HOAs originating from the corneal surface).

The CIPTA-generated ablation plan is then transferred to the iRES excimer laser, which employs a synchronized x,y and cyclotorsional tracking. To reduce the high-frequency laser's thermal effect and the ablation-rate difference between the corneal epithelium and the stroma, delivery of constant local frequency (number of pulses per second) per area is implemented into iRES, allowing the use of integrated transepithelial ablation as the system's recommended operative technique. The technique merges laser epithelium removal and stromal ablation into a single, uninterrupted custom ablation, termed "cTEN" (custom transepithelial "no-touch"). Such integrated, topography-guided ablation seems to be especially suited for therapeutic purposes for cases with irregular astigmatism, where epithelial remodeling plays a significant role and has to be addressed.[6]

The following case illustrates the use of iVIS Suite's topography-guided cTEN ablation in treatment of irregular astigmatism after decentered PRK/LASIK.

## Case 1

A 57-year-old woman had her right eye treated with PRK in 1997. She was retreated because of regression/undercorrection with LASIK in 1999. The baseline refractive error was -4.25 -0.25 x 90 degrees, and best-corrected distance visual acuity was 20/20. Blurred vision, starburst halos, and multiple images were noted after the PRK and increased after her LASIK. Irregular astigmatism due to decentered ablation and oblate asphericity were diagnosed. Topography-guided cTEN ablation with iVIS suite was planned and performed in October 2008.

Prior to corrective treatment, the patient's uncorrected distance visual acuity (UDVA) was 20/30, and subjective refraction of +1.50 -0.25 x 90 degrees failed to improve vision. Central ultrasound pachymetry (Corneo-Gage Plus, Sonogage Inc, Cleveland, OH) was 517 μm. Slit-lamp microscopy was unremarkable except for central grade 1 subepithelial haze within the LASIK flap. Precisio floating-elevation and axial curvature maps showed irregular astigmatism (Figure 11-7). Asymmetry within the central 3 mm was 1.5 D, while the Q-value was +0.56. Wavefront aberrometry measured at 6 mm with the Allegretto Analyzer (Wave-Light, Erlangen, Germany) showed total root-mean-square HOA of 0.95 μm (coma 0.67 μm and spherical aberration 0.44 μm). pMetrics dynamic pupillometry showed 3.95, 6.59, and 8.75 mm as photopic, "ideal," and scotopic pupil sizes.

The treatment goal was an aberration-free corneal surface and emmetropia using a single ablation involving the epithelium and the stroma (including the haze). After importing the patient's Precisio topography/tomography and manifest spherocylindrical refraction, the CIPTA software computed the desired regular aspheric postoperative surface with a curvature change, which compensated for the manifest spherocylindrical error within the optical zone, matching the "ideal" pupil size. The ablation plan showed maximum ablation depth of 34 μm and the outer transition zone of 8.75 mm. The ablation plan is shown on Figure 11-8. A detailed surgical protocol is described elsewhere.[7]

Twelve months after the treatment, slit-lamp microscopy showed a clear cornea, with no trace of haze. The patient's uncorrected and corrected visual acuity were 20/25 and 20/20, respectively, and manifest refraction was +0.50 -0.25 x 50 degrees in the right eye. Wavefront aberrometry showed total root-mean-square HOA of 0.33 μm (coma 0.22 μm and spherical aberration 0.18 μm) for 6-mm diameter. Floating elevation and axial curvature

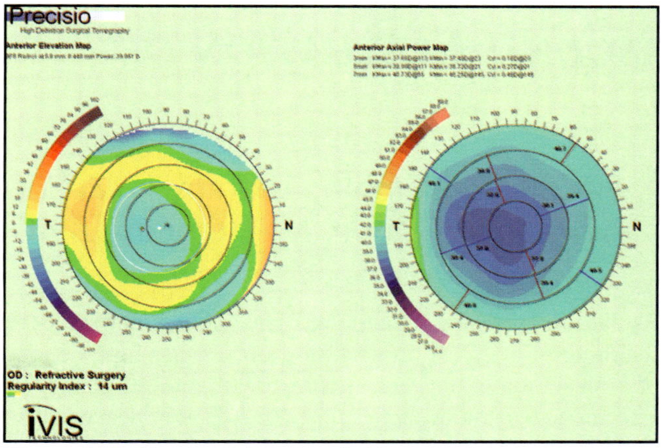


**Figure 11-7.** Floating elevation (left) and axial curvature map (right) before the topography-guided ablation using the iVIS Suite.

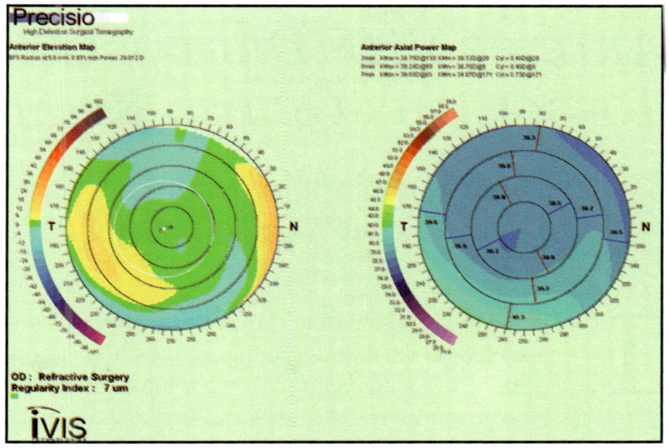


**Figure 11-9.** Floating elevation (left) and axial curvature map (right) 12 months after the topography-guided ablation with iVIS Suite.

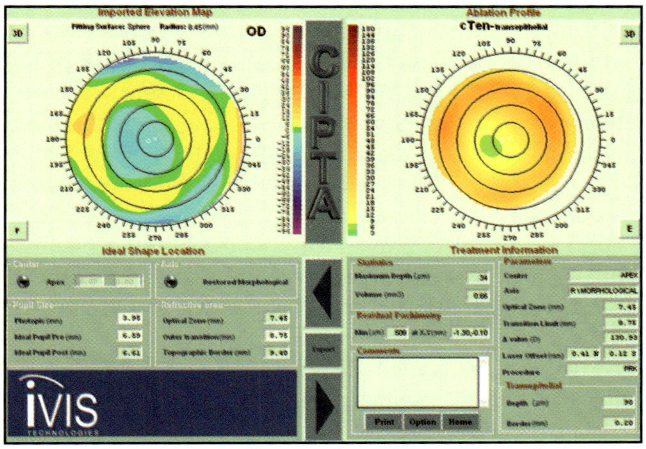


**Figure 11-8.** Ablation planning based on imported elevation topography (left) and the compiled ablation map (right).

maps showed significantly reduced irregular astigmatism (Figure 11-9) with asymmetry reduced to 0.7 D within the central 3 mm and prolate asphericity, with a Q value of -0.14. Most importantly, the patient's complaints of visual disturbances were fully resolved.

It may be undisputable that the corneal topography-guided custom ablation is the most logical approach in addressing iatrogenic corneal surface irregularity, but the choice of the operative technique to deliver the ablation and treat a post-LASIK case where visually disturbing pathology (eg, haze) resides within the flap may not be so clear. Flap relift, the most commonly used technique in LASIK retreatment, could not address the current case because the subepithelial haze residing within the flap would remain unaffected by an ablation on the stroma beneath the flap. Custom PRK on top of the flap would remove the subepithelial haze, but in that case, the epithelial remodeling could become an issue of concern. The epithelial remodeling, which would have most likely occurred in the current case due to the irregular astigmatism, would cause a mismatch between the epithelial surface morphology (the data source for topography-guided custom ablation planning) and the stromal morphology (the surface to be treated). In such a case, topography-guided ablation delivered on the stroma after the epithelial removal, as a part of PRK or other surface ablation technique that involves epithelial removal prior to the ablation, would lead to a potentially significant ablation error caused by the mentioned mismatch.

With the current cTEN technique, the epithelial removal is programmed into a single ablation together with the stromal ablation and is executed as an integral part of an uninterrupted laser treatment, thanks to the similar ablation rates between the epithelium and the stroma, achieved by the iRES laser. This allows the topography-detected surface to be used as a true basis for custom ablation, circumventing the problem of the epithelial remodeling and the stromal mismatch. Moreover, the area of the epithelial ablation in cTEN fits exactly the outer edges of the stromal ablation area, and therefore only the absolutely necessary amount of epithelium is removed, minimizing the trauma to the cornea and increasing the speed of re-epithelialization. One important desired improvement to the cTEN approach would be the use and integration of technology that would accurately measure the epithelial thickness, such as Artemis VHF scanner (ArcScan Inc, Golden, CO), mentioned elsewhere in this book.

# Artemis VHF Digital Ultrasound Evaluation of Topography-Guided Repair

Dan Z. Reinstein, MD, MA(Cantab), FRCSC, FRCOphth; Timothy J. Archer, MA(Oxon), DipCompSci(Cantab); and Marine Gobbe, MST(Optom), PhD

Topography-guided ablation profiles are derived from front surface corneal topography, and the algorithms are designed to calculate the tissue removal required to return the cornea to a regular aspheric shape. Therefore, the ablation profiles are usually irregular and nonsymmetric. The results of topography-guided treatments are usually evaluated by inspection of the change in front surface corneal topography; however, the shape of ablated stromal tissue has not been confirmed by direct measurement of stromal change. The Artemis very high-frequency digital ultrasound arc-scanner (ArcScan Inc, Morrison, CO) is capable of obtaining a map of the stromal thickness across the central 10-mm diameter in vivo.[8-10] The change in stromal thickness can be calculated as the difference in stromal thickness before and after surgery to evaluate the achieved central ablation depth in conventional myopic ablations,[11-13] as demonstrated by the following case.

A 45-year-old man was referred to our clinic complaining of ghosting and increasing blur in both eyes, but more pronounced in the right eye. Prior to undergoing radial keratotomy, the preoperative refraction was approximately -9.50 D in both eyes. The left eye was treated first using the "American" method, and the right eye was treated 2 weeks later using the "Russian" method. Sixteen incisions were created in both eyes. Clinical records were not available postoperatively, but the patient explained that he did not need to wear glasses for the first 10 years and was able to obtain a private pilot's license. After 4 years, the patient noticed his vision deteriorating, and the patient sought surgical correction of the right eye.

Uncorrected distance visual acuity of 20/40+1 improved with a manifest refraction of +0.75 -2.00 x (20/32+2). Further testing included topography, whole eye wavefront using the WASCA aberrometer (Carl Zeiss Meditec, Jena, Germany) both undilated and after cycloplegia using tropicamide 1%, pupillometry, corneal biomechanical analysis, handheld ultrasonic pachymetry, and tonometry. Vertical sinusoidal grid contrast sensitivity testing was obtained at 3, 6, 12, and 18 cycles per degree (cpd) using the CSV-1000 (VectorVision Inc, Greenville, OH). The Artemis 1 VHF digital ultrasound arc-scanner was used to determine the thickness profile of each corneal layer. The reproducibility of pachymetric topography of the Artemis has been shown to be 0.58 μm for the epithelium, 1.78 μm for the stroma, and 1.68 μm for the cornea.[10] Pachymetric profiles were calculated based on data from 4 meridional B-scans, comprising 8 hemimeridians. This is our standard scanning protocol as it provides a sufficiently high density of information in the central cornea with a lower density of information in the periphery, where it is less needed. The Artemis has been described in detail previously.[8-14]

Contrast sensitivity was well below the normal range; the patient was not able to see more than 2 patches at 3, 6, 12, or 18 cpd. Analysis of front surface topography showed that the optical zone was decentered inferotemporally relative to the visual axis; the Atlas axial map is presented in Figure 11-10. Wavefront analysis showed significant HOAs with a higher-order RMS of 1.63 μm and spherical aberration of 1.30 μm (OSA notation[15]). The Artemis epithelial thickness profile showed that the epithelium was up to 84-μm thick centrally, significantly thicker than normal,[14] surrounded by an annulus of thinner epithelium (down to 44 μm) at a radius of 5 mm. This annulus of thinner epithelium, over the midperipheral "knee" characteristic of radial keratotomy, was also decentered inferotemporally, matching the irregularity seen on topography.

A topography-guided PRK procedure was performed using the MEL80 excimer laser and CRS-Master custom ablation programming software (version 2.1), which has been described previously.[1] The CRS-Master algorithm uses corneal elevation data, captured by the Atlas topographer, to calculate the ablation required to obtain an aspheric surface. The algorithm also analyzes the corneal wavefront, derived from the corneal topography data, together with the clinical manifest refraction to calculate the refractive error correction. The algorithm takes into account that the manifest refraction possesses a component that compensates for corneal HOAs and is able to discriminate this component to determine the HOA-free manifest refractive error.

Numerous Atlas examinations were obtained, and the exam to use for treatment was selected by the surgeon (DZR). The criteria for selecting the examination to use for treatment were for the exam to a) be in focus, b) have smooth, regular mires rings, and c) have continuous data within sufficient diameter. The Atlas topographic data were imported into the CRS-Master. The CRS-Master automatically selects the center of the pupil as found by the Atlas to use as the center for the ablation generation algorithms. The CRS-Master also allows the surgeon to shift this location, and the corneal vertex was chosen for this case according to our standard protocol of centering all ablations on the corneal vertex.[1,16,17] The corneal vertex was determined

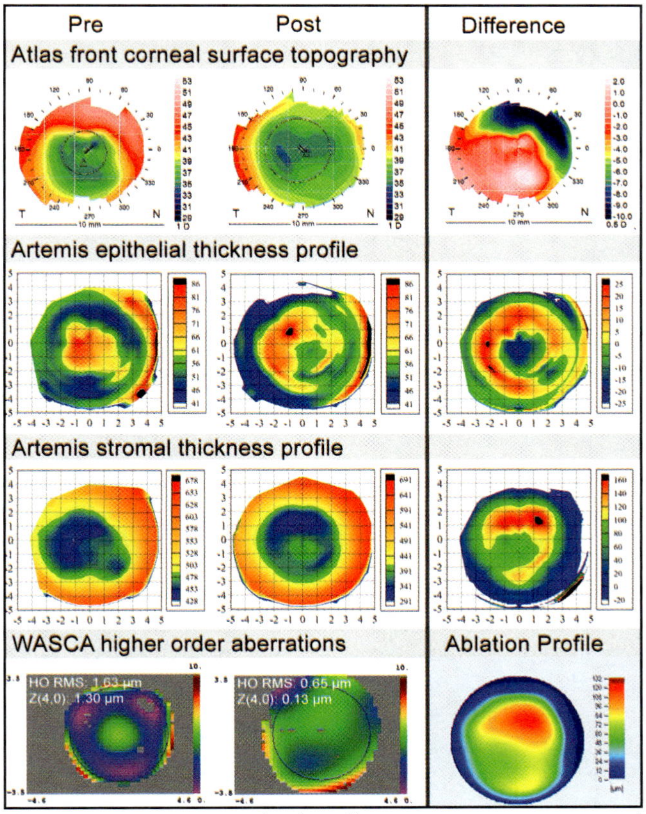


**Figure 11-10.** Artemis display illustrating preoperative and postoperative axial maps (top row), epithelial thickness profiles (second row), stromal thickness (third row), and wavefront aberrations (bottom row).

as the center of the topography mires, which is calculated automatically by the Atlas and displayed in the CRS-Master software. During surgery, the corneal vertex was determined as the first Purkinje reflex, seen as the patient fixated coaxially with the aiming beam and the view of the surgeon's contralateral eye through the Carl Zeiss operating microscope in the MEL 80. A 6.50-mm optical zone was used with a transition zone out to 8.50 mm. The ablation profile was irregular with an area of deepest ablation superiorly and a tongue of ablation inferiorly. The maximum ablation depth was 120 µm located 1.4-mm superiorly and 0.8-mm nasally, where the Artemis pachymetry was 518 µm, which resulted in a predicted postoperative corneal thickness of 398 µm. The ablation depth at the corneal vertex was 86 µm, where the Artemis pachymetry was 532 µm, which resulted in a predicted postoperative corneal thickness of 446 µm.

The ablation profile included a pre-ablation of 6-µm phototherapeutic keratectomy (PTK), which was programmed into the same treatment profile, to homogenize the hydration of the corneal surface in advance of the asymmetric ablation being performed. After the ablation was performed, a series of 3 "wet" 20-µm PTK ablations were performed to smooth out the incisional scarring; this involved flooding the exposed stroma with BSS solution to isolate ablation selectively only on the steep ridges of the edges of the radial keratotomy incisions and keratin plugs jutting above the general stromal surface. Typical postoperative treatment followed, including a bandage lens and topical medications.

Nine months after the procedure, the uncorrected distance visual acuity in the patient's right eye was 20/32 with a manifest refraction of +0.75 -0.75 x 20, and the CDVA had improved to 20/20-1. The slit-lamp examination showed no haze. Figure 11-10 demonstrates the Atlas topography, WASCA HOAs, and Artemis epithelial and stromal thickness, as well as difference maps for each. Front corneal surface topography showed that the corneal surface was significantly more regular and the optical zone was centered on the corneal vertex. The Atlas difference map demonstrated an area of flattening superiorly, which was the location of maximum ablation. WASCA showed that a significant reduction in HOAs had been achieved, with the higher-order RMS reduced by 60% from 1.63 µm to 0.65 µm, and spherical aberration reduced by 90% from 1.30 µm to 0.13 µm. The Artemis epithelial thickness profile showed that the epithelium had remodeled according to the new stromal surface; the effective optical zone on the epithelial thickness map was centered about the corneal vertex, and the diameter of the annulus of thin epithelium had increased to just over 6 mm. The epithelial change map showed that the epithelium had become thinner centrally and thicker in a paracentral annulus to achieve the new profile. The Artemis stromal thickness change map represented the profile of stromal tissue removed by the irregular topography-guided ablation; there was an area of maximum tissue removal superiorly with a tongue of tissue removed inferiorly, which matched the intended ablation profile. The maximum change in stromal thickness was 160 µm, which was 40 µm more than the predicted ablation. It is unlikely that the difference between the predicted ablation depth and the measured stromal thickness change was due to the wet PTK ablation.

Despite the dramatic changes in topography and HOAs, there was very little change in contrast sensitivity, which was still below the normal range.

In summary, evaluation of the change in stromal thickness using Artemis VHF digital ultrasound demonstrated excellent agreement with the pattern of the theoretical planned ablation.

# Scheimpflug-Based Topography-Guided Custom Ablation Treatment

Renato Ambrósio Jr, MD, PhD; Frederico P. Guerra, MD; and Cristiana de Moraes Ramalho, MD

The use of OCULUS tomography with Allegretto excimer treatment has reportedly been successful in cases of irregular astigmatism.[4] A 42-year-old female physician with a corneal scar following contact lens-related Acanthamoeba keratitis presented with uncorrected distance visual acuity of 20/400 and manifest refraction of +0.50 -4.50 x 20, improving the vision to 20/60 in the left eye.

Advanced Therapeutic Surface Ablation was performed with the Alcon-WaveLight Allegretto Eye Q. Epithelial removal was accomplished using a 50-µm PTK ablation with a 7.0-mm optical zone and transition to 8.9 mm. Topography-guided ablation was planned based on Oculyzer data. Mitomycin C at 0.005% was applied for 1 minute, followed by 50 cc of chilled BSS irrigation. A soft contact lens was placed, and the patient was instructed to use a fourth-generation fluoroquinolone and prednisolone acetate 1% six times a day until complete epithelialization. One week after surgery, uncorrected distance visual acuity was 20/30, the contact lens was removed, and the patient started topical cyclosporine twice daily and was instructed for steroid tapering.

One month after surgery, uncorrected distance visual acuity was 20/25+. Four months after surgery, uncorrected distance visual acuity was 20/25, and manifest refraction was plano -1.25 x 165, giving 20/20.

Figure 11-11 illustrates the subtraction sagittal curvature map from preoperatively and 4 months postoperatively. Note the reduction of keratometric astigmatism from 5.4@178 to 0.7@55. Note the subtraction map is very similar as the ablation TCAT plan (Figure 11-12).

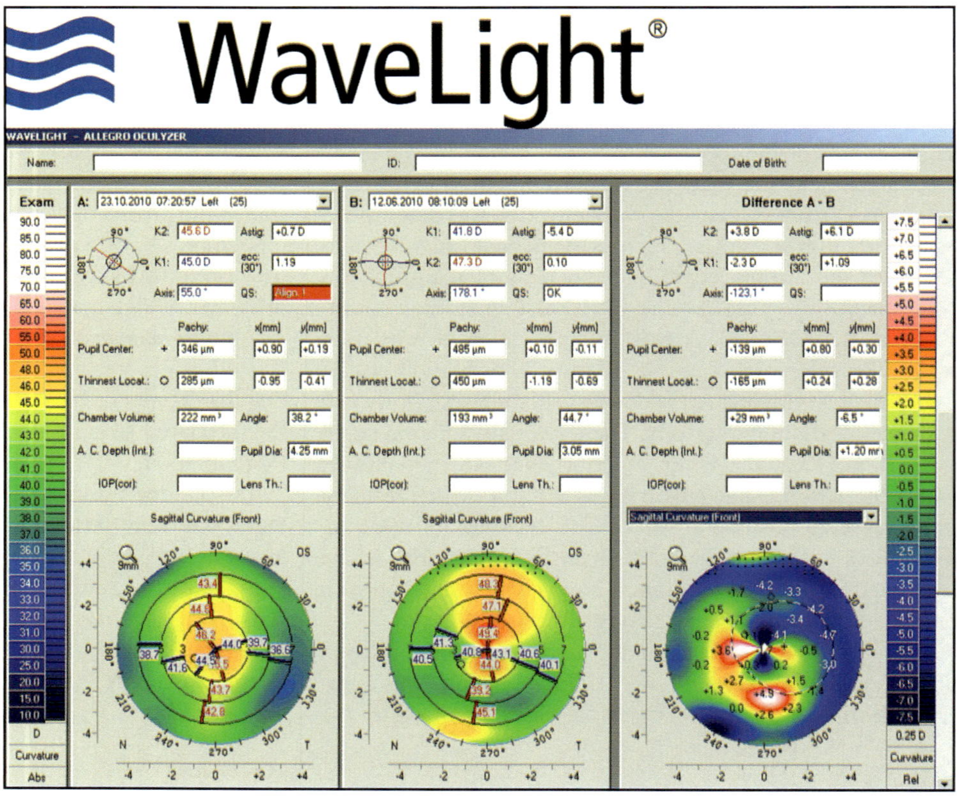


**Figure 11-11.** The difference in the sagittal curvature map from preoperative (B) and 4 months postoperative (A) corrective treatment. Note the reduction of astigmatism on the cornea from -5.40 D to 0.70 D.

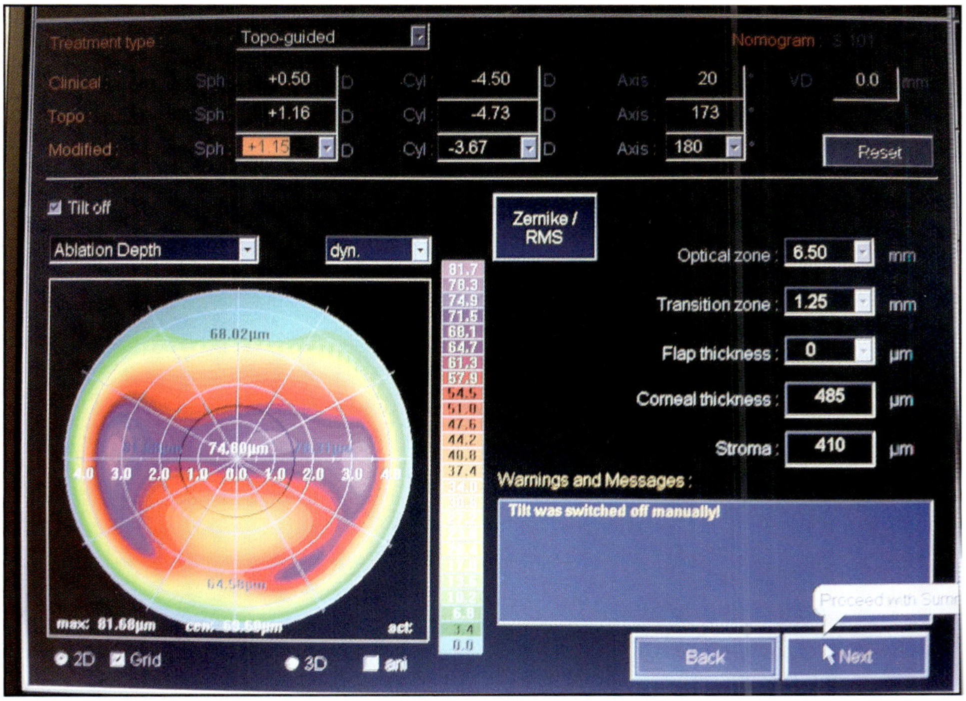


**Figure 11-12.** Ablation profile demonstrating the irregular ablation to address the variable astigmatism.

# REFERENCES


1. Reinstein DZ, Archer TJ, Gobbe M. Combined corneal topography and corneal wavefront data in the treatment of corneal irregularity and refractive error in LASIK or PRK using the Carl Zeiss Meditec MEL 80 and CRS-Master. *J Refract Surg*. 2009;25(6):503-515.
2. Wu L, Zhou X, Ouyang Z, Weng C, Chu R. Topography-guided treatment of decentered laser ablation using LaserSight's excimer laser. *Eur J Ophthalmol*. 2008;18(5):708-715.
3. Lin DT, Holland SR, Rocha KM, Krueger RR. Method for optimizing topography-guided ablation of highly aberrated eyes with the ALLEGRETTO WAVE Excimer Laser. *J Refract Surg*. 2008;24(4):S439-S445.
4. Jankov MR 2nd, Panagopoulou SI, Tsiklis NS, Hajitanasis GC, Aslanides M, Pallikaris G. Topography-guided treatment of irregular astigmatism with the WaveLight excimer laser. *J Refract Surg*. 2006;22(4):335-344.
5. Toda I, Yamamoto T, Ito M, Hori-Komai Y, Tsubota K. Topography-guided ablation for treatment of patients with irregular astigmatism. *J Refract Surg*. 2007;23(2):118-125.
6. Reinstein DZ, Silverman RH, Sutton HF, Coleman DJ. Very high-frequency ultrasound corneal analysis identifies anatomic correlates of optical complications of lamellar refractive surgery: anatomic diagnosis in lamellar surgery. *Ophthalmology*. 1999;106:474-482.
7. Stojanovic A, Jankov MR. Treatment of irregular astigmatism: developing an ideal corneal surface with the iVIS suite. In: Wang M, ed. *Irregular Astigmatism: Diagnosis and Treatment*. Thorofare, NJ: SLACK Incorporated; 2008:211-218.
8. Reinstein DZ, Silverman RH, Raevsky T, et al. Arc-scanning very high-frequency digital ultrasound for 3D pachymetric mapping of the corneal epithelium and stroma in laser in situ keratomileusis. *J Refract Surg*. 2000;16:414-430.
9. Reinstein DZ, Archer TJ, Gobbe M, Silverman R, Coleman DJ. Stromal thickness in the normal cornea: three-dimensional display with Artemis very high-frequency digital ultrasound. *J Refract Surg*. 2009;25:776-786.
10. Reinstein DZ, Archer TJ, Gobbe M, Silverman RH, Coleman DJ. Repeatability of layered corneal pachymetry with the Artemis very high-frequency digital ultrasound arc-scanner. *J Refract Surg*. 2009;Nov:1-14.
11. Reinstein DZ, Srivannaboon S, Archer TJ, Silverman RH, Sutton H, Coleman DJ. Probability model of the inaccuracy of residual stromal thickness prediction to reduce the risk of ectasia after LASIK part I: quantifying individual risk. *J Refract Surg*. 2006;22:851-860.
12. Reinstein DZ, Srivannaboon S, Archer TJ, Silverman RH, Sutton H, Coleman DJ. Probability model of the inaccuracy of residual stromal thickness prediction to reduce the risk of ectasia after LASIK part II: quantifying population risk. *J Refract Surg*. 2006;22:861-870.
13. Reinstein DZ, Archer TJ, Gobbe M. Corneal ablation depth readout of the MEL80 excimer laser compared to Artemis three-dimensional very high-frequency digital ultrasound stromal measurements. *J Refract Surg*. 2010;26(12):949-959.
14. Reinstein DZ, Archer TJ, Gobbe M, Silverman RH, Coleman DJ. Epithelial thickness in the normal cornea: three-dimensional display with Artemis very high-frequency digital ultrasound. *J Refract Surg*. 2008;24:571-581.
15. Applegate RA, Thibos LN, Bradley A, et al. Reference axis selection: subcommittee report of the OSA Working Group to establish standards for measurement and reporting of optical aberrations of the eye. *J Refract Surg*. 2000 16:S656-S658.

16. Reinstein DZ, Couch DG, Archer TJ. LASIK for hyperopic astigmatism and presbyopia using micro-monovision with the Carl Zeiss Meditec MEL80. *J Refract Surg*. 2009;25:37-58.

17. Reinstein DZ, Archer TJ, Gobbe M. LASIK for myopic astigmatism and presbyopia using non-linear aspheric micro-monovision with the Carl Zeiss Meditec MEL 80 Platform. *J Refract Surg*. 2011;27(1):23-37.

Chapter 12

# Planning Keratorefractive Treatments Using Wavefront and Corneal Topography Data

Noel Alpins, FRANZCO, FRCOphth, FACS
and George Stamatelatos, BScOptom

The differences that frequently exist between corneal parameters measured by keratometry or topography and the refractive astigmatism values, as measured by manifest or wavefront techniques, have become increasingly evident to the practicing refractive surgeon. The importance of preoperatively quantifying this parameter is a key ingredient in successful refractive astigmatism treatment. The ocular residual astigmatism (ORA), defined as the vectorial difference between the corneal and refractive astigmatism, singly takes into account the angular as well as the magnitude difference.[1-5] This should form part of any routine eye assessment prior to performing refractive surgery that includes astigmatism treatment.

In the excimer laser field, the perplexing decision whether to treat based on refractive, topographic, or a combination of both parameters continues to be of relevance.[6-8] This is because treatment by refractive parameters alone will leave the neutralization of this internal optical aberration (ORA) on the cornea. In approximately 7% of cases, this amount can be worse than the preoperative corneal astigmatism,[1] potentially leading to increased aberrations and associated visual symptoms, particularly under mesopic conditions. Equally, treatment by topographic parameters alone will leave all the ORA postoperatively remaining in the manifest refraction, again reducing the potential satisfactory visual outcome.

Ideally, a treatment paradigm incorporating both refractive and topographic parameters in a systematic manner would leave the minimum possible total astigmatism in the eye, distributed in an optimal proportion between the cornea and refraction.



Wang M. Corneal Topography: A Guide for Clinical Application in the Wavefront Era, Second Edition (pp. 253-258)

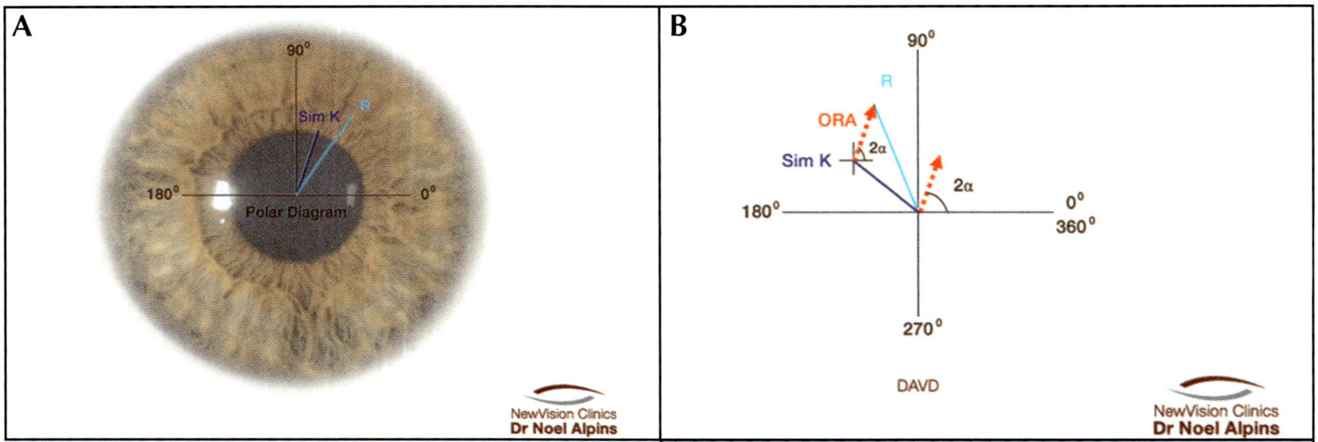


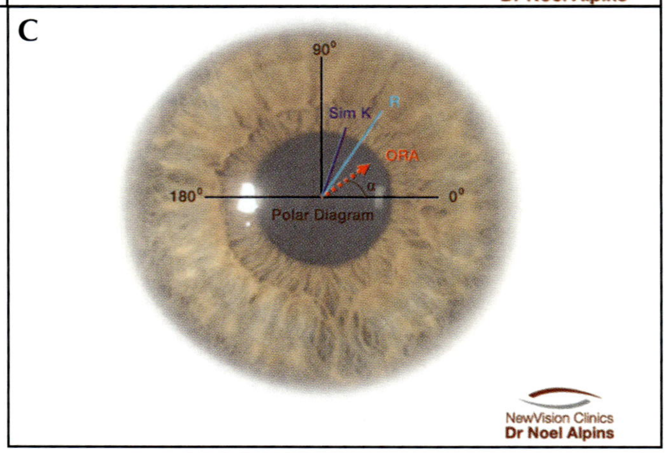


**Figure 12-1.** (A) Polar diagram of refractive cylinder (corneal plane) at positive axis and simulated keratometry. (B) Double angle vector diagram (DAVD) showing a "doubling" of the positive cylinder axes without a change in the astigmatic magnitudes. (C) Polar diagram displaying the ORA as it would appear on the eye.

# Calculation of ORA

Figure 12-1A shows on a polar display the second-order spherocylinder of the wavefront or the positive cylinder of the manifest refraction measurements, together with the topography or keratometry measurements for corneal astigmatism. Doubling the axes of the astigmatism while leaving the magnitudes unchanged allows for the conversion of polar coordinates to Cartesian coordinates (Figure 12-1B). The ORA, determined on the double-angle plot, is then transferred to the origin (x=0, y=0) and halved to simulate how it would exist within the eye (Figure 12-1C—polar diagram). This vectorial difference, measured in diopters and degrees and calculated using simple trigonometric principles, has a proportional relationship to astigmatism—meaning that, while the astigmatic differences between refractive and corneal astigmatism increases in either magnitude and/or angle difference, so too increases the magnitude of the ORA. As a result, treatment using refractive parameters alone neutralizes the internal ocular astigmatism quantified by the ORA on the front corneal surface, leading to increased aberrations and a reduction in the quality of vision achieved.[9,10]

There are currently software programs available that will calculate the ORA (Figure 12-2, www.assort.com) from simulated keratometry parameters exported directly from topography and refractive cylinder at the corneal plane. Conveniently, these can be used directly from the analytical outputs generated within the topography device.

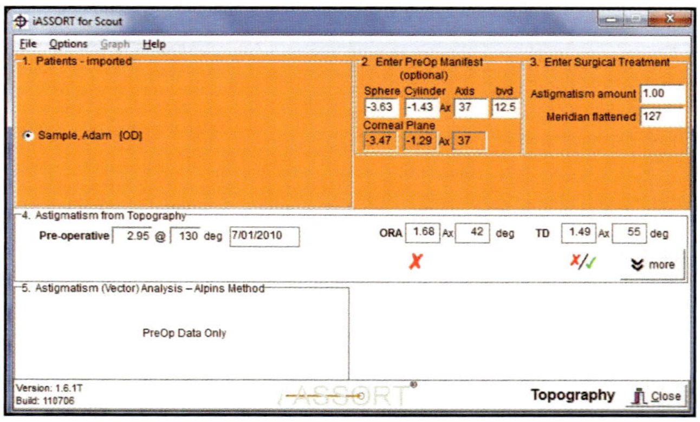


**Figure 12-2.** The iAssort software program for corneal astigmatism analysis. Simulated keratometry parameters are exported from the topography system (in this example, 2.95 D @ 130) and are compared to the refractive astigmatism (-1.29 D x 37 at the corneal plane) to calculate the ORA, which in this case is 1.68 D Ax 42. This is high in magnitude as displayed by the red cross, which indicates that it lies outside the normal range of 0.00 D to 1.00 D.

By quantifying the vectorial difference between the corneal and the refractive astigmatism using the ORA, the maximum possible correction of astigmatism can be determined. The distribution of the remaining ORA, which is the best outcome possible for an individual eye, needs to be considered carefully. Caution needs to be given to whether to treat the eye as is customary practice, leaving the astigmatism totally on the cornea by treating with manifest or wavefront refraction, or ascertaining if it is better to distribute the unavoidable remaining astigmatism between the two in an optimized manner to achieve the most favorable outcome.

## Vector Planning

The Alpins method of vector planning directs the treatment closer to the principal corneal meridian, thereby correcting a greater amount of corneal astigmatism. This results in less corneal induced aberrations and a greater potential for improvement in best-corrected visual acuity.[5,9,11,12] The reduction in corneal astigmatism substantially exceeds the increase in measurable refractive cylinder that might theoretically occur. This has the overall effect of minimizing the total amount of astigmatism (refractive plus topographic) remaining after laser surgery, effectively gaining "something for nothing."

This method of vector planning can be used employing any combination, either of keratometry or topography values and manifest wavefront or cycloplegic refraction parameters, to determine the ORA amount present. The importance of vector planning when preoperatively assessing an astigmatic patient for refractive laser surgery cannot be overemphasized. In cases where the ORA is high (>1.00 D), the patient needs to be advised that all of the astigmatism in the optical system cannot be corrected no matter how perfect the surgical treatment applied so that expectations of a perfect outcome are adjusted to a realistic level.

There are several limitations of wavefront-guided treatments. Wavefront-guided treatments do not address the excessive and unnecessary amount of corneal astigmatism that would be left remaining (equal to the ORA) on the cornea postoperatively. This would potentially compromise visual acuity and contrast sensitivity outcomes, particularly under mesopic conditions. No recognition of topographic astigmatism values are taken into account during treatment with this approach.

They also do not consider the patient's subjective appreciation of astigmatism. The inclusion in the treatment of a patient's conscious perception of his or her refractive astigmatism is likely to benefit satisfaction.[3,13]

Wavefront-guided treatments could result in corneal surface irregularities[3] if all aberrations measured are corrected on the corneal surface. It is important to note that even eyes with normal (emmetropic) vision can suffer from aberrations that affect functional vision.[14]

Alternatively, topography-guided treatments do not consider that the amount of corneal astigmatism often differs from the refractive (second-order) astigmatism. Omitting this phenomenon during planning can result in refractive astigmatism surprises.

The advantages of preoperatively addressing both corneal and refractive astigmatism reduces the level of astigmatism that is left on the cornea compared to using refractive parameters alone, and, as a result, fewer second- and third-order aberrations are likely to remain.[2,3,9]

### Vector Planning Studies Applied to Keratoconus and Wavefront-Guided Treatments

Two studies have shown the benefits of combining corneal and refractive parameters.[9,12] The first is a retrospective study of 45 eyes with forme fruste and mild keratoconus. These patients underwent surface ablation laser surgery.[12] All photoastigmatic refractive keratectomy (PARK) treatments were optimized to leave minimum remaining corneal astigmatism, favoring a bias to a with-the-rule orientation. Postoperative results at 12 months showed that, on average, for every eye in the group, the corneal cylinder was reduced by an additional 0.59 D compared to results that would have been attained by treating refractive values alone. A mean 1.61 D for each patient in the study group would have remained on the cornea postoperatively compared to the 1.02 D achieved. This was achievable without compromising the refractive outcome. In fact, it was enhanced with a better-than-predicted refractive astigmatism reduction. The expected mean refractive target was 0.59 D compared to the mean achieved at 12 months postoperatively of 0.43 D, demonstrating a clear net gain when assessing both corneal and refractive modes.

No problems or adverse signs such as increase in corneal irregularity and curvature or progression of ectasia resulting in a reduction of uncorrected or best-corrected visual acuity were detected.

In the second study, 21 eyes of 14 patients were distributed into 2 groups in a prospective double-masked study.[9] One group was treated by wavefront parameters alone, the other by wavefront combined with topography values (WF&VP) using vector planning. For the WF&VP combined group, the treatment profile was calculated using simulated keratometry readings from the topography (Humphrey Atlas) and second-order Zernike coefficients Defocus 4, Astigmatism 3, and 5 from the wavefront display (WaveScan Wavefront) of the entire eye.

Results showed a trend to greater correction of corneal astigmatism in the WF&VP combined group, with better visual outcomes in low-contrast mesopic conditions, a

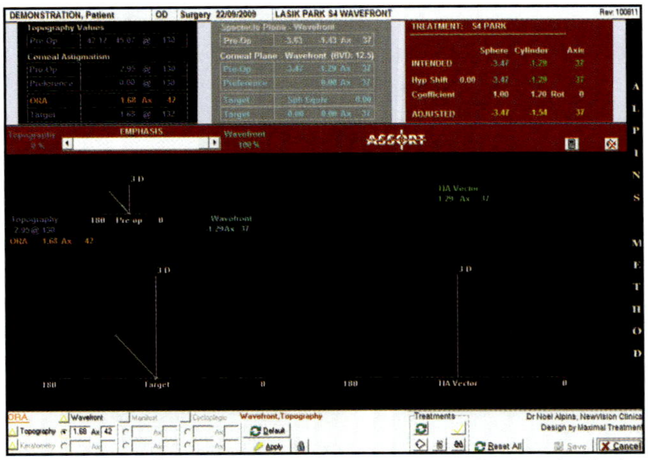

**Figure 12-3.** The ASSORT treatment screen displays both the manifest refraction and the corneal astigmatism by topography. The emphasis shown here is that of conventional treatment, 0% topography/100% wavefront refraction leaving all the ORA on the cornea as displayed by the "Target = 1.68 @ 132."

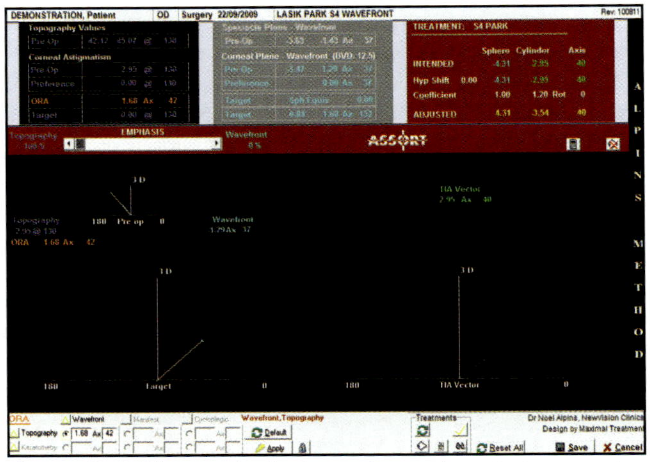

**Figure 12-4.** The emphasis shown here relates to topography-guided treatment where all the ORA (1.68 D) remains in the manifest refraction (100% topography/0% wavefront refraction), shown as the "Target = 0.84/-1.68 x 132."

greater reduction in horizontal coma, and greater potential for improvement in best-corrected visual acuity.

# Vector Planning: A Case Study

The Alpins Statistical System for Ophthalmic Refractive Surgery Techniques (ASSORT) program developed at NewVision Clinics uses vector planning and analysis in a paradigm that maximally reduces overall astigmatism and has the option to favor a bias to with-the-rule astigmatism. This software has been used in this chapter for all calculations.

Using the example referred to in Figure 12-2, the ASSORT laser treatment module in Figure 12-3 displays the second-order spherocylindrical wavefront refraction, as measured using aberrometry, to be -3.63 DS/-1.43 DC x 37 at vertex distance of 12.5 mm and -3.47 DS/-1.29 DC x 37 at the corneal plane.

The topographic data of the same astigmatic eye display a simulated keratometry value of 2.95 D of astigmatism at the steepest meridian of 130 degrees. The total of corneal and refractive (corneal plane) together is 4.24 D, the corneal astigmatism making up 70% of it.

The amount of uncorrectable astigmatism in this patient's eye is 1.68 D Ax 42 (ORA). The distribution of this is reflected in the "emphasis" bar, where 100% indicates a goal of completely eliminating refractive astigmatism and 0% shows the emphasis on completely reducing topographic astigmatism by the treatment.

If we treat conventionally, that is, with 100% reduction of manifest refractive astigmatism as shown in Figure 12-3, all of this (ocular) residual astigmatism will remain neutralized on the cornea. This is shown as the "Target" 1.68 D at a meridian of 132 degrees, which is 90 degrees away from the ORA axis to neutralize the internal (noncorneal) error and results in the calculated zero astigmatism in the postoperative refraction (shown as the light blue "Target"). The target-induced astigmatism vector (TIA) is the amount of astigmatism that we are attempting to correct, and for this treatment to sphericize the refraction is 1.29 D Ax 37.

At the other extreme in the planning process, if we treat this eye emphasizing the complete reduction of topographic astigmatism values alone (Figure 12-4), 1.68 D of the unavoidable residual ORA will theoretically remain in the postoperative refraction in conjunction with a spherical cornea. However, taking an optimized view of the situation and incorporating a proportion of each into the overall treatment by shifting the emphasis for astigmatism reduction "to the left" increases the proportion of a preference for complete corneal astigmatism correction, resulting in the maximum ablation of treatment being more closely aligned to the principal corneal meridian. Consequently, there is less "off axis" effect to the corneal astigmatism, with more astigmatism reduction and less torque and meridian shift.[15]

Figure 12-5 shows the optimal treatment as determined from the surgical emphasis graph (Figure 12-6), which displays a linear relationship between the emphasis and the orientation of the target astigmatism. Figure 12-6 is based on the notion that with-the-rule corneal astigmatism is favorable and against-the-rule astigmatism is relatively unfavorable, so that more corneal astigmatism is reduced when its orientation is not favorable, which might also include oblique astigmatism. The placement of the emphasis on total corneal or refractive astigmatism correction is a decision that is guided by the surgeon.

In this example, the meridian of the target topography is 132 degrees. As it lies 42 degrees from a favorable with-the-rule orientation of 90 degrees, 42/90 or 47% can preferentially be apportioned to a topography-based goal of zero astigmatism. By the same process, the refractive

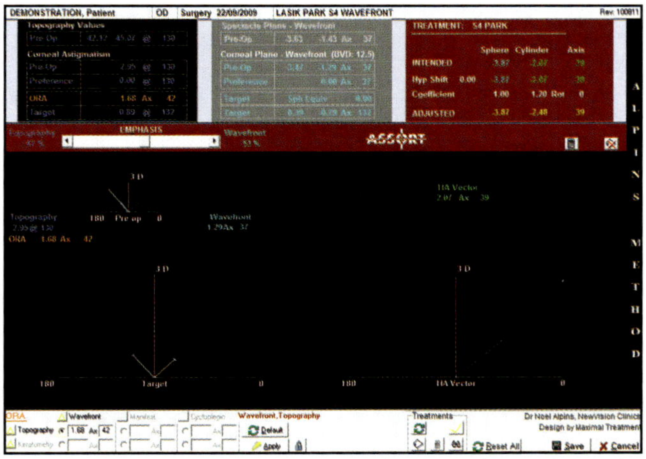


**Figure 12-5.** ASSORT Treatment Planning shows how the ORA of 1.68 D Ax 42 is apportioned 47% to eliminating the topography astigmatism and 53% to the refractive cylinder. The ORA is neutralized by an equivalent 0.89 D at the cornea and -0.79 DC at the spectacle refraction but at an orientation 90 degrees away of 132 degrees.

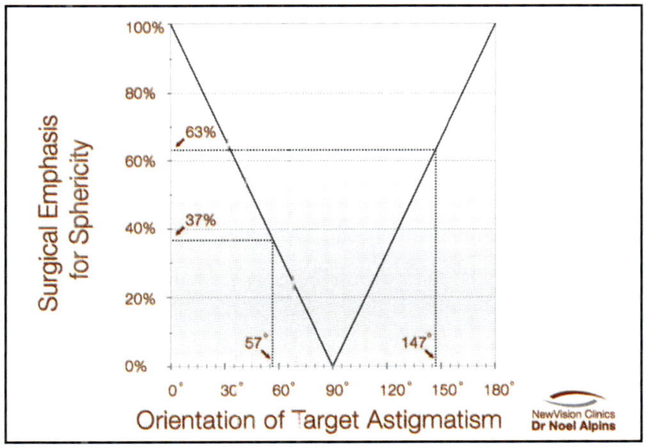


**Figure 12-6.** Linear relationship of surgical emphasis for sphericity versus orientation of target topography based on the notion that with-the-rule astigmatism is favorable and against-the-rule is unfavorable. This graph displays that, as the targeted corneal astigmatism approaches 90 degrees, the target refractive cylinder is reduced, so if the targeted corneal astigmatism is at 90 degrees, all the ORA will be corrected on the cornea.

astigmatism power axis of 42 degrees is 48 degrees away from 90 degrees and hence places 53% emphasis to a correction of refractive astigmatism. The TIA here is greater than before at 2.07 D Ax 39.

The overriding surgical principle is to approach corneal sphericity when the orientation of the target corneal astigmatism to remain becomes increasingly unfavorable. It is a surgical decision guided by which orientation is more favorable than others. Thus, the surgical emphasis needs to be apportioned accordingly, using a linear relationship or other formula. For most astigmatism treatment, the emphasis of 60% to refractive astigmatism (rather than 100% conventional) is a safe choice, gaining a reduction in remaining corneal astigmatism of 40%. In some cases, another option is maintaining the proportion of corneal to refractive astigmatism (70%/30%) after the surgery as existed before surgery was undertaken with an emphasis of 70% to refractive astigmatism.

The patient's ORA is still 1.68 D but is now apportioned between the refraction and the corneal parameters. The corneal astigmatism targeted in this example is 53% of 1.68 D (0.89 D) and the remaining 47% (0.79 DC) of the emphasis placed refractively in a spherical equivalent of zero (+0.39 DS/-0.79 DC Ax 132). This remaining refractive astigmatism with a spherical equivalent of zero may not be fully perceptually evident to the patient, as shown in a previous study,[12] providing a net benefit of less remaining astigmatism.

It is important to highlight that no matter what the percentage chosen on the "emphasis" bar, the maximal treatment enables the minimum amount of astigmatism to be targeted, equal to the ORA. If the combined magnitude of the targeted remaining astigmatism is greater than the initial ORA, the surgery then fails to achieve the maximum astigmatism treatment, and the astigmatism is either under- or overtreated, leaving an excess amount of astigmatism remaining.[1]

As technology advances with future possibilities, each and every point that is measurable on the cornea by topography, together with wavefront aberrometry, could be "vector planned," resulting in the ultimate ablation profile with smooth, even transitions and an optimized amount of corneal astigmatism remaining with the maximal treatment.

## CONCLUSION

Refractive treatments based completely on either extreme of topographic or refractive data alone can not attain the same optimal results in most astigmatic patients as vector planning, which combines both parameters in a balanced optimized manner. Wavefront-guided laser refractive surgery has certainly been of benefit in correcting, on the cornea, the internal aberrations of the eye. However, the correction of higher-order aberrations in cases where there is a significant ORA needs to be more fully explored to increase overall patient satisfaction, The ORA is the key parameter that quantifies the amount of excess corneal astigmatism to neutralize the internal ocular second-order aberrations.

Topographic-guided lasers provide comprehensive mapping in situations of corneal irregularity where manifest and wavefront refractions may be inadequate to provide a smoother corneal surface.

Using the Alpins method of vector planning to combine information from the refraction (manifest or wavefront) as well as the topography can help minimize astigmatism remaining on the cornea and in the optical system of the eye. This optimizes visual outcomes, particularly in low light and reduced-contrast environments. The ORA and the resultant astigmatism remaining on the cornea are the essential parameters to guide the astigmatism optimization in the vector planning process.

## REFERENCES


1. Alpins NA. New method of targeting vectors to treat astigmatism. *J Cataract Refract Surg.* 1997;23:65-75.
2. Alpins NA. Astigmatism analysis by the Alpins method. *J Cataract Refract Surg.* 2001;27:31-49.
3. Alpins NA. Wavefront Technology: a new advance that fails to answer old questions on corneal vs. refractive astigmatism correction. *J Cataract Refract Surg.* 2002;18:737-739.
4. Alpins NA, Walsh G. Aberrometry and topography in the vector analysis of refractive laser surgery. In: Boyd BF, Agarwal A, eds. *Wavefront Analysis, Aberrometers and Corneal Topography.* Panama: Highlights of Ophthalmology; 2003:313-322.
5. Alpins NA, Schmid L. Combining vector planning with wavefront analysis to optimize laser in-situ keratomileusis outcomes. In: Krueger RR, Applegate RA, MacRae SM, eds. *Wavefront Customized Visual Correction; The Quest for Super Vision II.* Thorofare, NJ: SLACK Incorporated; 2004:317-328.
6. Holladay JT, Bains HS. Optimized prolate ablations with the NIDEK CXII excimer laser. *J Refract Surg.* 2005;21(5 Suppl):S595-S597.
7. Mrochen M, Jankov M, Bueeler M, Seiler T. Correlation between corneal and total wavefront aberrations in myopic eyes. *J Refract Surg.* 2003;19(2):104-112.
8. Kohnen T. Combining wavefront and topography data for excimer laser surgery: the future of customized ablation? *J Cataract Refract Surg.* 2004;30:285-286.
9. Alpins NA, Stamatelatos G. Clinical outcomes of laser in situ keratomileusis using combined topography and refractive wavefront treatments for myopic astigmatism. *J Cataract Refract Surg.* 2008;34:1250-1259.
10. Kugler L, Cohen I, Haddad W, Wang MX. Efficacy of laser in situ keratomileusis in correcting anterior and non-anterior corneal astigmatism: comparative study. *J Cataract Refract Surg.* 2010;36(10):1745-1752.
11. Alpins NA, Stamatelatos G. Combined wavefront and topography approach to refractive surgery treatments. In: Wang M, ed. *Corneal Topography in the Wavefront Era: A Guide for Clinical Application.* Thorofare, NJ: SLACK Incorporated; 2006:139-143.
12. Alpins NA, Stamatelatos G. Customized PARK treatment of myopia and astigmatism in forme fruste and mild keratoconus using combined topographic and refractive data. *J Cataract Refract Surg.* 2007;33:591-602.
13. Lipshitz I. Thirty-four challenges to meet before excimer laser technology can achieve super vision. *J Refract Surg.* 2002;18:740-743.
14. Williams D, Yoon GY, Porter J, Guirao A, Hofer H, Cox I. Visual benefit of correcting higher-order aberrations of the eye. *J Refract Surg.* 2000;16:S554-S559.
15. Alpins NA. Vector analysis of astigmatism changes by flattening, steepening, and torque. *J Cataract Refract Surg.* 1997;23:1503-1514.

Chapter 13

# Corneal Topography
## What Will the Upcoming Decade Bring?

Lance J. Kugler, MD and Ming Wang, MD, PhD

In the 5 years since the first edition of this book was published, there have been tremendous advances in the technology used and understanding of corneal topography, wavefront analysis, ocular biometry, and biomechanics. Such advances have led to our ability to determine the anatomical shape and optical behavior of the eye in unprecedented detail. The volume of data generated by modern diagnostic instruments is staggering and, at times, overwhelming. By combining technologies, such as wavefront with topography or biomechanics with Scheimpflug imaging, we increase the value and clinical relevance of the data. Despite the volume of diagnostic data at our disposal, the precision with which we can surgically alter the optical performance of the cornea has not kept up with our ability to define its shape. It seems archaic in this era of advanced topography, tomography, aberrometry, biometry, and biomechanics that the major determination of an ablation profile remains refraction. Modern excimer lasers are remarkably precise, yet when used perioperatively, modern corneal topographers and aberrometers illustrate the limitations of current excimer laser surgery. Postoperative aberrometry reminds us of our limited ability to remove higher-order aberrations (HOAs) so beautifully described preoperatively by our devices.

The technology gap is partly due to the speed by which diagnostic devices gain clinical and regulatory acceptance relative to surgical devices. However, it has been suggested that excimer lasers have reached their peak in terms of precision of laser-tissue interaction, and wound healing remains the largest and least-controllable barrier to a predictable result. Despite these limitations, there is still room for improvement in the precision of excimer laser ablation profiles. Such improvement will depend upon our ability to combine preoperative topographic, wavefront, and biomechanical data to generate enhanced ablation profiles and then link such profiles to excimer lasers that can deliver the profile in a consistent, reproducible manner.

## Refinement of Measurement

Devices that combine corneal topography with wavefront aberrometry are uniquely able to define the source of an optical aberration (Figure 13-1).[1,2] AMO's iDesign platform is another example of this technology that has not yet been released commercially. These systems subtract the corneal aberrations from the total or whole eye aberrations measured to precisely identify the source of the optical aberration and guide the clinician as to the best approach for surgical correction. In the context of refractive surgery screening, current devices are dependent upon relatively crude pattern recognition on the part of the clinician and are not able to reliably quantify the magnitude of the aberrations in question to the degree required for precise surgical correction. The future will undoubtedly lead to further refinement of these combined devices.



Wang M. *Corneal Topography: A Guide for Clinical Application in the Wavefront Era, Second Edition (pp. 259-262)*

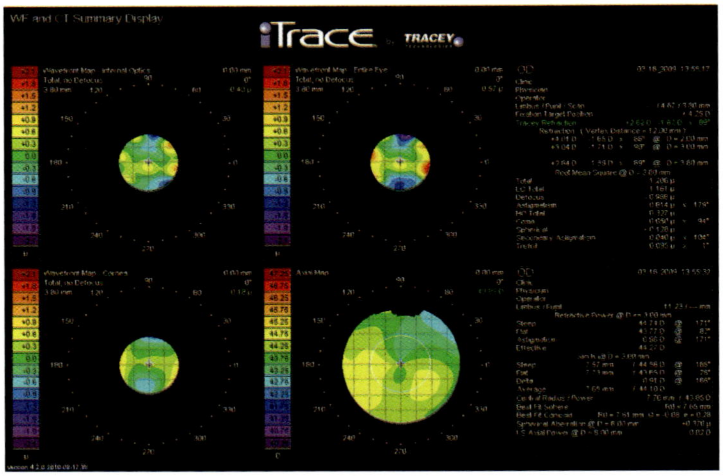


**Figure 13-1.** Combination of topography and wavefront aberrometry allows location of aberrations.

## Specificity of Screening

Posterior corneal surface analysis using tomography is increasingly used to screen patients for subclinical ectatic disease. Modern tomographers such as the Pentacam (OCULUS, Wetzlar, Germany) are able to detect subclinical keratoectatic disease[3-5] and measure corneal power[6] with increasing sensitivity. As with any new diagnostic technology, however, increased sensitivity brings with it an important limitation, namely decreased specificity. Despite the attention it receives in the literature and lay media, postkeratorefractive ectasia remains a rare condition and one that drives further investigation using biomechanics. The danger of increased sensitivity in screening prior to refractive surgery is that we may inadvertently deny refractive surgery to patients who do not carry significantly increased risk.

Future advancements in the field of corneal topography will include enhancing efficiency by which we identify clinically relevant trends and outliers within the massive volume of data at our disposal. Doing so will increase the specificity of our technology, thus improving our ability to separate patients at increased risk from those who are not. Important work is already being done in this area, as exemplified by the BAD (Belin-Ambrosia) Enhanced Ectasia scale on the OCULUS Pentacam. Future work in the area of refractive surgery screening will continue to further refine the specificity of screening parameters.

## Integration of Corneal Topography and Biomechanical Properties

Instruments that evaluate biomechanical characteristics of the cornea are currently evolving. The Ocular Response Analyzer first identified characteristics of elasticity, and others are currently being developed to analyze corneal stiffness and physical shape changes induced by applanation. Prior to the advent of these devices, we relied upon corneal architectural characteristics to approximate corneal biomechanical strength. For example, corneal thickness is an approximate representation of corneal strength in the assessment of keratoconus. By incorporating measured biomechanical properties with physical measurements, an enhanced understanding of an eye's response to keratorefractive surgery may more accurately be defined, and candidacy better determined.

Dynamic measurement of deformation may be performed using rasterstereographic corneal topography (RCT), Scheimpflug imaging, and anterior segment OCT. RCT employs a grid projected onto the fluorescein-covered corneal surface. The changes to the grid pattern induced by an air puff similar to NCT are monitored by an imaging camera. The images are then processed by a computer to generate data regarding the stiffness of the cornea.

Dynamic ultra high-speed Scheimpflug corneal imaging of the CorVis (Oculus, Wetzlar, Germany) combines air-puff tonometry with dynamic Scheimpflug images to measure various descriptors, including applanation time, applanation lengths, highest deformation, central concave curvature at the highest concavity point, and central thickness (Figure 13-2). Similar methods are being investigated using AS-OCT. Our approach to treatment of keratoconus may change as well as we gain understanding regarding the use of various surgical procedures to improve biomechanical properties.

## Customizing IOL Calculations

As cataract surgery continues to evolve and merge with refractive surgery, so must the instruments at our disposal. A simple K reading and axial length is no longer sufficient to provide the precise results required for success with presbyopic lenses. Eyes that have undergone keratorefractive

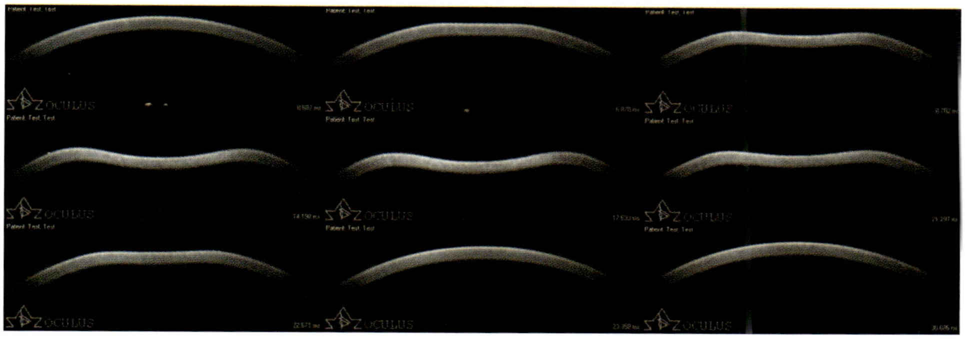

**Figure 13-2.** An image composite of CorVis ST measurements. Frames are captured around the monitored the air jet pulse. (Reprinted with permission of Renato Ambrósio Jr, MD, PhD, and Diogo Caldas, MD).

surgery now needing cataract extraction present further challenges in the realm of IOL calculations. It is becoming increasingly clear that our traditional methods of IOL calculation are not robust enough to handle postkeratorefractive eyes.[7-10] Traditional formulas require a few measured biometry values and derive the rest of the anatomy based upon assumptions. These assumptions are no longer valid following keratorefractive surgery and result in refractive surprises following surgery.

As our understanding of ocular biometry and its relationship to IOL power and IOL position continue to improve, so must our ability to accurately measure these values. For example, the refractive power of the posterior cornea becomes clinically relevant for IOL calculations in eyes that are postkeratorefractive surgery. Initial attempts at incorporating posterior corneal power in the determination of corneal power, such as the Holladay EKR report on the Oculus Pentacam, will continue to be refined as the instruments allow for more reliable and reproducible posterior power measurements. Biometry may be incorporated into topographic systems, and tomographers will likely develop improved algorithms for IOL power calculation.

## Topography-Driven Keratorefractive Surgery

Wavefront-guided excimer laser surgery continues to be a popular and well-established treatment modality. However, this technology suffers from an important limitation in that all aberrations of the entire visual system are treated on the anterior corneal surface, regardless of their site of origin. For example, treatment of a spherical cornea with lenticular astigmatism results in an astigmatic cornea. Similarly, HOAs arising from the crystalline lens or posterior cornea are treated on the anterior corneal surface. This approach may not provide ideal optical performance postoperatively.[11] Furthermore, the excimer laser treatment required to correct HOAs is calculated based on wavefront analysis rather than direct measurement of the curvature or irregularity of the corneal surface. In general, data that are directly measured are more reliable and robust than mathematically derived data.

Direct measurement of the structure in question is the goal of topography-guided excimer ablation. As the ocular structure most responsible for refraction of light, the anterior cornea is the surface from which the majority of HOAs arise. By directly measuring this surface with corneal topography, and applying treatment based on the results, an optically superior surgical result is possible. Topography-guided ablations are promising for the treatment of irregular astigmatism, which remains one of the most elusive post-LASIK complications to correct. A valiant effort was made toward this treatment modality by the Topolink system in the late 1990s; however, results were disappointing. A more recent generation of topography-guided platforms, including the iVIS (LIGI Tecnologie Medicali, Taranto, Italy), Allegretto WaveLight (Alcon, Fort Worth, TX), and Zeiss MEL 80 (Carl Zeiss Meditec, Jena, Germany) show promise toward refinement of topo-guided technology.

As promising as topography-guided treatments may be, excimer ablation guided by a combination of corneal topography and wavefront aberrometry will be the treatment approach of the future.

Overall, the theme of the next decade will be integration. As cataract surgery merges with refractive surgery, so will the devices and technology we use to achieve the best possible outcomes. Diagnostic equipment will continue to merge with excimer lasers to deliver more refined ablation patterns. In order to manage the vast amount of data that will result from these instruments, improved methods of data analysis and risk assessment will continue to be an important area of research and development.

## References

1. Won JB, Kim SW, Kim EK, Ha BJ, Kim TI. Comparison of internal and total optical aberrations for 2 aberrometers: iTrace and OPD scan. *Korean J Ophthalmol*. 2008;22(4):210-213.
2. Fontes BM, Ambrósio R Jr, Jardim D, Velarde GC, Nosé W. Ability of corneal biomechanical metrics and anterior segment data in the differentiation of keratoconus and healthy corneas. *Arq Bras Oftalmol*. 2010;73(4):333-337.
3. Fu J, Wang X, Li S, Wu G, Wang N. Comparative study of anterior segment measurement with Pentacam and anterior segment optical coherence tomography. *Can J Ophthalmol*. 2010;45(6):627-631.

4. Oliveira CM, Ribeiro C, Franco S. Corneal imaging with slit-scanning and Scheimpflug imaging techniques. *Clin Exp Optom.* 2011;94(1):33-42.
5. Tang M, Chen A, Li Y, Huang D. Corneal power measurement with Fourier-domain optical coherence tomography. *J Cataract Refract Surg.* 2010;36(12):2115-2122.
6. Rosa N, De Bernardo M, Borrelli M, Lanza M. New factor to improve reliability of the clinical history method for intraocular lens power calculation after refractive surgery. *J Cataract Refract Surg.* 2010;36(12):2123-2128.
7. Ghanem AA, El-Sayed HM. Accuracy of intraocular lens power calculation in high myopia. *Oman J Ophthalmol.* 2010;3(3):126-130.
8. Naseri A, McLeod SD. Cataract surgery after refractive surgery. *Curr Opin Ophthalmol.* 2010;21(1):35-38.
9. Savini G, Hoffer KJ, Carbonelli M, Barboni P. Intraocular lens power calculation after myopic excimer laser surgery: clinical comparison of published methods. *J Cataract Refract Surg.* 2010;36(9):1455-1465.
10. **Kugler L, Cohen I, Haddad W, Wang MX. Efficacy of laser in situ keratomileusis in correcting anterior and non-anterior corneal astigmatism: comparative study. *J Cataract Refract Surg.* 2010;36(10):1745-1752.**
11. Alpins N, Stamatelatos G. Clinical outcomes of laser in situ keratomileusis using combined topography and refractive wavefront treatments for myopic astigmatism. *J Cataract Refract Surg.* 2008;34(8):1250-1259.

# Financial Disclosures

*Dr. Ashkan M. Abbey* has no financial or proprietary interest in the materials presented herein.

*Dr. Amar Agarwal* is a paid consultant to Abott Medical Optics, STAAR Surgical, and Bausch & Lomb.

*Dr. Noel Alpins* is part of the ASSORT outcome and analyses program.

*Dr. Renato Ambrósio Jr* is a consultant for OCULUS and Alcon.

*Dr. Dianne Anderson* has no financial or proprietary interest in the materials presented herein.

*Dr. Timothy J. Archer* has no financial or proprietary interest in the materials presented herein.

*Dr. Amin Ashrafzadeh* is a consultant to Carl Zeiss Meditec.

*Dr. Harkaran S. Bains* is a consultant for NIDEK.

*Dr. Michael W. Belin* is a consultant to OCULUS GmbH.

*Dr. Megan Buliano* has no financial or proprietary interest in the materials presented herein.

*Dr. Phillip M. Buscemi* is a paid consultant for Nidek Co, Ltd.

*Dr. Diogo L. Caldas* has no financial or proprietary interest in the materials presented herein.

*Dr. Massimo Camellin* has no financial or proprietary interest in the materials presented herein.

*Dr. Ana Laura C. Canedo* has no financial or proprietary interest in the materials presented herein.

*Dr. Shihao Chen* has no financial or proprietary interest in the materials presented herein.

*Dr. Xiangjun Chen* has no financial or proprietary interest in the materials presented herein.

*Dr. Y. Ralph Chu* has no financial or proprietary interest in the materials presented herein.

*Dr. Ilan Cohen* has no financial or proprietary interest in the materials presented herein.

*Ms. Sonya M. Dakin* is a contracted employee of Tracey Technologies.

*Dr. Michael J. Endl* has no financial or proprietary interest in the materials presented herein.

*Dr. Zhengjun Fan* has no financial or proprietary interest in the materials presented herein.

*Dr. Claus M. Fichte* has no financial or proprietary interest in the materials presented herein.

*Dr. Marine Gobbe* has no financial or proprietary interest in the materials presented herein.

*Dr. Frederico P. Guerra* has no financial or proprietary interest in the materials presented herein.

*Dr. Doug Horner* has no financial or proprietary interest in the materials presented herein.

*Dr. Mirko R. Jankov II* is a consultant for Alcon.

*Dr. Jason Jedlicka* has no financial or proprietary interest in the materials presented herein.

*Dr. Paul M. Karpecki* is a consultant for Topcon and on the speaker's bureau for Oculus.

*Dr. Stephen S. Khachikian* has no financial or proprietary interest in the materials presented herein.

*Dr. Stephen D. Klyce* has no financial or proprietary interest in the materials presented herein.

*Dr. Randy Kojima* is Director of Technical Affairs for Precision Technology Services. This is a GP manufacturing company and distributor of the Medmont topographer in North America.

*Dr. Lance J. Kugler* is a consultant for Alcon, Allergan, and Refocus Group.

*Dr. Matthew Lampa* has no financial or proprietary interest in the materials presented herein.

*Mr. Sissimos Lemonis* is an employee of Wavelight GmbH.

*Dr. Ray-Ann Lin* has not disclosed any relevant financial relationships.

*Dr. Bing Liu* has no financial or proprietary interest in the materials presented herein.

*Dr. David D. Liu* is Chief Technology Officer for LaserSight Technologies, Inc.

*Dr. Naoyuki Maeda* has a research grant from Topcon.

*Dr. Renzo Mattioli* is a full time employee of Optikon 2000.

*Dr. Murray McFadden* has no financial or proprietary interest in the materials presented herein.

*Dr. Cristiana de Moraes Ramalho* has no financial or proprietary interest in the materials presented herein.

*Dr. Katherine E. Paton* has no financial or proprietary interest in the materials presented herein.

*Dr. Leonardo N. Pimentel* has no financial or proprietary interest in the materials presented herein.

*Dr. Gaurav Prakash* has no financial or proprietary interest in the materials presented herein.

*Dr. Jia Qu* has no financial or proprietary interest in the materials presented herein.

*Dr. J. Bradley Randleman* has no financial or proprietary interest in the materials presented herein.

*Dr. Dan Z. Reinstein* is a consultant for Carl Zeiss Meditec and has a propietary interest in the Artemis technology (ArcScan, Inc) through patents administered by the Cornell Center for Technology Enterprise and Commercialization (CCTEC).

*Dr. Karolinne Maia Rocha* has no financial or proprietary interest in the materials presented herein.

*Dr. George Stamatelatos* is a consultant for ASSORT.

*Dr. Aleksandar Stojanovic* has no financial or proprietary interest in the materials presented herein.

*Dr. Tracy Schroeder Swartz* is a consultant for Tracey Technologies.

*Dr. Bradford L. Tannen* has no financial or proprietary interest in the materials presented herein.

*Dr. Nancy K. Tripoli* is a parttime consultant for Optikon.

*Dr. Bruno F. Valbon* has no financial or proprietary interest in the materials presented herein.

*Dr. Shawna Hill Vanderhoof* has no financial or proprietary interest in the materials presented herein.

*Dr. Joe S. Wakil* has financial interest in Tracey Technologies and Eyesys Vision.

*Dr. Ming Wang* has no financial or proprietary interest in the materials presented herein.

*Dr. Junhua Xiao* has no financial or proprietary interest in the materials presented herein.

*Dr. Sonia H. Yoo* has no financial or proprietary interest in the materials presented herein.

# Index